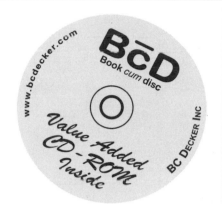
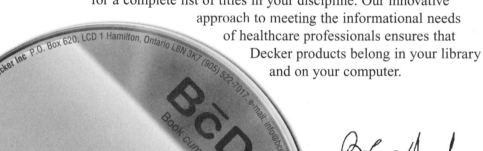

VIRAL AND IMMUNOLOGICAL MALIGNANCIES

Clinical Oncology Series

VIRAL AND IMMUNOLOGICAL MALIGNANCIES

Paul A. Volberding, MD

Professor and Vice Chair
Department of Medicine
University of California, San Francisco
Chief of the Medical Service
San Francisco Veterans Affairs Medical Center
Co-Director, UCSF-GIVI Center for AIDS Research
San Francisco, California

Joel M. Palefsky, MD, CM, FRCP(C)

Professor of Medicine
University of California, San Francisco
San Francisco, California

Carrie Clark Walsh, ELS

Assistant Editor
University of California, San Francisco
San Francisco, California

BC Decker Inc
Hamilton

BC Decker Inc
P.O. Box 620, L.C.D. 1
Hamilton, Ontario L8N 3K7
Tel: 905-522-7017; 800-568-7281
Fax: 905-522-7839; 888-311-4987
E-mail: info@bcdecker.com
www.bcdecker.com

ISBN 1-55009-256-1
Printed in the United States of America by Walsworth Publishing Company
Production Editor: Maria L. Reyes; Typesetter: Jansom; Cover Designer: Lisa Mattinson

Sales and Distribution

United States
BC Decker Inc
P.O. Box 785
Lewiston, NY 14092-0785
Tel: 905-522-7017; 800-568-7281
Fax: 905-522-7839; 888-311-4987
E-mail: info@bcdecker.com
www.bcdecker.com

Canada
BC Decker Inc
50 King St. E.
P.O. Box 620, LCD 1
Hamilton, Ontario L8N 3K7
Tel: 905-522-7017; 800-568-7281
Fax: 905-522-7839; 888-311-4987
E-mail: info@bcdecker.com
www.bcdecker.com

Foreign Rights
John Scott & Company
International Publishers' Agency
P.O. Box 878
Kimberton, PA 19442
Tel: 610-827-1640; Fax: 610-827-1671
E-mail: jsco@voicenet.com

Japan
Igaku-Shoin Ltd.
Foreign Publications Department
3-24-17 Hongo
Bunkyo-ku, Tokyo, Japan 113-8719
Tel: 3 3817 5680; Fax: 3 3815 6776
E-mail: fd@igaku-shoin.co.jp

UK, Europe, Scandinavia, Middle East
Elsevier Science
Customer Service Department
Foots Cray High Street
Sidcup, Kent
DA14 5HP, UK
Tel: 44 (0) 208 308 5760
Fax: 44 (0) 181 308 5702
E-mail: cservice@harcourt.com

*Singapore, Malaysia, Thailand, Philippines,
Indonesia, Vietnam, Pacific Rim, Korea*
Elsevier Science Asia
583 Orchard Road
#09/01, Forum
Singapore 238884
Tel: 65-737-3593; Fax: 65-753-2145

Australia, New Zealand
Elsevier Science Australia
Customer Service Department
STM Division
Locked Bag 16
St. Peters, New South Wales, 2044
Australia
Tel: 61 02 9517-8999
Fax: 61 02 9517-2249
E-mail: stmp@harcourt.com.au
www.harcourt.com.au

Mexico and Central America
ETM SA de CV
Calle de Tula 59
Colonia Condesa
06140 Mexico DF, Mexico
Tel: 52-5-5553-6657
Fax: 52-5-5211-8468
E-mail:
editoresdetextosmex@prodigy.net.mx

Brazil
Tecmedd Importadora E Distribuidora
De Livros Ltda.
Avenida Maurílio Biagi, 2850
City Ribeirão, Ribeirão Preto – SP –
Brasil
CEP: 14021-000
Tel: 0800 992236; Fax: (16) 3993-9000
E-mail: tecmedd@tecmedd.com.br

India, Bangladesh, Pakistan, Sri Lanka
Elsevier Health Sciences Division
Customer Service Department
17A/1, Main Ring Road
Lajpat Nagar IV
New Delhi – 110024, India
Tel: 91 11 2644 7160-64
Fax: 91 11 2644 7156
E-mail: esindia@vsnl.net

Notice: The authors and publisher have made every effort to ensure that the patient care recommended herein, including choice of drugs and drug dosages, is in accord with the accepted standard and practice at the time of publication. However, since research and regulation constantly change clinical standards, the reader is urged to check the product information sheet included in the package of each drug, which includes recommended doses, warnings, and contraindications. This is particularly important with new or infrequently used drugs. Any treatment regimen, particularly one involving medication, involves inherent risk that must be weighed on a case-by-case basis against the benefits anticipated. The reader is cautioned that the purpose of this book is to inform and enlighten; the information contained herein is not intended as, and should not be employed as, a substitute for individual diagnosis and treatment.

Contents

Preface

Viruses can cause cancer and cancers are more common in the setting of immune deficiency. Examples of these relationships have been known for decades, but newer molecular tools and the human immunodeficiency virus (HIV) epidemic have shed vital new light on this active and interesting area of research. Rarely, in humans, viruses can be directly oncogenic. Much more commonly, the role of viruses in human cancer is indirect, requiring an interaction with a second infection, chronic inflammation, or other host factor. In many cases, the precise relationship between viral infection and malignancy remains an epidemiologic association and the subject of active investigation. Nonmalignant hematologic disorders have a similarly complex relationship with cancer-associated viruses and may offer insight into the pathogenesis of oncogenesis. This book explores the relationships between viral infections, immune impairments, and hematologic and malignant diseases, particularly against the backdrop of the HIV epidemic.

Cancers were among the earliest recognized manifestations of acquired immune deficiency syndrome (AIDS), and efforts to understand them helped lead to the discovery of HIV infection. Prior to the AIDS epidemic, Kaposi's sarcoma (KS) was a rare cancer in most areas, usually confined to very elderly men in whom it typically followed a slowly progressive course. Because KS often is immediately visible involving the skin, and has a characteristic histology, its appearance in young previously healthy men in the early 1980s was a striking alert to the onset of the AIDS epidemic. Not long thereafter, non-Hodgkin's lymphomas were also appreciated to be part of the clinical spectrum of AIDS.

In the early stages of HIV infection, lymphatic proliferation causes diffuse generalized lymphadenopathy. HIV was, in fact, first isolated from an excised node, and the clinical description of generalized adenopathy was instrumental in understanding that AIDS as initially defined did not capture the full spectrum of HIV disease, later shown to include even completely asymptomatic individuals.

The lymphomas associated with AIDS are themselves complex and instructive. Peripheral lymphomas often arise in extranodal sites rarely affected in non–HIV-infected persons and follow an aggressive clinical course. Lymphomas in the central nervous system (CNS) in HIV-infected persons are a marker of extremely advanced immune deficiency and are almost always associated with evidence of Epstein-Barr virus (EBV) coinfection. Primary effusion lymphomas, first recognized in HIV-infected patients, follow an aggressive clinical course.

The theme of viral coinfection is a recurring one in AIDS-associated malignancies. The striking epidemiology of KS led to the identification of a novel human herpes virus, HHV-8. This virus is associated with all groups affected by KS, but dramatically so with HIV coinfection. Viral coinfections are also studied in HIV-infected persons with respect to cancers associated with EBV (non-Hodgkin's lymphoma), HHV-8 (KS and primary effusion lymphoma), and human papillomavirus (anal and cervical cancers), as well as coinfection with hepatitis viruses B and C (hepatocellular cancer).

The immune impairment of HIV infection is also an important setting in which to explore potential oncogenesis of other viral infections long suspected to be linked to human cancer. Here, studies of simian virus 40 and human T-lymphotropic virus infections come to mind, as well as cancers suspected but not proven to be virally induced, including those arising in immunosuppressed patients after organ transplantation.

HIV infection clearly causes hematologic and oncologic sequelae, but the immune restoration seen in HIV treatment offers further insight. Antiretroviral therapy differentially alters the incidence of associated malignancies and can even cause tumor regression. KS incidence is relatively more decreased in treated HIV-infected populations than peripheral non-Hodgkin's lymphomas, whereas CNS lymphomas have nearly disappeared. HIV therapy can lead to KS regression and is, in fact, now the preferred treatment for that formerly aggressive cancer. HIV therapy does not typically cause lymphoma regression, but has substantially improved overall treatment response and survival. Even more interesting are the reports of clinical flares in KS after antiretroviral therapy initiation. This immune response inflammatory syndrome is well described in those with underlying opportunistic infection and presumably follows the recovery of antigen-driven immune response.

The hematology of HIV infection is similarly revealing of biologic insights. HIV infection itself causes anemia, probably in the majority of patients during their disease course. Anemia is, in fact, an important and independent survival predictor along with CD4 cell count and HIV viral load. As in other patient groups, anemia adversely affects quality of life. Whether the reversal of anemia prolongs survival is unproven, but it clearly reduces associated symptoms. Thrombocytopenia is also seen in HIV infection. Interestingly, thrombocytopenia may decrease in severity as HIV disease stage advances. Clinically significant coagulopathies are uncommon in HIV infection, but thrombotic thrombocytopenic purpura is substantially increased in incidence, as are serologic abnormalities, including the lupus-like anticoagulants.

Clearly, our understanding of the intricate interrelationships between immune surveillance, immune deficiency, and human cancer biology has been advanced through the study of HIV infection. In many cases, the specific pathogenesis relationship between HIV, coincident infections, and the host immune response still requires further investigation. It is hoped that the monographs collected in this volume will serve as an effective overview of current research and clinical consequences.

Finally, creating this book benefitted enormously from the talented editorial assistance of Ms. Carrie Clark Walsh. The editors also gratefully acknowledge the contributions of Dr. Susan Krown for providing key clinical illustrations.

PAUL A. VOLBERDING
JOEL M. PALEFSKY

Contributors

KELTY R. BAKER, MD
Baylor College of Medicine
Houston, Texas
*Abnormalities of the Coagulation System
Associated with HIV Infection*

GIANNA BALLON, MD
Weill Medical College of Cornell University
New York, New York
Castleman's Disease

MARK A. BEILKE, MD
Tulane University Health Sciences Center
New Orleans, Louisiana
*The Human T-Lymphotropic Leukemia
Viruses 1 and 2*

CAROLINE BEHLER, MD, MS
University of California, San Francisco
San Francisco, California
Anemia in HIV Infection

MITCHEL S. BERGER, MD
University of California, San Francisco
San Francisco, California
*Management of Primary Central Nervous System
Lymphoma and Primary Intraocular Lymphoma*

ETHEL CESARMAN, MD, PhD
Weill Medical College of Cornell University
New York, New York
Castleman's Disease

ANTHONY T.C. CHAN, MD, FRCP(UK)
The Chinese University of Hong Kong
Shatin, Hong Kong
*Nasopharyngeal Cancer Diagnosis
and Management*

AJAI CHARI, MD
University of California, San Francisco
San Francisco, California
*Diagnosis and Management of Non-Hodgkin's
Lymphoma and Hodgkin's Lymphoma*

ELIZABETH Y. CHIAO, MD, MPH
Baylor College of Medicine
Houston, Texas
*Non–AIDS-Defining Cancers in HIV-Infected
Individuals*

PETER V. CHIN-HONG, MD
University of California, San Francisco
San Francisco, California
*Human Papillomavirus–Related Malignancies
With and Without HIV: Epidemiology,
Diagnosis, and Management*

RAYMOND T. CHUNG, MD
Massachusetts General Hospital
Boston, Massachusetts
Viral Hepatitis and Hepatocarcinogenesis

ROBERTA CINELLI, MD
National Cancer Institute
Aviano, Italy
*Clinical Features and Management of
Kaposi's Sarcoma*

PATRICIA A. CORNETT, MD
University of California, San Francisco
San Francisco, California
Anemia in HIV Infection

ILKA ENGELMANN, MD
Hannover Medical School
Hannover, Germany
Human Herpesvirus 8/Kaposi's
  Sarcoma–Associated Herpesvirus Biology

ERIC A. ENGELS, MD
National Cancer Institute
Rockville, Maryland
Simian Virus 40 and Human Malignancy

CORNELIA HENKE-GENDO, MD
Hannover Medical School
Hannover, Germany
Human Herpesvirus 8/Kaposi's
  Sarcoma–Associated Herpesvirus Biology

NANCY A. HESSOL, MSPH
University of California, San Francisco
San Francisco, California
Epidemiology of Cancer in the Pre-HAART
  and HAART Eras

KENNETH HIRSCH, MD
Washington DC Veterans Medical Administration
Washington, District of Columbia
Hepatocellular Cancer: Diagnosis and
  Management

PHILIP J. JOHNSON, MD, FRCP
University of Birmingham
Birmingham, United Kingdom
Nasopharyngeal Cancer Diagnosis and
  Management

LAWRENCE KAPLAN, MD
University of California, San Francisco
San Francisco, California
Diagnosis and Management of Non-Hodgkin's
  Lymphoma and Hodgkin's Lymphoma

JEFF KOHLWES, MD
University of California, San Francisco
San Francisco, California
Screening for Hepatocellular Cancer:
  Current Strategies and Controversies

SUSAN E. KROWN, MD
Memorial Sloan-Kettering Cancer Center
New York, New York
Non–AIDS-Defining Cancers in
  HIV-Infected Individuals

ANNETTE Y. KWON, MD
Massachusetts General Hospital
Boston, Massachusetts
Viral Hepatitis and Hepatocarcinogenesis

LEWIS L. LANIER, PhD
University of California, San Francisco
San Francisco, California
Immune Surveillance in Cancer

NATALIE LEE, MD
University of California, San Francisco
San Francisco, California
Screening for Hepatocellular Cancer:
  Current Strategies and Controversies

SING-FAI LEUNG, FRCR (UK)
The Chinese University of Hong Kong
Shatin, Hong Kong
Nasopharyngeal Cancer Diagnosis and
  Management

JEFFREY N. MARTIN, MD, MPH
University of California, San Francisco
San Francisco, California
Epidemiology of Kaposi's Sarcoma–Associated
  Herpesvirus Infection

EDWARD L. MURPHY, MD, MPH
University of California, San Francisco
San Francisco, California
The Human T-Lymphotropic Leukemia
  Viruses 1 and 2

PAUL G. MURRAY, PhD
University of Birmingham
Birmingham, United Kingdom
Epstein-Barr Virus Infection and the
  Pathogenesis of Cancer: Lymphomas
  and Nasopharyngeal Carcinoma

JOEL M. PALEFSKY, MD, CM, FRCP(C)
University of California, San Francisco
San Francisco, California
*Human Papillomavirus–Related Malignancies
With and Without HIV: Epidemiology,
Diagnosis, and Management*

SAMIR PAREKH, MD
Montefiore Medical Center
Bronx, New York
*Primary Effusion Lymphomas: Biology
and Management*

JAMES L. RUBENSTEIN, MD, PhD
University of California, San Francisco
San Francisco, California
*Management of Primary Central Nervous System
Lymphoma and Primary Intraocular Lymphoma*

SUSAN SCHEER, MD, MPH
San Francisco Department of Public Health
San Francisco, California
*Epidemiology of Cancer in the Pre-HAART
and HAART Eras*

THOMAS F. SCHULZ, MD, FRCPATH
Hannover Medical School
Hannover, Germany
*Human Herpesvirus 8/Kaposi's
Sarcoma–Associated Herpesvirus Biology*

KAREN SMITH-MCCUNE, MD, PhD
University of California, San Francisco
San Francisco, California
*Pathogenesis of Human Papillomavirus–Related
Malignancies*

JOSEPH A. SPARANO, MD
Montefiore Medical Center
Bronx, New York
*Primary Effusion Lymphomas: Biology
and Management*

RAYNA TAKAKI
University of California, San Francisco
San Francisco, California
Immune Surveillance in Cancer

UMBERTO TIRELLI, MD
National Cancer Institute
Aviano, Italy
*Clinical Features and Management of
Kaposi's Sarcoma*

EMANUELA VACCHER, MD
National Cancer Institute
Aviano, Italy
*Clinical Features and Management of
Kaposi's Sarcoma*

LAWRENCE S. YOUNG, PhD
University of Birmingham
Birmingham, United Kingdom
*Epstein-Barr Virus Infection and the
Pathogenesis of Cancer: Lymphomas and
Nasopharyngeal Carcinoma*

Epidemiology of Cancer in the Pre-HAART and HAART Eras

SUSAN SCHEER
NANCY A. HESSOL

In the 1970s, the increasing use of immune suppressive drugs for organ transplantation led to the discovery that the risk of certain cancers was elevated in transplant recipients. A decade later, scientists recognized that the risk of some cancers was also elevated in people with severe immunodeficiency owing to HIV infection. With the advent of more powerful anti-HIV treatment, termed highly active anti-retroviral therapy (HAART), in the mid-1990s, a noticeable decline in the incidence of AIDS-defining cancers occurred.

Unquestionably, the introduction and widespread use of HAART has led to reduced AIDS morbidity and mortality among people with HIV infection (Figure 1–1). However, longer life expectancy may also lead to the development of diseases that require a longer latency period, such as cancer. Under these conditions, it is important to closely monitor for emerging epidemiologic trends to accurately determine the risks of malignancy in this population. Implementation of appropriate cancer prevention, screening, and treatment recommendations requires a better understanding of the etiology, epidemiology, and natural history of AIDS defining and non–AIDS-defining malignancies.

After briefly reviewing cancers found to be associated with immunosuppression in non–HIV-infected patients, this chapter will focus on those cancers, both AIDS-defining and non–AIDS-defining, that have an increased occurrence in people with HIV infection. Particular attention will be given to con-

trasting the risk of cancer in the time period prior to HAART and in the HAART era. The majority of the data cited for this chapter draws upon results from large cohort studies and linkage studies between HIV/AIDS and cancer registries that quantified cancer risk and survival. The mainly descriptive data from case reports were used to assess change in cancer presentation.

CANCERS ASSOCIATED WITH IMMUNOSUPPRESSION PRIOR TO HIV

Independent of HIV infection, the occurrence of a number of cancers is associated with severe immunodeficiency.[1,2] Cancers resulting from congenital

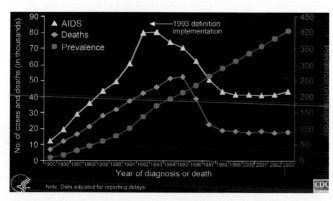

Figure 1–1. Estimated number of AIDS cases, deaths, and persons living with AIDS, 1985–2003, United States. Data adjusted for reporting delays. From Centers for Disease Control & Prevention, National Center for HIV, STD, and TB Prevention. Last updated: July 15, 2003. Available at: http://www.cdc.gov/hiv/graphics/surveill.htm (accessed Aug 22, 2005).

immunosuppression related to autoimmune diseases have long been found in children. Increases in organ and tissue transplantation in the 1970s, and the resulting use of immunosuppressive drugs, have caused the relative risk of a number of cancers, specifically non-Hodgkin's lymphoma (NHL), Kaposi's sarcoma (KS), hepatocellular carcinoma, and squamous cell carcinoma of the skin, to increase dramatically.[1] Cancers associated with immunosuppression in transplant recipients appear to be more aggressive than in the general population. However, discontinuation of the immunosuppressive therapy can stop or even reverse tumor growth. In addition, the same risk factors that predict cancers in the general population also influence the development of a malignancy among those with immunosuppression. For example, transplant recipients who are fair skinned and/or have high lifetime exposures to the sun are at greater risk for developing skin cancer than other transplant recipients.[1] Cancers associated with immunodeficiency are summarized in Table 1–1. As survival among persons with AIDS increases, the role of immunosuppression and its association with malignancies will become increasingly important.

AIDS-DEFINING CANCERS, PRE-HAART VERSUS HAART ERA

Current estimates are that 30 to 40% of persons with HIV infection develop a malignancy at some point in the course of their disease.[3] As people with HIV live longer, especially with advances in anti-retroviral therapies, more people are expected to develop malignancies, including cancers not currently associated with HIV or AIDS.

The Centers for Disease Control and Prevention (CDC) currently considers three cancers to be AIDS-defining conditions: (1) KS, (2) intermediate or high-grade B-cell NHL, and (3) invasive cervical cancer.[4] For each of these three cancers, the etiologic agent, risk groups and geography, incidence and presentation, and survival time are discussed below.

Kaposi's Sarcoma

KS is a multifocal endothelial tumor that can involve skin, mucous membranes, lymph nodes, and internal organs. In 1872, Moritz Kaposi reported odd skin tumors in five men in their sixties and seventies.[5] Commonly referred to as "classic KS," it was characterized as a benign tumor usually occurring in men between the ages of 50 and 60 who were of Eastern European and Mediterranean ancestry. Tumor progression tended to be slow, and lesions were usually confined to the skin of the lower extremities with no internal organ involvement. It was common for people to survive 8 to 10 years with KS and then die of an unrelated cause.

Etiologic Agent

Prior to 1994, the cause of KS among persons with HIV infection was unknown. However, the pattern of occurrence in persons with AIDS suggested that KS had an infectious etiology and was sexually transmitted in the same manner but less efficiently than HIV. In 1994, a newly identified virus, human herpesvirus type 8 (HHV-8) was determined to be the etiologic agent for KS.[6] HHV-8 has been found in over 90% of KS lesions, supporting the role of HHV-8 in the development of KS.[2]

The mode of HHV-8 transmission is not clearly understood. Given the early detection of KS in men who have sex with men (MSM) in the United States,

Table 1–1. IMMUNODEFICIENCY-ASSOCIATED CANCERS		
Type of Cancer	**Type of Immunosuppression**	**Infectious Agent or Underlying Condition**
KS (transplant or iatrogenic)	Resulting from tissue/organ transplant	Human herpesvirus 8
NHL		Epstein-Barr virus
Hepatocellular carcinoma		Hepatitis B and C viruses
Squamous cell carcinoma of the skin		Human papillomavirus types
Anogenital cancer		Human papillomavirus types
Lymphoma	Congenital defect	X-linked gamma globulinemia or ataxia telangiectasia

KS = Kaposi's sarcoma; NHL = non-Hodgkin's lymphoma.

KS was originally thought to be sexually transmitted, particularly through oral anal contact. Recent studies[7] have found that HHV-8 DNA is more readily detected in saliva than in genital secretions. Supporting this theory is the occurrence of KS among families in areas where HHV-8 is endemic, such as Africa and Israel.[8]

Numerous studies now indicate that HHV-8 is necessary but not sufficient for the development of KS.[8,9] The risk of KS is increased by the detection of HHV-8 DNA in peripheral blood and is correlated with HHV-8 viral load. Additionally, both KS and HHV-8 are inversely correlated with immune competence.[8] Clearly, underlying host immunosuppression plays a role in development of KS among persons with HHV-8 infection.

It has also been suggested that Tat, a protein expressed by HIV, is associated with increased KS incidence, but again, incidence is only increased in those who are immunocompromised.[10,11]

Risk Group and Geography

With the establishment of cancer registries in the 1950s, KS was found to be endemic in Central and Eastern Africa. Following advances in transplant medicine, another form of KS associated with immune deficiency was found. Patients who took immunosuppressive regimens to prevent graft rejections after a transplant began to develop KS. This form of KS, also known as post-transplant or iatrogenic KS, often resolves when immunosuppressive therapy is stopped.[8]

Prior to the onset of the HIV/AIDS epidemic, KS was extremely rare in the United States,[12] with an expected rate in men of 0.29 cases per 100,000 annually.[13] In the late 1970s and early 1980s, an outbreak of KS was identified in young homosexual men.[14] These men had an observed rate of KS more than 2,000 times higher than the expected rate among never-married men of the same ages. As a result, KS became one of the first recognized indicators of AIDS.[14,15]

Since the risk of KS increases as immunosuppression increases,[8] people infected with HIV have a higher risk of developing KS than those not infected with HIV. By destroying CD4+ T lymphocytes and compromising the host immune system,[16] HIV

increases one's susceptibility to KS. Among persons with HIV/AIDS, KS tumors most commonly involve mucocutaneous sites. KS may also involve visceral organs, including the lungs, in about one-third to one-half of persons with KS.

KS became the first malignancy identified as an AIDS-defining illness when it was incorporated into the original CDC AIDS case definition.[14] The number of KS cases continued to increase rapidly, and KS continues to be the most common HIV-associated malignancy.[17]

The risk of KS among HIV-infected MSM is five- to 10-fold higher than in other risk groups for HIV and AIDS.[3] In Spain and Italy where injection drug users (IDUs) make up the majority of AIDS cases, the occurrence of KS is much lower than in the United States and Northern Europe, where MSM account for the majority of AIDS cases.

Women with KS have a poorer survival and generally present with more advanced KS than men.[18] Women also have an increased incidence of lymphedema, lymph node disease, and visceral disease. The increased proportion of women with KS with visceral disease and their poorer survival has been found independent of adjustment for CD4 lymphocyte count.[18–20]

Incidence and Presentation

Significant declines in the incidence of KS as a presenting AIDS diagnosis were seen prior to the widespread use of HAART (Figure 1–2). A number of possible factors, including a decreased exposure to HHV-8 through the use of safer sex practices to prevent HIV, an expansion of the AIDS case definition to include conditions that usually precede KS, use of antiviral drugs that have anti-herpetic properties, and/or a decrease in the identification or the reporting of KS, could explain these declines.[17]

To examine whether increased HAART use was primarily responsible for a decrease in the incidence of KS and a decrease in HHV-8 virus prevalence and transmission rates, Osmond and colleagues tested stored blood samples from MSM in San Francisco in three time periods, 1978 to 1979, 1984 to 1985, and 1995 to 1996.[21] They did not find any significant declines in the prevalence of HHV-8

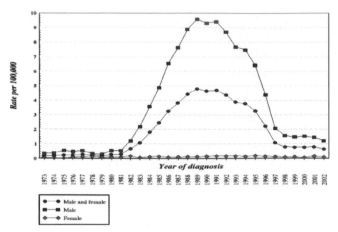

Figure 1–2. Age-adjusted incidence rates for Kaposi's sarcoma, by sex, 1973–2002, United States SEER 9 registries. From Surveillance, Epidemiology, and End Results (SEER) Program SEER*Stat Database: Incidence – SEER 9 Regs Public-Use, (1973–2002). National Cancer Institute, DCCPS, Surveillance Research Program, Cancer Statistics Branch, released April 2005, based on the November 2004 submission. Available at: http://www.cdc.gov/hiv/graphics/surveill.htm (accessed Aug 22, 2005).

during these time periods and also reported that the proportion of men practicing unprotected oral sex remained the same during these periods. They concluded that the decline in KS was, therefore, not a result of HHV-8 prevalence or changes in sexual behaviors, but instead was due to improvements in immune function and decreases in HIV-1 viral load as a result of HAART use, and that prior to HAART use, immune function improvement could be attributed to zidovudine monotherapy.

One of the most dramatic changes in the AIDS epidemic has been the decline in KS among persons with AIDS associated with their use of HAART. When the period before HAART was compared to 1996 and beyond, the incidence of KS declined by about two-thirds, with KS now being a relatively uncommon diagnosis in people with AIDS.[11]

Numerous studies have reported significant declines in the incidence of KS. The Multicenter AIDS Cohort Study (MACS) reported rates of KS declining by 66% between the pre-HAART years 1989 to 1994 and the years 1996 to 1997, after HAART became readily available.[22] The International Collaboration on HIV and Cancer pooled data from 47,936 HIV-infected persons in 23 prospective studies and found that the overwhelming majority of cancers (more that 90%) during the period of 1992 to 1999 were either KS or NHL.

They reported that KS incidence declined from 15.2 per 1,000 person-years in the period 1992 through 1996 (1,489 cases) to 4.9 per 1,000 person-years in 1997 through 1999 (190 cases).[23] In addition, analyses looking individually at the 23 studies found that KS incidence declined in each, with many of the declines statistically significant.

Investigators from the Swiss HIV Cohort Study reported that KS incidence substantially decreased immediately following the initiation of HAART.[24] When the period before HAART was compared with the 15 months after HAART initiation, KS risk decreased by 66% ($p = .001$), suggesting that the impact of HAART is rapid. A population-based linkage of the HIV and cancer registries in Australia found that KS started declining between July 1990 and June 1994 (a pre-HAART period when zidovudine monotherapy was standard practice) and that there was a significant overall decline ($p = .045$) over the four time periods covered (prior to July 1990, July 1990–June 1994, July 1994–July 1996, and July 1996–December 1998).[25]

A linkage study between the San Francisco, California, AIDS registry and the California state cancer registry identified 3,407 cases of KS between 1988 and 2000 and found a statistically significant decreased adjusted rate ratio (RR) for KS in the HAART versus the pre-HAART time period (RR = 0.55, 95% CI 0.51–0.59).[26]

KS as the initial AIDS-defining illness has continued to decrease, but as people live longer on HAART, KS as a secondary AIDS diagnosis has increased from 23% in the 1980s to 50% in 1996 to 1997.[17,27] Nonetheless, overall the incidence of KS has significantly declined in the era following the introduction of HAART.

Survival

In addition to declining incidence, survival with KS has significantly improved with HAART use. The MAC Study reported an 81% reduced risk of death among KS patients who received HAART.[28] Additionally, survival with pulmonary KS, the most severe form of KS, has improved with HAART. Prior to HAART, 90% of AIDS patients who developed pulmonary KS progressed and died, whereas after the introduction of HAART, only 47% of patients with pulmonary KS died.[29]

In the linkage study between the San Francisco, California, AIDS registry and the California state cancer registry, median survival among persons with KS in the pre-HAART time period was 19 months (95% CI 18–20 months) and during the HAART era median survival increased to 93 months (95% CI 79 –upper bound not achieved), a statistically significant difference (*p* < .001)[30] (Figure 1–3).

Recent studies have found that both protease inhibitor–based and non-nucleoside reverse transcriptase inhibitor–based anti-retroviral treatment combinations may lead to an undetectable HIV-8 viral load, which is in turn associated with KS regression.[31]

Persons with pulmonary KS generally live about 4 to 6 months; with chemotherapy, median survival may increase to 9 to 11 months.[32]

Non-Hodgkin's Lymphoma

The first cases of AIDS-related NHL, specifically advanced stage Burkitt's-like lymphoma, were identified about one year after the first reports of AIDS in MSM.[33] As a result, in 1985, the CDC added diffuse, undifferentiated Burkitt's and Burkitt's-like lymphoma to the list of AIDS-defining illnesses.[34,35] As the AIDS epidemic progressed, a number of studies of NHL in persons with AIDS reported that the incidence of NHL and, specifically, clinically aggressive, high-grade NHL was increasing.[33,36] Again, the CDC expanded the AIDS-defining illnesses to include diffuse aggressive, intermediate-grade or high-grade NHL or B-cell or indeterminant phenotype occurring in an HIV-seropositive individual.[37,38]

Almost all AIDS-related NHLs derive from B cells. AIDS-related NHLs are extremely aggressive and are located in sites usually not found in other lymphomas.[39] AIDS-related NHLs tend to develop later in the course of HIV infection when compared to other AIDS-defining conditions, such as KS, and are characterized by clinical and histological heterogeneity.

AIDS-related NHLs are divided into three broad groups based on the anatomic site of origin: (1) systemic (nodal or extranodal), (2) primary central ner-

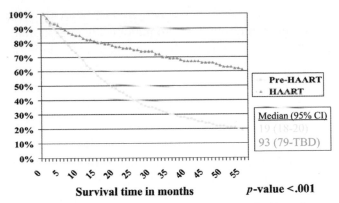

Figure 1–3. Kaplan-Meier survival time estimates for Kaposi's sarcoma, stratified by HAART time period, San Francisco AIDS cases, 1990–2000. Reproduced with permission from Hessol and Scheer.[30]

vous system (CNS), and (3) body-cavity–based or primary effusion lymphomas.[38]

Systemic NHLs make up approximately 80% of all AIDS-related NHLs. Approximately 85% of systemic NHLs have extranodal involvement, usually occurring in the central nervous system, the gastrointestinal tract, bone marrow, or the liver.[38] These include Burkitt's and Burkitt's-like lymphomas. Primary CNS lymphomas include immunoblastic lymphomas that present most commonly in the brain. They are usually large and multifocal occurring in the cerebrum, but they also occur in the cerebellum, basal ganglia, and the brain stems; they account for approximately 20% of AIDS-related NHLs.[38] Primary effusion lymphomas account for approximately 3% of all AIDS-related NHLs. These lymphomas are referred to as body cavity lymphomas because they usually remain localized in the body cavity of origin and usually do not spread to the lymph nodes or to distant sites.[38]

Etiologic Agent

NHL is associated with a viral pathogen, the Epstein-Barr virus (EBV). However, unlike KS and its association with the Kaposi's sarcoma herpesvirus (KSHV), EBV is not uniformly present in NHLs. EBV sequences are estimated to be present in approximately 30% of Burkitt's lymphoma and 80% of large-cell immunoblastic lymphomas.[40] Primary CNS lymphoma, however, is strongly associated with the presence of EBV, which is present in almost 100% of CNS lymphomas.[38,41–43] A study by MacMahon found that the majority of CNS lymphomas studied were large cell lymphomas or immunoblastic lymphoma, and EBV is preferentially associated with both of these histopathologies.[38,42] Another subset of NHLs, body cavity–based lymphomas, is strongly associated with the presence of KSHV.

The reactivation of latent EBV infection along with immune stimulation by the HIV virus is thought to lead to stimulation and proliferation of B-lymphocytes.[35] Even without EBV infection, HIV infection induces the production of inflammatory cytokines that cause B-cell stimulation, proliferation and activation.[35] Evidence also suggests that chronic simulation of B cells may be a risk factor for NHL.[35,40,44,45]

In addition, NHL is associated with both primary congenital immunodeficiency as well as iatrogenic secondary immunosuppression.[35] However, although the development of NHLs is related to immune deficiency, it does not seem to be as closely affected by immune status as other AIDS-related conditions.[40] Other than primary CNS lymphoma, the development of which is closely related to severe immune deficiency, NHLs occur in persons with AIDS when immune deficiency is moderate rather than profound. Primary CNS lymphoma most commonly occurs at the end stages of AIDS when CD4 counts fall below 50 cells per cubic millimeter.[41]

Risk Group and Geography

Unlike KS that overwhelmingly affects MSM with AIDS, NHL is distributed fairly evenly among the various AIDS risk groups.[3,39] Although the risk of developing AIDS-related NHL is relatively similar across geographic areas, the risk of NHL in industrialized countries is higher than in less industrialized countries. However, this is probably owing to competing mortality from other AIDS-related conditions in less industrialized countries. In the United States, approximately 80% of persons with AIDS-related NHL are MSM, a reflection of the epidemiology of the US AIDS epidemic. In Western Europe, IDUs make up a greater proportion of those with AIDS and account for approximately two-thirds of the persons with AIDS-related NHL.[38] NHL occurs more frequently in men than in women and occurs in all age groups,[46] with

lymphoma being the most common malignancy among children with HIV infection. NHL continues to be the second most common malignancy, after KS, found among persons with HIV infection. And, with the declining incidence of KS, NHL may become the most common malignancy among persons with AIDS.

Incidence and Presentation

Prior to the introduction of HAART, NHL occurred in HIV-positive persons 60 to 200 times more frequently than in the general population.[35,38,47,48] The incidence of NHL in AIDS patients is between 4 and 10%.[38] The risk of developing lymphoma among persons with symptomatic HIV infection has been estimated to be approximately 1.6% per year, and the risk among persons with AIDS on HAART for 3 years is approximately 19%.[3,49] There is a broad range in frequency estimates, which is likely due to the underreporting of NHL.

Underreporting of NHL occurs for a number of reasons; most significantly, many AIDS agencies and registries collect information on only the initial AIDS-defining condition.[3,38] However, 5% of persons with AIDS will develop NHL as a secondary AIDS diagnosis.[39] Many NHLs occur most commonly in the end stages of AIDS, when immune system deterioration has taken place and after an initial AIDS-defining condition has been recorded. Central nervous system lymphomas are often not recognized until death and even then may go undiagnosed owing to failure to conduct a postmortem examination on persons with other AIDS diagnoses.[38] Primary CNS lymphoma is approximately 1,000 times more frequent in persons with AIDS than in the general population.[38] As such, AIDS is the most common risk factor for primary CNS lymphoma. Primary CNS lymphoma has historically affected approximately 1% of persons with AIDS; however, as discussed below, primary CNS lymphoma has become increasingly unusual since the advent of HAART.[41]

The effect of HAART on systemic AIDS-related NHL is less dramatic than other AIDS-defining conditions and less clear,[35] with studies reporting mixed results. Most studies report no significant declines in the incidence of systemic NHL since the introduction of HAART,[39] and as people live longer with AIDS, the risk of NHL, a late complication of AIDS, is likely to increase. Only CNS lymphoma has shown a dramatic reduction in incidence (see below).

Ledergerber and colleagues reported results from a cohort in Switzerland with more than 18,000 person-years of follow-up. Comparing the pre-HAART period (1992–1994) with the post-HAART period (July 1997–June 1998), they found no significant decrease in lymphoma (relative hazard [RH] = 0.61; 95% CI 0.31–1.20).[24] In addition, no significant decline in primary CNS lymphoma was observed in this cohort.

Data from the San Francisco City Clinic Cohort found that among 622 HIV-infected MSM, the incidence of systemic NHL was not significantly different (p = .2) in the pre-HAART era (14 per 1,000 patient years) compared to the HAART era (18 per 1,000 patient years).[50]

Analyses of data among patients (n = 3,677) attending a hospital in London found that incidence of systemic NHL (CNS lymphoma and Hodgkin's disease cases were excluded) remained unchanged when the pre-HAART time frame (before 1996) was compared to the HAART time frame (1996 to 1999) (0.53% versus 0.47%, p = .73).[51] However, although the incidence remained unchanged, the proportion of NHL cases as a first AIDS-defining illness increased in the HAART era (1.3% versus 5.6%, p ≤ .0001).[51]

Trends in HIV-associated cancers were examined in the Adult/Adolescent Spectrum of HIV Disease Project Group representing nine US cities, 19,684 HIV-infected persons, and 26,638 years of follow-up.[52] When trends in incidence of NHL (excluding primary brain lymphoma) were calculated from January 1994 to June 1997, there was no significant trend over time (p = .070). However, there was a significant declining trend for primary brain lymphoma (p = .025). When the analyses were repeated and stratified by prescription of antiretroviral therapy, there was no significant trend in incidence of NHL among those receiving anti-retroviral therapy (p = .162) and those not receiving anti-retroviral therapy (p = .249). For primary brain lymphoma, there was a significant decline in incidence (p = .012) among those receiving anti-retroviral therapy, but not among those who did not receive anti-retroviral therapy (p = .937).[52]

On the other hand, the EuroSIDA cohort study group reported that among all subtypes of NHL studied, incidence decreased from 1.99 events per 100 person-years of follow-up (95% CI 1.51–2.47) before September 1995 to 0.30 per 100 person-years of follow-up after March 1999 (p < .001). Comparing the same time periods, the most significant decrease was found in primary brain lymphoma (0.83 to 0.04 cases per 100 person-years of follow-up [p < .001]). For the following other subtypes, the decreases were also significant: Burkitt's lymphoma declined from 0.18 to 0.03 (p < .018), immunoblastic lymphoma declined from 0.50 to 0.10 (p < .001) and for other/unknown histology 0.48 to 0.19 (p = .008). Furthermore, the incidence of NHL decreased from 0.88 (95% CI 0.60–1.16) cases per 100 person-years of follow-up within the first 12 months of starting HAART to 0.45 (95% CI 0.31–0.60) cases per 100 person-years of follow-up after more than 24 months on HAART.[53]

Another study evaluating incidence of systemic and primary CNS lymphoma from 1988 to 1997 in 17 Western European countries found that lymphoma incidence among AIDS patients steadily rose from 1988 until 1996, and then slightly declined in 1997. However, systemic lymphoma as a percentage of all AIDS cases rose to 4.9% in 1997, compared with 3.6% in 1994.[54] No significant declines in CNS lymphoma were reported.

In a population-based linkage of the HIV and cancer registries in Australia, NHL increased (p = .012) over the four time periods (prior to July 1990, July 1990–June 1994, July 1994–July 1996, and July 1996–December 1998), but incidence rates in the last period (post-HAART) were significantly lower than in the three previous periods (incidence rate ratio, 0.58; 95% CI 0.36–0.92).[25] To evaluate whether the increases over the first three time periods were due to the increasing immune deficiency among people in the HIV registry, the investigators also looked at the incidence of NHL among recent seroconverters (n = 1,101) for three time periods (prior to July 1994, July 1994–June 1996, and June 1996–December 1998). They found that among recent seroconverters, there was a non-significant decrease in incidence (p = .662) across the study time frames.[25]

A linkage study between the San Francisco, California, AIDS registry and the California state cancer registry identified 1,225 cases of NHL (including 184 cases of CNS NHL) between 1988 and 2000 and found a statistically significant decreased adjusted rate ratio for NHL in the HAART versus the pre-HAART time period (RR = 0.49, 95% CI 0.43–0.56).[26]

A study of 1,5549 HIV-infected women in the US Women's Interagency HIV Study (WIHS) also found a significant decrease of NHL in the HAART period (1997–2001) compared to the pre-HAART era (1994–1996) (RR = 0.15, 95% CI 0.03–0.61, p = .005).[9]

Clearly, the use of HAART has not had as significant an impact on systemic NHL rates as it has on KS rates. A number of factors may account for this. Since systemic NHL is not uniformly associated with a viral pathogen, partial immune restoration may be less effective in preventing the occurrence of systemic NHL.[25] Furthermore, when compared to other AIDS-defining illnesses, including CNS lymphomas, systemic NHL occurs before immune deficiency is as severe. Because systemic NHL tends to occur prior to severe immunodeficiency, HAART may not be as effective at preventing systemic disease or may not even be indicated and therefore prescribed at the time of occurence.[52] Chronic immune stimulation has also been shown to be a risk factor for the development of AIDS-related NHL, and HAART may not be fully effective at reversing the immune stimulation.[25] In addition, incidence trends may vary based on whether the analyses include CNS lymphomas with all other NHLs or not.

In contrast to the conflicting data on systemic NHLs, one subset of NHL, primary CNS lymphomas, seem to have had significant declines in incidence since the introduction of HAART.[39,43,52] However, accurate data on CNS lymphomas are often lacking owing to incorrect or missing diagnoses. Since CNS lymphomas do not occur as frequently compared to other NHLs, many studies do not have the power to analyze CNS lymphomas separately. However, it does appear that, as a result of HAART use, primary CNS lymphomas are now becoming increasingly rare among persons with HIV infection.[41] Although the reasons for this are not entirely clear, preserved immune function as a result of HAART must account for some portion of the declines seen.[39]

Survival

Except for multifocal encephalopathy, NHL limits the life expectancy of persons with AIDS more than any other AIDS-defining condition.[3] Prior to HAART, the median survival for persons with NHL was fewer than 18 months, and survival with primary CNS lymphoma was even poorer. The EuroSIDA cohort study group reported that median survival time with primary brain lymphoma (1 month; 95% CI 1–2 months) was significantly worse than other NHLs ($p < .001$). Survival time for Burkitt's, immunoblastic, and unknown/other histology were 6 months (95% CI 2–16 months), 6 months (95% CI 4–10 months), and 5 months (95% CI 2–7 months), respectively.[53]

Chemotherapy regimens used for NHL in non–HIV-infected persons have not been as successful when used in persons with HIV infection,[3,55] and opportunistic infections associated with aggressive chemotherapy increase in persons with HIV infection. Twenty to 80% of persons with HIV-related NHL developed opportunistic infections following chemotherapy treatment.[3] Efforts to improve chemotherapy tolerance by trying low-dose chemotherapy have not been successful. In one large, randomized trial, the incidence of opportunistic infections in the standard-dose and low-dose arms were the same, and the low-dose arm failed to show improved survival.[56]

Some studies have indicated that HAART may be influencing not only the incidence of but also the clinical presentation and treatment outcomes of AIDS-related NHL.[41] HAART may improve survival among persons with AIDS-related NHL by limiting the damage to the immune system during chemotherapy and possibly permitting the development of antitumor immune responses,[3]

In the linkage study between the San Francisco, California, AIDS registry and the California state cancer registry, median survival among persons with NHL (excluding CNS NHL) in the pre-HAART time period was 7 months (95% CI 6–8 months) compared to 27 months in the HAART era (95% CI 17–37 months), a statistically significant difference ($p < .001$)[30] (Figure 1–4). Looking specifically at CNS NHL, median survival in the pre-HAART time

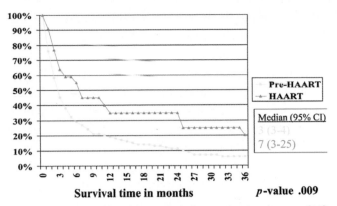

Figure 1–4. Kaplan-Meier survival time estimates for non-CNS NHL, stratified by HAART time period, San Francisco AIDS cases, 1990–2000. Reproduced with permission from Hessol and Scheer. [30]

period was 3 months (95% CI 3–4 months) versus 7 months during the HAART era (95% CI 3–25 months) (p = .009)[30] (Figure 1–5).

Vaccher and colleagues reported on the effect of HAART on three measures of survival: progression-free, disease-free, and overall survival among patients with HIV-related systemic NHL in an Italian cohort study. For each measure of survival, no-HAART use was a significant predictor of poorer survival; hazard ratios were 17.42 (95% CI 17.42–40.25), 9.11 (95% CI 3.71–22.32), and 8.54 (95% CI 1.19–61.11), respectively, when comparing no-HAART use to HAART use greater than or equal to 24 months.[57]

However, the EuroSIDA cohort study group did not find a significant increase in median survival over time for patients with primary brain lymphoma or other types of NHL. For primary brain lymphoma, the median survival time before 1997, in 1997, and after 1997 was 1 month (95% CI 1–2 months),

1 month (95% CI 1–2 months), and 3 months (95% CI 1–4 months), respectively (p = .80).[53] Combining Burkitt's, immunoblastic, or unknown/other histology for the same three time periods, median survival time was 4 months (95% CI 3–6 months), 12 months (95% CI 5–32 months), and 5 months (95% CI 3–9 months), respectively (p = .08).

Post-HAART survival has somewhat improved for CNS lymphoma as more treatment options have become available. The restorative impact of HAART on the immune system has made the use of systemic chemotherapy more feasible among persons with AIDS-related CNS lymphoma.

Invasive Cervical Cancer

AIDS-related cancers occurring in HIV-infected men have been identified and studied extensively. However, less is known about cancers occurring among women with HIV infection. Invasive cervical cancer (squamous cell carcinoma) clearly occurs in excess (as much as a fourfold excess[52]) among women with AIDS as compared to the general population and was added to the CDC AIDS case definition in 1993.[58]

Squamous neoplasia of the cervix can be viewed as a continuum of a single disease, beginning with mild dysplasia, followed by moderate and then severe dysplasia, and eventually invasive carcinoma.[3] Owing to this broad spectrum of cervical disease, with invasive carcinoma being the rarest manifestation, it is very important to avoid misclassification of lesser disease with invasive cancer when quantifying the effect of HAART or HIV infection on cervical cancer. Especially given the higher rate of precancerous lesions, even a small amount of misclassification of these as cancers can dramatically alter study results.

Etiologic Agent

Like KS and NHL, cervical cancer is associated with a viral pathogen, the human papillomavirus (HPV). HPV is a small DNA virus that can cause both benign and malignant epithelial proliferations. HPV viral sequences play a key role in the pathogenesis of cervical cancer[59] and are found in 99% of cervical cancers.[59,60]

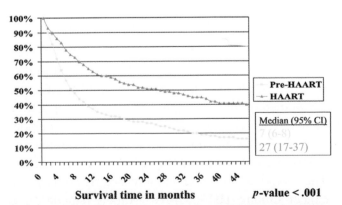

Figure 1–5. Kaplan-Meier survival time estimates for CNS NHL, stratified by HAART time period, San Francisco AIDS cases, 1990–2000. Reproduced with permission from Hessol and Scheer. [30]

However, it remains controversial as to whether or not HIV infection and resulting immune deficiency influences the development of cervical cancer in women. Instead, it may be that the same sexual risk factors that place women at risk of the HPV may also place them at risk of sexually acquired HIV infection. In addition, other similar risk behaviors among women at risk for HPV and HIV infection, such as smoking, may also confound the association between HIV and cervical cancer.

Risk Group and Geography

HIV and HPV share many of the same risk factors or predictors. These include multiple sex partners, smoking, early age at first intercourse, sex with men who have had multiple sex partners, low socioeconomic status, and low usage of barrier contraceptives. In addition, infection with either HPV or HIV may be enhanced by the presence of the other infection.[60]

In countries with routine cervical cytologic screening, the incidence and mortality of cervical cancer is low.[61] However, the incidence and prevalence of cervical intraepithelial neoplasia (CIN), a cervical cancer precursor lesion, are high in HIV-infected women. In developed countries, HIV-infected women with CIN are more likely to be carefully monitored and treated before lesions progress to invasive cancer. However, studies in developing countries have also been unable to find an association between HIV infection and invasive cervical cancer, in spite of the increased incidence of HPV and cervical dysplasia among women with HIV infection.[60] A possible explanation for this could be that, in developing countries, death from other HIV-related causes often occurs before cervical cancer develops among women with CIN.[60,61]

Incidence and Presentation

There is conflicting evidence that the risk of cervical cancer is greater among women with HIV than those without HIV,[62,63] and data on how HAART have affected cervical cancer incidence is sparse and ambiguous. However, HIV-infected women are more likely to be infected with multiple HPV subtypes, to have lower regression rates, and at the time of presen-

tation are more likely to have multifocal and advanced lesions that are less responsive to treatment.[64–68]

In Africa, cervical cancer is the most common form of cancer in women; however, although HIV is widely prevalent in central and southern Africa, there has not been an epidemic of cervical cancer.[1] Three studies from Africa failed to find an increased risk of cervical cancer when HIV-positive women were compared to HIV-seronegative women. When the overall risk was calculated for all three studies, comprising 363 HIV-seropositive women, the overall relative risk was 0.8 (95% CI 0.5–1.4).[1,69–71]

There are also very few studies from North America and Europe owing to the low prevalence of cervical cancer in these geographic areas. Since women in these areas tend to have regular Pap smears, preclinical cervical neoplasia is most often detected and treated early. The few studies that have looked at the incidence of cervical cancer among women with HIV-infection have found mixed results regarding cervical cancer incidence in this population.

Some cohort studies have, however, reported an increased incidence of cervical cancer among women with AIDS. A study from Rome, Italy, reported that among 483 women, the relative hazard of invasive cervical cancer for 1996 to 1998 was 7.41% (95% CI 1.21–45.44) when compared to 1981 through 1995.[72] This study also found that invasive cervical cancer was the only AIDS-defining condition with an increasing trend during 1981 to 1995. The decline in incidence of all other AIDS-defining diseases since 1996 suggests that the increased relative hazard of cervical cancer may be due to decrease in mortality from other AIDS-defining conditions in HIV-infected women.[72]

The number of observed cases of cervical cancer among women from the Italian HIV Seroconverter Study and the DMI-2 study in Southeastern France was compared with the expected number of cases for women of the same age in the general population of these two countries.[73] There were 9,070 person-years of follow-up among HIV-positive women and 2,310 person-years among HIV-negative women. The investigators found an increased risk of cervical cancer among HIV-positive women (standardized incidence rate [SIR] = 12.8) especially among women who were injection drug users (SIR = 16.7), perhaps reflecting a lack of access to medical care and screening in this high-risk population.

Researchers with the HIV Epidemiology Research Study (HERS) analyzed cancer incidence data from 871 HIV-positive women (contributing 4,180 person-years) and 439 HIV-negative women (contributing 2,308 person-years) enrolled in four urban sites in the United States. These women had a high prevalence of smoking history (85%) as well as injection drug use (50%). Using medical record review and death certificates for cancer ascertainment, investigators reported an increased rate of cancers among HIV-infected women, including five cervical cancers. They concluded that counseling regarding smoking cessation and access to Pap smear screening is crucial among HIV positive women, especially as they live longer with HAART.[74]

Another US cohort study compared the number of incident cancer cases among HIV-infected women and at-risk HIV-uninfected women from the WIHS with expected number of cases based on the population-based US Surveillance, Epidemiology, and End Results (SEER) registry. They did not find an excess number of cervical cancer cases (one case among HIV-infected women and no cases among HIV-uninfected women).[9] The authors concluded that this may be due to cancer screening services in this cohort that are not as easily available to other at-risk women, including cytologic surveillance and treatment of precursor lesions. However, they also note that another analysis from the WIHS data found that after pathology review, a substantial number of invasive cervical cancer cases in regional cancer registries were misclassified and were actually cervical dysplasia.[75] As a result, studies that rely solely on registry matches may find higher rates of cervical cancer among HIV-infected women than do those that include other forms of cancer ascertainment.

Analysis of the International Collaboration on HIV and Cancer data found 36 cervical cancer cases detected between 1992 and 1999. There was no significant change in incidence rates of cervical cancer between 1992 to 1996 and 1997 to 1999 (rate ratio 1.87; 99% CI 0.77–4.56; based on 19 and 17 cases, respectively; $p = .07$). The authors noted that since the introduction of HAART, cervical cancer screening among women with HIV infection may be increasing. Given the small number of cervical cancer cases detected, they could only conclude that cervical cancer does not appear to be common in HIV-infected women.[23]

Survival

The use of HAART may influence the relationship between HIV and the incidence of and/or survival with cervical cancer or cervical cancer precursors in two ways. First, HAART prolongs survival among persons with HIV and, therefore, may also prolong exposure to HPV. This increases the likelihood that genetic somatic mutations occur and thus the risk of cervical disease.[76] In contrast, immune system improvements on HAART may mitigate the effect of HIV on HPV disease.[76]

Surprisingly, little epidemiologic data are available on the treatment and outcomes of HIV-infected patients with invasive cervical cancer. In the few studies that have been done, stage of disease rather than HIV status appeared to be the most important determinant of survival.[77] A study using cancer registry data from Kampala, Uganda, evaluated survival in 261 patients with invasive cervical cancer between 1995 and 1997.[78] Only 63 cases (24.1%) had been treated by radiotherapy. They found an overall survival at three years of 52.4%, and there was no difference in survival among HIV-infected patients compared to HIV-uninfected patients at 1, 3, and 4 years after diagnosis.[78]

Although reliable studies on cervical cancer survival changes in the era of HAART are not available yet, HAART clearly extends the survival of HIV-infected women with CIN and, therefore, may increase the risk of CIN progressing to cervical cancer. As such, screening for, and treatment of, CIN in HIV-infected women is crucial.

NON–AIDS-DEFINING CANCERS, PRE-HAART VERSUS HAART ERA

In addition to the AIDS-defining malignancies, there are several other malignancies that may be associated with HIV infection but are not considered AIDS defining. Below is a review of the most frequently reported malignancies found in excess among people with HIV and AIDS. Like the AIDS-defining cancers, many of these cancers are associated with viruses other than HIV, leading to the theory that the effects of HIV may directly or indirectly predispose individuals to virally induced malignancies. Because individuals with HIV infection often present with advanced stage of disease and unusually aggressive clinical courses, at the least it appears that the natural history of many malignancies may be altered by HIV infection.[79]

Hodgkin's Disease

Not long after non-Hodgkin's lymphoma was added to the AIDS case definition, several clinical studies reported that an unusually high proportion of HIV-infected patients with Hodgkin's disease were presenting with high histologic grade (mixed cellularity and lymphocyte depletion subtypes) and advanced stage (III and IV) disease.[80–84] These patients also demonstrated poor responses to therapy and short survival times.[84–87]

These initial reports were followed by epidemiologic studies, including evaluations of cancer[88] and AIDS[89] registry data and epidemiologic cohort studies[15,90–92] that suggested there might be an increased incidence of Hodgkin's disease in HIV-infected individuals. However, the increased incidence of the disease was considerably lower than the incidence seen for non-Hodgkin's lymphoma.[89–94] This low-magnitude increase of Hodgkin's disease is probably the reason it was not detected earlier in the HIV epidemic. Nonetheless, once the association between Hodgkin's disease and HIV infection was demonstrated, Hodgkin's disease became the most commonly and consistently found excess cancer among the non–AIDS-defining malignancies.

Etiologic Agent

As with non-Hodgkin's lymphoma, the EBV has also been linked to the development of Hodgkin's disease, especially among HIV-infected individuals. In HIV-infected Hodgkin's disease patients, a large majority (80–100%) of the Hodgkin's disease tumors carry the EBV genome.[95–98] In HIV-uninfected Hodgkin's disease patients, approximately 30 to 40%

have detectable EBV.[97–99] The EBV subtypes A and B are found in equal frequency in non-Hodgkin's lymphoma tumors, whereas subtype A is more common in Hodgkin's disease tumors.[95]

Risk Groups and Geography

Among the general population, the crude incidence rate of Hodgkin's disease is greater in men (27.0 per 1,000,000) than women (18.1 per 1,000,000) and the sex ratio is estimated at approximately 1.5 males to females.[100] This increased risk in men is also seen in those individuals with HIV infection,[101,102] although not all studies have demonstrated a significant sex difference among HIV-infected people.[94,103,104]

Among HIV-uninfected individuals in developed countries, Hodgkin's disease has a bimodal age distribution, with the first peak occurring at 15 to 34 years and another among people over 55 years.[105] Histologically, nodular sclerosis is primarily diagnosed in young Hodgkin's disease patients, whereas mixed cellularity predominates in the older age groups. Among HIV-infected individuals, despite a younger median age at diagnosis of Hodgkin's disease, mixed cellularity and lymphocyte depletion are the predominant histological features.[106]

Early in the AIDS epidemic, a few European studies of HIV-infected adults noted a greater increase in the incidence of Hodgkin's disease among IDUs compared with other HIV risk groups.[86,107] However, since then most studies, including those in Europe,[102–104] have not found IDUs to have a higher incidence of Hodgkin's disease compared to other HIV risk groups.

Incidence and Presentation

As stated above, there are a large number of published reports that have found an increased incidence of Hodgkin's disease among people with HIV[90,102,108] and AIDS.[63,103,109] In addition, the risk increases with immunodeficiency, especially around the time of an initial AIDS-defining event.[15,101,104]

One study that evaluated the risk of Hodgkin's disease in the pre-HAART and HAART eras found that those diagnosed in the HAART era had less aggressive disease (70 versus 87% of stage III/IV disease, p = .03).[98] Two other studies found no change in the incidence of Hodgkin's disease during the HAART era compared to the pre-HAART time period.[23,52] However, a large French cohort study of 77,025 HIV-infected patients found the standardized incidence ratio (SIR) for Hodgkin's disease in the pre-HAART time period to be 22.75 (95% CI 17.27–29.40) in men and 9.62 (95% CI 3.10–22.44) in women. This increased in the HAART period, with a SIR for men of 31.66 (95% CI 25.79–38.47) and a SIR for women of 14.29 (95% CI 6.84–26.27).[102]

A linkage study between the San Francisco, California, AIDS registry and the California state cancer registry identified 76 cases of Hodgkin's disease between 1988 and 2000 and found that the increased, but not statistically different, adjusted rate ratio for Hodgkin's disease in the HAART versus the pre-HAART time period was 1.47 (95% CI 0.94–2.30).[26]

Survival

A few studies have suggested that Hodgkin's disease survival time is increasing in the HAART era. One of two population-based linkage studies in the greater San Francisco Bay area found that HIV-infected individuals diagnosed with Hodgkin's disease in the HAART era (n = 31) had a marginally better survival (p = .07) compared to those diagnosed in the pre-HAART era (n = 87).[98] The 1-year, 2-year, and 5-year survival probabilities were 74 versus 68%, 64 versus 53%, and 58 versus 33%, respectively. Another AIDS-cancer registry linkage study in San Francisco found the Hodgkin's disease median survival time in the pre-HAART era to be 30 months (95% CI 21–50 months) and the median survival time in the HAART era to be 103 months (95% CI 28–upper bound not achieved), p = .10[30] (Figure 1–6).

One study that had direct measures for HAART use found that when evaluating the survival time for Hodgkin's disease using calendar period, there was no statistical difference in the HAART versus pre-HAART time period.[110] However, when the investigators stratified the data by response to HAART, there was a significant difference. In multivariate analyses of risk factors for overall survival, response to HAART (RH = 0.19, 95% CI 0.06–0.60),

age ≤ 45 years (RH = 0.23, 95% CI 0.09–0.60), and complete remission (RH = 0.30, 95% CI 0.13–0.72) were all associated with improved survival.

Anal Cancer

Prior to the HIV/AIDS epidemic, the incidence of anal cancer was increasing in Sweden, Denmark, and the United States.[111–113] Secular changes in sexual behavior were likely the reason for this increase.[114] Studies of behavioral risk factors for anal cancer identified anal intercourse and number of sexual partners to be associated with this outcome.[115]

Once HIV was identified as the etiologic agent for the development of AIDS, there was concern that HIV-infected MSM were at an even higher risk for anal cancer than HIV-uninfected MSM. This prompted additional investigations into the risk of cancer among those at risk for AIDS.[88,116–118]

Etiologic Agent

Both anal and cervical cancer are strongly associated with lifestyles that increase exposure to sexually transmissible diseases,[119] and both are HPV-related.[115] The oncogenic HPV subtype most strongly associated with both in situ and invasive anal cancer is HPV 16,[115,120] and, to a lesser extent, HPV 18, 31, and 33.[115] The natural history of anal cancer mimics other neoplasms where HPV plays an etiological role.[119] A fair number of non-regressing anal and genital warts become dysplastic, and a

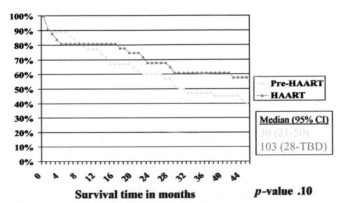

Figure 1–6. Kaplan-Meier survival time estimates for Hodgkin's disease, stratified by HAART time period, San Francisco AIDS cases, 1990–2000. Reproduced with permission from Hessol and Scheer.[30]

small percentage of these will become malignant, with invasion into the subjacent stroma.

Risk Groups and Geography

Prior to the 1980s, the increased risk of anal cancer was more pronounced in women than in men and more evident in urban than in rural areas.[112,113] Furthermore, Blacks were at higher risk than Whites and never-married men were at higher risk than ever-married men,[113] The increased risk of anal cancer among never-married men dates back to the 1940s and 1950s and suggests that important behavioral changes, specifically sexual practices, were taking place in that population. Before the HIV epidemic, the incidence of anal cancer among men with a history of receptive anal intercourse was estimated to be as high as 35 per 100,000,[113] a rate comparable with the incidence of cervical cancer prior to the introduction of routine cervical cytology screening.

In the United States prior to the 1980s, the rates of invasive and in situ anal carcinoma were higher in women than in men.[121] This began to change in the 1980s and 1990s when the rates in men (presumably MSM) began to equal those in women. Between 1973 and 2000, men had poorer overall survival than did women with anal cancer (relative 5-year survival, 58 versus 64%), and black men had worse 5-year survival than white men (38 versus 61%). More advanced disease stage was inversely associated with survival, and in each disease stage category, men had poorer survival than did women.

Incidence and Presentation

In the general population, anal cancer is a rare disease, occurring in approximately 1 per 100,000 persons.[121,122] Whereas anal cancer incidence is clearly higher in MSM and adults with AIDS than in the general population (10–35 times higher),[15,63,88,101,109,118] it is not clear how much of this excess is due to HIV infection. Other risk factors for the development of anal cancer besides HIV infection include sexual practices that increase HPV exposure and cigarette smoking.[114,123]

One large AIDS and cancer registry linkage study in the United States evaluated the incidence of both in situ and invasive anal cancer in women with AIDS and found a relative risk of 6.8 (95% CI 2.7–14.0) for invasive disease and 7.8 (95% CI 0.2–43.6) for in situ anal cancer.[124] The comparable rates in men were 37.9 (95% CI 33.0–43.4) and 60.1 (49.2–72.7), respectively. Among MSM, the rates were even higher: a relative risk of 59.5 (95% CI 51.5–68.4) for invasive cancers and 99.8 (95% CI 81.4–121.2) for in situ cancers.

Although HPV-associated invasive anal cancer may not be a direct consequence of HIV-mediated immunosuppression, HPV-associated low grade and high grade anal squamous intraepithelial lesions (ASIL) and in situ anal carcinomas are likely associated with HIV immunosuppression.[124] Two prospective studies in homosexual men found that after adjustment for HPV status, HIV-infected men with CD4 cell counts < 200 at baseline were at highest risk for ASIL, followed by those with CD4 cell counts 200 to 500 and those with baseline CD4 cell counts of > 500.[125,126] Data from an AIDS and cancer registry linkage study found a high incidence of both in situ and invasive anogenital cancers among patients with low CD4 cell counts but showed no indication of a further increase in risk among patients with CD4 cell counts < 100 compared with those having CD4 cell counts ≥ 200.[124]

Several studies have evaluated the effect of HAART on ASIL, but few have examined the impact of HAART on anal cancer. In an anal neoplasia natural history cohort study of a subgroup of 202 HIV-infected MSM participants for whom the dates of continuous HAART use were known, HPV infection and HPV levels remained unchanged in the first 6 months after HAART initiation. Moreover, the rates of progression or regression of anal neoplasia, despite a considerable increase in CD4+ lymphocyte count,[127] also remained constant. Another study, this one in France, of 120 HIV-infected MSM patients who had previously received HAART for a median of 32 months, found a high prevalence of ASIL, including high grade SIL, and anal HPV infection despite immune restoration.[128] A third prospective study of anal intraepithelial neoplasia (AIN) in 23 HIV-infected homosexual men in London, England, with symptomatic AIN found no evidence of a correlation between the successful treatment of HIV-infection and improvements in AIN.[129] The results of these three studies indicate that the future rates of invasive cancer may continue to rise in the HIV population because HAART appears to have little to no effect on anal HPV infection or on the rates of anal SIL.

One AIDS and cancer registry linkage study that did examine the temporal effects of HAART on anal cancer in San Francisco, California, identified 88 anal cancers (all in men) between 1988 and 2000 and found a significant increase in incidence; the adjusted rate ratio in the HAART versus the pre-HAART time period was 3.35 (95% CI 2.13–5.27).[26] Another study, this time of HIV-infected patients in a French database network, found the SIR for colon, rectum, and anal cancer in the pre-HAART period (1992–1995) for homosexual men to be 2.59 (95% CI 1.54–4.10) and 1.74 (1.10–2.61) in the HAART period (1996–1999).[102] Although the first study found an increase in anal cancer in the HAART era and the second study did not, it should be noted that the second study included colon and rectum cancers with the anal cancers. Since it is generally known that the pathology of colon and rectum cancers is quite distinct from anal cancers, combining them may result in the loss of pertinent information.

Survival

Prior to the widespread use of HAART, HIV-infected patients with anal carcinoma had a poorer tolerance to combined therapy (chemotherapy and radiation) and a shorter time to cancer-related death than HIV-uninfected patients. The median time to cancer-related death was 1.4 years in the HIV-infected patients compared to 5.3 years in the HIV-uninfected patients ($p = .02$).[130]

One study that failed to show a change in the anal cancer survival time was a San Francisco linkage study, which found the anal cancer survival time in the pre-HAART era (median 52 months; 95% CI 39–90) to be similar to the survival time in the HAART era (median time not yet reached) ($p = .84$)[30] (Figure 1–7).

Longer follow-up of anal cancer patients in the HAART era is needed to determine if there is truly an increase in survival time.

Lung Cancer

The data on lung cancer incidence among people with HIV vary, with most studies reporting a higher risk,[9,101,104,109] and a few reporting an equal risk or lower risk than that of the general population.[94,106,108,131] Several studies that found an increased risk of lung cancer among people with HIV and AIDS attribute this increase to cigarette smoking rather than HIV itself.[9,101,102,104,132,133] Whereas some studies have demonstrated an association between the degree and/or duration of immunosuppression and lung cancer,[104,134] others have failed to find this association.[101]

Etiologic Agent

There is little doubt that cigarette smoking is the most common risk factor for the development of lung cancer; cigarette smoking accounts for 79 to 90% of all lung cancers.[135,136] Among smokers, the risk for lung cancer is estimated to be 1,200 to 2,000 times higher than for non-smokers, and the risk increases with age, number of cigarettes smoked per day, and duration of smoking.

Risk Groups and Geography

Besides cigarette smoking, other factors that may account for the increased risk of lung cancer among people with HIV infection include opportunistic lung infections and intravenous drug use.[132,133] Preexisting scar tissue from pulmonary infections, including TB, may also elevate lung cancer risk. IDUs who may

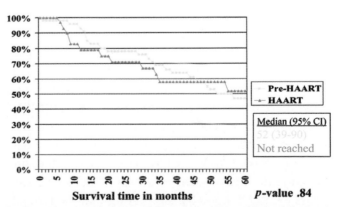

Figure 1–7. Kaplan-Meier survival time estimates for invasive anal cancer, stratified by HAART time period, San Francisco AIDS cases, 1990–2000. Reproduced with permission from Hessol and Scheer.[30]

have drug-induced changes in the pulmonary stroma from recurrent pulmonary infections could have increased production of growth factors, which would lead to the development of lung cancer.

Lung cancer was the most common cancer in the world in 2000, and it causes greater mortality in the developed (22% of cancer deaths) than developing (14.6% of deaths) countries.[137] Geographic patterns for lung cancer reflect past exposure to tobacco smoking, and the geographic patterns in women differ from those in men. In men, the areas with the highest incidence and mortality are Europe (especially Eastern Europe), North America, Australia/New Zealand, and South America. The rates in China, Japan, and Southeast Asia are moderately high, whereas the lowest rates are found in Southern Asia (India, Pakistan) and sub-Saharan Africa (excluding Zimbabwe and South Africa). Among women, the highest lung cancer rates are in the United States, Canada, the United Kingdom, and Denmark.[137]

Incidence and Presentation

A large French hospital database was used to evaluate the incidence of lung cancer in the pre-HAART and HAART time periods. In the pre-HAART time period, the standardized incidence ratios for both HIV-infected men ($n = 22$) and women ($n = 1$) with lung cancer were not significantly elevated (SIR = 1.13, 95% CI 0.71–1.72 for men; SIR = 1.08, 95% CI 0.01–5.98 for women) but were elevated in the HAART era (SIR = 2.12, 95% CI 1.67–2.65 for men [$n = 77$]; SIR = 6.59, 95% CI 3.40–11.52 for women [$n = 12$]).[102]

A study in southeast England evaluated the age- and sex-adjusted rates of lung cancer in the general population with the rates in HIV patients in the pre-HAART ($n = 2$) and HAART eras ($n = 9$). Investigators found that in the pre-HAART time period, the age- and sex-adjusted incidence of lung cancer was estimated to be 0.8 per 10,000 person-years (95% CI 0.2–1.4) among people with HIV and was similar to the population rate of 0.75 per 10,000 person-years (95% CI 0.63–0.87).[138] In the HAART era, the lung cancer rate was higher at 6.7 per 10,000 person-years (95% CI 3.5–9.9), suggesting that the risk has increased since the introduction of HAART. Interestingly, the patients in the HAART era presented

with lung cancer at a similar age, smoked as many cigarettes, and had a similar level of immunosuppression when compared with pre-HAART studies.

A large prospective study of HIV-infected and at-risk women in the United States found an increased age- and race-adjusted SIR for lung cancer in both the HIV-infected women (SIR = 6.3, 95% CI 2.7–11.3; $n = 8$) and the HIV-uninfected women (SIR = 6.9, 95% CI 0.8–19.3; $n = 2$).[9] The SIR among HIV-infected women in the pre-HAART time period was 6.8 (95% CI 0.8–18.9) and 6.2 (95% CI 2.3–12.1) in the HAART era. The adjusted rate ratio for lung cancer in the HAART versus the pre-HAART time period was not significant (RR = 1.38, 95% CI 0.25–13.98).

A linkage study between the San Francisco, California, AIDS registry and the California state cancer registry identified 75 lung/bronchial cancers between 1988 and 2000 and found no statistical difference in incidence; the adjusted rate ratio for lung cancer in the HAART versus the pre-HAART time period was 1.09 (95% CI 0.69–1.72).[26]

Although there are conflicting findings on whether HIV increases the risk of lung cancer, there is agreement that the presentation and severity of disease is different in people with HIV infection than those without. Lung cancer patients with HIV are more likely to present with advanced disease (stage IIIB/IV) and adenocarcinomas than lung cancer patients without HIV.[133,138]

Survival

A few European studies have shown that lung cancer survival is shorter for people with concomitant HIV infection compared to those without HIV.[87,133] This is likely influenced by the fact that people with HIV present with more advanced disease and have a higher risk of mortality owing to other causes.

Although there is little evidence to show that the lung cancer incidence has declined in the HAART era, lung cancer survival may be increasing, but these results are not uniform. One study that failed to show a change in the lung cancer survival time includes a San Francisco linkage study, which found the lung cancer median survival time in the pre-HAART era to be 14 months (95% CI 10–21 months) and the median survival time in the HAART era to be 13 months (95%

CI 7–26 months).[30] Of note, the survival times reported in this study are similar to the reported median survival times for lung cancer patients without HIV infection in the European studies.[87,133]

A summary of the changes in incidence and survival in the HAART era, for the most common HIV-related malignancies, is shown in Table 1–2.

Other Potentially HIV-Related Malignancies

Since the beginning of the AIDS epidemic, additional cancers have been linked to HIV infection, but the incidence is either inconsistently reported across studies or potential confounders exist. For the following cancers, little, if anything, has been reported on the effect of HAART on the incidence or survival.

Testicular Cancer. There have been case reports and small case series of testicular cancer in HIV-infected men. Since the incidence of both testicular germ-cell tumors and infection with HIV is highest in men aged 20 to 40 years, this is not a surprising finding. Two population-based cancer registry studies evaluating testicular cancer over time in never-married men in San Francisco and Manhattan

failed to find any increase.[116,117] One prospective study reported an increase in seminoma cases in HIV-infected MSM,[91] although another failed to show an increased incidence between testicular cancer and HIV infection.[15] Similarly, some HIV/AIDS and cancer registry linkage studies found a slight increase in testicular seminomas,[101,104] whereas other linkage studies have not.[89,108,109,139]

Skin Cancer. In addition to KS, other primary skin cancers have been found in excess in people with HIV/AIDS, including basal cell carcinoma,[103] squamous cell carcinoma,[94,103] and melanoma.[101] Complicating the evaluation of skin cancer and its association with HIV infection is (1) the possibility of misclassification of KS as a non-KS skin cancer, and (2) the fact that basal and squamous cell skin cancers are likely to be under-reported (these cancers are not required to be reported to the US SEER program). However, melanoma is a reportable malignancy to cancer registries, and most studies that have used cancer registries to verify cases have failed to find any increase over time in never-married men,[116,117] in people with HIV,[9,15,108] or in people with AIDS.[104,109]

Table 1–2. THE EFFECT OF HAART ON THE INCIDENCE AND SURVIVAL TIME FOR SELECT CANCERS				
Cancer	Change in Incidence	Possible Reason for Change	Change in Survival	Possible Reason for Change
KS	Decrease[22–26]	Immune reconstitution	Increase[28–30,32]	Immune reconstitution/ less comorbidity
Systemic NHL	None[24,39,50–52]/ decrease[9,26,53]	Immune reconstitution	None[53]/increase[30,57]	Immune reconstitution/ less comorbidity/ changes in treatment
CNS NHL	None[24,54]/ decrease[26,39,52,53]	Immune reconstitution	None[53]/increase[30]	Immune reconstitution/ less comorbidity/ changes in treatment
Invasive cervical cancer	None[23]	Improved screening for cervical cancer	?	
Hodgkin's Disease	None[23,52]/ increase[26,102]	Living longer/ less comorbidity	Increase[30,98,110]	Immune reconstitution/ less comorbidity/ less advanced disease/ decreased HIV RNA
Anal	None[102]/increase[26]	Living longer/ less comorbidity	None[30]	—
Lung	None[9,26]/increase[102,138]	Living longer/ less comorbidity	None[30]	—

CNS = central nervous system; KS = Kaposi's sarcoma; NHL = non-Hodgkin's lymphoma.

Conjunctival Carcinoma. Squamous cell carcinoma of the conjunctiva (SCCC) has been associated with chronic, intense ultraviolet light exposure, typically near the equator, and with HPV infection.[140] Prior to the AIDS epidemic, the incidence of SCCC in Uganda was 6 per million per year and increased to 35 per million per year in 1992,[141] a six-fold increase. A 10-fold rise in incidence of eye tumors was also noted in the general population of Kyadondo County, Uganda, from 0.3 to 0.4 per 100,000 (1960–1966) to 3.0 to 3.4 (1995–1997), with the proportion owing to SCCC increasing over this period from 23.5 to 71% in men and 0 to 85% in women.[142] In the African countries of Rwanda, Uganda, and Zimbabwe, several case-control studies have shown a higher rate of HIV infection among patients with SCCC and in situ carcinoma of the conjunctiva when compared to those with non-malignant eye conditions.[141,143–145] The first case-control study on SCCC and HIV infection was done during 1989 to 1990 in Kigali, Rwanda, and investigators found 82% of the 11 patients with SCCC and in situ carcinoma of the conjunctiva were HIV-infected, whereas only 27% of the 22 matched controls were HIV-positive (odds ratio [OR] = 13; 95% CI 2.2–7.9).[143] A hospital-based case-control study of patients seen during 1990 to 1991 in Kampala, Uganda, found a relative risk for SCCC among people with HIV to be 13.0 (95% CI 4.5–39.4) and that the HIV-infected patients were younger and had more aggressive lesions than the HIV-uninfected patients.[141] In 1994, a case-control study of patients from Uganda and Malawi found a higher prevalence of HIV infection among SCCC patients (71% in Uganda and 86% in Malawi) compared to 16% of the control patients (OR = 13.1).[144] A subset of subjects from a large cross-sectional study of cancer in Uganda, from 1994 to 1998, were evaluated for the risk of SCCC and found a 10-fold risk (OR 10.1, 95% CI 5.2–19.4) among patients with HIV infection.[145] Another hospital-based case control study, this time in Mashonalad Central, Zimbabwe, found that the most common (92%) clinical finding in the HIV-infected patients was corneal overriding and that conjunctival malignancy was the first presenting sign for AIDS in 50% of the patients.[146] In addition to case studies in Africa, a US AIDS and cancer registry linkage study also found an excess of SCCC among people with AIDS. Although there appeared to be an association with advanced immune deficiency rather than HIV alone, the total number of cases was four and too few for more rigorous analysis.[147]

Multiple Myeloma. Hematological malignancies, including multiple myeloma and leukemia, have been reported in people with HIV and AIDS, but only multiple myeloma has consistently shown an excess occurrence in large-scale studies of people with AIDS. This increased risk ranges from 1.7 to 12.1 among persons who have developed AIDS[63,101,104,109,148] to 0 to 4.2 among people with HIV infection.[9,15,94,102,108,131,132,149] Among the studies that evaluated the risk of multiple myeloma in relation to AIDS onset, conflicting evidence exists as to whether there is an increasing trend with advancing immunodeficiency.[63,101,109]

In the general population, the median age at diagnosis is 68 years, and the incidence is twice as high in Blacks than in Whites, 2 versus 1%, respectively.[150] The incidence in the United States is around 4 per 100,000 per year, and men are more frequently affected than women. In one review of HIV-infected patients with multiple myeloma, the median age at diagnosis of plasma cell disorders was 31 years.[151] In addition to younger age at diagnoses, many cases reported in the literature present with extramedullary sites of disease.[151,152]

Although some have speculated that multiple myeloma has a viral association with HHV-8,[153] current evidence has failed to confirm this.[12,154]

Leiomyomas/Leiomyosarcomas. Leiomyosarcomas (or leiomyomas) are extremely rare tumors of the smooth muscle that have been reported with increased frequency in people with AIDS, primarily in children.[8] Among US children with HIV infection in the 1980s and 1990s, NHL was the most common malignancy,[155–160] and leiomyosarcoma was the second leading cancer.[155,160] In Africa, however, KS has been the second leading cause of cancer among HIV-infected children,[156,157] Since leiomyosarcomas are exceptionally rare in children (< 1 per 100,000 person-years),[161] even the occurrence of one or two cases can result in an SIR of well over 1,000.[155,159] One retrospective study in the United States of cancers in HIV-infected children for the period 1982 to

1997 identified 64 children with cancer, of whom 65% had NHL and 17% had leiomyosarcomas.[155] A case-control study of risk factors for malignancy in HIV-infected children identified 43 children with cancer diagnosed between 1992 and 1998, of whom 77% had NHL and 19% had leiomyosarcoma.[160] However, since the blood supply is now screened for HIV and anti-retroviral drugs have been effectively used to prevent vertical transmission from mother to child, reports of this cancer in HIV-infected children have decreased dramatically.[158]

There has been one report of an excess of leiomyosarcomas in adults with AIDS,[101] but the risk did not increase with time since HIV infection. Most studies have failed to find an excess risk of leiomyosarcomas in adults with HIV or AIDS.[12]

EFFECT OF HAART ON ONCOGENESIS AND IMMUNOSUPPRESSION

As with both HIV-infection and organ transplantation, chronic immunosuppression increases the risk of some, but not all, cancers. Among the cancers that have a higher incidence in people with HIV infection, most have a viral agent associated with their pathology. Thus, impaired viral immunity caused by HIV infection, rather than impaired response to tumor cells, may be the primary etiologic factor.

Several researchers have hypothesized that differences in the degree of immunosuppression at which various cancer types typically arise in people with AIDS could explain the differential influence of HAART on lymphomas and KS.[23,79,162] For example, the median CD4 cell count at diagnosis of Burkitt's lymphoma (177) or Hodgkin's disease (141) is higher than for primary brain lymphoma (24) or KS (30).[52] Thus, the partial immune reconstitution induced by HAART may be sufficient to prevent those cancers that occur at very low CD4 cell counts (such as primary brain lymphoma and KS) but not those cancers that occur at higher CD4 cell counts (such as Burkitt's lymphoma and Hodgkin's disease).

There has been much debate about when to initiate HAART. The benefit of starting treatment early and preventing damage to the immune system must be weighted against the increased risk of HIV-related diseases when treatment is delayed until evidence of immunosuppression exists. Because of the potential risk of serious side effects, viral resistance, and difficulties with adherence to HAART regimens, the current guidelines recommend starting treatment when an individual is symptomatic or has CD4 cell counts ≤ 350 or plasma HIV viral load of > 55,000 copies.[163]

Immune reconstitution has been observed in many individuals treated with HAART, but it is unlikely that such individuals truly recover normal immune function. Qualitative studies of immune function suggest that the T-cell gamut may not be completely restored once significant damage has occurred.[79,164,165]

FUTURE DIRECTIONS

New Antiviral Drugs

New AIDS drugs are just around the corner, and they may be more potent at viral suppression and immune reconstitution, less toxic, with fewer side effects, and easier to administer. Several new HAART drugs in clinical trials include integrase inhibitors, entry and fusion inhibitors, and second-generation protein inhibitors. Evidence of the benefits of HAART on HIV-related malignancies presents a promising future for further improvement in treatments. Other more experimental areas of treatment include immuno-modulation and gene therapy.[166]

New Chemotherapeutics and Treatment Guidelines

As later chapters will discuss, the clinical management of malignancies in HIV-infected individuals is also evolving and will likely result in improved cancer survival time. The feasibility and toxicity, including drug–drug interactions, of using the combination of HAART and chemotherapy is an important consideration. Yet most of the treatment strategies now recommend continuing HAART during cancer treatments, including chemotherapy, until unacceptable toxicity occurs. By possibly limiting immune damage inflicted by HIV, HAART administration during chemotherapy may even allow the development of antitumor responses, thereby reducing HIV-associated production of proinflammatory cytokines.[3]

Preventive Vaccines

Until there is an effective vaccine to prevent HIV infection, HIV-related cancers may be effectively prevented by vaccines that protect against other oncogenic viruses. Research into new vaccine development continues, and one of the most promising areas are vaccines to prevent HPV infection and for controlling HPV-associated lesions. These vaccines are now in Phase I and II clinical trials.[167]

The development of a vaccine against EBV has also been under consideration.[168,169] EBV-associated malignancies arise in people years after their primary infection, and protection from these long-term consequences of EBV infection would require a vaccine that ideally confers sterile immunity and prevents the establishment of the carrier state.[170] Furthermore, a reduced virus replication during primary infection might result in a smaller reservoir of latent virus in the individual, thus limiting the risk of harmful virus reactivation and development of lympho-proliferative diseases in immunosuppressed people.

SUMMARY

We have presented a condensed review of the English language literature on the epidemiological effect of HAART on HIV-related malignancies. A few limitations should be noted about this review. First, we are still in the early years of the HAART era, and long-term effects are not likely to have manifested themselves. For instance, it is possible that metabolic side effects and toxicities owing to HAART medications may lead to the development of new cancers in people with HIV and AIDS. Conversely, we may see an even more drastic reduction in the incidence of HIV-related cancers and an increase in cancer survival, as time goes on. Another limitation of the studies we reviewed is that many of them relied on calendar period to assess the effect of HAART on cancer incidence and survival time. This is, at best, an indirect measure and has been heavily relied upon since direct data on HAART use are limited and may be confounded by selection by indication. Lastly, there may be other temporal effects contributing to a change in incidence of HIV-related cancers in the era of HAART. It is possible that improved and more widespread screening practices for both cervical and anal cancer may be preventing the development of invasive disease in HIV-infected individuals.

The declines in incidence for KS and NHL and improved survival for KS, NHL, and HD, with a corresponding lack of an increase in other HIV-related malignancies since the widespread use of HAART, should be reassuring for people with HIV infection. The non-HIV related cancers that do appear to be increasing in the era of HAART, such as lung and multiple myeloma, are likely a result of longer life expectancy and aging rather than immune reconstitution or metabolic toxicities owing to HAART. Close monitoring of epidemiologic trends in HIV-related cancers is necessary to implement appropriate cancer prevention, screening, and treatment for people with HIV infection.

ACKNOWLEDGMENTS

This work was partially supported by the National Institute of Allergy and Infectious Diseases: grant numbers U01-AI-34989 and RO3-AI-005270. We are grateful to Ms Michelle Barry for her help with the preparation of this chapter.

REFERENCES

1. Beral V, Newton R. Overview of the epidemiology of immunodeficiency-associated cancers. J Natl Cancer Inst Monogr 1998:1–6.
2. Hessol NA. The changing epidemiology of HIV-related cancers. AIDS Read 1998;(Spring):45–9, 68.
3. Berretta M, Cinelli R, Martellotta F, et al. Therapeutic approaches to AIDS-related malignancies. Oncogene 2003;22:6646–59.
4. 1993 revised classification system for HIV infection and expanded surveillance case definition for AIDS among adolescents and adults. MMWR Morb Mortal Wkly Rep 1992;41(RR-17):1–19.
5. Kaposi M. Classics in oncology: idiopathic multiple pigmented sarcoma. CA Cancer J Clin 1982;32:342–7.
6. Chang Y, Cesarman E, Pessin MS, et al. Identification of herpes-virus-like DNA sequences in AIDS-associated Kaposi's sarcoma. Science 1994;266:1865–9.
7. Plancoulaine S, Abel L, van Beveren M, et al. Human herpesvirus 8 transmission from mother to child and between

siblings in an endemic population. Lancet 2000; 356:1062–5.

8. Mbulaiteye SM, Parkin DM, Rabkin CS. Epidemiology of AIDS-related malignancies an international perspective. Hematol Oncol Clin North Am 2003;17:673–96.

9. Hessol NA, Seaberg EC, Preston-Martin S, et al. Cancer risk among participants in the Women's Interagency HIV Study. J Acquir Immune Defic Syndr 2004;36:978–85.

10. Buonaguro L, Buonaguro FM, Tornesello ML, et al. Role of HIV-1 Tat in the pathogenesis of AIDS-associated Kaposi's sarcoma. Antibiot Chemother 1994;46:62–72.

11. Biggar RJ. AIDS-related cancers in the era of highly active antiretroviral therapy. Oncology 2001;15:439–48.

12. Goedert JJ. The epidemiology of acquired immunodeficiency syndrome malignancies. Semin Oncol 2000;27:390–401.

13. Biggar R, Horm J, Fraumeni J. Incidence of Kaposi's sarcoma and mycosis fungoides in the United States including Puerto Rico, 1973–1981. J Natl Cancer Inst 1984;73:89–94.

14. Kaposi's sarcoma and Pneumocystis pneumonia among homosexual men—New York City and California. Morb Mortal Wkly Rep 1981;30:305–8.

15. Koblin BA, Hessol NA, Zauber AG, et al. Increased incidence of cancer among homosexual men, New York City and San Francisco, 1978–1990. Am J Epidemiol 1996; 144:916–23.

16. Engels EA. Human immunodeficiency virus infection, aging, and cancer. J Clin Epidemiol 2001;54(Suppl 1): S29–34.

17. Von Roenn JH. Clinical presentations and standard therapy of AIDS-associated Kaposi's sarcoma. Hematol Oncol Clin North Am 2003;17:747–62.

18. Dezube BJ. Acquired immunodeficiency syndrome-related Kaposi's sarcoma: clinical features, staging, and treatment. Semin Oncol 2000;27:424–30.

19. Nasti G, Serraino D, Ridolfo A, et al. AIDS-associated Kaposi's sarcoma is more aggressive in women: a study of 54 patients. J Acquir Immune Defic Syndr Hum Retrovirol 1999;20:337–41.

20. Cooley TP, Hirschhorn LR, O'Keane JC. Kaposi's sarcoma in women with AIDS. AIDS 1996;10:1221–5.

21. Osmond DH, Buchbinder S, Cheng A, et al. Prevalence of Kaposi sarcoma-associated herpesvirus infection in homosexual men at beginning of and during the HIV epidemic. JAMA 2002;287:221–5.

22. Palella F, Delaney K, Moorman A, et al. Declining morbidity and mortality among patients with advanced human immunodeficiency virus infection. N Engl J Med 1998; 338:853–60.

23. Highly active antiretroviral therapy and incidence of cancer in human immunodeficiency virus-infected adults. International Collaboration on HIV and Cancer. J Natl Cancer Inst 2000;92:1823–30.

24. Ledergerber B, Telenti A, Egger M. Risk of HIV related Kaposi's sarcoma and non-Hodgkin's lymphoma with potent antiretroviral therapy: prospective cohort study. Swiss HIV Cohort Study. BMJ 1999;319(7201):23–4.

25. Grulich AE, Li Y, McDonald AM, et al. Decreasing rates of Kaposi's sarcoma and non-Hodgkin's lymphoma in the era of potent combination anti-retroviral therapy. AIDS 2001;15:629–33.

26. Scheer S, Hessol NA. Cancer incidence among adults with AIDS in the pre-HAART and HAART eras. Proceedings of the 8th International Conference on Malignancies in AIDS and Other Immunodeficiencies; 2004 April 29–30; Bethesda, MD.

27. Jacobson LP, Yamashita TE, Detels R, et al. Impact of potent antiretroviral therapy on the incidence of Kaposi's sarcoma and non-Hodgkin's lymphomas among HIV-1-infected individuals. Multicenter AIDS Cohort Study. J Acquir Immune Defic Syndr 1999;21(Suppl 1):34–41.

28. Tam HK, Zhang ZF, Jacobson LP, et al. Effect of highly active antiretroviral therapy on survival among HIV-infected men with Kaposi sarcoma or non-Hodgkin lymphoma. Int J Cancer 2002;98:916–22.

29. Holkova B, Takeshita K, Cheng DM, et al. Effect of highly active antiretroviral therapy on survival in patients with AIDS-associated pulmonary Kaposi's sarcoma treated with chemotherapy. J Clin Oncol 2001;19:3848–51.

30. Hessol N, Scheer S. Increased cancer survival time for some but not all cancers, among adults with AIDS, in the era of HAART. Proceedings of the 8th International Conference on Malignancies in AIDS and Other Immunodeficiencies; 2004 April 29–30; Bethesda, MD.

31. Gill J, Bourboulia D, Wilkinson J, et al. Prospective study of the effects of antiretroviral therapy on Kaposi sarcoma–associated herpesvirus infection in patients with and without Kaposi sarcoma. J Acquir Immune Defic Syndr 2002;31:384–90.

32. Aboulafia DM. Regression of acquired immunodeficiency syndrome-related pulmonary Kaposi's sarcoma after highly active antiretroviral therapy. Mayo Clin Proc 1998; 73:439–43.

33. Ziegler JL, Beckstead JA, Volberding PA, et al. Non-Hodgkin's lymphoma in 90 homosexual men. Relation to generalized lymphadenopathy and the acquired immunodeficiency syndrome. N Engl J Med 1984;311:565–70.

34. Revision of the case definition of acquired immunodeficiency syndrome for national reporting—United States. Centers for Disease Control, Department of Health and Human Services. Ann Intern Med 1985;103:402–3.

35. Bower M. Acquired immunodeficiency syndrome-related systemic non-Hodgkin's lymphoma. Br J Haematol 2001; 112:863–73.

36. Knowles DM, Chamulak GA, Subar M, et al. Lymphoid neoplasia associated with the acquired immunodeficiency syndrome (AIDS). The New York University Medical Center experience with 105 patients (1981–1986). Ann Intern Med 1988;108:744–53.

37. Revision of the CDC surveillance case definition for acquired immunodeficiency syndrome. Council of State and Territorial Epidemiologists; AIDS Program, Center for Infectious Diseases. MMWR Morb Mortal Wkly Rep 1987;36(Suppl 1):1–15.

38. Knowles DM. Etiology and pathogenesis of AIDS-related non-Hodgkin's lymphoma. Hematol Oncol Clin North Am 2003;17:785–820.

39. Tirelli U, Spina M, Gaidano G, et al. Epidemiological, biological and clinical features of HIV-related lymphomas in the era of highly active antiretroviral therapy. AIDS 2000; 14:1675–88.

40. Grulich AE. AIDS-associated non-Hodgkin's lymphoma in the era of highly active antiretroviral therapy. J Acquir Immune Defic Syndr 1999;21(Suppl 1):S27–30.

41. Gates AE, Kaplan LD. Biology and management of AIDS-associated non-Hodgkin's lymphoma. Hematol Oncol Clin North Am 2003;17:821–41.

42. MacMahon EM, Glass JD, Hayward SD, et al. Epstein-Barr virus in AIDS-related primary central nervous system lymphoma. Lancet 1991;338:969–73.

43. Scadden DT. AIDS-related malignancies. Ann Rev Med 2003;54:285–303.

44. Pluda JM, Venzon DJ, Tosato G, et al. Parameters affecting the development of non-Hodgkin's lymphoma in patients with severe human immunodeficiency virus infection receiving antiretroviral therapy. J Clin Oncol 1993;11:1099–107.

45. Lane HC, Masur H, Edgar LC, et al. Abnormalities of B-cell activation and immunoregulation in patients with the acquired immunodeficiency syndrome. N Engl J Med 1983;309:453–8.

46. Levine AM, Seneviratne L, Tulpule A. Incidence and management of AIDS-related lymphoma. Oncology (Huntingt) 2001;15:629–39.

47. Biggar R, Rosenberg P, Cote T. Kaposi's sarcoma and non-Hodgkin's lymphoma following the diagnosis of AIDS. Int J Cancer 1996;68:754–8.

48. Beral V. Epidemiology of Kaposi's sarcoma. In: Beral V, Jaffe H, Wiess R, editors. Cancer, HIV and AIDS. Cold Spring Harbor, NY: Cold Spring Harbor Press; 1991. p. 5–22.

49. Tulpule A, Levine A. AIDS-related lymphoma. Blood Rev 1999;13:147–50.

50. Buchbinder SP, Holmberg SD, Scheer S, et al. Combination antiretroviral therapy and incidence of AIDS-related malignancies. J Acquir Immune Defic Syndr 1999; 21(Suppl 1):23–6.

51. Matthews GV, Bower M, Mandalia S, et al. Changes in acquired immunodeficiency syndrome-related lymphoma since the introduction of highly active antiretroviral therapy. Blood 2000;96:2730–4.

52. Jones JL, Hanson DL, Dworkin MS, et al. Effect of antiretroviral therapy on recent trends in selected cancers among HIV-infected persons. Adult/Adolescent Spectrum of HIV Disease Project Group. J Acquir Immune Defic Syndr 1999;21(Suppl 1):S11–7.

53. Kirk O, Pedersen C, Cozzi-Lepri A, et al. Non-Hodgkin lymphoma in HIV-infected patients in the era of highly active antiretroviral therapy. Blood 2001;98:3406–12.

54. Dal Maso L, Serraino D, Hamers F, et al. Non-Hodgkins lymphoma and primary brain lymphoma as AIDS-defining illness in Western Europe, 1988-1997. Proceedings of the Third National AIDS Malignancy Conference, May 26–27 1999; Bethesda, MD.

55. Sparano JA, Wiernik PH, Hu X, et al. Pilot trial of infusional cyclophosphamide, doxorubicin, and etoposide plus didanosine and filgrastim in patients with human immunodeficiency virus-associated non-Hodgkin's lymphoma. J Clin Oncol 1996;14:3026–35.

56. Kaplan LD, Straus DJ, Testa MA, et al. Low-dose compared with standard-dose m-BACOD chemotherapy for non-Hodgkin's lymphoma associated with human immunodeficiency virus infection. National Institute of Allergy and Infectious Diseases AIDS Clinical Trials Group. N Engl J Med 1997;336:1641–8.

57. Vaccher E, Spina M, Talamini R, et al. Improvement of systemic human immunodeficiency virus-related non-Hodgkin lymphoma outcome in the era of highly active antiretroviral therapy. Clin Infect Dis 2003;37:1556–64.

58. 1993 revised classification system for HIV infection and expanded surveillance case definition for AIDS among adolescents and adults. The Centers for Disease Control and Prevention. JAMA 1993;269:729–30.

59. Del Mistro A, Chieco Bianchi L. HPV-related neoplasias in HIV-infected individuals. Eur J Cancer 2001;37: 1227–35.

60. Clarke B, Chetty R. Postmodern cancer: the role of human immunodeficiency virus in uterine cervical cancer. Mol Pathol 2002;55:19–24.

61. Palefsky JM. Cervical human papillomavirus infection and cervical intraepithelial neoplasia in women positive for human immunodeficiency virus in the era of highly active antiretroviral therapy. Curr Opin Oncol 2003;15:382–8.

62. Rabkin C, Biggar R, Baptiste M, et al. Cancer incidence trends in women at risk of human immunodeficiency virus (HIV) infection. Int J Cancer 1993;55:208–12.

63. Goedert JJ, Cote TR, Virgo P, et al. Spectrum of AIDS-associated malignant disorders. Lancet 1998;351:1833–9.

64. Maiman M, Fruchter RG, Serur E, et al. Human immunodeficiency virus infection and cervical neoplasia. Gynecol Oncol 1990;38:377–82.

65. Adachi A, Fleming I, Burk RD, et al. Women with human immunodeficiency virus infection and abnormal Papanicolaou smears: a prospective study of colposcopy and clinical outcome. Obstet Gynecol 1993;81:372–7.

66. Maiman M, Fruchter RG, Serur E, et al. Recurrent cervical intraepithelial neoplasia in human immunodeficiency virus-seropositive women. Obstet Gynecol 1993;82:170–4.

67. Sun XW, Kuhn L, Ellerbrock TV, et al. Human papillomavirus infection in women infected with the human immunodeficiency virus. N Engl J Med 1997;337:1343–9.

68. Bellan C, De Falco G, Lazzi S, Leoncini L. Pathologic aspects of AIDS malignancies. Oncogene 2003;22:6639–45.

69. Newton R, Grulich A, Beral V, et al. Cancer and HIV infection in Rwanda. Lancet 1995;345:1378–9.

70. Sitas F, Bezwoda WR, Levin V, et al. Association between human immunodeficiency virus type 1 infection and cancer in the black population of Johannesburg and Soweto, South Africa. Br J Cancer 1997;75:1704–7.

71. Ziegler JL, Newton R, Katongole-Mbidde E, et al. Risk factors for Kaposi's sarcoma in HIV-positive subjects in Uganda. AIDS 1997;11:1619–26.

72. Dorrucci M, Suligoi B, Serraino D, et al. Incidence of invasive cervical cancer in a cohort of HIV-seropositive women before and after the introduction of highly active antiretroviral therapy. J Acquir Immune Defic Syndr 2001;26:377–80.

73. Serraino D, Carrieri P, Pradier C, et al. Risk of invasive cervical cancer among women with, or at risk for, HIV infection. Int J Cancer 1999;82:334–7.

74. Phelps RM, Smith DK, Heilig CM, et al. Cancer incidence in women with or at risk for HIV. Int J Cancer 2001;94: 753–7.

75. Massad LS, Seaberg EC, Watts DH, et al. Low incidence of invasive cervical cancer among HIV-infected US women in a prevention program. AIDS 2004;18:109–13.

76. Minkoff H, McCalla S. Uterine rupture among women with a prior cesarean delivery. N Engl J Med 2002;346:134–7.

77. Orem J, Otieno MW, Remick SC. AIDS-associated cancer in developing nations. Curr Opin Oncol 2004;16:468–76.

78. Wabinga H, Ramanakumar AV, Banura C, et al. Survival of cervix cancer patients in Kampala, Uganda: 1995–1997. Br J Cancer 2003;89:65–9.

79. Gates AE, Kaplan LD. AIDS malignancies in the era of highly active antiretroviral therapy. Oncology (Huntingt) 2002;16:441–59.

80. Robert NJ, Schneiderman H. Hodgkin's disease and the acquired immunodeficiency syndrome. Ann Intern Med 1984;101:142–3.

81. Ioachim HL, Cooper MC, Hellman GC. Hodgkin's disease and the acquired immunodeficiency syndrome. Ann Intern Med 1984;101:876–7.

82. Temple JJ, Andes WA. AIDS and Hodgkin's disease. Lancet 1986;2:454–5.

83. Scheib RG, Siegel RS. Atypical Hodgkin's disease and the acquired immunodeficiency syndrome. Ann Intern Med 1985;102:554.

84. Tirelli U, Vaccher E, Rezza G, et al. Hodgkin's disease in association with acquired immunodeficiency syndrome (AIDS). A report on 36 patients. Gruppo Italiano Cooperativo AIDS and Tumori. Acta Oncol 1989;28:637–9.

85. Kaplan LD. AIDS-associated lymphoma. Baillieres Clin Haematol 1990;3:139–51.

86. Rubio R. Hodgkin's disease associated with human immunodeficiency virus infection. A clinical study of 46 cases. Cooperative Study Group of Malignancies Associated with HIV Infection of Madrid. Cancer 1994;73:2400–7.

87. Spina M, Sandri S, Serraino D, et al. Therapy of non-small-cell lung cancer (NSCLC) in patients with HIV infection. GICAT. Cooperative Group on AIDS and Tumors. Ann Oncol 1999;10(Suppl 5):S87–90.

88. Rabkin CS, Yellin F. Cancer incidence in a population with a high prevalence of infection with human immunodeficiency virus type 1. J Natl Cancer Inst 1994;86:1711–6.

89. Reynolds P, Saunders LD, Layefsky ME, Lemp GF. The spectrum of acquired immunodeficiency syndrome (AIDS)-associated malignancies in San Francisco, 1980–1987. Am J Epidemiol 1993;137:19–30.

90. Hessol NA, Katz MH, Liu JY, et al. Increased incidence of Hodgkin disease in homosexual men with HIV infection. Ann Intern Med 1992;117:309–11.

91. Lyter DW, Bryant J, Thackeray R, et al. Incidence of human immunodeficiency virus-related and nonrelated malignancies in a large cohort of homosexual men. J Clin Oncol 1995;13:2540–6.

92. Rabkin CS, Hilgartner MW, Hedberg KW, et al. Incidence of lymphomas and other cancers in HIV-infected and HIV-uninfected patients with hemophilia. JAMA 1992;267:1090–4.

93. Serraino D, Pezzotti P, Dorrucci M, et al. Cancer incidence in a cohort of human immunodeficiency virus serconverters. Cancer 1997;79:1004–8.

94. Cooksley CD, Hwang LY, Waller DK, Ford CE. HIV-related malignancies: community-based study using linkage of cancer registry and HIV registry data. Int J STD AIDS 1999;10:795–802.

95. Boyle MJ, Sculley TB, Penny R, et al. The role of Epstein-Barr virus subtypes in human immunodeficiency virus-associated lymphoma. Leuk Lymphoma 1993;10:17–23.

96. Herndier BG, Sanchez HC, Chang KL, et al. High prevalence of Epstein-Barr virus in the Reed-Sternberg cells of HIV-associated Hodgkin's disease. Am J Pathol 1993;142:1073–9.

97. Tirelli U, Errante D, Dolcetti R, et al. Hodgkin's disease and human immunodeficiency virus infection: clinicopathologic and virologic features of 114 patients from the Italian Cooperative Group on AIDS and Tumors. J Clin Oncol 1995;13:1758–67.

98. Glaser SL, Clarke CA, Gulley ML, et al. Population-based patterns of human immunodeficiency virus-related Hodgkin lymphoma in the Greater San Francisco Bay Area, 1988-1998. Cancer 2003;98:300–9.

99. Dolcetti R, Boiocchi M. Epstein-Barr virus in the pathogenesis of Hodgkin's disease. Biomed Pharmacother 1998;52:13–25.

100. Cartwright RA, Gurney KA, Moorman AV. Sex ratios and the risks of haematological malignancies. Br J Haematol 2002;118:1071–7.

101. Frisch M, Biggar RJ, Engels EA, Goedert JJ. Association of cancer with AIDS-related immunosuppression in adults. AIDS-Cancer Match Registry Study Group. JAMA 2001;285:1736–45.

102. Herida M, Mary-Krause M, Kaphan R, et al. Incidence of non-AIDS–defining cancers before and during the highly active antiretroviral therapy era in a cohort of human immunodeficiency virus-infected patients. J Clin Oncol 2003;21:3447–53.

103. Franceschi S, Dal Maso L, Arniani S, et al. Risk of cancer other than Kaposi's sarcoma and non-Hodgkin's lymphoma in persons with AIDS in Italy. Cancer and AIDS Registry Linkage Study. Br J Cancer 1998;78:966–70.

104. Gallagher B, Wang Z, Schymura MJ, et al. Cancer incidence in New York State acquired immunodeficiency syndrome patients. Am J Epidemiol 2001;154:544–56.

105. Medeiros LJ, Greiner TC. Hodgkin's disease. Cancer 1995;75(1 Suppl):357–69.

106. IARC Working Group on the Evaluation of Carcinogenic Risks to Humans: Human Immunodeficiency Viruses and Human T-Cell Lymphotropic Viruses. Lyon, France, 1-18 June 1996. IARC Monogr Eval Carcinog Risks Hum 1996;67:1–424.

107. Roithmann S, Tourani JM, Andrieu JM. Hodgkin's disease in HIV-infected intravenous drug abusers. N Engl J Med 1990;323:275–6.

108. Grulich AE, Li Y, McDonald A, et al. Rates of non-AIDS–defining cancers in people with HIV infection before and after AIDS diagnosis. AIDS 2002;16:1155–61.

109. Grulich AE, Wan X, Law MG, et al. Risk of cancer in people with AIDS. AIDS 1999;13:839–43.

110. Hoffmann C, Chow KU, Wolf E, et al. Strong impact of highly active antiretroviral therapy on survival in patients with human immunodeficiency virus-associated Hodgkin's disease. Br J Haematol 2004;125:455–62.

111. Goldman S, Glimelius B, Nilsson B, Pahlman L. Incidence of anal epidermoid carcinoma in Sweden 1970–1984. Acta Chir Scand 1989;155:191–7.

112. Frisch M, Melbye M, Moller H. Trends in incidence of anal cancer in Denmark. BMJ 1993;306:419–22.

113. Melbye M, Rabkin C, Frisch M, Biggar RJ. Changing patterns of anal cancer incidence in the United States, 1940–1989. Am J Epidemiol 1994;139:772–80.

114. Daling JR, Madeleine MM, Johnson LG, et al. Human papillomavirus, smoking, and sexual practices in the etiology of anal cancer. Cancer 2004;101:270–80.

115. Frisch M, Glimelius B, van den Brule AJ, et al. Sexually transmitted infection as a cause of anal cancer. N Engl J Med 1997;337:1350–8.

116. Biggar RJ, Horm J, Goedert JJ, Melbye M. Cancer in a group at risk of acquired immunodeficiency syndrome (AIDS) through 1984. Am J Epidemiol 1987;126:578–86.

117. Biggar RJ, Burnett W, Mikl J, Nasca P. Cancer among New York men at risk of acquired immunodeficiency syndrome. Int J Cancer 1989;43:979–85.

118. Melbye M, Cote TR, Kessler L, et al. High incidence of anal cancer among AIDS patients. The AIDS/Cancer Working Group. Lancet 1994;343:636–9.

119. Melbye M, Sprogel P. Aetiological parallel between anal cancer and cervical cancer. Lancet 1991;338:657–9.

120. Palefsky JM, Holly EA, Gonzales J, et al. Detection of human papillomavirus DNA in anal intraepithelial neoplasia and anal cancer. Cancer Res 1991;51:1014–9.

121. Johnson LG, Madeleine MM, Newcomer LM, et al. Anal cancer incidence and survival: The Surveillance, Epidemiology, and End Results experience, 1973–2000. Cancer 2004;101:281–8.

122. Greenlee RT, Murray T, Bolden S, Wingo PA. Cancer statistics, 2000. CA Cancer J Clin 2000;50:7–33.

123. Frisch M, Glimelius B, Wohlfahrt J, et al. Tobacco smoking as a risk factor in anal carcinoma: an antiestrogenic mechanism? J Natl Cancer Inst 1999;91:708–15.

124. Frisch M, Biggar RJ, Goedert JJ. Human papillomavirus-associated cancers in patients with human immunodeficiency virus infection and acquired immunodeficiency syndrome. J Natl Cancer Inst 2000;92:1500–10.

125. Critchlow CW, Surawicz CM, Holmes KK, et al. Prospective study of high grade anal squamous intraepithelial neoplasia in a cohort of homosexual men: influence of HIV infection, immunosuppression and human papillomavirus infection. AIDS 1995;9:1255–62.

126. Palefsky JM, Holly EA, Ralston ML, et al. High incidence of anal high-grade squamous intra-epithelial lesions among HIV-positive and HIV-negative homosexual and bisexual men. AIDS 1998;12:495–503.

127. Palefsky JM, Holly EA, Ralston ML, et al. Effect of highly active antiretroviral therapy on the natural history of anal squamous intraepithelial lesions and anal human papillomavirus infection. J Acquir Immune Defic Syndr 2001; 28:422–8.

128. Piketty C, Darragh TM, Heard I, et al. High prevalence of anal squamous intraepithelial lesions in HIV-positive men despite the use of highly active antiretroviral therapy. Sex Transm Dis 2004;31:96–9.

129. Fox P, Stebbing J, Portsmouth S, et al. Lack of response of anal intra-epithelial neoplasia to highly active antiretroviral therapy. AIDS 2003;17:279–80.

130. Kim JH, Sarani B, Orkin BA, et al. HIV-positive patients with anal carcinoma have poorer treatment tolerance and outcome than HIV-negative patients. Dis Colon Rectum 2001;44:1496–1502.

131. Sitas F, Pacella-Norman R, Carrara H, et al. The spectrum of HIV-1 related cancers in South Africa. Int J Cancer 2000; 88:489–92.

132. Serraino D, Boschini A, Carrieri P, et al. Cancer risk among men with, or at risk of, HIV infection in southern Europe. AIDS 2000;14:553–9.

133. Tirelli U, Spina M, Sandri S, et al. Lung carcinoma in 36 patients with human immunodeficiency virus infection. The Italian Cooperative Group on AIDS and Tumors. Cancer 2000;88:563–9.

134. Powles T, Bower M. HIV and the risk of lung cancer. J Clin Oncol 2004;22:1348–9.

135. Shopland DR. Changes in tobacco consumption and lung cancer risk: evidence from studies of individuals. IARC Sci Publ 1990:77–91.

136. Shopland DR, Eyre HJ, Pechacek TF. Smoking-attributable cancer mortality in 1991: is lung cancer now the leading cause of death among smokers in the United States? J Natl Cancer Inst 1991;83:1142–8.

137. Parkin DM. International variation. Oncogene 2004;23: 6329–40.

138. Bower M, Powles T, Nelson M, et al. HIV-related lung cancer in the era of highly active antiretroviral therapy. AIDS 2003;17:371–5.

139. Petruckevitch A, Del Amo J, Phillips AN, et al. Risk of cancer in patients with HIV disease. London African HIV/AIDS Study Group. Int J STD AIDS 1999;10:38–42.

140. Newton R, Ferlay J, Reeves G, et al. Effect of ambient solar ultraviolet radiation on incidence of squamous-cell carcinoma of the eye. Lancet 1996;347:1450–1.

141. Ateenyi-Agaba C. Conjunctival squamous-cell carcinoma associated with HIV infection in Kampala, Uganda. Lancet 1995;345(8951):695–6.

142. Wabinga HR, Parkin DM, Wabwire-Mangen F, Nambooze S. Trends in cancer incidence in Kyadondo County, Uganda, 1960–1997. Br J Cancer 2000;82:1585–92.

143. Kestelyn P, Stevens AM, Ndayambaje A, et al. HIV and conjunctival malignancies. Lancet 1990;336:51–2.

144. Waddell KM, Lewallen S, Lucas SB, et al. Carcinoma of the conjunctiva and HIV infection in Uganda and Malawi. Br J Ophthalmol 1996;80:503–8.

145. Newton R, Ziegler J, Ateenyi-Agaba C, et al. The epidemiology of conjunctival squamous cell carcinoma in Uganda. Br J Cancer 2002;87:301–8.

146. Porges Y, Groisman GM. Prevalence of HIV with conjunctival squamous cell neoplasia in an African provincial hospital. Cornea 2003;22:1–4.

147. Goedert JJ, Cote TR. Conjunctival malignant disease with AIDS in USA. Lancet 1995;346:257–8.

148. Biggar RJ, Kirby KA, Atkinson J, et al. Cancer risk in elderly persons with HIV/AIDS. J Acquir Immun Defic Syndr 2004;36:861–8.

149. Johnson CC, Wilcosky T, Kvale P, et al. Cancer incidence among an HIV-infected cohort. Pulmonary Complications

of HIV Infection Study Group. Am J Epidemiol 1997; 146:470–5.

150. Sirohi B, Powles R. Multiple myeloma. Lancet 2004; 363:875–87.

151. Kumar S, Kumar D, Schnadig VJ, et al. Plasma cell myeloma in patients who are HIV-positive. Am J Clin Pathol 1994;102:633–9.

152. Gold JE, Schwam L, Castella A, et al. Malignant plasma cell tumors in human immunodeficiency virus-infected patients. Cancer 1990;66:363–8.

153. Rettig MB, Ma HJ, Vescio RA, et al. Kaposi's sarcoma-associated herpesvirus infection of bone marrow dendritic cells from multiple myeloma patients. Science 1997;276:1851–4.

154. Cannon MJ, Flanders WD, Pellett PE. Occurrence of primary cancers in association with multiple myeloma and Kaposi's sarcoma in the United States, 1973–1995. Int J Cancer 2000;85:453–6.

155. Granovsky MO, Mueller BU, Nicholson HS, et al. Cancer in human immunodeficiency virus-infected children: a case series from the Children's Cancer Group and the National Cancer Institute. J Clin Oncol 1998;16:1729–35.

156. Parkin DM, Wabinga H, Nambooze S, Wabwire-Mangen F. AIDS-related cancers in Africa: maturation of the epidemic in Uganda. AIDS 1999;13:2563–70.

157. Mueller BU. Cancers in children infected with the human immunodeficiency virus. Oncologist 1999;4:309–17.

158. Caselli D, Klersy C, de Martino M, et al. Human immunodeficiency virus-related cancer in children: incidence and treatment outcome—report of the Italian Register. J Clin Oncol 2000;18:3854–61.

159. Biggar RJ, Frisch M, Goedert JJ. Risk of cancer in children with AIDS. AIDS-Cancer Match Registry Study Group. JAMA 2000;284:205–9.

160. Pollock BH, Jenson HB, Leach CT, et al. Risk factors for pediatric human immunodeficiency virus-related malignancy. JAMA 2003;289:2393–9.

161. Linet MS, Ries LA, Smith MA, et al. Cancer surveillance series: recent trends in childhood cancer incidence and mortality in the United States. J Natl Cancer Inst 1999;91:1051–8.

162. Dal Maso L, Franceschi S. Epidemiology of non-Hodgkin lymphomas and other haemolymphopoietic neoplasms in people with AIDS. Lancet Oncol 2003;4:110–9.

163. Guidelines for the Use of Antiretroviral Agents in HIV-1-Infected Adults and Adolescents. Dept of Health and Human Services; March 23, 2004.

164. Lange CG, Xu Z, Patterson BK, et al. Proliferation responses to HIVp24 during antiretroviral therapy do not reflect improved immune phenotype or function. AIDS 2004; 18:605–13.

165. Ye P, Kirschner DE, Kourtis AP. The thymus during HIV disease: role in pathogenesis and in immune recovery. Curr HIV Res 2004;2:177–83.

166. Robertson P, Scadden DT. Immune reconstitution in HIV infection and its relationship to cancer. Hematol Oncol Clin North Am 2003;17:703–716.

167. Fife KH, Wheeler CM, Koutsky LA, et al. Dose-ranging studies of the safety and immunogenicity of human papillomavirus Type 11 and Type 16 virus-like particle candidate vaccines in young healthy women. Vaccine 2004;22:2943–52.

168. Spring SB, Hascall G, Gruber J. Issues related to development of Epstein-Barr virus vaccines. J Natl Cancer Inst 1996;88:1436–41.

169. Khanna R, Moss DJ, Burrows SR. Vaccine strategies against Epstein-Barr virus-associated diseases: lessons from studies on cytotoxic T-cell–mediated immune regulation. Immunol Rev 1999;170:49–64.

170. Arico E, Robertson KA, Belardelli F, et al. Vaccination with inactivated murine gammaherpesvirus 68 strongly limits viral replication and latency and protects type I IFN receptor knockout mice from a lethal infection. Vaccine 2004;22:1433–40.

2

Immune Surveillance in Cancer

RAYNA TAKAKI

LEWIS L. LANIER

THE IMMUNOSURVEILLANCE HYPOTHESIS

The concept that the immune system can recognize and eliminate nascent transformed cells was first conceived over a century ago by Paul Ehrlich but has gained wide acceptance only in recent years. In the 1950s, Burnet and Thomas formally hypothesized this concept of immune surveillance and put forward the idea that lymphocytes could prevent neoplastic malignancies by monitoring and destroying "potentially dangerous mutant cells."[1] In the following years, experimental mouse models were used to investigate whether immunocompromised hosts were more susceptible to developing malignancies, spontaneous or chemically induced. Because of the inconclusive and often conflicting results of these studies, the validity of the cancer immunosurveillance hypothesis was fiercely debated and eventually disregarded. A major set of experiments that led to the abandonment of the hypothesis was performed using immunocompromised athymic nude mice, which lack T cells because of a genetic mutation causing aberrant epithelial morphogenesis in the thymus. These experiments showed that nude mice treated with the chemical carcinogen 3-methylcholanthrene (MCA) did not have higher incidences of malignancies or accelerated tumor development compared to their wild-type controls.[2] Additionally, when monitored over a 7-month period, the nude mice did not develop a greater number of spontaneous tumors compared to their wild-type counterparts.[3] These findings, along with others that conflicted with the immune surveillance hypothesis, led scientists to conclude for many years that the immune system did not play an important role in preventing the development of cancer. As Dunn and colleagues[4] noted, even in a major review in the year 2000, immune surveillance was still not regarded as a significant obstacle that a transformed cell had to overcome to develop into a cancer.

Further characterization of the CBA/H strain of nude mice used in these earlier experiments has shown, however, that these studies are not as conclusive as originally believed. It is now known the CBA/H nude mice are not completely immunocompromised and still have a small population of functional $\alpha\beta$-T cell antigen receptor (TcR)-bearing T cells.[5,6] The presence of these $\alpha\beta$-TcR$^+$ T cells, in conjunction with $\gamma\delta$-TcR$^+$ T cells, B cells, and natural killer (NK) cells, which develop normally in athymic mice, may have allowed the nude mice to reject the MCA-induced tumors with efficiency comparable to wild-type mice. Studies have also shown that different strains of mice have variable sensitivity to chemical carcinogens.[7] Specifically, the CBA/H strain of nude mice is more sensitive to MCA, owing to its ability to metabolize the pro-form of the chemical into its carcinogenic form more rapidly. It has been proposed that this increased sensitivity to the carcinogen creates a larger population of transformed cells in the CBA/H strain and can overpower even a fully functional immune system; thus, differences in immunosurveillance between nude mice and wild-type mice may not be evident. Additionally, if the mice had been observed for a longer time period, a difference in the frequency of spontaneous tumors may have resulted. Recent studies by Shankaran and colleagues[8] have shown that spontaneous malignancies often do not arise until 15 to 20 months of age in immunocompromised RAG2-/- mice (which completely lack B and T cells). Looking retrospectively, although the immunocompromised CBA/H strain nude mice did not succumb to tumors more readily than wild-type mice, in light of the important caveats of these experiments, the findings do not necessarily negate the importance of immunosurveillance in cancer prevention.

IMMUNE SURVEILLANCE IN HUMANS

Although researchers initially had difficulty demonstrating the existence of immunosurveillance in certain mouse models, there have been examples of immunosurveillance in immunocompromised humans for decades; two of the most extensively documented groups have been patients receiving a transplant and patients with AIDS.

Organ transplantation patients are placed on long-term immunosuppressive regimens to ensure successful graft function. Immunosuppressive drugs, such as cyclosporine A (CsA) or OKT3 (an anti-human CD3 monoclonal antibody), block T-cell signaling and inhibit the immune system by preventing vital co-stimulatory and effector functions. Treatment with these types of drugs has improved the success rate of organ transplantation, but the resulting immunosuppressive state has been correlated with an increased risk of developing various cancers, particularly those of viral origin.[9] Among the various documented cancers that arise in patients posttransplant, skin cancers are among the most prevalent.[10–12] The frequency of squamous-cell carcinoma in transplant patients is 65 to 250 times higher than in the general population.[13–15] Although it has not been definitively resolved, it is likely that human papillomavirus (HPV) infection causes the development of squamous cell carcinomas in transplant patients. Squamous cell carcinomas share physical and histological characteristics associated with HPV infection,[16] and HPV DNA can be detected in 65 to 95% of squamous cell carcinoma patient samples.[17]

Lymphoproliferative diseases are also among the most common cancers that develop in immunosuppressed transplant patients. Transplant patients can have up to an 8- to 12-fold higher risk of developing lymphomas than in an age-matched non-transplanted population.[18,19] Most cases of post-transplant lymphoproliferative disease (PTLD) correlate with infection by Epstein-Barr virus (EBV).[20] Interestingly, over 90% of the population is infected with EBV[21]; but after the primary infection, EBV persists latently in resting memory B cells and is carried by a majority of individuals as a lifelong asymptomatic infection.[22] It has been proposed that the latent phase of EBV is regulated by EBV-specific cytotoxic T lymphocytes (CTL),[23] which are crucial for the clearance of the initial infection and prevention of developing PTLD. Studies have shown that transplant patients with EBV-PTLD can be successfully treated with infusions of in vitro cultured EBV-specific CTLs, resulting in the regulation of EBV-infected cells and even clearance of lymphomas in the treated patients.[24–26] Thus, in the presence of functional immune surveillance, infected cells are properly regulated, and EBV-related lymphomas are unable to develop.

The risk of developing cancer after organ transplantation has been shown to be directly proportional to the intensity and duration of immunosuppression required to prevent graft rejection. Patients receiving lower doses of immunosuppressants have a decreased risk of developing cancers compared with patients receiving higher doses.[27–29] In renal transplants, immunosuppressed patients with lower levels of CD4+ T cells have a greater risk of developing skin cancers compared to transplant patients who have higher CD4+ T-cell counts.[30] Thus, transplant patients with more functional immune systems have a lower likelihood of developing cancer.

Patients with AIDS also suffer from an increased risk of developing cancer owing to their immunocompromised state. Similar to transplant recipients, the cancers that develop in the immunocompromised patients with AIDS are rare in the general population and are associated with viral infection.[31] Kaposi's sarcoma (KS), high-grade B-cell non-Hodgkin's lymphoma (NHL), and invasive cervical cancer are common AIDS-defining malignancies. With the advent of highly active anti-retroviral therapy (HAART), however, the incidences of these malignancies have decreased. Patients treated with HAART who have restored immune function are able to resolve cancers, such as KS[32–34] and AIDS-related lymphoma,[35,36] indicating that proper immune function can play a role in the protection against cancer.

REEVALUATION OF IMMUNE SURVEILLANCE IN EXPERIMENTAL MODELS OF CANCER

Early studies testing the hypothesis of immune surveillance in mice were hampered by the lack of appropriate experimental tools to critically evaluate the potential role of both innate and adaptive immunity in the prevention of cancer. Recent advancements in the development of mice with defined genetic alterations (ie, "gene knockout" mice) have permitted selective disruption of critical cell types, immune receptors, and soluble mediators of both the innate and adaptive immune response. Here, we will review briefly the potential role for the different cell types of the immune system to recognize transformed cells, the receptors used in this process, and the effector molecules used to mediate tumor rejection.

EFFECTOR CELLS OF IMMUNOSURVEILLANCE

Immunity is mediated by an early or "innate" response, followed by an adaptive response that pro-vides antigen-specific recognition, a more rapid response upon reexposure to the original antigen, and long-term memory. Leukocytes responsible for the immediate response include myeloid cells (eg, granulocytes, monocytes, macrophages, and dendritic cells), and NK cells, whereas adaptive immunity is conferred by B and T lymphocytes (Figure 2–1). From studies of transplantable tumors, there is evidence that all of these cell types may participate in the recognition and elimination of tumors.

Considering the innate immune system, cytokine-activated granulocytes and macrophages have clearly been shown to kill certain tumor cell lines, by as-yet-undefined recognition mechanisms. For example, eosinophils were the predominate cells responsible for the rejection of a transplantable mouse renal cell carcinoma in response to treatment with interleukin-4 (IL-4).[37] Similarly, cytokine-activated macrophages have also been shown to kill tumor cells in vitro, although this is more difficult to establish in vivo because there are no efficient methods to deplete macrophages in vivo. NK cells comprise the lymphoid component of innate immunity, and these cells were first identified by their ability to kill certain tumor cell lines without prior immunization or deliberate activation of the host.[38,39] NK cells have been implicated in the rejection of transplantable tumors in several mouse models, and there has been

Figure 2–1. Effector cells of immunosurveillance. The early or "innate" response during tumor immunity is mediated by myeloid cells (granulocytes, monocytes, macrophages, and dendritic cells) and NK cells. The effector mechanisms of many of these innate effector cells have yet to be clearly determined. Immediately following the innate response is an antigen-specific adaptive immune response, mediated by B and T lymphocytes.

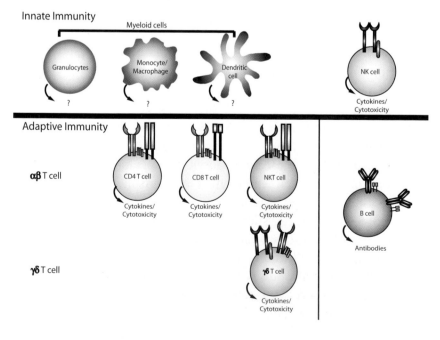

considerable progress in understanding the recognition mechanisms and mediators of this activity (reviewed by Smyth and colleagues).[40] It has been shown that mice depleted of NK cells (by using an anti-asialo-GM1 antibody that recognizes a glycolipid on the NK cell surface) are two to three times more susceptible to tumors induced by MCA than in non-NK depleted counterparts.[41]

B and T cells are responsible for adaptive immunity and are distinguished by their ability to generate an infinitely diverse repertoire of receptors that recognize antigens with exquisite specificity. Furthermore, these antigen-specific cells are able to expand clonally in a very rapid fashion and, more importantly, confer long-term protection by an accelerated response upon encountering an antigen after the initial immunization. There is extensive literature on the presence of tumor-specific antibodies in tumor-bearing animals and humans. Moreover, the administration of passive antibodies against antigens overexpressed by tumor cells, compared with normal tissues, has therapeutic benefit in many types of cancer in humans and experimental model systems (reviewed by Carter).[42] As yet, whether mice selectively lacking B cells, but having normal T cells and innate immune cells, have a higher incidence of spontaneous or carcinogen–induced tumors has not been addressed. Nonetheless, tumor-specific antibodies, whether naturally occurring or passively delivered, are likely important in rendering tumors susceptible to phagocytosis or killing by Fc receptor-bearing myeloid cells and NK cells.

Several types of T cells are involved in antitumor immunity. Two sub-lineages of T cells are defined by the type of antigen receptor expressed, $\alpha\beta$-TcR$^+$ T cells and $\gamma\delta$-TcR$^+$ T cells, with the former comprising the majority of T cells in the circulation and lymphoid tissues. $\alpha\beta$-TcR$^+$ T cells can be further subdivided into CD4$^+$ and CD8$^+$ populations that have been categorized as "helper" and "cytotoxic" T cells. Within the $\alpha\beta$-TcR$^+$ T-cell population, there exists a small subset often called "NKT cells" because they frequently co-express several cell surface receptors in common with NK cells. NKT cells express an invariant TcR[43]; therefore, they have a limited recognition repertoire, rather than the diverse repertoire of $\alpha\beta$-TcR$^+$ T cells.

Because they generate their receptors by somatic genetic recombination, NKT cells and $\gamma\delta$-TcR$^+$ T cells are considered members of the adaptive immune system. However, they share many characteristics in common with cells of the innate immune system (eg, rapid responses and a lack of long-term memory after encountering antigen).

NKT cells have been proposed to play an important role in tumor immunity. Their innate capacity allows a rapid secretion of important immunoregulating cytokines, such as IL-4 and IFN-γ, upon antigen recognition through the TcR. The importance of NKT cells in tumor immune surveillance was supported when mice lacking Vα14Jα281-expressing invariant NKT cells were treated with MCA and succumbed to tumors at a rate higher than control wild-type mice.[44]

Included in the small subset of unconventional T cells that play an important role in tumor immunity are $\gamma\delta$-TcR$^+$ T cells. Like NKT cells, these cells have a rearranged TCR, but their functional properties are more characteristic of the innate immune system.[45] These cells have a disproportional representation in specific tissues; $\gamma\delta$-TcR$^+$ T cells are found in large numbers in the intestinal epithelium of humans and in the skin of mice.[46–48] $\gamma\delta$-TcR$^+$ T cells respond rapidly to transformed cells and can mount a significant immune response within the first few days of encountering a tumor,[49–52] unlike conventional T cells, which require a longer activation period to permit clonal expansion. Recently, Gao and colleagues[53] demonstrated that $\gamma\delta$-TcR$^+$ T cells provide an important early source of IFN-γ, which plays a critical role in tumor immunosurveillance and prevents the development of MCA-induced or transplanted B16 melanoma tumor cells.

Although the innate immune system provides an important initial line of defense for eliminating nascent transformed cells, complete rejection of a developing tumor often requires the involvement of the adaptive immune system. $\alpha\beta$-TcR$^+$ T cells are the principal cells of the adaptive immune system that play a critical role in the tumor rejection process. After being activated in a peripheral lymph node, tumor-antigen specific CD4$^+$ and CD8$^+$ T cells migrate to the tumor site and assist in the elimination of antigen-positive tumor cells. Tumor-infiltrating CD4$^+$ T cells secrete IL-2, which in conjunction with

IL-15 produced by non-lymphoid host cells, is important for sustaining and promoting the cytotoxic functions of CD8[+] T cells. Additionally, CD4[+] T-cell help has been shown to be crucial for developing long-term tumor specific immunity.[54] Infiltrating CD8[+] T cells can eliminate transformed cells directly through cell–cell mediated mechanisms, or indirectly through cytokine-mediated mechanisms, such as the production of IFN-γ. Treatment of αβ-TcR[+] T-cell–deficient mice with MCA resulted in significantly higher incidences of tumors in the immunocompromised mice compared with control mice.[55] Strikingly, when RAG2-/- mice, a strain that is completely deficient in the adaptive immune system (lacking all types of T cells as well as B cells), were monitored for an extended period, an increased incidence of tumor malignancies was observed in the immunocompromised mice compared to age-matched, wild-type mice.[8] Thus, in the absence of a functional immune system, mice were much more susceptible to the development of tumors.

EFFECTOR RECOGNITION OF TUMOR CELLS

What distinguishes transformed cells from healthy cells, thereby allowing the immune system to respond? With regard to innate immunity, we will first consider tumor recognition by NK cells. Although NK cells were first discovered by their ability to kill certain tumors, the initial hints about their recognition process came from studies performed by Klas Kärre and colleagues using RMA, a transplantable mouse T-lymphoma cell line. His experiments demonstrated that NK cells recognized and rejected lymphomas that lacked expression of major histocompatibility complex (MHC) class I (Figure 2–2).[56] According to the "missing self" hypothesis first proposed by Kärre, NK cells recognize and kill transformed cells that have lost self-MHC class I, while sparing healthy cells.[56] The presence of self-MHC class I protects healthy cells by engaging inhibitory NK cell receptors, thereby preventing cytotoxic activity.[57,58]

Although tumors may evade detection by CD8[+] cytotoxic T cells by failing to express MHC class I, the ability of NK cells to detect cells and respond to

cells lacking class I would provide a complementary immune mechanism to prevent this occurrence. These observations may have relevance to cancer because a common event that follows transformation or viral infection of a cell is the loss of surface MHC class I expression.[59] Whereas the loss of MHC class I renders tumors more susceptible to NK cell attack, it is not absolutely required for an NK cell-mediated response. NK cell responses are determined by the integration of signals transmitted by inhibitory receptors for MHC class I and a variety of activating receptors that induce cell-mediated cytotoxicity and cytokine production.[60] Several activating NK cell receptors have been implicated in the recognition of tumors, including the NKp30, NKp44, NKp46, and NKG2D.[60–62] NKG2D is the best characterized NK receptor that is involved in antitumor immunity, and its ligands are preferentially expressed on many types of cancer.[60,63]

Expressed on NK cells, γδ-TcR[+] T cells, and CD8[+] αβ-TcR[+] T cells, NKG2D is an activating receptor that can bind to ligands present on the surface of tumor cells, resulting in NK cell-mediated lysis of tumor cells, even if they express high levels of MHC class I (Figure 2–3). The NKG2D receptor is a type II disulfide-linked homodimer that must associate with the adapter proteins DAP10 (in

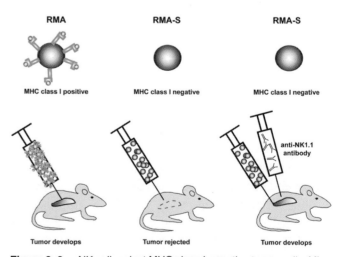

Figure 2–2.   NK cells reject MHC class I negative tumor cells. Mice injected with RMA, an MHC class I expressing tumor cell line, are unable to efficiently reject the transplanted cells and develop tumors. In contrast, when injected with RMA-S, a mutant RMA cell line lacking MHC class I expression, mice efficiently reject the tumor cells and remain tumor free. This has been shown to be a NK cell-dependent process by depleting mice with anti-NK1.1 monoclonal antibody, a surface molecule expressed on NK cells.

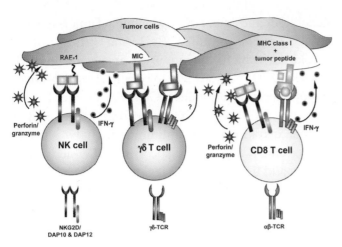

Figure 2–3. NK cells and CD8+ T cells detect upregulated NKG2D ligands on tumors. NKG2D is a primary activating receptor for NK cells and on T cells acts as a co-stimulatory receptor augmenting the activation signal received through the TcR. NKG2D binds to MICA and MICB (also ULBP1-4 and RAET1G, not shown) on human tumors and binds to RAE-1 (also H60 and MULT1, not shown) on mouse tumors. This interaction activates NK cell effector functions, including perforin and IFN-γ–mediated killing.

humans and mice) or DAP12 (only in mice) to signal through the PI3 kinase pathway or the Syk-ZAP70 tyrosine kinase pathway, respectively.[64] In mice, NKG2D binds to several cell surface glycoproteins (Figure 2–4) frequently expressed on tumors, including retinoic acid early-inducible-1 (RAE-1) proteins,[65,66] a minor histocompatibility antigen H60,[65,66] and MULT1.[67,68] There are at least five *RAE-1* genes (*RAE-1α, β, γ, δ, ε*) currently identified, and these are polymorphic and differentially expressed in various mouse strains. Although RAE-1 is expressed during embryonic development, its expression is downregulated in adult mice and is not present on most normal healthy cells. RAE-1 is expressed on many tumor cell lines[65,66] and is induced on virally infected cells.[69] Girardi and colleagues[55] have shown that RAE-1 and H60 transcripts, which are absent in normal skin, are upregulated in carcinomas and papillomas induced by 12-*O*-tetradecanoylphorbol (TPA), a chemical carcinogen, on mouse skin. Moreover, other studies have shown that ectopic expression of RAE-1 rendered NK-insensitive tumor cells susceptible to NKG2D-dependent NK cell-mediated killing. Mice injected with RAE-1–transfected cells had a much lower incidence of tumor development compared to mice injected with mock-transfected

cells; this protection could be abrogated by depleting the mice of NK and NKT cells.[70,71]

The human orthologs of the mouse RAE-1 molecules are known as UL16-binding proteins (ULBP) (also called RAET1). Similar to the RAE-1 proteins, there are at least five functional *ULBP* genes (*ULBP1,2,3,4,* and *RAET1G*) encoding proteins that can specifically bind to human NKG2D.[72–74] Like RAE-1, ULBP glycoproteins are frequently expressed on the cell surface of human tumors.[75–77] Another family of proteins that bind to NKG2D with high affinity is the human MHC class I chain-related proteins A and B (MICA and MICB).[78] These nonclassical MHC class I molecules are highly polymorphic and do not require association with β2-microglobulin or peptide.[79–81] They do not function as ligands for αβ-TcR, although they do appear to be recognized by some γδ-TcR.[82] Thus, in γδ-TcR+ T cells, MICA/B can activate tumor cell killing through both TcR and NKG2D-mediated pathways.[78,82] In healthy individuals, MICA and MICB are normally expressed only in the gastrointestinal epithelium of the stomach and large and small intestines; however, increased MICA/B expression has been detected in various primary tumor samples of the lung, breast, kidney, ovary, prostate, and colon.[83] The upregulation of MICA/B has also been documented in melanomas[84] and hepatocarcinomas.[85] Like RAE-1, expression of MICA/B sensitizes tumor cells to

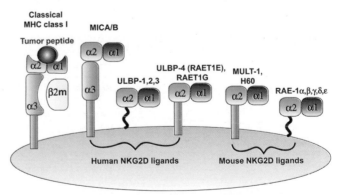

Figure 2–4. NKG2D ligands are distantly related to classical MHC class I, but functionally distinct. Human NKG2D binds to MICA, MICB, ULBP-1, ULBP-2, ULBP-3, ULBP-4 (also called RAET1E or Letal) and RAET1G in humans; and to H60, MULT1, and RAE-1α,β,γ,δ,ε in mice. The mouse RAE-1 genes are orthologs of the human ULBP genes. There is no known mouse ortholog of MICA orMICB. MULT1, H60, ULBP-4, RAET1G are transmembrane bound proteins. ULBP1,2,3 and RAE-1 are GPI-linked proteins.

NKG2D-dependent NK cell-mediated cytotoxicity. It is also possible that MICA/B expression in tumors can influence the migration of tumor-infiltrating lymphocytes. In various tumor tissue samples examined, Groh and colleagues[83] showed that an increased frequency of γδ-TcR[+] T cells infiltrated into the tissues of tumors expressing MICA/B compared to tissues negative for MICA/B. In summary, NKG2D has been implicated as an important activating receptor in tumor recognition by both NK cells and T cells. However, because NK cells efficiently kill tumors lacking NKG2D ligands, other as-yet-undefined receptors are also critical for NK cell-mediated surveillance against cancer.

Adaptive immunity against tumors is predominantly mediated by αβ-TcR[+] T cells. Thus, tumor recognition is antigen-specific, and the TcR functions by binding to tumor-associated peptides bound to MHC class I or MHC class II molecules. The initial priming of a T-cell response against tumors likely occurs by "cross-presentation," whereby dendritic cells in the tumor environment ingest fragments of apoptotic tumors. NK cells and other innate immune effector cells may participate by killing the nascent tumor cells to provide cellular fragments for uptake by the dendritic cells.[86–88] Dendritic cells bearing antigen migrate to the draining lymph node[89] and present these antigens to naïve CD4[+] and CD8[+] T cells.[90,91] Provided that antigenic peptides are made by the tumor and can bind to the host's MHC molecules, antigen-specific T cells are generated and clonally expanded. Tumor-specific CD4[+] T cells produce IL-2 and other critical cytokines, which can augment responses by NK cells and CD8[+] T cells and may help B cells produce tumor-specific antibodies. CD8[+] cytotoxic T lymphocytes (CTL) can directly kill tumors, as well as secrete cytokines with antitumor activity, such as TNFα and IFNγ. Tumor-specific CD4[+] and CD8[+] T cells and tumor-specific IgG antibodies have been detected in animals and humans, demonstrating that immune responses are elicited in the tumor-bearing host (although in these cases the tumors have prevailed despite the immune response).

In order to elicit a T-cell response, a tumor must express a peptide that can bind to the host's MHC class I or II molecule but that does not induce T-cell tolerance, either by deleting reactive immature T cells in the thymus or causing anergy in mature T cells in the peripheral lymphoid tissues. This is not a problem when the tumor antigen is a viral protein encoded by an oncogenic virus, such as EBV or HHV8. Eliciting a robust adaptive immune response against tumor antigens, however, is often very difficult because most antigens expressed on tumors are self-antigens. Other than viral antigens, several human tumor antigens that induce T-cell responses have been characterized and fall into different categories (Table 2–1): "cancer testis" antigens, mutated self proteins, and overexpressed self proteins.[92–94] T cells recognizing these tumor antigens have been detected in the circulation of cancer patients by

Table 2–1. IDENTIFIED HUMAN TUMOR ANTIGENS		
	Antigen Type	**Examples**
Differentiation antigens	Melan-A/MART-1, tyrosinase, gp-100	Components of melanin biosynthesis pathway
	PSA, PSMA, PAP	Commonly upregulated in prostate cancer patients
Unique antigens (often caused by mutations)	Mutated tumor suppressor gene *TP53*	Detected in about 50% of human malignancies
	Mutated ras	Oncogene, associated with 15% of malignancies
	Mutated β-catenin	Mutated adhesion molecule commonly found in melanoma patients
Overexpressed/Amplified antigens	*HER2/neu*	Commonly overexpressed in breast cancer patients
	EGFR	Commonly overexpressed in colorectal cancer patients
	CD20	Commonly overexpressed in lymphoma patients
Cancer testis (CT) antigens	MAGE, BAGE, GAGE, NY-ESO-1	Male germ cell antigen, normally not expressed on somatic cells, but detected on various tumors
Viral antigens	EBV	Commonly detected in post-transplant lymphoproliferative diseases and nasopharyngeal cancer
	HPV	Commonly detected in cervical cancers

using soluble MHC molecules loaded with the tumor peptide, which can be visualized by immunofluorescence and flow cytometry.[95,96] However, it must be noted that in these cancer patients, these tumor-specific T cells apparently are incapable of eliminating the tumor, raising the question whether these antigens are relevant for cancer immune surveillance or, alternatively, whether the tumor has evolved other mechanisms to escape immune elimination.

EFFECTOR CELL MECHANISMS

Immune effector cells can kill tumor cells by various pathways, including cytokine or cell–cell mediated mechanisms (Figure 2–5). The perforin/granzyme pathway is a primary pathway used by CTL and NK cells to eliminate transformed cells.[97] The expression of perforin is constitutive in NK cells and can be induced in T cells and enhanced in NK cells by IL-2[98]; it has also been shown that IL-12 is a key activator of perforin-mediated NK killing of target

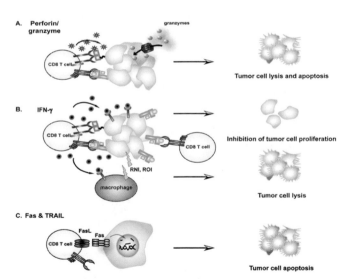

Figure 2–5. Effector Mechanisms. *A,* Perforin that is released from effector cells forms pores in the tumor cells, through which granzymes can rapidly enter to induce apoptosis. *B,* IFN-γ secreted by NK cells and T cells binds to IFN-γ receptors on tumor cells and surrounding leukocyte effector cells (eg, T cells, NK cells, and macrophages). IFN-γ inhibits tumor cell proliferation and upregulates MHC class I presentation of antigen to CD8+ T cells. In addition to the NK and T cells that are activated by the secreted IFN-γ, tumor-infiltrating macrophages become activated and kill tumor cells by releasing reactive nitrogen intermediates (RNI) and reactive oxygen intermediates (ROI). *C,* Fas or TRAIL receptors expressed on tumor cells bind to Fas ligand or TRAIL, respectively, expressed on activated effector cells, resulting in apoptosis of the tumor cell.

cells.[99] Upon activation of the effector cell, perforin is released from cytolytic granules present in the cytoplasm of the NK cell and is secreted and inserted into the membrane of the tumor cells.[98,100] The perforin pores that develop on the membrane of the tumor disrupt the cell integrity, allowing the entry of DNA-damaging granzymes (proteases) into the cell, thereby killing the cell by the initiation of caspase-induced apoptosis.[97,101] Currently, the importance of granzymes in this process is being debated; there is conflicting experimental evidence demonstrating that either perforin alone is sufficient to mediate efficient tumor rejection,[102] or that a combination of perforin and granzymes is required.[103] It is clear, however, that perforin plays a critical role in NK and CTL cell–cell mediated cytotoxicity against certain tumors. Mice deficient in perforin (*pfp-/-*) have reduced ability to reject RMA-S (a MHC class I–negative variant of the RMA T-cell lymphoma) which is normally efficiently rejected in wild-type mice.[104] Additionally, *pfp-/-* mice have increased sensitivity to viruses[105] or MCA-induced[44,105,106] tumors compared to wild-type mice.[107] Smyth and colleagues[108] have shown that NK cell-mediated perforin mechanisms are necessary for preventing lung metastasis of the prostate carcinoma (RM1) and mammary carcinoma (DA3) cell lines; *pfp-/-* mice are 10- to 100-fold less proficient than wild-type mice. Perforin-deficient mice also develop more spontaneous tumors than wild-type mice.[109]

In addition to the perforin pathway, CTL and NK cells also inhibit tumor development through IFN-γ–dependent mechanisms, which can act on both host effector cells and tumor cells.[110] The effects of IFN-γ include the upregulation of MHC class I expression on tumors,[8] inhibition of tumor proliferation,[111] and suppression of tumor angiogenesis.[112–114] When mice were treated with a neutralizing antibody against IFN-γ, tumor cell recognition and lipopolysaccharide-induced elimination of transplanted tumors were significantly inhibited, and tumors that developed in treated mice grew much more aggressively than those that developed in untreated mice.[115] The importance of IFN-γ–mediated tumor surveillance in preventing the development of primary tumors was demonstrated using mice insensitive to IFN-γ. Mice deficient for functional IFN-γ receptors[116] or the

IFN-γ gene itself[106] developed MCA-induced tumors at an appreciably faster rate and with greater incidence compared to mice sensitive to IFN-γ mediated tumor rejection. Additionally, IFN-γ has been observed to be required for the prevention of spontaneous tumors; C57BL/6 mice or BALB/c mice deficient in IFN-γ were observed to develop a greater number of disseminated lymphomas or lung adenocarcinomas, respectively.[117]

Another important effector mechanism involved in tumor immunosurveillance is the induction of tumor cell apoptosis. Key pathways used by effector lymphocytes in tumor immunosurveillance to induce apoptosis include those mediated through members of the tumor necrosis factor (TNF) super-family, such as TNF apoptosis-inducing ligand (TRAIL), Fas ligand (FasL), and possibly TNF. Constitutively expressed on some NK cells, TRAIL is upregulated on all NK cells after stimulation with IL-2, IFN-γ, or IL-15.[118–120] When mice treated with a neutralizing anti-TRAIL antibody[121] or lacking the *TRAIL* gene[122] were injected with MCA, the incidences of sarcomas were substantially higher in the TRAIL-deficient mice compared to wild-type mice. Smyth and colleagues[123] have demonstrated that, in NK cells, TRAIL is an important alternative cytotoxic pathway to the perforin pathway, and mice deficient in both effector mechanisms are less proficient at inhibiting tumor metastasis. FasL expression by activated αβ-TcR[+] and γδ-TcR[+] T cells has been shown to suppress the development of spontaneous lymphomas[124] and plasmacytoid tumors.[125] Upon transformation, many tumor cells upregulate the expression of Fas and become susceptible to apoptosis-induced death.[126,127]

EVADING IMMUNE SURVEILLANCE

During the development of a tumor, transformed cells are genetically unstable and continually altering their phenotype in response to the environment. Schreiber and colleagues[4] have coined the term "immunoediting" to describe the selective pressure that the immune system imposes on the developing tumor. Elegant studies have shown that tumors arising in immunocompetent mice are less immunogenic than tumors developing in mice lacking IFN-γ

and an adaptive immune system.[8] In particular, tumors from the immunocompetent mice could be easily transplanted into syngeneic mice, whereas tumors of the immunodeficient mice were inherently antigenic and rejected by immunocompetent syngeneic mice. This clearly demonstrates that developing tumors are shaped by the immune system. Further, it suggests that tumors that occur in immunocompetent mice have evolved to evade immune effector cells.

Tumor evasion may occur at any one of the many steps that are necessary for the immune system to mount an effective attack (Figure 2–6). In order for an immune effector cell to kill a tumor, adhesion and conjugate formation is required, a process which can occur, for example, through interactions between LFA-1 on a NK cell or CTL and intercellular adhesion molecules (ICAMs) on the tumor. Loss of ICAMs or other molecules involved in cell–cell adhesion may render tumors less susceptible to cell-mediated cytotoxicity. Escape from CD8[+] T-cell recognition could occur either by loss of the antigenic peptide in the tumor or down-regulation of MHC class I. Such abnormalities in MHC class I expression[128] and defects in the key components of

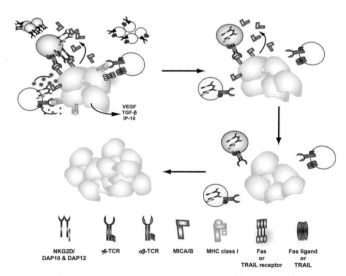

Figure 2–6. Tumor evasion of immune effector mechanisms. Depicted above are a few means by which tumor cells can escape immune recognition, including the down-regulation of MHC class I, the down-regulation of Fas or TRAIL, secretion of soluble MICA or MICB, and the secretion of immune inhibitory cytokines. The secretion of soluble MICA/B can induce the down-modulation of NKG2D on effector cells and can prevent NKG2D-mediated activation. Tumor cells that have evaded the immune system can rapidly proliferate and eventually overwhelm the immune system.

the MHC class I antigen presentation pathway[129] are frequently observed in tumors. Mice deficient in LMP2, a critical subunit of the antigen processing pathway, have a higher frequency of developing neoplasms than wild-type mice.[130] Thus, alterations in the adhesion, co-stimulatory molecules or MHC class I molecules on tumors are effective means of escape.

Another avenue of escape is by acquiring resistance to immune effector molecules. For example, although many cells upregulate Fas upon transformation, throughout tumor progression many tumor cells can selectively lose Fas expression or become insensitive to Fas-mediated killing, as reviewed by French and colleagues.[131] Similar mechanisms may result in the loss of sensitivity to granzymes,[132] TRAIL,[107] or other death mediators. This can be achieved by loss of the relevant death receptor or upregulation in the tumor of anti-apoptotic cellular components, such as Bcl-2, Bcl-xl, serpin protease inhibitors, and others.

Tumor cells can also evade immune surveillance through direct mechanisms, such as the secretion of inhibitory cytokines or the secretion of decoy ligands for immune-activating receptors. A cytokine commonly secreted by tumor cells is vascular endothelial growth factor, which has been shown to inhibit dendritic cell (DC) differentiation and maturation.[133] IL-10 is also frequently detected in cancer patients, and it can exert immunosuppressive effects by inhibiting DC differentiation, IL-12–mediated activation of T cells,[134] and antigen presentation.[135,136] The presence of transforming growth factor-β (TGF-β), which can potently inhibit NK and T-cell activation, is also correlated with poor prognosis and is often detected in high concentrations in the serum of cancer patients.[137,138] These cytokines may augment tumor formation by acting as growth factors and promoters of angiogenesis for the tumor cells, while also inhibiting of the immune system. Recent studies have shown that some human tumors also shed or secrete soluble forms of the NKG2D ligands, which cause internalization or inactivation of the NKG2D receptors on NK cells and CTLs.[75,139,140] Of particular note, Groh and colleagues[139] have detected soluble MICA in the serum of certain cancer patients, and this correlates with down-regulation of NKG2D on their tumor-infiltrating and peripheral lymphocytes. NKG2D and other activating NK receptors are also diminished on NK cells exposed to TGF-β[141,142] providing another potential mechanism that tumors may use to avoid immune attack. Thus, suppressive cytokines and soluble receptor ligands likely play an important role in tumor avoidance of immune effector cells.

CONCLUSIONS

Based on substantial evidence from animal models and observation of human patients, the immune surveillance hypothesis is regaining popularity. Numerous laboratories have shown that, in the presence of a compromised innate or adaptive immune system, mice have an increased susceptibility to transplantable, chemically induced, and spontaneous tumors. While providing a protective effect, the immune response is also selecting for transformed cells that can eventually evade effector mechanisms and develop into an aggressively growing tumor. Thus, some tumor cells that develop in immunocompromised hosts are more immunogenic than those derived in immunocompetent hosts.[8,117,121]

Whereas there is growing support for a protective role of the immune system in cancer, there is solid evidence that, in some circumstances, the immune system may actually be augmenting tumor growth. Although there is an extensive literature on this phenomenon,[143] a clear example is provided by the finding that CD4+ T cells can enhance skin carcinogenesis in a mouse transgenic model in which the E6 and E7 HPV oncogenes are expressed by a keratinocyte-specific promoter.[144] In addition, the secretion of matrix metalloproteinases by myeloid cells has been shown to promote tumor growth in a mouse model system by aiding in the restructuring of the tumor environment.[145,146] Collectively, it appears that a Darwinian relationship exists between the tumor and the host immune system, with each attempting to gain advantage. Unlike microbial pathogens, tumors may have the advantage in that they are essentially "self" cells, and the immune system has evolved to avoid autoimmunity. Thus, many tumors may never evoke a host immune response because, like healthy tissues, they fail to express sufficiently strong antigens to initiate the process. The challenge of cancer immunotherapy is to break tolerance to these cell antigens, while not inducing a prolonged or systemic autoimmune reaction.

REFERENCES

1. Burnet FM. Immunological aspects of malignant disease. Lancet 1967;1:1171–4.

2. Stutman O. Tumor development after 3-methylcholanthrene in immunologically deficient athymic-nude mice. Science 1974;183:534–6.

3. Rygaard J, Povlsen CO. The mouse mutant nude does not develop spontaneous tumours. An argument against immunological surveillance. Acta Pathol Microbiol Scand [B] Microbiol Immunol 1974;82:99–106.

4. Dunn GP, Old LJ, Schreiber RD. The three Es of cancer immunoediting. Annu Rev Immunol 2004;22:329–60.

5. Maleckar JR, Sherman LA. The composition of the T cell receptor repertoire in nude mice. J Immunol 1987;138: 3873–6.

6. Ikehara S, Pahwa RN, Fernandes G, et al. Functional T cells in athymic nude mice. Proc Natl Acad Sci U S A 1984; 81:886–8.

7. Heidelberger C. Chemical carcinogenesis. Annu Rev Biochem 1975;44:79–121.

8. Shankaran V, Ikeda H, Bruce AT, et al. IFNgamma and lymphocytes prevent primary tumour development and shape tumour immunogenicity. Nature 2001;410:1107–11.

9. Penn I. Posttransplant malignancies. Transplant Proc 1999;31:1260–2.

10. Sanchez EQ, Marubashi S, Jung G, et al. De novo tumors after liver transplantation: a single-institution experience. Liver Transpl 2002;8:285–91.

11. Webb MC, Compton F, Andrews PA, et al. Skin tumours posttransplantation: a retrospective analysis of 28 years' experience at a single centre. Transplant Proc 1997; 29:828–30.

12. Hiesse C, Rieu P, Kriaa F, et al. Malignancy after renal transplantation: analysis of incidence and risk factors in 1700 patients followed during a 25-year period. Transplant Proc 1997;29:831–3.

13. Lindelof B, Sigurgeirsson B, Gabel H, et al. Incidence of skin cancer in 5356 patients following organ transplantation. Br J Dermatol 2000;143:513–9.

14. Jensen P, Hansen S, Moller B, et al. Skin cancer in kidney and heart transplant recipients and different long-term immunosuppressive therapy regimens. J Am Acad Dermatol 1999;40:177–86.

15. Hartevelt MM, Bavinck JN, Kootte AM, et al. Incidence of skin cancer after renal transplantation in the Netherlands. Transplantation 1990;49:506–9.

16. Euvrard S, Chardonnet Y, Pouteil-Noble C, et al. Association of skin malignancies with various and multiple carcinogenic and noncarcinogenic human papillomaviruses in renal transplant recipients. Cancer 1993;72:2198–206.

17. Harwood CA, Surentheran T, McGregor JM, et al. Human papillomavirus infection and non-melanoma skin cancer in immunosuppressed and immunocompetent individuals. J Med Virol 2000;61:289–97.

18. Opelz G, Dohler B. Lymphomas after solid organ transplan-

tation: a collaborative transplant study report. Am J Transplant 2004;4:222–30.

19. Domingo-Domenech E, de Sanjose S, Gonzalez-Barca E, et al. Post-transplant lymphomas: a 20-year epidemiologic, clinical and pathologic study in a single center. Haematologica 2001;86:715–21.

20. Rondinara GF, Muti G, De Carlis L, et al. Posttransplant lymphoproliferative diseases: report from a single center. Transplant Proc 2001;33:1832–3.

21. Cohen JI. Epstein-Barr virus infection. N Engl J Med 2000; 343:481–92.

22. Babcock GJ, Decker LL, Volk M, et al. EBV persistence in memory B cells in vivo. Immunity 1998;9:395–404.

23. Callan MF, Tan L, Annels N, et al. Direct visualization of antigen-specific CD8+ T cells during the primary immune response to Epstein-Barr virus In vivo. J Exp Med 1998; 187:1395–402.

24. Rooney CM, Smith CA, Ng CY, et al. Use of gene-modified virus-specific T lymphocytes to control Epstein-Barr–virus-related lymphoproliferation. Lancet 1995;345:9–13.

25. Heslop HE, Ng CY, Li C, et al. Long-term restoration of immunity against Epstein-Barr virus infection by adoptive transfer of gene-modified virus-specific T lymphocytes. Nat Med 1996;2:551–5.

26. Boyle TJ, Berend KR, DiMaio JM, et al. Adoptive transfer of cytotoxic T lymphocytes for the treatment of transplant-associated lymphoma. Surgery 1993;114:218–26.

27. Bouwes Bavinck JN, Hardie DR, Green A, et al. The risk of skin cancer in renal transplant recipients in Queensland, Australia. A follow-up study. Transplantation 1996;61: 715–21.

28. Boubenider S, Hiesse C, Goupy C, et al. Incidence and consequences of post-transplantation lymphoproliferative disorders. J Nephrol 1997;10:136–45.

29. Ho M. Risk factors and pathogenesis of posttransplant lymphoproliferative disorders. Transplant Proc 1995;27:38–40.

30. Ducloux D, Carron PL, Rebibou JM, et al. CD4 lymphocytopenia as a risk factor for skin cancers in renal transplant recipients. Transplantation 1998;65:1270–2.

31. Frisch M, Biggar RJ, Engels EA, et al. Association of cancer with AIDS-related immunosuppression in adults. JAMA 2001;285:1736–45.

32. Dupin N, Rubin De Cervens V, Gorin I, et al. The influence of highly active antiretroviral therapy on AIDS-associated Kaposi's sarcoma. Br J Dermatol 1999;140:875–81.

33. Brander C, Suscovich T, Lee Y, et al. Impaired CTL recognition of cells latently infected with Kaposi's sarcoma-associated herpes virus. J Immunol 2000;165:2077–83.

34. Wilkinson J, Cope A, Gill J, et al. Identification of Kaposi's sarcoma-associated herpesvirus (KSHV)-specific cytotoxic T-lymphocyte epitopes and evaluation of reconstitution of KSHV-specific responses in human immunodeficiency virus type 1-infected patients receiving highly active antiretroviral therapy. J Virol 2002;76:2634–40.

35. Kirk O, Pedersen C, Cozzi-Lepri A, et al. Non-Hodgkin lymphoma in HIV-infected patients in the era of highly active antiretroviral therapy. Blood 2001;98:3406–12.

36. Oksenhendler E, Clauvel JP, Jouveshomme S, et al. Complete remission of a primary effusion lymphoma with antiretroviral therapy. Am J Hematol 1998;57:266.

37. Golumbek PT, Lazenby AJ, Levitsky HI, et al. Treatment of established renal cancer by tumor cells engineered to secrete interleukin-4. Science 1991;254:713–6.

38. Kiessling R, Klein E, Wigzell H. "Natural" killer cells in the mouse I. Cytotoxic cells with specificity for mouse Moloney leukemia cells. Specificity and distribution according to genotype. Eur J Immunol 1975;5:112–7.

39. Herberman RB, Nunn ME, Lavrin DH. Natural cytotoxic reactivity of mouse lymphoid cells against syngeneic and allogeneic tumors. I. Distribution of reactivity and specificity. Int J Cancer 1975;16:216–29.

40. Smyth MJ, Hayakawa Y, Takeda K, et al. New aspects of natural-killer–cell surveillance and therapy of cancer. Nat Rev Cancer 2002;2:850–61.

41. Smyth MJ, Crowe NY, Godfrey DI. NK cells and NKT cells collaborate in host protection from methylcholanthrene-induced fibrosarcoma. Int Immunol 2001;13:459–63.

42. Carter P. Improving the efficacy of antibody-based cancer therapies. Nat Rev Cancer 2001;1:118–29.

43. Bendelac A, Bonneville M, Kearney JF. Autoreactivity by design: innate B and T lymphocytes. Nat Rev Immunol 2001;1:177–86.

44. Smyth MJ, Thia KYT, Street SEA, et al. Differential tumor surveillance by natural killer (NK) and NKT cells. J Exp Med 2000;191:661–8.

45. Hayday A, Tigelaar R. Immunoregulation in the tissues by gammadelta T cells. Nat Rev Immunol 2003;3:233–42.

46. Itohara S, Farr AG, Lafaille JJ, et al. Homing of a gamma delta thymocyte subset with homogeneous T-cell receptors to mucosal epithelia. Nature 1990;343:754–7.

47. Asarnow DM, Kuziel WA, Bonyhadi M, et al. Limited diversity of gamma delta antigen receptor genes of Thy-1+ dendritic epidermal cells. Cell 1988;55:837–47.

48. Goodman T, Lefrancois L. Expression of the gamma-delta T-cell receptor on intestinal CD8+ intraepithelial lymphocytes. Nature 1988;333:855–8.

49. Moore TA, Moore BB, Newstead MW, et al. Gamma delta-T cells are critical for survival and early proinflammatory cytokine gene expression during murine Klebsiella pneumonia. J Immunol 2000;165:2643–50.

50. Kasper LH, Matsuura T, Fonseka S, et al. Induction of gammadelta T cells during acute murine infection with Toxoplasma gondii. J Immunol 1996;157:5521–7.

51. Tsuji M, Mombaerts P, Lefrancois L, et al. Gamma delta T cells contribute to immunity against the liver stages of malaria in alpha beta T-cell-deficient mice. Proc Natl Acad Sci U S A 1994;91:345–9.

52. Mombaerts P, Arnoldi J, Russ F, et al. Different roles of alpha beta and gamma delta T cells in immunity against an intracellular bacterial pathogen. Nature 1993;365:53–6.

53. Gao Y, Yang W, Pan M, et al. Gamma delta T cells provide an early source of interferon gamma in tumor immunity. J Exp Med 2003;198:433–42.

54. Topalian SL. MHC class II restricted tumor antigens and the role of CD4+ T cells in cancer immunotherapy. Curr Opin Immunol 1994;6:741–5.

55. Girardi M, Oppenheim DE, Steele CR, et al. Regulation of cutaneous malignancy by γδ T cells. Science 2001;605–9

56. Karre K, Ljunggren HG, Piontek G, et al. Selective rejection of H-2–deficient lymphoma variants suggests alternative immune defense strategy. Nature 1986;319:675–8.

57. Karlhofer FM, Ribuado RK, Yokoyama WM. MHC class I alloantigen specificity of Ly-49+ IL-2- activated natural killer cells. Nature 1992;358:66–70.

58. Ravetch JV, Lanier LL. Immune inhibitory receptors. Science 2000;290:84–9.

59. Cabrera T, Lopez-Nevot MA, Gaforio JJ, et al. Analysis of HLA expression in human tumor tissues. Cancer Immunol Immunother 2003;52:1–9.

60. Lanier LL. NK cell recognition. Annu Rev Immunol 2005; 23:1.

61. Moretta A, Bottino C, Vitale M, et al. Activating receptors and coreceptors involved in human natural killer cell-mediated cytolysis. Annu Rev Immunol 2001;19:197–223.

62. Smyth MJ, Godfrey DI, Trapani JA. A fresh look at tumor immunosurveillance and immunotherapy. Nat Immunol 2001;2:293–9.

63. Raulet DH. Roles of the NKG2D immunoreceptor and its ligands. Nat Rev Immunol 2003;3:781–90.

64. Gilfillan S, Ho EL, Cella M, et al. NKG2D recruits two distinct adapters to trigger NK cell activation and costimulation. Nat Immunol 2002;3:1150–5.

65. Diefenbach A, Jamieson AM, Liu SD, et al. Ligands for the murine NKG2D receptor: expression by tumor cells and activation of NK cells and macrophages. Nature Immunology 2000;1:119–26.

66. Cerwenka A, Bakker AB, McClanahan T, et al. Retinoic acid early inducible genes define a ligand family for the activating NKG2D receptor in mice. Immunity 2000;12:721–7.

67. Carayannopoulos LN, Naidenko OV, Fremont DH, et al. Cutting edge: murine UL16-binding protein-like transcript 1: A newly described transcript encoding a high-affinity ligand for murine NKG2D. J Immunol 2002;169:4079–83.

68. Diefenbach A, Hsia JK, Hsiung MY, et al. A novel ligand for the NKG2D receptor activates NK cells and macrophages and induces tumor immunity. Eur J Immunol 2003;33: 381–91.

69. Lodoen M, Ogasawara K, Hamerman JA, et al. NKG2D-mediated natural killer cell protection against cytomegalovirus is impaired by viral gp40 modulation of retinoic acid early inducible 1 gene molecules. J Exp Med 2003;197:1245–53.

70. Diefenbach A, Jensen ER, Jamieson AM, et al. Rae1 and H60 ligands of the NKG2D receptor stimulate tumour immunity. Nature 2001;413:165–71.

71. Cerwenka A, Baron JL, Lanier LL. Ectopic expression of retinoic acid early inducible-1 gene (RAE-1) permits natural killer cell-mediated rejection of a MHC class I-bearing tumor in vivo. Proc Natl Acad Sci U S A 2001;98:11521–6.

72. Cosman D, Fanger N, Borges L, et al. A novel immunoglobulin superfamily receptor for cellular and viral MHC class I molecules. Immunity 1997;7:273–82.

73. Jan Chalupny N, Sutherland CL, Lawrence WA, et al. ULBP4 is a novel ligand for human NKG2D. Biochem Biophys Res Commun 2003;305:129–35.

74. Bacon L, Eagle RA, Meyer M, et al. Two human ULBP/RAET1 molecules with transmembrane regions are ligands for NKG2D. J Immunol 2004;173:1078–84.

75. Salih HR, Antropius H, Gieseke F, et al. Functional expression and release of ligands for the activating immunoreceptor NKG2D in leukemia. Blood 2003;102:1389–96.

76. Pende D, Rivera P, Marcenaro S, et al. Major histocompatibility complex class I-related chain A and UL16-binding protein expression on tumor cell lines of different histotypes: analysis of tumor susceptibility to NKG2D-dependent natural killer cell cytotoxicity. Cancer Res 2002;62:6178–86.

77. Conejo-Garcia JR, Benencia F, Courreges MC, et al. Ovarian carcinoma expresses the NKG2D ligand Letal and promotes the survival and expansion of CD28-antitumor T cells. Cancer Res 2004;64:2175–82.

78. Bauer S, Groh V, Wu J, et al. Activation of natural killer cells and T cells by NKG2D, a receptor for stress-inducible MICA. Science 1999;285:727–30.

79. Groh V, Bahram S, Bauer S, et al. Cell stress-regulated human major histocompatibility complex class I gene expressed in gastrointestinal epithelium. Proc Natl Acad Sci U S A 1996;93:12445–50.

80. Li P, Morris DL, Willcox BE, et al. Complex structure of the activating immunoreceptor NKG2D and its MHC class I-like ligand MICA. Nat Immunol 2001;2:443–51.

81. Li P, Willie ST, Bauer S, et al. Crystal structure of the MHC class I homolog MIC-A, a gammadelta T cell ligand. Immunity 1999;10:577–84.

82. Groh V, Steinle A, Bauer S, et al. Recognition of stress-induced MHC molecules by intestinal epithelial γδ T cells. Science 1998;279:1737–40.

83. Groh V, Rhinehart R, Secrist H, et al. Broad tumor-associated expression and recognition by tumor-derived gamma delta T cells of MICA and MICB. Proc Natl Acad Sci U S A 1999;96:6879–84.

84. Vetter CS, Groh V, Straten Pt P, et al. Expression of stress-induced MHC class I related chain molecules on human melanoma. J Invest Dermatol 2002;118:600–5.

85. Jinushi M, Takehara T, Tatsumi T, et al. Expression and role of MICA and MICB in human hepatocellular carcinomas and their regulation by retinoic acid. Int J Cancer 2003;104:354–61.

86. Fernandez NC, Lozier A, Flament C, et al. Dendritic cells directly trigger NK cell functions: cross-talk relevant in innate anti-tumor immune responses in vivo. Nat Med 1999;5:405–11.

87. Piccioli D, Sbrana S, Melandri E, et al. Contact-dependent stimulation and inhibition of dendritic cells by natural killer cells. J Exp Med 2002;195:335–41.

88. Gerosa F, Baldani-Guerra B, Nisii C, et al. Reciprocal activating interaction between natural killer cells and dendritic cells. J Exp Med 2002;195:327–33.

89. Sallusto F, Mackay CR, Lanzavecchia A. The role of chemokine receptors in primary, effector, and memory immune responses. Annu Rev Immunol 2000;18:593–620.

90. Albert ML, Sauter B, Bhardwaj N. Dendritic cells acquire antigen from apoptotic cells and induce class I-restricted CTLs. Nature 1998;392:86–9.

91. Schoenberger SP, Toes RE, van der Voort EI, et al. T-cell help for cytotoxic T lymphocytes is mediated by CD40-CD40L interactions. Nature 1998;393:480–3.

92. Van den Eynde BJ, van der Bruggen P. T cell defined tumor antigens. Curr Opin Immunol 1997;9:684–93.

93. Wang RF, Rosenberg SA. Human tumor antigens for cancer vaccine development. Immunol Rev 1999;170:85–100.

94. Houghton AN. Cancer antigens: immune recognition of self and altered self. J Exp Med 1994;180:1–4.

95. Yee C, Savage PA, Lee PP, et al. Isolation of high avidity melanoma-reactive CTL from heterogeneous populations using peptide-MHC tetramers. J Immunol 1999;162:2227–34.

96. Yee C, Thompson JA, Roche P, et al. Melanocyte destruction after antigen-specific immunotherapy of melanoma: direct evidence of T cell-mediated vitiligo. J Exp Med 2000;192:1637–44.

97. Russell JH, Ley TJ. Lymphocyte-mediated cytotoxicity. Annu Rev Immunol 2002;20:323–70.

98. Podack ER, Hengartner H, Lichtenheld MG. A central role of perforin in cytolysis? Ann Rev Immunol 1991;9:129–57.

99. Kodama T, Takeda K, Shimozato O, et al. Perforin-dependent NK cell cytotoxicity is sufficient for anti-metastatic effect of IL-12. Eur J Immunol 1999;29:1390–6.

100. Trapani JA, Smyth MJ. Functional significance of the perforin/granzyme cell death pathway. Nat Rev Immunol 2002;2:735–47.

101. Liu C-C, Walsh CM, Eto N, et al. Morphologic and functional characterization of perforin-deficient lymphokine-activated killer cells. J Immunol 1995;155:602–8.

102. Davis JE, Smyth MJ, Trapani JA. Granzyme A- and B-deficient killer lymphocytes are defective in eliciting DNA fragmentation but retain potent in vivo anti-tumor capacity. Eur J Immunol 2001;31:39–47.

103. Pardo J, Balkow S, Anel A, et al. Granzymes are essential for natural killer cell-mediated and perf-facilitated tumor control. Eur J Immunol 2002;32:2881–7.

104. van den Broek MF, Kagi D, Zinkernagel RM, et al. Perforin dependence of natural killer cell-mediated tumor control in vivo. Eur J Immunol 1995;25:3514–6.

105. van den Brock MF, Kagi D, Ossendorp F, et al. Decreased tumor surveillance in perforin-deficient mice. J Exp Med 1996;184:1781–90.

106. Street SE, Cretney E, Smyth MJ. Perforin and interferon-gamma activities independently control tumor initiation, growth, and metastasis. Blood 2001;97:192–7.

107. Hersey P, Zhang XD. How melanoma cells evade trail-induced apoptosis. Nat Rev Cancer 2001;1:142–50.

108. Smyth MJ, Thia KYT, Cretney E, et al. Perforin is a major contributor to NK cell control of tumor metastasis. J Immunol 1999;162:6658–62.

109. Smyth MJ, Thia KY, Street SE, et al. Perforin-mediated cytotoxicity is critical for surveillance of spontaneous lymphoma. J Exp Med 2000;192:755–60.

110. Boehm U, Klamp T, Groot M, et al. Cellular responses to interferon-gamma. Annu Rev Immunol 1997;15:749–95.

111. Bromberg JF, Horvath CM, Wen Z, et al. Transcriptionally active Stat1 is required for the antiproliferative effects of both interferon alpha and interferon gamma. Proc Natl Acad Sci U S A 1996;93:7673–8.

112. Qin Z, Blankenstein T. CD4+ T cell–mediated tumor rejection involves inhibition of angiogenesis that is dependent on IFN gamma receptor expression by nonhematopoietic cells. Immunity 2000;12:677–86.

113. Coughlin CM, Salhany KE, Gee MS, et al. Tumor cell responses to IFNgamma affect tumorigenicity and response to IL-12 therapy and antiangiogenesis. Immunity 1998;9:25–34.

114. Angiolillo AL, Sgadari C, Taub DD, et al. Human interferon-

inducible protein 10 is a potent inhibitor of angiogenesis in vivo. J Exp Med 1995;182:155–62.

115. Dighe AS, Richards E, Old LJ, et al. Enhanced in vivo growth and resistance to rejection of tumor cells expressing dominant negative IFN gamma receptors. Immunity 1994;1: 447–56.

116. Kaplan DH, Shankaran V, Dighe AS, et al. Demonstration of an interferon gamma-dependent tumor surveillance system in immunocompetent mice. Proc Natl Acad Sci U S A 1998;95:7556–61.

117. Street SE, Trapani JA, MacGregor D, et al. Suppression of lymphoma and epithelial malignancies effected by interferon gamma. J Exp Med 2002;196:129–34.

118. Kashii Y, Giorda R, Herberman RB, et al. Constitutive expression and role of the TNF family ligands in apoptotic killing of tumor cells by human NK cells. J Immunol 1999;163:5358–66.

119. Kayagaki N, Yamaguchi N, Nakayama M, et al. Expression and function of TNF-related apoptosis-inducing ligand on murine activated NK cells. J Immunol 1999;163:1906–13.

120. Zamai L, Ahmad M, Bennett IM, et al. Natural killer (NK) cell-mediated cytotoxicity: differential use of TRAIL and fas ligand by immature and mature primary human NK cells. J Exp Med 1998;188:2375–80.

121. Takeda K, Smyth MJ, Cretney E, et al. Critical role for tumor necrosis factor-related apoptosis-inducing ligand in immune surveillance against tumor development. J Exp Med 2002;195:161–9.

122. Cretney E, Takeda K, Yagita H, et al. Increased susceptibility to tumor initiation and metastasis in TNF-related apoptosis-inducing ligand-deficient mice. J Immunol 2002;168: 1356–61.

123. Smyth MJ, Cretney E, Takeda K, et al. Tumor necrosis factor-related apoptosis-inducing ligand (TRAIL) contributes to interferon gamma-dependent natural killer cell protection from tumor metastasis. J Exp Med 2001;193:661–70.

124. Peng SL, Robert ME, Hayday AC, et al. A tumor-suppressor function for fas (CD95) revealed in T cell-deficient mice. J Exp Med 1996;184:1149–54.

125. Davidson WF, Giese T, Fredrickson TN. Spontaneous development of plasmacytoid tumors in mice with defective Fas-Fas ligand interactions. J Exp Med 1998;187:1825–38.

126. Kondo E, Yoshino T, Yamadori I, et al. Expression of Bcl-2 protein and Fas antigen in non-Hodgkin's lymphomas. Am J Pathol 1994;145:330–7.

127. Rosen D, Li JH, Keidar S, et al. Tumor immunity in perforin-deficient mice: a role for CD95 (Fas/APO-1). J Immunol 2000;164:3229–35.

128. Marincola FM, Jaffee EM, Hicklin DJ, et al. Escape of human solid tumors from T-cell recognition: molecular mechanisms and functional significance. Adv Immunol 2000;74:181–273.

129. Seliger B, Wollscheid U, Momburg F, et al. Coordinate down-regulation of multiple MHC class I antigen processing genes in chemical-induced murine tumor cell lines of distinct origin. Tissue Antigens 2000;56:327–36.

130. Hayashi T, Faustman DL. Development of spontaneous uterine tumors in low molecular mass polypeptide-2 knockout mice. Cancer Res 2002;62:24–7.

131. French LE, Tschopp J. Defective death receptor signaling as a cause of tumor immune escape. Semin Cancer Biol 2002;12:51–5.

132. Lieberman J. Cell death and immunity: The ABCs of granule-mediated cytotoxicity: new weapons in the arsenal. Nat Rev Immunol 2003;3:361–70.

133. Oyama T, Ran S, Ishida T, et al. Vascular endothelial growth factor affects dendritic cell maturation through the inhibition of nuclear factor-kappa B activation in hemopoietic progenitor cells. J Immunol 1998;160:1224–32.

134. Sharma S, Stolina M, Lin Y, et al. T cell-derived IL-10 promotes lung cancer growth by suppressing both T cell and APC function. J Immunol 1999;163:5020–8.

135. Salazar-Onfray F, Charo J, Petersson M, et al. Down-regulation of the expression and function of the transporter associated with antigen processing in murine tumor cell lines expressing IL-10. J Immunol 1997;159:3195–202.

136. Zeidler R, Eissner G, Meissner P, et al. Downregulation of TAP1 in B lymphocytes by cellular and Epstein-Barr virus-encoded interleukin-10. Blood 1997;90:2390–7.

137. Gorsch SM, Memoli VA, Stukel TA, et al. Immunohistochemical staining for transforming growth factor beta 1 associates with disease progression in human breast cancer. Cancer Res 1992;52:6949–52.

138. Doran T, Stuhlmiller H, Kim JA, et al. Oncogene and cytokine expression of human colorectal tumors responding to immunotherapy. J Immunother 1997;20:372–6.

139. Groh V, Wu J, Yee C, et al. Tumour-derived soluble MIC ligands impair expression of NKG2D and T-cell activation. Nature 2002;419:734–8.

140. Doubrovina ES, Doubrovin MM, Vider E, et al. Evasion from NK cell immunity by MHC class I chain-related molecules expressing colon adenocarcinoma. J Immunol 2003;171:6891–9.

141. Castriconi R, Cantoni C, Della Chiesa M, et al. Transforming growth factor beta 1 inhibits expression of NKp30 and NKG2D receptors: consequences for the NK-mediated killing of dendritic cells. Proc Natl Acad Sci U S A 2003;100:4120–5.

142. Lee JC, Lee KM, Kim DW, et al. Elevated TGF-beta1 secretion and down-modulation of NKG2D underlies impaired NK cytotoxicity in cancer patients. J Immunol 2004;172: 7335–40.

143. Coussens LM, Werb Z. Inflammation and cancer. Nature 2002;420:860–7.

144. Daniel D, Meyer-Morse N, Bergsland EK, et al. Immune enhancement of skin carcinogenesis by CD4+ T cells. J Exp Med 2003;197:1017–28.

145. Coussens LM, Raymond WW, Bergers G, et al. Inflammatory mast cells up-regulate angiogenesis during squamous epithelial carcinogenesis. Genes Dev 1999;13:1382–97.

146. Coussens LM, Tinkle CL, Hanahan D, et al. MMP-9 supplied by bone marrow-derived cells contributes to skin carcinogenesis. Cell 2000;103:481–90.

3

Human Herpesvirus 8/Kaposi's Sarcoma–Associated Herpesvirus Biology

ILKA ENGELMANN
CORNELIA HENKE-GENDO
THOMAS F. SCHULZ

It has been just over 10 years since two small DNA fragments with sequence homologies to two herpesviruses, Epstein-Barr virus (EBV) and herpesvirus saimiri (HVS) of squirrel monkeys, were identified in a Kaposi's sarcoma (KS) biopsy, leading to the discovery of a new tumor virus and member of the human γ_2-herpesvirus family, termed Kaposi's sarcoma–associated herpesvirus (KSHV) or human herpesvirus 8 (HHV-8).[1] Further analysis of this newly discovered virus revealed a causative role not only for KS, for which the involvement of a transmissible agent was long suggested by multiple epidemiologic studies, but also its association with a very rare form of B-cell lymphoma, body-cavity–associated lymphoma (BCBL), or primary effusion lymphoma (PEL), as well as the plasma cell variant of multicentric Castleman's disease (MCD).[2,3] Apart from neoplastic diseases, KSHV may also play a role in occasional cases of bone marrow failure in immunosuppressed individuals.[4] Over the last decade, a substantial body of information has accumulated about the biology of KSHV/HHV-8 and its role in the pathogenesis of these diseases.

VIRUS MORPHOLOGY AND GENOME STRUCTURE

Following the discovery of KSHV in primary effusion lymphomas, several groups succeeded in establishing persistently infected cell lines from such lymphomas, and subsequently to visualize KSHV virions after chemical induction of the lytic replication cycle.[2,5,6] KSHV virions exhibit the characteristic morphologic appearance of herpesviruses: 100- to 150-nm particles with a lipid envelope, an icosahedral capsid with a 110 nm diameter, and an electron-dense central core, consisting of a complex of double-stranded DNA and protein.[6] In this context, it is worth noting that the presence of herpesvirus-like structures in a short-term tissue culture of a KS lesion had been described as early as 1972, long before the discovery of the virus. These structures had been, probably erroneously, attributed to cytomegalovirus.[7,8] Similar to other herpesvirus genomes, the KSHV genome is stably maintained in infected cells as circular monomeric episomes during latency, whereas in cells undergoing the production of new virions ("lytic" replication cycle), viral genomes are replicated by "rolling circle."[9,10] The KSHV genome contains a long unique region (LUR) of a 140.5 kb double-stranded DNA with 53.5% of GC content. The LUR is flanked by multiple tandem 801 bp terminal repeats, which show a much higher GC proportion of 84.5%.[11,12] Sequencing of the whole genome of KSHV revealed at least 90 putative open reading frames (ORFs) within the LUR (Figure 3–1). These ORFs are named and numbered following the nomenclature initially adopted for HVS, the prototype of γ_2-herpesviruses. Genes without homology to those found in HSV are designated

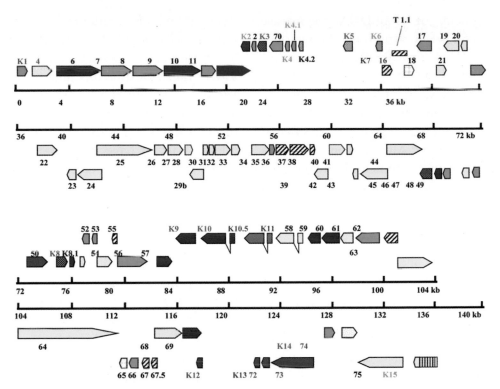

Figure 3–1. The genome of Kaposi's sarcoma–associated herpesvirus. Individual open reading frames (viral genes) are shown in their transcriptional orientation and are color coded to reflect their expression patterns during latency and lytic reactivation. The color coding of the names of selected viral genes reflects their functional role, as discussed in the text. Genes encoding viral proteins with transforming activity in transfection studies are shown in *red*, those for proteins involved in cell cycle regulation in *blue*, those for proteins affecting angiogenesis or B-cell proliferation in *green*, those modulating apoptosis in *purple*, and those contributing to immune escape in *brown*. As outlined in the text, several viral proteins have multiple functions; this is not reflected in the color coding used here. (KS = Kaposi's sarcoma; PAA = phosphonoacetic acid.)

The genome of KSHV. Individual open reading frames (viral genes) are shown in their transcriptional orientation and color – coded to reflect their expression patterns during latency and lytic reactivation: The color coding of the names of selected viral genes reflects their functional role, as discussed in the text. Genes encoding viral proteins with transforming activity in transfection studies are shown in red, those for proteins involved in cell cycle regulation in blue, those for proteins affecting angiogenesis or B-cell proliferation in green, those modulating apoptosis in purple, those contributing to immune escape in brown. As outlined in the text, several viral proteins have multiple functions – this is not reflected in the colour coding used here.

by the letter "K" followed by a number. The KSHV genome contains many genes with homology to cellular genes that are implicated in signaling transduction, cell cycle control, and apoptosis regulation. The same feature has also been found in many other known γ2-herpesviruses. It is believed that these genes were acquired, from host cells, by the virus in the distant past of herpesviral evolution, a process sometimes referred to as "viral piracy." The presence of cytokine signaling genes in the KSHV genome is intriguing because the involvement of cellular cytokines in the pathogenesis of KS has been suspected for a long time.

CLASSIFICATION, ORIGIN, AND EVOLUTION OF KSHV

As mentioned above, phylogenetic analysis of its genomic sequence classified KSHV as presently the only human member of the γ2 subgroup of herpesviruses, also called rhadinoviruses.[11,12] Rhadinoviruses have been found not only in primates but also in other mammals (eg, equine herpesvirus 2 [EHV-2] and murine herpesvirus 68 [MHV-68]).[13,14] Among primates, several additional rhadinoviruses have been identified by consensus polymerase chain reaction (PCR) in recent years. Thus, as shown in

Figure 3–2, fragments of viral DNA polymerase genes (ORF9) have been found in chimpanzees (PtRV-1 or PanRHV-1 and PanRHV-2), gorillas (GoRHV-1), mandrills (MnRHV-1 and MnRHV-2), African Green monkeys (ChRV-1 and ChRV-2), baboons (PapRV-2), and macaques (RFHVMm, RFHVMn, RRV), as well as in squirrels (HSV) and spider monkeys (HVA).[15–23] Although only based on relatively short sequence fragments, phylogenetic analysis shows the subdivision into New World and Old World viruses, and among the latter, the existence of two separate lineages of Old World rhadinoviruses, termed RV-1 and RV-2. KSHV is the human representative of the first lineage (RV-1). Whether a human RV-2 remains to be discovered, or whether it has died out during evolution, is not known at present.

KSHV strains from different geographic regions show minor sequence divergence, usually below 3%, throughout most of the viral genome. However, much more substantial variability is found in the *K1* gene at the left end of the KSHV genome (Figure 3–3) and the *K15* gene at the opposite genomic end. *K1* encodes a type I transmembrane protein with an immunoglobulin superfamily-like extracellular domain, which contains two highly variable regions, VR-1 and VR-2, and shows up to 30% variability at the amino acid level between different virus strains. Despite this high degree of interstrain variability, the virus does not change over time in a single individual.[24] Based on phylogenetic analysis of ORF *K1* (see Figure 3–3), five KSHV variants (clade A to E) have been identified, all of them diversified over the course of the last 65,000 years from one common ancestor, termed P ("prototype").[25] The separation of the different clades, most likely by isolation and founder effects, mirrors human evolution and supports the prevailing model of humankind migrating out of Africa and later subdividing into a European–West Asian and an Asian branch, which 50,000 years later parted to reach southern Asia and Australia as well as the Americas. Thus, clade B is found in Africa and in individuals of African descent, whereas clade D was found in samples from old Asian populations such as the Ainu, an old population on Hokkaido in the North of Japan.[26–31] Clade E, observed in Amerindian populations of Brazil, is most closely related to clade D, supporting the model of migration of ancient Amerindian populations to the New World via the

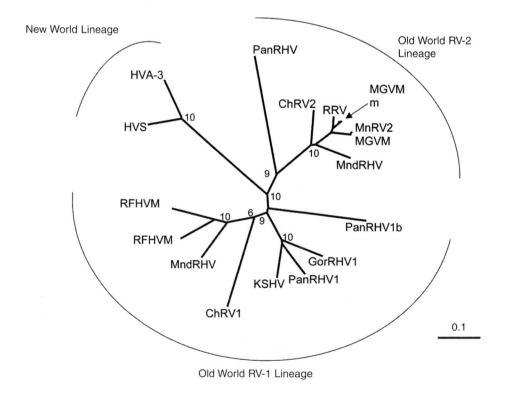

Figure 3–2. Phylogenetic relationships among primate γ_2-herpesviruses. The phylogenetic tree shown here was created by the Neighbour-Joining method of partial DNA polymerase gene sequences of the γ_2-herpesviruses shown. Numbers at branch points denote bootstrap values to indicate the reliability of this analysis (values over 75% are generally taken to indicate a robust assignment to a branch). The figure shows that Kaposi's sarcoma–associated herpesvirus belongs to the RV1 subgroup of γ_2-herpesviruses, with closely related viruses being found in many Old World primate species. In addition, a second group, RV2, comprises slightly more distantly related γ_2-herpesviruses in many primate species. The New World primate γ_2-herpesviruses form a third branch.

Figure 3–3. Evolution of the *K1* gene of Kaposi's sarcoma–associated herpesvirus (KSHV): *K1*, located at the "left" end of the KSHV genome (see Figure 3–1), exists in five different, but closely related variants, A through E. Some of these are associated with particular geographic regions or populations, indicating a possible coevolution of *K1* with human populations. Genotype B is found in Africa or in individuals of African descent, whereas genotype D was found in samples from old Asian populations. Genotype E, most closely related to genotype D, was observed in South American Indians, an observation that would be consistent with the migration of the ancient Native American population to the New World via the Behring Straits. Genotypes A and C are now found in many parts of the world and can be further subdivided to C' and C'', or A' and A5, respectively. Genotype A5 is frequently found in Africa and Italy, presumably as result of the trading contacts of people in ancient time.

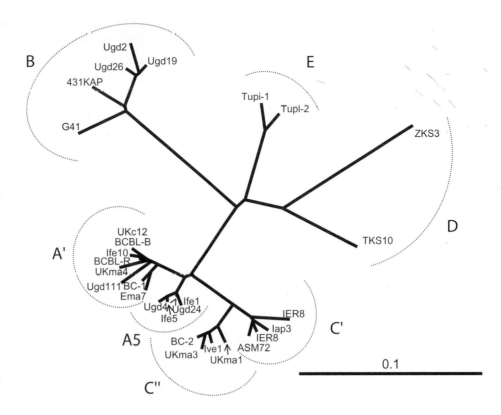

Behring Straits.[32] In contrast, genotypes A and C are now found in most parts of the world, presumably as a result of the mixing of populations over the last three millenia.[27,31] The wide distribution of the A5 subtype in Africa and its presence on the east coast of Italy could be the result of old trading links.[27,28] The same clades can be broadly recognized in other regions of the KSHV genome, although the variability between them is much less than in the *K1* gene. The pattern of variability in *K1* indicates some evolutionary selective pressure, as nucleotide substitutions that alter the protein sequence ("nonsynonymous" mutations) are found more frequently in this region than those that do not ("synonymous" mutations).[27]

There is also evidence of extensive recombination among the "P-derived" clades A through E of different KSHV genomes, suggesting that recombination has been an important factor in the evolution of this virus.[25,28,29,33] In addition, there is also evidence of recombination with at least three more distantly related rhadinoviruses. One, the M type, has recombined into P-type variants at the right end of the viral genome. Both the fact that this M type has been seen in isolates from different parts of the world, and the observation of two separate lineages of the M type, indicate that this recombination event took place a long time ago, possibly in the order of 100,000 years.[25,28,29,33] The other types, Q and N, also originated from a recombination event with other γ2-herpesviruses at the right end of the KSHV genome, but have so far only been seen in South Africa.[25,34]

PATHOGENESIS

KSHV Infection of the Cell: Tissue Culture Models

In vitro, KSHV can infect a broad spectrum of different cells, including permanent cell lines and multiple primary endothelial or keratinocyte cultures.[9,35–37] Several endothelial-based models of KSHV infection have been described.[38–40] Infection of these cells results in morphologic changes: early-passage bone-marrow microvascular endothelial cells (BMEC) and human umbilical vein endothelial cells (HUVEC) tend to lose their cobblestone morphology and adopt a spindle cell morphology reminiscent of the KS spindle cell. They also display anchorage-independent growth in soft agar, indicating a transformed phenotype. Furthermore, KSHV infection confers long-term proliferation and survival of those cells, possibly by paracrine signaling, since only a fraction of cells still harbor the viral genome.[35] However, different tissue culture systems vary significantly in response to KSHV infection. Stable persistence of KSHV has been found in the HPV-immortalized endothelial cell line.[38] In contrast, KSHV persists inefficiently in the majority of infected endothelial or epithelial cells, reflecting the rapid loss of KSHV from primary cultures of KS biopsies, which tend to lose the KSHV genome after in vitro passage.[41,42] This inefficient persistence of the viral genome in most cultured cell lines contrasts with its stable long-term persistence in primary effusion lymphoma (PEL)-derived cell lines. Remarkably, most of the infected cells in tissue culture are strictly latently infected, with lytic viral replication likely restricted to a much smaller subpopulation of cells.[39]

Cell Entry

KSHV has been shown to attach to peripheral blood B cells, T cells, and monocytes, as well as to different primary endothelial culture cells.[37] Electron microscopy studies have provided visual evidence that viral envelope either rapidly fuses with the plasma membrane or cytoplasmic vesicles or endosomes after internalization.[37,43–45] Thus, with respect to cell entry, KSHV behaves like a typical herpesvirus. Ubiquitously expressed host cell surface heparan sulfate-like molecules might serve as possible attachment sites, as these molecules have been shown to interact with glycoprotein B (ORF8) and glycoprotein K8.1 of KSHV virions.[43,44] $\alpha 3\beta 1$ integrin molecules are thought to be one of the cellular receptors used by KSHV to enter into the cell. KSHV glycoprotein B contains an RGD (arginine-glycine-aspartate) motif, which has been shown to be important for interaction with cell surface integrins.[43,44,46,47]

Binding of KSHV virions to $\alpha 3\beta 1$ integrins not only initiates viral entry into the target cells, but also induces integrin-mediated activation of preexisting host signaling pathways. As a first step, the focal adhesion kinase is phosphorylated and the MEK-ERK1/2 pathway is activated, both crucial steps in the outside-in signaling necessary for integrin-mediated cytoskeletal rearrangements, cell adhesion, motility, and proliferation[48,49] However, the mechanism by which these signaling pathways overcome several host-mediated obstacles and thus facilitate successful infection is still unknown and under intensive research. It is now believed that endocytosis of KSHV is clathrin mediated, and a low pH environment for KSHV entry is needed.[45] There is also evidence that upon infection, KSHV can induce Rho guanosine triphosphatases (GTPases), and in doing so, modulates microtubule formation and thus promotes the trafficking of viral capsids.[50] Once at the nucleus, viral DNA is assumed to be injected into the nucleus, the capsid to be disintegrated, and the linear KSHV genome is circularized, a process believed to happen only a few hours after infection.[37] To date, nothing is known about a putative regulatory role of many other (tegument) proteins that are associated with KSHV virions (eg, ORF45 or ORF21).[51,52]

Viral and Cellular Gene Expression Profiles in the Viral Life Cycle

Herpesviruses, and thus KSHV, can establish a latent or a productive (lytic) infection. The productive (or lytic) infection is characterized by the production and the release of new virions. Latent infection is noncytolytic and is characterized by (1) the maintenance of the viral genome in the nucleus at low copy number, (2) a dramatic restriction of viral gene expression, and (3) the lack of virion production.[53] However, because latently infected cells harbor the entire viral genome, they retain the capacity to initiate lytic viral replication upon receipt of the appropriate signal. Then, an ordered cascade of lytic gene expression is switched on. Depending on the time of expression of a viral gene during the herpesvirus life cycle, it is classified into 1 of 4 different groups: latent, immediate-early, early, and late lytic genes. In the case of KSHV, several genes are known to be expressed during latency; the most prominent is ORF73/*LANA* (latency-associated nuclear antigen), which among other things is required for the persistence of the viral episomal genome in the host cells.[54,55] Furthermore, ORF71 and ORF72 encode latently expressed proteins: the antiapoptotic v-FLIP (Fas-ligand interleukin-1β–converting enzyme inhibitory protein) and v-cyc, a homologue of a D-cyclin, which is known to disturb cell cycle regulation at the G1/S checkpoint (see "Angiogenesis and B-Cell Proliferation," below). Next, a group of short membrane-associated proteins encoded by ORF *K12* have been found to be expressed during latency, and one of these, kaposin A, has transforming properties in rodent fibroblasts (see "Transformation," below).[53] Finally, ORF *K10.5*/v-*IRF*-3, an interferon regulatory factor homologue (v-*IRF*; see below), is only expressed in latently infected B cells, but not in endothelial cells (see "Latent Persistence of KSHV," below).[56–59] Lytic transcripts are markedly increased in abundance after experimental stimulation of latently infected PEL cell lines with sodium butyrate or phorbol myristate acetate. A lytic cycle gene is categorized as immediate early, if no protein synthesis is required to produce the messenger RNA (mRNA); that is, it is induced as a result of the interaction of preexisting host cell and viral components. *RTA* (regulator of transcription and activation), encoded by ORF50, is an important immediate-early gene, which functions in the earliest phases of reactivation from latency.[56–58,60] Expression of *RTA* becomes detectable within the first 4 hours after induction of the lytic cycle, and upon transfection, it is able to drive early and late lytic KSHV gene expression.[60] Other immediate-early genes might be ORF57/*MTA*, ORF45, *K4.2*, *K5*, and *K8*.[61,62] Some of them (ORF57, ORF *K8*) are thought to have a regulatory role in the lytic cycle.

Viral genes are defined as early lytic, if their expression is abolished by inhibition of host protein synthesis, but is not blocked by phosphonoacetic acid (PAA), a specific inhibitor of herpesvirus-encoded DNA polymerase. Late lytic gene expression can be inhibited by PAA. Genes involved in DNA replication can be detected at significant levels by 14 h after induction, followed by those presumed to function in DNA repair and nucleotide metabolism at 20 h. Genes encoding proteins that form part of the virus particle (tegument, capsid, and envelope glycoproteins) and those involved in virus assembly are not expressed until later in the virus life cycle (~ 34 h, for late lytic genes).[58] Surprisingly, several chemokines, proinflammatory cytokines, and putative cytokine receptors also behaved as early lytic genes. These included v-*IL-6*/*K2*, viral macrophage inflammatory proteins I and II (v-*MIP-I* and v-*MIP-II*), and the G protein coupled receptor as well as the 1.1 kb polyadenylated nuclear (PAN) RNA, the most abundant nucleic RNA, which is however not translated.[53,56,58,61] Detailed functions of these viral proteins will be reviewed in the following sections.

Following de novo infection of primary tissue culture cells, not only is latent gene expression (ORF72, ORF72, ORF *K13*) initiated, but a few lytic genes, including the main lytic cycle activator ORF50/*RTA*, are also transiently expressed. Interestingly, this gene expression does not lead to the production of full virus progeny, since viral DNA synthesis and the production of structural proteins are not initiated. Only the lytic cycle proteins *K2*, *K4*, *K5*, and *K6*, and v-*IRF2* genes, which all modulate different aspects of the immune response (see below), and the antiapoptotic *K7* gene are expressed, presumably indicating their requirement in establishing latency.[63]

Not only does viral gene expression change within the viral life cycle, the expression pattern of cellular genes is also altered following infection with KSHV. Several groups reported a significant up-regulation of a large number of interferon (IFN)-induced genes, when analyzing the expression profile of KSHV-infected tissue cultures.[64,65] There were also significant changes in the expression of some cellular genes involved in cell cycle arrest, in alterations of cell morphology, and in the process of tumor formation, angiogenesis, and immune regulation. During the KSHV lytic cycle, there is a profound shut-off of host gene expression, mediated by the viral shut-off exonuclease (SOX, encoded by ORF37), 10 to 12 h after lytic reactivation of KSHV, which promotes degradation of cellular mRNA.[66] However, a few cellular genes (eg, interleukin-6 [*IL-6*]) can escape the host shut-off and are potently upregulated during lytic KSHV growth.[66,67]

The transcriptional profile of infected B cells (BJAB) 2 and 4 hours after infection differs from that of primary endothelial and fibroblast cells (HMVECd and HFF), suggesting a degree of cell-type specificity in the cellular gene expression patterns following viral infection. In contrast to antiapoptotic regulators induced in the latter, proapoptotic regulators were induced in B cells. Furthermore, as in longer-established infection, a robust increase in the expression of IFN-induced genes suggestive of innate immune response induction was observed in HMVECd and HFF, whereas there was a total lack of immunity-related protein induction in B cells.[63]

Latent Persistence of KSHV

Similar to other herpesviruses, KSHV can persist in some infected cells in a latent state during which only a minimal number of viral genes is transcriptionally active. Among these are ORF73, the gene for LANA-1, ORF72/v-cyc, ORF71/*K13*/v-FLIP, and transcripts in the *K12*/"kaposin" gene locus. In addition, *K10.5*/v-*IRF-3*/*LANA-2* is expressed in latently infected B cells in PEL and MCD but not in the KSHV-infected endothelial and spindle cells of KS.[68–72] An additional distinguishing feature of latency is the circular nature of the episomal viral genome. KSHV adopts this latent stage in the majority of infected cells in KS, PEL, and MCD.[10,73] However, a small percentage of infected cells express immediate-early or early proteins, indicating a small number of cells undergoing virus production. In KS, < 1 to 5% of spindle cells express ORF59/*PF-8*, *K8*/k-*bZIP*, or ORF74/v-*GCR*, markers of the early lytic cycle.[70,71,74] Similarly, in uncultured PEL samples, the majority of cells express *LANA-1*, but < 5% of *LANA-1*–expressing cells stain with antibodies to v-IL-6, and < 1% with antibodies to ORF59/PF-8, K8/K-bZIP, or v-IRFs.[70,71] In contrast, the viral gene expression pattern appears to be less restricted in MCD, at least in some cases, with 3 to 25% of B cells expressing v-*IL-6* or v-*IRF-1* or *K8*/k-*bZIP*.[70,71] Taken together, these observations indicate that KSHV adopts a restrictive viral gene expression pattern consistent with latency in the majority of infected cells in vitro, but that a minority of cells at any given time point may switch into lytic replication. The propensity toward a less restricted gene expression pattern that involves not only the production of paracrine factors such as v-IL-6 (see "Mechanisms of Oncogenesis," below) but also the expression of viral genes essential for the lytic replication cycle, such as *K8*/k-*bZIP*, or ORF59/*PF-8*, appears to be stronger in MCD. MCD can therefore be viewed as the first example of a human malignancy resulting from the paracrine effects of a lytically replicating virus.

Of the viral proteins expressed during latency, ORF73/LANA-1 is essential for the extrachromosomal replication of the circular viral genome, and is also sufficient for mediating this replication in short-term replication assays involving dividing cells and transient transfection of a plasmid containing the latent origin of replication in the KSHV terminal repeat region, together with an expression vector for *LANA-1*.[54,55,75–77] In these transient assays, there appears to be no need for ORF72/v-*cyc* and ORF71/*K13*/v-*FLIP*, which are translated from an alternatively spliced mRNA expressed, like the LANA-1 transcript, from the latent LANA-1 promoter.[68,78,79] Although the latent expression of v-*cyc*, together with its biochemical properties, in particular its ability to promote S-phase entry (see "Angiogenesis and B-Cell Proliferation," below), could suggest an involvement during latent replication, this issue has not yet been addressed experimentally.

LANA-1 binds to the latent KSHV origin of replication, located in the terminal repeat region, via its carboxy (C)-terminal domain.[54,75,76] The LANA-1 amino (N)-terminal region binds to mitotic chromosomes, thus ensuring the tethering of KSHV episomes to mitotic chromosomes during mitosis.[55,77,80] It is thought that this ensures the efficient distribution of KSHV genomes to daughter cells during cell division and hence their retention in dividing cells.[55] However, the retention of KSHV genomes in dividing cells in cultured cell lines is very inefficient, with most KSHV genomes lost after a few passages of infected or transfected cultures.[42] This is in line with the old observation that cultures established from KS biopsies rapidly lose their KSHV genomes.[41,81] Although the association of LANA-1 with mitotic chromosomes is well established, its role in retaining viral episomes therefore appears to be limited.

Our understanding of how LANA-1 mediates the replication of latent viral genomes is only at its beginning. LANA-1 recruits several nuclear proteins that have been linked to replication of chromosomal DNA or to chromatin architecture to the latent viral replication origin. Among these are the origin of recognition complex 2 protein (ORC-2) and brd-2/RING-3.[82–84] The latent viral replication origin is also associated with the minichromosome maintenance complex protein 3 (MCM-3) and the histone acetyltransferase HBO1 (histone acetyltransferase binding to ORC), and suppression of MCM-5, ORC-2, and HBO-1 using small/short interfering RNA (siRNA) inhibits LANA-1–dependent replication of a plasmid containing the latent origin.[84] These observations indicate that, by binding to the terminal repeat region, LANA-1 recruits several components of the cellular DNA replication machinery, may modify the chromatin architecture, and thus initiates replication from the latent origin.

LANA-1 also regulates transcription from a variety of cellular and viral promoters, including an enhancer/promoter located in the terminal repeat region.[54,83,85–87] Its effect on several cellular promoters may be linked to modulate E2F-dependent gene expression, likely as a result of its interaction with the retinoblastoma protein (pRB) or brd-2/RING-3, which has also been linked to E2F-containing transcriptional complexes.[82,88]

Control of the Lytic Replication Cycle

The mechanism that determines the reactivation of KSHV from its latent stage and the initiation of the lytic replication cycle is also only partially understood. Central to the activation of the lytic cycle is the immediate-early protein RTA, encoded by ORF50.[89]

In the experimental model commonly used to study the early stages of the lytic cycle (ie, the induction of PEL cells by tetradecanoyl phorbol acetate [TPA] or sodium butyrate), the immediate-early ORF50 gene, encoding RTA, is the earliest viral gene to be expressed. The ORF50/*RTA* promoter contains several transcription factor-binding sites, including *AP-1, Oct-1, CEBP/α*.[90–92] RTA activates its own promoter through 2 of 3 *CEBP/α* binding sites, most likely by physically associating with *CEBP/α*.[92] *RTA* also increases the expression of *CEBP/α*, thereby generating an amplification loop that leads to the expression of not only the immedi-

ate-early ORF50/*RTA* gene, but also of other early genes (see below).

In persistently infected PEL cell lines, biopsies of PEL, MCD, and KS, as well as in KSHV-infected B cells in vivo, the ORF50/*RTA* promoter appears to be methylated, with an inverse correlation between the expression of lytic viral proteins and the methylation status of the ORF50 promoter in individual samples.[93] Treatment of persistently infected PEL cell lines with TPA or 5-azacytidine reduces the number of methylated CpG residues in the ORF50 promoter and activates the lytic cycle.[93] It is therefore conceivable that methylation of the ORF50 promoter during viral persistence regulates, at least in part, the spontaneous activation of the lytic cycle in persistently infected cells. In addition, the *RTA* promoter contains a number of transcription factor sites that are targeted by components of signaling pathways known to be induced by TPA or sodium butyrate (eg, *AP-1*) and these could also contribute to the activation of the lytic cycle.

RTA activates a number of viral early promoters, including those of ORF *K8* (*KbZIP*), nut-1 (*PAN/T1.1*), ORF57 (*MTA*), ORF *K2* (v-*IL-6*), v-*MIP*, ORF *K12* (*kaposin*), ORF74 (v-*OX-2/GPCR*). In at least some target promoters (ie, nut-1, ORF *K12*, v-*IL-6*), *RTA* binds to specific DNA sequence elements (type II *RTA* responsive elements; RRE).[92,94–96] In contrast, the promoters for ORF50 (*RTA*), ORF *K8* (*KbZIP/RAP*), nut-1 (*PAN*), and ORF57 (*MTA*) contain *CEBP/α* binding sites, and their activation by *RTA* involves an interaction of *RTA* with DNA-bound *CEBP/α*.[92] In addition, *RTA* also binds to the transcriptional repressor RBP-Jk and can thus be targeted to promoters containing the RBP-Jk site, such as the promoters for *PAN*, ORF57, and *SSB*. Thus, *RTA*-mediated redirection of RBP-Jk activity from repression to activation may be critical for lytic viral replication.[97,98]

Several clinical observations suggest that reactivation of KSHV could be mediated by environmental factors, injury, immune suppression, or inflammation. Thus, the frequent localization of classic KS lesions on the feet has been linked to an exposure to volcanic soil or to reduced blood flow and poor oxygenation of the lower extremities in elderly individuals.[99] Experimentally, hypoxia has been shown to activate KSHV lytic replication in PEL cell lines.[100] Recently, Haque and colleagues reported the presence of functional hypoxia response elements in the ORF50/*RTA* and ORF34 promoter.[101] These elements are activated by either HIF-2α (ORF50/*RTA* promoter) or by both HIF-1α and HIF-2α (ORF34 promoter), and hypoxia induces the transcription of ORF34 and ORF50/*RTA* mRNAs.[101]

Zoeteweij and colleagues reported that agents that mobilize intracellular calcium, such as ionomycin and thapsigargin, can activate the lytic replication cycle in PEL cells.[102]

That KS lesions can arise in scar tissue or regions of traumatized skin (Köbner phenomenon) is another well-established clinical observation. In addition, an extensive body of experimental work has suggested that inflammatory cytokines may accelerate the development of KS lesions in acquired immune deficiency syndrome (AIDS) patients (for a review, see Ensoli B, et al[103]). There is some direct evidence that inflammatory cytokines can activate the lytic replication cycle of KSHV. Thus Monini and colleagues showed that inflammatory cytokines, and in particular interferon-γ, can increase the viral load in cultured peripheral blood mononuclear cells of KSHV-infected individuals.[104] A similar study identified oncostatin M, hepatocyte growth factor/scatter factor, and interferon-α as cytokines that are released from HIV-1–infected T cells and can induce the expression of ORF *K12* and ORF26 mRNA, as well as ORF59 and K8.1 proteins, in the BCBL-1 cell line.[105]

Mechanisms of Oncogenesis

Prompted by the strong epidemiologic evidence for a causative role of KSHV in KS, and its association with PEL and MCD (see Chapter 7 "Primary Effusion Lymphomas: Biology and Management," and Chapter 6 "Castleman's Disease"), intensive research efforts over the last 10 years have focused on identifying the KSHV genes responsible for, or contributing to, its oncogenic potential. These efforts have been hampered by the lack of a suitable animal model that could serve as a model for the in vivo oncogenicity of KSHV. In addition, unlike in the case of its γ-herpesvirus relative EBV, there is no convincing in vitro assay to test for the transformation of

cultured cells by KSHV, although the induction of spindle cells in primary endothelial cell cultures (see "KSHV Infection of the Cell: Tissue Culture Models," above) is widely regarded as a surrogate marker for the formation of spindle cells in vivo. In contrast, there is no shortage of KSHV genes that can be shown, when tested in isolation, to have transforming activity in transfection assays in vitro, or even in in vivo models, or whose cell biologic or biochemical properties would make them interesting candidates for "pathogenicity factors." These will be discussed in the following sections. It needs to be stressed that in most cases, KSHV genes contribution to KSHV pathogenicity in the context of the complete viral genome is currently still unknown.

Transformation

Three immediate-early or early genes (ORF *K1*, ORF *K9*, and ORF74, encoding VIP, v-IRF-1, and v-GCR, respectively) and one viral gene expressed during latency (ORF *K12*, encoding the kaposin family of transcripts) have transforming properties and can induce intracellular signaling pathways. In addition, biochemical properties that could contribute to cellular transformation have been reported for *LANA-1* and v-*FLIP*, both expressed during latency.

Although the oncogenic properties of a viral protein that is expressed in latently infected tumor cells point to a directly transforming role, similar in vitro properties of a lytic protein are more difficult to reconcile with a direct oncogenic effect. It has therefore been postulated that indirect paracrine effects may be responsible for the contribution, if any, of lytic viral proteins that have been shown to have transforming potential in vitro or when tested in isolation in animal models.

ORF **K1/VIP.** VIP (*v*ariable *I*TAM-containing *p*rotein), the protein expressed from ORF *K1*, is a transmembrane protein that signals constitutively through its cytoplasmic immunoreceptor tyrosine activation motif (ITAM). It thereby activates the cellular nuclear factor of activated transcription (NFAT) growth control pathway.[106,107] K1 transforms rodent fibroblasts and can replace the saimiri transforming protein in the HVS genome in its immortalizing effect on T lymphocytes.[108] K1-expressing transgenic mice develop KS-like tumors and plasmablastic lymphomas exhibiting constitutive activation of NF-κB, Oct-2, and Lyn.[109] *K1* was shown to be expressed during the early lytic cycle of viral replication in primary effusion lymphoma cells, and was detected in MCD tissues, whereas it was undetectable in KS lesions, in accordance with the view that *K1* is preferentially expressed in lymphoid cells.[110]

Furthermore, K1 was shown to induce expression and secretion of vascular endothelial growth factor (VEGF) in epithelial and endothelial cells and expression of matrix metalloproteinase 9 in endothelial cells.[111]

ORF K9/vIRF-1. Expression of v-*IRF-1* inhibits IFN signal transduction in reporter assays, downregulates expression of the cell cycle inhibitor p21$^{WAF-1CIP-1}$, transforms NIH 3T3 cells in culture, and is tumorigenic in nude mice.[112] Activation of the c-*myc* promoter is a prerequisite for transformation by v-IRF-1. c-*myc* transcription is increased up to 15-fold by v-*IRF-1* and the CREB-binding protein (CBP) binds v-*IRF-1* and functions as a coactivator of c-*myc*.[113]

Despite all these reports, expression of *K1/VIP* or *K9*/v-*IRF-1* has not been documented in the majority of tumor cells of KS, MCD, or PEL. Northern blot analysis revealed that v-*IRF-1* is weakly expressed in KSHV-infected B cells, and is absent from spindle KS cells.[112] Consequently, the relevance of the in vitro transforming properties of *K1* and *K9* for the oncogenicity of KSHV in vivo is not yet clearly defined.[112]

ORF 74/v-GCR. v-GCR transforms murine cells and induces angiogenesis mediated by upregulation of VEGF. In vivo KSHV v-*GCR* expression in the hematopoietic cell lineage of transgenic mice has been shown to result in the development of angioproliferative lesions in multiple organs, resembling KS lesions.[114–118]

The expression of v-*GCR* in PEL and MCD tumors and in KS lesions has been observed by immunohistochemistry, but only a small proportion of the tumor cells expressed v-*GCR*, suggesting that the principal mode of action of this membrane signaling protein is via paracrine effects.[74,115,118,119] v-GCR activates several intracellular signaling pathways and cellular cytokines (see "Angiogenesis and

B-Cell Proliferation," below). Its ability to transform rodent fibroblasts has been linked to its ability to activate the JAK2-STAT3 pathway.[120]

K12/Kaposin. A group of transcripts originating in the *K12/kaposin* locus has been reported to encode several proteins.[121] Among these, kaposin A (T0.7), a type II transmembrane protein, transforms rodent fibroblasts and induces lymphocyte aggregation and adhesion, possibly mediated through its direct interaction with cytohesin 1, a guanine nucleotide exchange factor for adenosine diphosphate ribosylation factor (ARF) GTPases and regulator of integrin-mediated cell adhesion.[122–124] Injection of these transformed cells into nude mice led to high-grade, highly vascular, undifferentiated sarcomas. Expression of kaposin A protein was also detected in the PEL cell lines BCBL-1 and KS-1.[125] Localization studies showed that kaposin A is localized perinuclearly and at the cell membrane.[124]

Other transcripts from the *K12* locus involve upstream sequences with GC-rich direct repeats (DRs: DR1 and DR2) and are expressed during latency and after induction of the lytic cycle in PEL cell lines and KS tumors. The major part of kaposin B is encoded by the repeats terminating before the *K12* sequence and has been shown to be abundantly translated in the PEL cell line BCBL-1. Other translation products include a DR-K12 fusion protein termed kaposin C.[121,126] Kaposin B has recently been shown to bind to the kinase MK2, a target of the p38 mitogen-activated protein kinase signaling pathway, and to thereby stabilize cytokine mRNAs containing AU-rich elements in their 3' noncoding regions.[127]

LANA-1. LANA-1 mediates the episomal replication of the KSHV genome during latency and is expressed in all latently infected cells (see "Latent Persistence of KSHV," above). With regard to a role in tumorigenesis, LANA-1 can transform rodent cells in cotransfection assays with a constitutively active Ha-ras.[88] LANA-1 binds several proteins involved in transcriptional regression, including pRB and mSin3a, and modulates the transcriptional activity of *TP53*.[88,128,129]

LANA-transduced HUVEC were shown to proliferate faster and exhibit a more greatly prolonged life span than cells not expressing LANA.[130] Furthermore, LANA upregulates human telomerase reverse transcriptase promoter activity, mediated through direct interaction of LANA with Sp1. This potentially contributes to the prolonged life span of KSHV-infected primary endothelial cells.[131,132] However, no immortalization of transfected or transduced cells has so far been achieved with LANA-1 alone.

K13/v-FLIP. *K13* encodes a FADD (Fas-associated death-domain-like) IL-1β–converting enzyme–like or caspase 8 (FLICE) inhibitory protein (FLIP). K13/v-FLIP is the only viral FLIP that has been shown to possess transforming ability: Rat-1 cells expressing HHV-8 v-*FLIP* form colonies in soft agar and induce tumors in nude mice. Activation of the NF-κB pathway is necessary for this effect.[133] v-FLIP has been postulated to act as a tumor progression factor by interfering with apoptotic signals induced by virus-specific T killer cells (see "Angiogenesis and B-Cell Proliferation," below).[134]

Interference with Cell Cycle Regulation

ORF72/v-cyc. Cell cycle transitions are controlled by the activation of cyclin-dependent kinases (CDKs), which are regulated through binding of cyclin proteins. Several γ-herpesviruses encode homologues of cellular cyclins that interfere with normal cell cycle regulation (for a review, see Verschuren EW, et al[135]). ORF72 codes for v-cyc, a protein that resembles cellular D-type cyclins structurally and functionally. It binds to and activates CDK4 and CDK6 and thereby mediates phosphorylation and inactivation of pRb.[136–140] Other DNA tumor viruses, such as polyoma, papilloma, and adenovirus, also target the pRb pathway (for a review, see Helt AM and Galloway DA[141]).

PEL cell lines have been reported to be defective for p16INK4a expression, a protein that promotes arrest in G1 phase only upon the presence of pRb.[142] Ectopic expression of p16INK4a induces a pRb-dependent G1 cell cycle block in PEL, suggesting that pRb is functional in these KSHV-infected cells despite the presence of two proteins that target the pRb pathway, v-cyc and LANA-1.[142]

Interestingly, v-cyc preferentially interacts with CDK6, which is expressed at relatively high levels in lymphoid cells, the host cells for KSHV.[138] The v-cyc/CDK6 complexes show even enhanced

kinase activity compared with cellular cyclin D/CDK complexes.[138,139]

Inactivation of STAT3 seems to be one mechanism of action of v-cyc, which would prevent growth-suppressive effects.[143] Another mechanism might be the activation of the cyclin A promoter, a regulator of entry into S phase.[144]

Despite the homology with cellular D- and E-cyclins, KSHV v-cyc also shows distinct characteristics. For example, the v-cyc/CDK6 complex needed to phosphorylate pRb is resistant to the cellular CDK inhibitors p16, p21, and p27 and to p16INK4a, conferring resistance to the antiproliferative action of these inhibitors.[139,142] The same is true for the viral cyclin encoded by HVS.[139] Moreover, v-cyclin has been shown to phosphorylate and enhance degradation of p27, thereby enhancing constitutive cell cycling.[140,145]

The v-cyc/CDK6 complex can also phosphorylate and thereby inactivate BCL2, which leads to the activation of apoptotic pathways. However, the action of v-BCL2 (but not cellular BCL2) may counteract this effect (see "Inhibition of Apoptosis," below).[146,147] Furthermore, phosphorylation of the CDK T-loop by the CDK-activating kinase (CAK) cycH/CDK7 is dispensable for the stimulation of CDK6 activity by v-cyc, but then activation is incomplete because non–CAK-phosphorylated v-cyclin/CDK6 does not target the full range of pRb phosphorylation sites and does not enable S-phase entry.[148,149]

The viral and cellular cyclins also differ in their ability to phosphorylate certain proteins. KSHV v-cyc does not induce phosphorylation of p107—(a pRb-related protein) and cannot thereby induce dissociation of p107 from E2F.[144] However, it phosphorylates histone H1 and the CDK inhibitor p27[kip], which are not targeted by cellular cyclin.[137,140,145] These differences with respect to cellular D-type cyclins might explain why v-cyc avoids the CDK inhibitor–regulated checkpoints.

Furthermore, v-cyclin–expressing cells undergo continued DNA synthesis, but do not undergo cytokinesis, probably because of v-cyc–associated misexpression of mitotic regulators (eg, increase of E2F transcriptional targets).[150] The mitotic deregulation of v-*cyc*–expressing cells leads to TP53 activation, which triggers apoptosis and growth arrest.[150] TP53 normally triggers a G1 arrest via p21 induction and consequent G1/S CDK inhibition.[151] v-cyc/CDK complexes are resistant to CDK inhibition, however, and so lack functional G1 and G2 checkpoints, which might explain why these cells become polyploid and contain centromere amplifications contributing to genomic instability.[135] In the absence of functional TP53, these aneuploid cells can expand.[150,152]

The ability of v-cyc to promote the progression of resting cells into the S phase of the cell cycle may be essential to create suitable conditions for the replication of the viral genome.[139,140,143] Whether, as a consequence, it can also play a role in KSHV oncogenicity is unknown at present.

K8/K-bZIP. K-bZIP shows sequence homology to the central regulator of the EBV lytic regulator ZEBRA. However, in KSHV, the neighboring gene ORF50/*RTA* is the central player in the initiation of the lytic cycle. K-bZIP has been shown to bind to CCAAT/enhancer-binding protein alpha (C/EBPα) and p21^{CIP-1} and stabilize them by inhibiting proteasome-dependant degradation.[153] Through interaction with C/EBPα K-bZIP promotes p21^{CIP-1}-mediated inhibition of entry into S phase.[154] This probably creates a suitable environment for lytic viral replication by preventing competition with host-cell DNA synthesis for limited resources. C/EBPα, RTA, and K-bZIP form a complex that associates with and activates the K-bZIP promoter.[92,155] Therefore, both C/EBPα and K-bZIP are activating each other.

K-bZIP also associates with cyclin CDK2 and inhibits its activity resulting in a prolongation of G1 phase.[156]

LANA-1. The pRb plays a role in cell cycle control by repressing E2F-mediated transcription of genes required for cell cycle progression. LANA-1 has been shown to counteract pRB-mediated transcriptional repression of E2F and to activate E2F-regulated promoters, possibly by sequestering pRB.[88]

Recently, a role for LANA-1 in promoting entry into the S phase has been shown as a result of its interaction with GSK-3β, a kinase involved in phosphorylation and consequent degradation of β-catenin by the proteasome. Association of GSK-3β with LANA-1 leads to its transfer to the nucleus and the

stabilization and increased β-catenin levels in infected cells, which allows activation of promoters containing Lef/Tcf-binding sites and entry into the S phase.[157,158] Another recent report shows that LANA protects lymphoid cells from p16INK4a-induced cell cycle arrest and supports S-phase entry.[159]

Angiogenesis and B-Cell Proliferation

KSHV-associated disorders express high levels of vascular endothelial growth factor (VEGF) and its receptor, kinase insert domain-containing receptor, which induces angiogenesis (for a review, see Hayward GS[160]). In KS lesions, VEGF and other angiogenic factors stimulate the inflammatory and neovascular responses that determine spindle cell proliferation, the predominant cell type within these lesions.[115,161–163]

***ORF* K2/*v*-IL-6.** Human IL-6 is expressed in lymphocytes, macrophages, and endothelial cells. It can act on various cell types but is particularly important in inducing B-cell differentiation into plasma cells and is considered to be an important growth factor for multiple myeloma, lymphoma, and leukemia.[164]

v-IL-6 shows structural and functional homology to cellular IL-6. In contrast to its cellular homologue, v-IL-6 acts independently of IL-6 receptor alpha (gp80), but stimulates multiple cellular pathways through interaction with the gp130 coreceptor, resulting in cell proliferation and extrahepatic acute phase responses.[165–168] IL-6Rα and gp130 differ in expression patterns, with gp130 being more widely expressed.[169] This probably allows v-IL-6 to stimulate a broader spectrum of cells. On the other hand, N-linked glycosylation at site N89 of v-IL-6 markedly enhances binding to gp130, signaling through the JAK1-STAT1/3 pathway, and induction of cell proliferation, whereas human IL-6 does not need N-glycosylation to exert these functions.[170]

v-IL-6 has been shown to induce growth and proliferation of B cells and is expressed at higher levels in PEL and MCD than in KS lesions. It has been suggested that the v-*IL-6* gene has two promoters allowing differential regulation of v-*IL-6* gene expression in different tissues.[95] RTA binds to the v-IL-6 RTA-responsive element and activates the v-*IL-6* promoter.[95] LANA-1, on the other hand, has been shown to activate the activator protein 1 (AP1) response element (RE) within the cellular *IL-6* promoter, to stimulate binding of a c-Jun-Fos heterodimer to the AP1 RE, and thereby to induce expression of hIL-6.[171,172]

Furthermore, v-IL-6 has been shown to induce neurite outgrowth in the rat pheochromocytoma cell line PC12 and to promote colony formation of human CD34 positive bone marrow progenitor cells.[173]

There is evidence of v-IL-6 being involved in inducing proliferation of infected B cells (see Schulz TF[174]). Like its cellular counterpart, v-IL-6 is able to support the growth of IL-6–dependent B cells in vitro.[175]

v-IL-6 induces human IL-6 secretion and is an autocrine growth factor for PEL cells.[176,177] Expression of vascular endothelial growth factor type B in PEL cells is also induced by v-IL-6.[178] In vivo, v-IL-6–transfected fibroblasts inoculated into nude mice induced hepatosplenomegaly, lymphadenopathy, and polyclonal hypergammaglobulinemia, accompanied by increased hematopoiesis of the myeloid, erythroid, and megakaryocytic lineages and plasmacytosis in the spleen and lymph nodes.[162] Tumors developing in these animals showed more extensive vascularization than those in control animals, and expressed high levels of VEGF, which were correlated with the amount of v-IL-6 in these tumors.[162] VEGF is also expressed in PEL-derived cell lines, and a neutralizing antibody to VEGF blocked the formation of effusion lymphoma and bloody ascites in mice inoculated with PEL cell lines.[163] VEGF can also be detected in the malignant effusions of PEL patients.[179] VEGF-induced stimulation of vascular permeability may therefore be critical to the formation of the malignant ascites characteristic for this AIDS lymphoma.

v-IL-6 can activate STAT3, JAK1, and the MAP kinase and other pathways.[165–167] v-IL-6 is directly activated by interferon-α and blocks interferon signaling, indicating that one of its roles is to act as an interferon antagonist.[180]

Interestingly, it has been shown that renal transplant patients who are homozygous for the G allele in the *IL-6* promoter polymorphism G-174C, which is associated with increased IL-6 production, had increased KS incidence.[181]

ORF74/v-GCR. ORF74 of KSHV has early lytic kinetics and encodes a G-protein–coupled receptor (v-GCR). KSHV and HVS v-GCRs are homologues of the human IL-8 receptor.[182] Unlike its human homologue, KSHV v-GCR shows ligand-independent constitutive activity due to the presence of a point mutation in a sequence motif (DRY) that is highly conserved among GCRs.[114,183] v-GCR engages pathways downstream of multiple G protein subunits, including protein kinase C, protein kinase B, Akt, NF-κB, JAK2/STAT3, and mitogen-activated protein kinases, resulting in increased transcriptional activity of their nuclear targets, stimulation of cell proliferation, promotion of cell survival, and transformation.[114,115,184–190] More recently, it has been shown that v-GCR–induced activation of AP-1 and CREB is mediated cooperatively by a Gq-ERK-1/2 and a Gi-PI3K-Src axis. Unlike in other cell types, however, NF-κB activation by v-GPCR does not seem to be substantially mediated by Gi or PI3K/Akt in PEL cells.[191]

The stimulation of transcription factors like NF-κB, AP-1, and NFAT by v-GCR has been reported to be mediated through the activation of the small G protein Rac1.[192]

On the other hand, it is unclear to what extent de novo host gene expression induced by viral signaling can proceed during the lytic life cycle, as host gene expression is strongly inhibited 10 to 12 h after lytic reactivation of KSHV, and this host shut-off leads to a drastic limitation of the expression of most v-GCR targets. However, one of the rare cellular genes that can escape the host shut-off and is potently upregulated during lytic KSHV growth is human IL-6.[66]

v-GCR has been shown to transform murine fibroblasts (see "Transformation," above) and induce angiogenesis mediated by upregulation of VEGF. KSHV v-GCR expression in the hematopoietic cell lineage of transgenic mice results in the development of angioproliferative lesions in multiple organs, resembling KS lesions.[114–118]

Interestingly, despite its tumorigenic and angiogenic functions, v-GCR is only expressed in approximately 10% of the KS cells.[74] Expression of ORF74 conferred on primary endothelial cells a morphology that was strikingly similar to that of spindle cells present in KS lesions.[190] Similarly, infection of transgenic mice with a retroviral vector allowing endothelial cell-specific expression of v-GCR led to the development of KS-like lesions, but expression of v-GCR was limited to a small proportion of tumor cells. Expression of v-GCR appeared to lead to the recruitment of other endothelial cells, suggesting that v-GCR acts through paracrine mechanisms, probably by inducing secretion of angiogenic factors, a theory that is supported by the finding that supernatants from transfected KS cells activated NF-κB signaling in untransfected cells and elicited the chemotaxis of monocytoid and T-lymphoid cells.[118,190]

The role of v-GCR on disease progression in hematopoietic cells was analyzed by using PEL cell lines expressing v-*GCR* under the control of an inducible promoter.[193] Using this system, the authors observed activation of p38 and ERK-2, augmented transcription of several KSHV lytic genes (ie, ORF57), and increased production of v-IL-6 and VEGF due to v-*GCR*.[193] All these observations point to v-GCR as a major player in the angiogenesis and thereby pathogenesis of KSHV.

v-MIPs. KSHV possesses three homologues of human MIP-Iα: v-MIP-I through -III. These proteins are encoded by KSHV ORF *K6*, ORF4, and ORF4.1, respectively. v-MIPs are considered to be important in promoting leukocyte chemotaxis, eosinophil migration, and angiogenesis.

Among them, v-MIP-I has been reported to induce the expression of VEGF-A in PEL cell lines.[178] MIP-I, MIP-II, and MIP-III have been shown to be highly angiogenic in the chick chorioallantoic membrane assay as opposed to cellular MIP-Iα.[194,195] Other viruses, such as mouse and human cytomegalovirus, also encode functional chemokines.[196–198]

The v-MIPs are also required for evading the immune response and inhibiting apoptosis (see below).

***ORF* K15.** A family of alternatively spliced transcripts are transcribed late in the lytic replication cycle from 8 exons located between ORF75 and the terminal repeat. The corresponding proteins are predicted to contain up to 12 transmembrane domains and a common cytoplasmic domain containing SH2- and SH3-binding motifs and a putative TRAF (tumor necrosis factor receptor-associated factor) and Src kinase-binding motifs.[33,199,200] The largest *K15*-derived protein seems to share functional prop-

erties with LMP1 and LMP2A of EBV.[199] Phosphorylation of the cytoplasmic domain of this protein by *src* kinases leads to the activation of the NF-κB and of two MAPK (mitogen-activated kinase) pathways.[201] Recent gene expression array experiments have shown that K15 can also induce a range of cellular and inflammatory cytokines, as well as other cellular genes usually activated by VEGF (Brinkmann MM et al., in preparation). Intracellular localization studies have shown that K15 resides in the endoplasmic reticulum and mitochondria, where it interacts with HS 1–associated protein X-1 (HAX-1), a BCL2-related protein functioning as an inhibitor of Bax-induced apoptosis.[202]

Inhibition of Apoptosis

Programmed cell death or apoptosis is a complex process involving several cellular proteins. Viral infection can trigger apoptosis pathways as a defense mechanism against further virus propagation. However, several viruses have also developed mechanisms that interfere with apoptotic pathways to increase the survival rate of virus-infected cells, thus increasing the time available for viral replication and spread within the host and to other individuals. As inhibition of apoptotic pathways is also one of the hallmarks of tumor cells, viral proteins that interfere with apoptosis are thought to play a major role in virus-induced oncogenesis.[203] Two different apoptotic pathways in mammalian cells result in the activation of effector caspases.[204,205] The extrinsic pathway requires the activation of procaspases 8 and 10 by so-called death receptors, which belong to the tumor necrosis factor receptor gene superfamily, whereas in the intrinsic pathway, mitochondria release caspase-activating proteins.[206]

***ORF* K13/*v-FLIP*.** KSHV encodes a FLICE inhibitory protein (v-FLIP) that prevents death by receptor-mediated apoptosis by inhibiting the recruitment and activation of FLICE. The v-FLIP encoded by ORF *K13* is expressed on the same bicistronic transcript as v-cyc.[68] It can block Fas-induced apoptosis and has been postulated to act as a tumor progression factor by interfering with apoptotic signals induced by virus-specific T killer cells.[134,207,208] v-FLIP inhibits the protease activities of caspase-3, -8, and -9.[134,209] It also interacts directly with the cytosolic IκB kinase complex and thereby contributes to the continuous NF-κB activation observed in PEL cells.[210] More recent studies show that the activation of the NF-κB pathway is necessary for the inhibition of apoptosis induced by growth factor withdrawal, probably by upregulating antiapoptotic proteins like BCLx$_L$.[211] By transient and stable transfection experiments, it was demonstrated that v-FLIP activates the JNK/AP1 pathway in a TRAF-dependent fashion and induces gene expression from the *c-IL-6* promoter in a JNK/AP1-dependent fashion.[87]

The in vivo significance of v-FLIP expression has been shown by experiments, where murine B-lymphoma cells expressing v-FLIP developed into aggressive tumors when injected into immunocompetent mouse strains, largely because of v-FLIP-mediated prevention of death receptor-induced apoptosis triggered by T cells.[134] The amount of v-FLIP transcripts has been reported to be associated with a reduction in apoptosis in KS lesions.[72]

ORF K7/survivin. *K7/survivin* is the only currently known herpesviral inhibitor-of-apoptosis protein (IAP) homologue. It is a homologue of the cellular protein survivin, as revealed by computational analysis, and is expressed during the lytic cycle in PEL cells, as shown by Northern blot using a K7-specific probe.[212] Human survivin, a member of the IAPs family, protects cells from apoptosis, possibly by enhancing TP53 degradation.[213] Furthermore, it has been reported that human survivin associates with X-linked IAP (XIAP), thereby increasing XIAP stability and synergistically inhibiting caspase-9 activation.[214,215] K7 inhibits apoptosis induced by several stimuli.[212,216] It anchors to cellular membranes in the vicinity of BCL2 and binds to BCL2 (but not Bax) via its putative BH2 domain and to caspase-3 via its BIR domain.[212] Thus, K7 seems to be an adaptor molecule bringing together BCL2 and effector caspases, allowing the inhibition of the latter by BCL2.[212] Furthermore, K7 binds to the cellular calcium-modulating cyclophilin ligand, thereby enhancing cytosolic calcium flow and protecting cells from mitochondrial damage and apoptosis.[216]

ORF16/v-BCL2. BCL2 is a cellular antiapoptotic protein belonging to a family of proteins involved in the regulation of apoptosis (for a review, see Cory S and Adam JM[217]). Like all other γ-herpesviruses, for which genomic sequences are available, KSHV expresses a viral homologue of human BCL2.[218] v-BCL2 is expressed during the lytic life cycle and the protein has been detected in late stages of KS lesions.[219] v-BCL2 forms heterodimers with h-BCL2 and might inhibit apoptosis in KSHV-infected cells.[218,220,221] Although human BCL2 forms heterodimers with proapoptotic members of the BCL2 family (such as Bax and Bak), the viral homologue does not seem to do so.[218,221] Moreover, whereas many cellular antiapoptotic members of the BCL2 family can be converted into proapoptotic factors following proteolysis by caspases, calpain, and possibly by other mechanisms, v-BCL2, like other herpesviral BCL2 homologues, cannot be regulated in this way and therefore has exclusively anti-apoptotic properties.[218,221,222] As mentioned above (see "Interference with Cell Cycle Regulation," above), the v-cyc/CDK6 complex phosphorylates and inactivates human BCL2, which results in apoptosis. In contrast to human BCL2, v-BCL2 is not phosphorylated by the v-cyc/CDK6 complex, allowing KSHV to overcome the v-cyc–induced apoptosis.[147] These differences are thought to be due to variations in the protein structure between the viral and the human protein: v-BCL2 lacks a nonstructured loop where phosphorylation by the v-cyc/CDK6 complex takes place.[223] A possible mechanism of action of v-BCL2 is to inhibit apoptosis by interacting with the cellular proapoptotic protein Diva.[224]

Interferon regulatory factor homologues. Interferon regulatory factors (IRFs) are a family of interferon-responsive transcription factors that regulate expression of genes involved in pathogen response, cell proliferation, and immune modulation through binding to interferon-stimulated response elements (ISREs) in the promoters of interferon-responsive genes. Among the members of the IRF family, IRF-3 and IRF-7 seem to be the key regulators for the induction of type I IFNs, the primary response against viral infection (for a review, see Stark GR[225]). KSHV encodes four IRF homologues named v-IRFs.[12,226]

v-IRF-1 and v-IRF-2 inhibit IRF-1–induced expression of CD95-ligand (CD95L), an apoptosis-inducing ligand of CD95/Apo-1/Fas. The mechanism of action of v-IRF-1 seems to involve the inhibition of IRF-1 binding to the CD95L promoter, whereas v-IRF-2, might repress the induction of CD95L by interfering with NF-κB.[227]

ORF K9/v-IRF-1. v-IRF-1, encoded by ORF *K9*, is a multifunctional protein that inhibits apoptosis mediated by various death signals, such as IFN signaling and TP53.[112,175,228–231] v-IRF-1 binds to TP53 and inhibits its phosphorylation and acetylation and blocks its ability to transactivate transcription.[229,230] Another tumor suppressor protein inhibited by v-IRF-1 is retinoid-IFN–induced mortality 19 (GRIM-19), which is a nuclear protein responsive to IFN/all-*trans* retinoic acid (RA) that enhances caspase-9 activity and, consequently, apoptosis. HPV-16 E6 protein also binds to GRIM-19, suggesting that other viruses might target this apoptotic pathway.[231]

ORF K11/v-IRF-2. v-IRF-2 is encoded by ORF *K11*, spliced to a small upstream exon, and also inhibits IFN-mediated cell death.[227,232] The expression of CD95L is upregulated by IFN-γ-activated IRF-1.[227] It is conceivable that by blocking interferon-induced signal transduction and/or apoptosis, v-IRF-1 and v-IRF-2 allow KSHV-infected cells to escape the effect of virus-specific T cells (see "Modulation of the Host Immune Response" below).

ORF K10.5/v-IRF-3/LANA-2. ORF *K10.5* is a latent gene whose product is another KSHV IRF homologue (v-IRF-3).[59,233] As it is a nuclear protein expressed in B cells during latency, it has also been referred to as LANA-2. v-IRF-3 inhibits the activation of TP53-dependent promoters and thereby restrains TP53-mediated apoptosis. It also inhibits apoptosis triggered by the double-stranded RNA-activated protein kinase (PKR) by (partially) blocking downstream events of PKR activation like the PKR-mediated inhibition of protein synthesis, PKR-induced phosphorylation of eIF-2α, and activation of caspase-3 but not of caspase-9.[59,234] However, LANA-2 does not abrogate apoptosis or RNA degradation mediated by the 2-5A system.[234] Therefore, unlike LANA-1, which is essential for the replication of latent viral genomes, LANA-2 is mainly a defense protein against the effect of interferon.

v-MIPs. A role for v-MIP-I and -II (see above) in the inhibition of apoptosis has also been suggested, as they inhibit apoptosis either by chemical induction or by serum withdrawal in PEL cells, probably mediated through the chemokine receptor CCR8.[178,235]

ORF K1/VIP. ORF *K1* expression in B lymphocytes activates the Akt kinase leading to the phosphorylation and inhibition of members of the forkhead (FKHR) transcription factor family, which are key regulators of cell cycle progression and apoptosis. Thereby, K1 can inhibit apoptosis induced by the FKHR proteins and by stimulation of the Fas receptor.[236]

ORF 50/RTA. RTA has been reported to inhibit TP53-induced apoptosis through interaction with CBP.[237]

ORF K8/K-bZIP. K-bZIP also binds to TP53, and thereby represses TP53-mediated apoptosis, presumably to create a favorable environment for viral replication.[238]

ORF 73/LANA-1. LANA-1 binds to TP53 and pRb and inhibits the activation of TP53-dependent promoters and to induce the activation of E2F-dependent genes and thereby protects from apoptosis.[88,129]

Modulation of the Host Immune Response

The interaction between viruses and their hosts during evolution has probably shaped the host immune system and has resulted in the development of viral strategies to evade the immune response. Many viruses encode proteins that target essential pathways of the immune system. KSHV has also acquired several mechanisms to protect infected cells from an attack by the immune system.

The viral proteins involved in the manipulation of the host immune response are K3, K5, the v-MIPs, v-IRFs, ORF4/KCP, v-FLIP, and possibly v-IL-6, v-OX-2, and K1.

ORFs K3 and K5 (MIR1,2). The K3 and K5 proteins (also termed modulator of immune recognition (MIR) 1 and 2, respectively) are unique to KSHV and have been shown to be expressed as early and late lytic genes following reactivation in PEL cell lines, whereas K3 transcripts were not detected in KS lesions.[56,58,239]

The K3 and K5 proteins are involved in protecting virus-infected cells against natural killer (NK) cells or cytotoxic T lymphocytes.[240,241] These membrane proteins downregulate major histocompatibility (MHC) class I molecules. MIR1 targets HLA-A, -B, -C, and -E, whereas MIR2 does so primarily with HLA-A and -B.[240,242,243] The synthesis or transport of MHC class I molecules (at least until the medial-Golgi) is not affected, but a higher rate of endocytosis and degradation of MHC class I molecules has been observed.[242,244,245] The degradation is thought to occur by an ubiquitin/proteasome-dependent mechanism, as it has been reported that the expression of MIR1 and MIR2 leads to ubiquitination of the cytosolic tail of their target proteins and that ubiquitination is essential for their removal from the cell surface. MIR1 and MIR2 both contain an N-terminal zinc finger belonging to the plant homeodomain subfamily. This domain and the C-terminal region are responsible for MIR-mediated endocytosis, whereas the transmembrane region is required for target specificity.[246,247] In vitro, MIR2 has been shown to act as an E3 ubiquitin ligase.[246]

MHC class I down-regulation protects KSHV-infected cells from cytotoxic T-lymphocyte recognition. However, lack of MHC class I expression can render these cells susceptible to NK cell-mediated lysis. Interestingly, it has been shown that K5 also downregulates two ligands for NK cell-mediated cytotoxicity receptors; namely, ICAM-1 and B7-2. Thereby, K5 expression can inhibit NK cell-mediated cytotoxicity. The down-regulation of ICAM and B7-2 surface expression has been shown to be due to their enhanced endocytosis. This down-regulation will also affect the cellular immune response, as K5-transfected B cells are impaired in their ability to induce T cell activation.[241,248]

v-IRFs. As discussed above, the initial immune response against viral infection is regulated by IRFs through binding to ISREs in the promoters of interferon-responsive genes. The mechanism by which v-IRFs inhibit IFN signal transduction seems to involve direct binding to IRFs p300/CBP and other transcription factors impeding the formation of the transcriptional active complexes.[232,233,249–252] v-IRF-1 (ORF *K9*), v-IRF-2 (ORF *K11* spliced to a second upstream exon), and v-IRF-4 (ORF *K10* spliced to a second upstream exon) are expressed during the lytic life cycle of KSHV, whereas v-IRF-3 (ORF *K10.5* spliced to a second upstream exon) are expressed during latency.[253]

K9/v-IRF-1 is able to bind to the transcriptional coactivator CBP and inhibit its transcriptional activity.[251] It also interacts with the histone acetyl transferase p300, impeding its activity and modifying chromatin structure, and blocks IRF-3 recruitment of p300/CBP.[249,250,252] As a consequence, cellular cytokine expression is affected, and this could be a mechanism to evade certain aspects of the immune response.[250] More recent studies show that the low levels of v-IRF-1 that are expressed during latency are insufficient to block IFN-α–induced alterations in gene expression, whereas cells that expressed high levels of v-IRF-1 after induction of the lytic cycle were resistant to some changes induced by IFN-α. However, the transient expression of high levels of v-IRF-1 during lytic replication is insufficient to inhibit all of the antiviral effects of IFN-α.[254]

In a similar way as v-IRF-1, v-IRF-2 can also bind to IRFs and p300/CBP, and thereby inhibits virus-mediated induction of IFN type I gene transcription.[232] Another mechanism of action of v-IRF-2 involves the interaction with the IFN-induced double-stranded RNA-activated serine-threonine kinase (PKR), a main component of the host antiviral defense.[255,256] Such interaction blocks autophosphorylation of PKR and subsequent phosphorylation of PKR targets.[255]

K10.5/v-IRF-3, also called LANA-2, is a nuclear protein closely related to cellular IRF-4 and v-IRF-2. It directly interacts with cellular IRF-3 and IRF-7 through its C-terminal region. In transient transfection assays, v-IRF-3 functioned as a dominant-negative mutant of both IRF-3 and IRF-7 and inhibited virus-mediated transcriptional activity of the IFN-α promoter. Similarly, the overexpression of v-IRF-3 resulted in inhibition of virus-mediated synthesis of biologically active interferons. However, v-IRF-3 has also been shown to stimulate the IRF-3– and IRF-7–mediated activation of type I interferon (IFN-α and IFN-β) genes and the synthesis of biologically active type I interferons in infected B cells. Thus, v-IRF-3 has a corepressor activity, but it can also act as a transcriptional activator on genes controlled by cellular IRF-3 and IRF-7.[233,257]

Another mechanism of viral immune evasion is inhibition of cellular factors required for the expression of interferon gene expression. An example is the viral immediate-early protein ORF45, which blocks phosphorylation and nuclear translocation of cellular IRF-7 (which plays a key role in virus-induced IFN-α and IFN-β production).[258] IRF-7 and IRF-3 are also targeted by ORF50/RTA, which in addition to its role as a transcription factor in the activation of the lytic replication cycle (see "Control of the Lytic Replication Cycle," above), is an E3 ubiquitin ligase and specifically mediates the ubiquitination of IRF-7 and its destruction by the ubiquitin–proteasome system.[259]

v-MIPs. The three viral beta chemokines v-MIP-I through -III (see "Angiogenesis and B-Cell Proliferation," above) may also play a role in modulating the immune response. Other herpesviruses and poxviruses also encode homologues of chemokines (see Alcami A[198] and references cited therein).

v-MIP-II binds to several chemokine receptors either as an agonist or as an antagonist, including CC chemokine receptor (CCR) 1, CCR2, CCR5, CXCR4, and CXCR3, whereas v-MIP-I is more selective, binding exclusively to and acting as an agonist of CCR8.[194,260–262]

v-MIP-II reduced the infiltration of inflammatory leukocytes and suppressed the onset of the host inflammatory response in a rat model.[263] However, v-MIP-II has also been shown to act as a CCR3 agonist and drive a T helper (Th)2-type immune response.[194] The leukocyte infiltrate within KS lesions is composed mainly of mononuclear phagocytes and T cells, with the CD4[+] and CD8[+] cells having a marked type II cytokine profile.[264] This is probably due to the fact that both v-MIP-I and -II act as chemoattractants for monocytes and Th2 cells and not Th1, NK, or dendritic cells.[261,264,265] This may allow the virus to skew the immune response from a type I antiviral response pattern toward a type II pattern.[265]

v-MIP-III is an agonist for the cellular chemokine receptor CCR4, which is expressed by Th2-type T cells and has consistently been shown to preferentially chemoattract this cell type.[195]

ORF4/KCP. The product of ORF4, KSHV complement control protein (KCP), is expressed during the lytic replication cycle and specifically increases the decay of the classical C3-convertase.[58,266,267] It contains four complement control protein (CCP) domains. A cluster of positively charged amino acids in CCP1 stretching into CCP2 as well as positively and negatively charged areas at opposing faces of the border region between CCPs 2 and 3 are necessary to regulate the classical pathway. The regulation of the alternative pathway (via factor I–mediated C3b cleavage) was found to both overlap with classical pathway regulatory sites as well as to require unique, more C-terminal residues in CCPs 3 and 4.[268] It is conceivable that KCP could enhance virus pathogenesis through evasion of complement attack, opsonization, and anaphylaxis.[267]

ORF K2/v-IL-6. v-IL-6 has been implicated in the inhibition of IFN signaling. IFN-α directly activates a viral transcriptional program, leading to expression of the viral IL-6 gene, allowing the virus to modify its cellular environment by sensing and responding to levels of intracellular IFN signaling. Human IL-6 cannot mimic this effect because IFN-α downregulates the IL-6 receptor, gp80. Viral IL-6 bypasses the gp80 regulatory checkpoint by binding directly to the gp130 transducer molecule. v-IL-6 can thus protect PEL cells from the antiviral effects of IFN-α.[180]

ORF K14/v-OX-2. KSHV encodes a homologue of the immunoglobulin-related rat adhesion protein and immune regulator MRC OX-2, termed viral OX-2. Unlike its cellular counterpart, v-OX-2 stimulates production of proinflammatory cytokines, possibly leading to recruitment of lymphocytes to the site of infection and thereby to the enhanced dissemination of the virus.[269]

ORF K1/VIP. There is also some evidence for *K1* being involved in immune evasion as it was shown to inhibit transport of B-cell receptor complexes to the B-cell surface.[270]

SUMMARY AND OUTLOOK

Intensive research over the last 10 years has not only shown the strong epidemiologic link between KSHV and KS (see Chapter 5 "Clinical Features and Management of Kaposi's Sarcoma), but also identified many interesting cell biologic and biochemical properties of individual genes of this virus. These provide many possible explanations of how KSHV persists in infected individuals in the presence of the different effector mechanisms of the innate and adaptive immune system. As to the viral proteins responsible for its oncogenic properties, we are currently faced with a bewildering array of candidates. The lack of a suitable animal model limits our ability to study the contribution of candidate KSHV genes to oncogenicity in vivo in the context of the entire viral genome. Recently, reverse genetics has become available for KSHV and will enable us to begin to understand the contribution of individual viral proteins to KSHV-mediated effects that can be measured in tissue culture and that may represent surrogate markers of its oncogenic potential (eg, the induction of spindle cell formation in cultured primary endothelial cells).[271] KSHV has changed our thinking about how viruses can cause cancer. Specifically, whereas the classic concepts of viral oncogenesis involve a direct effect of one or several viral proteins, expressed during latent persistence on the infected cell (as in the case of HPV, EBV, HTLV-I), or an indirect effect as a result of uncontrolled regeneration (as for HBV and HCV), KSHV has put the spotlight on the possibility that indirect paracrine effects, occurring during lytic viral replication, might contribute to tumorigenicity. Mechanisms like these may inform our thinking when trying to understand the molecular basis for the increased cancer risk that is possibly associated with some other infectious agents.

REFERENCES

1. Chang Y, Cesarman E, Pessin MS, et al. Identification of herpesvirus-like DNA sequences in AIDS-associated Kaposi's sarcoma. Science 1994;266:1865–9.
2. Cesarman E, Chang Y, Moore PS, et al. Kaposi's sarcoma-associated herpesvirus-like DNA sequences in AIDS-related body-cavity-based lymphomas. N Engl J Med 1995;332:1186–91.
3. Soulier J, Grollet L, Oksenhendler E, et al. Kaposi's sarcoma-associated herpesvirus-like DNA sequences in multicentric Castleman's disease. Blood 1995;86:1276–80.
4. Luppi M, Barozzi P, Schulz TF, et al. Bone marrow failure associated with human herpesvirus 8 infection after transplantation. N Engl J Med 2000;343:1378–85.
5. Renne R, Zhong W, Herndier B, et al. Lytic growth of Kaposi's sarcoma-associated herpesvirus (human herpesvirus 8) in culture. Nat Med 1996;2:342–6.
6. Said W, Chien K, Takeuchi S, et al. Kaposi's sarcoma-associated herpesvirus (KSHV or HHV8) in primary effusion lymphoma: ultrastructural demonstration of herpesvirus in lymphoma cells. Blood 1996;87:4937–43.
7. Giraldo G, Beth E, Haguenau F. Herpes-type virus particles in tissue culture of Kaposi's sarcoma from different geographic regions. J Natl Cancer Inst 1972;49:1509–26.
8. Giraldo G, Beth E, Kourilsky FM, et al. Antibody patterns to herpesviruses in Kaposi's sarcoma: serological association of European Kaposi's sarcoma with cytomegalovirus. Int J Cancer 1975;15:839–48.
9. Renne R, Lagunoff M, Zhong W, Ganem D. The size and conformation of Kaposi's sarcoma-associated herpesvirus (human herpesvirus 8) DNA in infected cells and virions. J Virol 1996;70:8151–4.
10. Decker LL, Shankar P, Khan G, et al. The Kaposi sarcoma-associated herpesvirus (KSHV) is present as an intact latent genome in KS tissue but replicates in the peripheral blood mononuclear cells of KS patients. J Exp Med 1996;184:283–8.
11. Neipel F, Albrecht JC, Fleckenstein B. Cell-homologous genes in the Kaposi's sarcoma-associated rhadinovirus human herpesvirus 8: determinants of its pathogenicity? J Virol 1997;71:4187–92.
12. Russo JJ, Bohenzky RA, Chien MC, et al. Nucleotide sequence of the Kaposi sarcoma-associated herpesvirus (HHV-8). Proc Natl Acad Sci U S A 1996;93:14862–7.
13. Efstathiou S, Ho YM, Hall S, et al. Murine herpesvirus 68 is genetically related to the gammaherpesviruses Epstein-Barr virus and herpesvirus saimiri. J Gen Virol 1990;71(Pt 6):1365–72.
14. Telford EA, Studdenrt MJ, Agius CT, et al. Equine herpesviruses 2 and 5 are gamma-herpesviruses. Virology 1993;195:492–9.
15. Desrosiers RC, Sasseville VG, Czajak SC et al. A herpesvirus of rhesus monkeys related to the human Kaposi's sarcoma-associated herpesvirus. J Virol 1997;71:9764–9.
16. Lacoste V, Mauclere P, Dubreuil G, et al. Simian homologues of human gamma-2 and betaherpesviruses in mandrill and drill monkeys. J Virol 2000;74:11993–9.
17. Whitby D, Stossel A, Gamache C, et al. Novel Kaposi's sarcoma-associated herpesvirus homolog in baboons. J Virol 2003;77:8159–65.
18. Lacoste V, Mauclere P, Dubreuil G, et al. KSHV-like herpesviruses in chimps and gorillas. Nature 2000;407:151–2.
19. Lacoste V, Mauclere P, Dubreuil G, et al. A novel gamma 2-herpesvirus of the Rhadinovirus 2 lineage in chimpanzees. Genome Res 2001;11:1511–9.
20. Greensill J, Sheldon JA, Renwick NM, et al. Two distinct gamma2 herpesviruses in African green monkeys: a second gamma-2 herpesvirus lineage among old world primates? J Virol 2000;74:1572–7.
21. Greensill J, Sheldon JA, Murthy KK, et al. A chimpanzee rhadinovirus sequence related to Kaposi's sarcoma-associated herpesvirus/human herpesvirus 8: increased detection after HIV-1 infection in the absence of disease. AIDS 2000;14:F129–35.
22. Rose TM, Strand KB, Schultz ER, et al. Identification of two homologs of the Kaposi's sarcoma-associated herpesvirus (human herpesvirus 8) in retroperitoneal fibromatosis of different macaque species. J Virol 1997;71:4138–44.
23. Searles RP, Bergquam EP, Axthelm MK, Wong SW. Sequence and genomic analysis of a Rhesus macaque rhadinovirus with similarity to Kaposi's sarcoma-associated herpesvirus/human herpesvirus 8. J Virol 1999;73:3040–53.
24. Stebbing J, Wilder N, Ariad S, Abu-Shakra M. Lack of intra-

patient strain variability during infection with Kaposi's sarcoma-associated herpesvirus. Am J Hematol 2001;68: 133–4.

25. Zong J, Ciufo DM, Viscidi R, et al. Genotypic analysis at multiple loci across Kaposi's sarcoma herpesvirus (KSHV) DNA molecules: clustering patterns, novel variants and chimerism. J Clin Virol 2002;23:119–48.

26. Kasolo FC, Monze M, Obel N, et al. Sequence analyses of human herpesvirus-8 strains from both African human immunodeficiency virus-negative and -positive childhood endemic Kaposi's sarcoma show a close relationship with strains identified in febrile children and high variation in the K1 glycoprotein. J Gen Virol 1998;79(Pt 12):3055–65.

27. Cook PM, Whitby D, Calabro ML, et al. Variability and evolution of Kaposi's sarcoma-associated herpesvirus in Europe and Africa. International Collaborative Group. AIDS 1999;13:1165–76.

28. Lacoste V, Judde JG, Briere J, et al. Molecular epidemiology of human herpesvirus 8 in Africa: both B and A5 K1 genotypes, as well as the M and P genotypes of K14.1/K15 loci, are frequent and widespread. Virology 2000;278:60–74.

29. Kakoola DN, Sheldon J, Byabazzaire N, et al. Recombination in human herpesvirus-8 strains from Uganda and evolution of the K15 gene. J Gen Virol 2001;82:2393–404.

30. Meng YX, Sata T, Starney FR, et al. Molecular characterization of strains of human herpesvirus 8 from Japan, Argentina and Kuwait. J Gen Virol 2001;82:499–506.

31. Zong JC, Ciufo DM, Alcendor DJ, et al. High-level variability in the ORF-K1 membrane protein gene at the left end of the Kaposi's sarcoma-associated herpesvirus genome defines four major virus subtypes and multiple variants or clades in different human populations. J Virol 1999;73:4156–70.

32. Biggar RJ, Whitby D, Marshall V, et al. Human herpesvirus 8 in Brazilian Amerindians: a hyperendemic population with a new subtype. J Infect Dis 2000;181:1562–8.

33. Poole LJ, Zong JC, Ciufo DM, et al. Comparison of genetic variability at multiple loci across the genomes of the major subtypes of Kaposi's sarcoma-associated herpesvirus reveals evidence for recombination and for two distinct types of open reading frame K15 alleles at the right-hand end. J Virol 1999;73:6646–60.

34. Alagiozoglou L, Sitas F, Morris L. Phylogenetic analysis of human herpesvirus 8 in South Africa and identification of a novel subgroup. J Gen Virol 2000;81:2029–38.

35. Flore O, Raffi S, Bly S, et al. Transformation of primary human endothelial cells by Kaposi's sarcoma-associated herpesvirus. Nature 1998;394:588–92.

36. Cerimele F, Curreli F, Bly S, et al. Kaposi's sarcoma-associated herpesvirus can productively infect primary human keratinocytes and alter their growth properties. J Virol 2001;75:2435–43.

37. Dezube BJ, Zambela M, Sage DR, et al. Characterization of Kaposi sarcoma-associated herpesvirus/human herpesvirus-8 infection of human vascular endothelial cells: early events. Blood 2002;100:888–96.

38. Moses AV, Fish KN, Ruhl R, et al. Long-term infection and transformation of dermal microvascular endothelial cells by human herpesvirus 8. J Virol 1999;73:6892–902.

39. Ciufo DM, Cannon JS, Poole LJ, et al. Spindle cell conversion by Kaposi's sarcoma-associated herpesvirus: forma-tion of colonies and plaques with mixed lytic and latent gene expression in infected primary dermal microvascular endothelial cell cultures. J Virol 2001;75:5614–26.

40. Lagunoff M, Bechtel J, Venetsanalos E, et al. De novo infection and serial transmission of Kaposi's sarcoma-associated herpesvirus in cultured endothelial cells. J Virol 2002;76:2440–8.

41. Lebbe C, de Cremoux P, Millot G, et al. Characterization of in vitro culture of HIV-negative Kaposi's sarcoma-derived cells. In vitro responses to alfa interferon. Arch Dermatol Res 1997;289:421–8.

42. Grundhoff A, Ganem D. Inefficient establishment of KSHV latency suggests an additional role for continued lytic replication in Kaposi sarcoma pathogenesis. J Clin Invest 2004;113:124–36.

43. Akula SM, Pramod NP, Wang FZ, Chandran B. Human herpesvirus 8 envelope-associated glycoprotein B interacts with heparan sulfate-like moieties. Virology 2001;284: 235–49.

44. Akula SM, Wang FZ, Vieira J, Chandran B. Human herpesvirus 8 interaction with target cells involves heparan sulfate. Virology 2001;282:245–55.

45. Akula SM, Naranatt PP, Walia NS, et al. Kaposi's sarcoma-associated herpesvirus (human herpesvirus 8) infection of human fibroblast cells occurs through endocytosis. J Virol 2003;77:7978–90.

46. Akula SM, Pramod NP, Wang FZ, Chandran B. Integrin alpha3beta1 (CD 49c/29) is a cellular receptor for Kaposi's sarcoma-associated herpesvirus (KSHV/HHV-8) entry into the target cells. Cell 2002;108:407–19.

47. Birkmann A, Mahr K, Ensser A, et al. Cell surface heparan sulfate is a receptor for human herpesvirus 8 and interacts with envelope glycoprotein K8.1. J Virol 2001;75:11583–93.

48. Naranatt PP, Akula SM, Zien CA, et al. Kaposi's sarcoma-associated herpesvirus induces the phosphatidylinositol 3-kinase-PKC-zeta-MEK-ERK signaling pathway in target cells early during infection: implications for infectivity. J Virol 2003;77:1524–39.

49. Sharma-Walia N, Naranatt PP, Krishnan HH, et al. Kaposi's sarcoma-associated herpesvirus/human herpesvirus 8 envelope glycoprotein gB induces the integrin-dependent focal adhesion kinase-Src-phosphatidylinositol 3-kinase-rho GTPase signal pathways and cytoskeletal rearrangements. J Virol 2004;78:4207–23.

50. Naranatt PP, Krishnan HH, Smith MS, Chandran B. Kaposi's sarcoma-associated herpesvirus modulates microtubule dynamics via rhoA-GTP-diaphanous 2 signaling and utilizes the dynein motors To deliver Its DNA to the nucleus. J Virol 2005;79:1191–206.

51. Zhu FX, Yuan Y. The ORF45 protein of Kaposi's sarcoma-associated herpesvirus is associated with purified virions. J Virol 2003;77:4221–30.

52. Zhu FX, Chong JM, Wu L, Yuan Y. Virion proteins of Kaposi's sarcoma-associated herpesvirus. J Virol 2005;79:800–11.

53. Zhong W, Wang H, Herndier B, Ganem D. Restricted expression of Kaposi sarcoma-associated herpesvirus (human herpesvirus 8) genes in Kaposi sarcoma. Proc Natl Acad Sci U S A 1996;93:6641–6.

54. Garber AC, Shu MA, Hu J, Renne R. DNA binding and modulation of gene expression by the latency-associated

nuclear antigen of Kaposi's sarcoma-associated herpesvirus. J Virol 2001;75:7882–92.

55. Ballestas ME, Chatis PA, Kaye KM. Efficient persistence of extrachromosomal KSHV DNA mediated by latency-associated nuclear antigen. Science 1999;284:641–4.

56. Sun R, Lin SF, Staskus K, et al. Kinetics of Kaposi's sarcoma-associated herpesvirus gene expression. J Virol 1999; 73:2232–42.

57. Jenner RG, Maillard K, Cattini N, , et al. Kaposi's sarcoma-associated herpesvirus-infected primary effusion lymphoma has a plasma cell gene expression profile. Proc Natl Acad Sci U S A 2003;100:10399–404.

58. Jenner RG, Alba MM, Boshoff C, Kellam P. Kaposi's sarcoma-associated herpesvirus latent and lytic gene expression as revealed by DNA arrays. J Virol 2001;75:891–902.

59. Rivas C, Thlick AE, Parravicini C, et al. Kaposi's sarcoma-associated herpesvirus LANA2 is a B-cell-specific latent viral protein that inhibits *p53*. J Virol 2001;75:429–38.

60. Sun R, Lin SF, Gradoville L, et al. A viral gene that activates lytic cycle expression of Kaposi's sarcoma-associated herpesvirus. Proc Natl Acad Sci U S A 1998;95:10866–71.

61. Paulose-Murphy M, Ha NK, Xiang C, et al. Transcription program of human herpesvirus 8 (Kaposi's sarcoma-associated herpesvirus). J Virol 2001;75:4843–53.

62. Zhu FX, Cusano T, Yuan Y. Identification of the immediate-early transcripts of Kaposi's sarcoma-associated herpesvirus. J Virol 1999;73:5556–67.

63. Krishnan HH, Naranatt PP, Smith MS, et al. Concurrent expression of latent and a limited number of lytic genes with immune modulation and antiapoptotic function by Kaposi's sarcoma-associated herpesvirus early during infection of primary endothelial and fibroblast cells and subsequent decline of lytic gene expression. J Virol 2004;78:3601–20.

64. Moses AV, Jarvis MA, Raggo C, et al. Kaposi's sarcoma-associated herpesvirus-induced upregulation of the c-kit proto-oncogene, as identified by gene expression profiling, is essential for the transformation of endothelial cells. J Virol 2002;76:8383–99.

65. Poole LJ, Yu Y, Kim PS, et al. Altered patterns of cellular gene expression in dermal microvascular endothelial cells infected with Kaposi's sarcoma-associated herpesvirus. J Virol 2002;76:3395–420.

66. Glaunsinger B, Ganem D. Highly selective escape from KSHV-mediated host mRNA shutoff and its implications for viral pathogenesis. J Exp Med 2004;200:391–8.

67. Polson AG, Wang D, DeRisi J, Ganem D. Modulation of host gene expression by the constitutively active G protein-coupled receptor of Kaposi's sarcoma-associated herpesvirus. Cancer Res 2002;62:4525–30.

68. Rainbow L, Platt GM, Simpson GR, et al. The 222- to 234-kilodalton latent nuclear protein (LNA) of Kaposi's sarcoma-associated herpesvirus (human herpesvirus 8) is encoded by orf73 and is a component of the latency-associated nuclear antigen. J Virol 1997;71:5915–21.

69. Dupin N, Fisher C, Kellam P, et al. Distribution of human herpesvirus-8 latently infected cells in Kaposi's sarcoma, multicentric Castleman's disease, and primary effusion lymphoma. Proc Natl Acad Sci USA 1999;96:4546–51.

70. Katano H, Sato Y, Kurata T, et al. Expression and localization of human herpesvirus 8-encoded proteins in primary effu-

sion lymphoma, Kaposi's sarcoma, and multicentric Castleman's disease. Virology 2000;269:335–44.

71. Parravicini C, Chandran B, Corbellino M, et al. Differential viral protein expression in Kaposi's sarcoma-associated herpesvirus-infected diseases: Kaposi's sarcoma, primary effusion lymphoma, and multicentric Castleman's disease. Am J Pathol 2000;156:743–9.

72. Sturzl M, Hohenadl C, Zietz C, et al. Expression of K13/v-FLIP gene of human herpesvirus 8 and apoptosis in Kaposi's sarcoma spindle cells. J Natl Cancer Inst 1999; 91:1725–33.

73. Judde JG, Lacoste V, Briere J, et al. Monoclonality or oligoclonality of human herpesvirus 8 terminal repeat sequences in Kaposi's sarcoma and other diseases. J Natl Cancer Inst 2000;92:729–36.

74. Chiou CJ, Poole LJ, Kim PS, et al. Patterns of gene expression and a transactivation function exhibited by the vGCR (ORF74) chemokine receptor protein of Kaposi's sarcoma-associated herpesvirus. J Virol 2002;76:3421–39.

75. Komatsu T, Ballestas ME, Barbera AJ, et al. KSHV LANA1 binds DNA as an oligomer and residues N-terminal to the oligomerization domain are essential for DNA binding, replication, and episome persistence. Virology 2004;319:225–36.

76. Hu J, Garber AC, Renne R. The latency-associated nuclear antigen of Kaposi's sarcoma-associated herpesvirus supports latent DNA replication in dividing cells. J Virol 2002;76:11677–87.

77. Barbera AJ, Ballestas ME, Kaye KM. The Kaposi's sarcoma-associated herpesvirus latency-associated nuclear antigen 1 N terminus is essential for chromosome association, DNA replication, and episome persistence. J Virol 2004; 78:294–301.

78. Talbot SJ, Weiss RA, Kellam P, Boshoff C. Transcriptional analysis of human herpesvirus-8 open reading frames 71, 72, 73, K14, and 74 in a primary effusion lymphoma cell line. Virology 1999;257:84–94.

79. Jeong JH, Orvis J, Kim JW, et al. Regulation and autoregulation of the promoter for the latency-associated nuclear antigen of Kaposi's sarcoma-associated herpesvirus. J Biol Chem 2004;279:16822–31.

80. Piolot T, Tramier M, Coppey M, et al. Close but distinct regions of human herpesvirus 8 latency-associated nuclear antigen 1 are responsible for nuclear targeting and binding to human mitotic chromosomes. J Virol 2001;75:3948–59.

81. Flamand L, Zeman RA, Bryant JL, et al. Absence of human herpesvirus 8 DNA sequences in neoplastic Kaposi's sarcoma cell lines. J Acquir Immune Defic Syndr Hum Retrovirol 1996;13:194–7.

82. Platt GM, Simpson GR, Mittnacht S, Schulz TF. Latent nuclear antigen of Kaposi's sarcoma-associated herpesvirus interacts with RING3, a homolog of the Drosophila female sterile homeotic (fsh) gene. J Virol 1999;73:9789–95.

83. Lim C, Sohn H, Lee D, et al. Functional dissection of latency-associated nuclear antigen 1 of Kaposi's sarcoma-associated herpesvirus involved in latent DNA replication and transcription of terminal repeats of the viral genome. J Virol 2002;76:10320–31.

84. Stedman W, Deng Z, Lu F, Lieberman PM. ORC, MCM, and histone hyperacetylation at the Kaposi's sarcoma-

associated herpesvirus latent replication origin. J Virol 2004;78:12566–75.

85. Renne R, Barry C, Dittmer D, et al. Modulation of cellular and viral gene expression by the latency-associated nuclear antigen of Kaposi's sarcoma-associated herpesvirus. J Virol 2001;75:458–68.

86. Viejo-Borbolla A, Kati E, Sheldon JA, et al. A domain in the C-terminal region of latency-associated nuclear antigen 1 of Kaposi's sarcoma-associated herpesvirus affects transcriptional activation and binding to nuclear heterochromatin. J Virol 2003;77:7093–100.

87. An J, Sun Y, Sun R, Rettig MB. Kaposi's sarcoma-associated herpesvirus encoded vFLIP induces cellular IL-6 expression: the role of the NF-kappaB and JNK/AP1 pathways. Oncogene 2003;22:3371–85.

88. Radkov SA, Kellam P, Boshoff C. The latent nuclear antigen of Kaposi sarcoma-associated herpesvirus targets the retinoblastoma-E2F pathway and with the oncogene Hras transforms primary rat cells. Nat Med 2000;6:1121–7.

89. Schulz TF, Chang Y. KSHV gene expression. In: Arvin A, Mocarski ES, Moore P, Roizman B, editors. The Human Herpesviruses Cambridge Press; 2005. [In press]

90. Deng H, Young A, Sun R. Auto-activation of the rta gene of human herpesvirus 8/Kaposi's sarcoma-associated herpesvirus. J Gen Virol 2000;81:3043–8.

91. Sakakibara S, Ueda K, Chen J, et al. Octamer-binding sequence is a key element for the autoregulation of Kaposi's sarcoma-associated herpesvirus ORF50/Lyta gene expression. J Virol 2001;75:6894–900.

92. Wang SE, WU FY, Fujimuro M, et al. Role of CCAAT/enhancer-binding protein alpha (C/EBPalpha) in activation of the Kaposi's sarcoma-associated herpesvirus (KSHV) lytic-cycle replication-associated protein (RAP) promoter in cooperation with the KSHV replication and transcription activator (RTA) and RAP. J Virol 2003;77:600–23.

93. Chen J, Ueda K, Skakibara S, et al. Activation of latent Kaposi's sarcoma-associated herpesvirus by demethylation of the promoter of the lytic transactivator. Proc Natl Acad Sci U S A 2001;98:4119–24.

94. Chang PJ, Shedd D, Gradoville L, et al. Open reading frame 50 protein of Kaposi's sarcoma-associated herpesvirus directly activates the viral PAN and K12 genes by binding to related response elements. J Virol 2002;76:3168–78.

95. Deng H, Chu JT, Rettig MB, et al. Rta of the human herpesvirus 8/Kaposi sarcoma-associated herpesvirus upregulates human interleukin-6 gene expression. Blood 2002;100:1919–21.

96. Song MJ, Li X, Brown HJ, Sun R. Characterization of interactions between RTA and the promoter of polyadenylated nuclear RNA in Kaposi's sarcoma-associated herpesvirus/human herpesvirus 8. J Virol 2002;76:5000–13.

97. Liang Y, Chang J, Lynch SJ, et al. The lytic switch protein of KSHV activates gene expression via functional interaction with RBP-Jkappa (CSL), the target of the Notch signaling pathway. Genes Dev 2002;16:1977–89.

98. Liang Y, Ganem D. Lytic but not latent infection by Kaposi's sarcoma-associated herpesvirus requires host CSL protein, the mediator of Notch signaling. Proc Natl Acad Sci U S A 2003;100:8490–5.

99. Ziegler JL. Endemic Kaposi's sarcoma in Africa and local volcanic soils. Lancet 1993;342:1348–51.

100. Davis DA, Rinderknecht AS, Zoeteweij JP, et al. Hypoxia induces lytic replication of Kaposi sarcoma-associated herpesvirus. Blood 2001;97:3244–50.

101. Haque M, Davis DA, Wang V, et al. Kaposi's sarcoma-associated herpesvirus (human herpesvirus 8) contains hypoxia response elements: relevance to lytic induction by hypoxia. J Virol 2003;77:6761–8.

102. Zoeteweij JP, Moses AV, Rinderknecht AS, et al. Targeted inhibition of calcineurin signaling blocks calcium-dependent reactivation of Kaposi sarcoma-associated herpesvirus. Blood 2001;97:2374–80.

103. Ensoli B, Sgadari C, Barillari C, et al. Biology of Kaposi's sarcoma. Eur J Cancer 2001;37:1251–69.

104. Monini P, Carlini F, Sturzl M, et al. Alpha interferon inhibits human herpesvirus 8 (HHV-8) reactivation in primary effusion lymphoma cells and reduces HHV-8 load in cultured peripheral blood mononuclear cells. J Virol 1999;73:4029–41.

105. Mercader M, Taddeo B, Panella JR, et al. Induction of HHV-8 lytic cycle replication by inflammatory cytokines produced by HIV-1-infected T cells. Am J Pathol 2000;156:1961–71.

106. Lee H, Guo J, Li M, et al. Identification of an immunoreceptor tyrosine-based activation motif of K1 transforming protein of Kaposi's sarcoma-associated herpesvirus. Mol Cell Biol 1998;18:5219–28.

107. Lagunoff M, Majeti R, Weiss A, Ganem D. Deregulated signal transduction by the K1 gene product of Kaposi's sarcoma-associated herpesvirus. Proc Natl Acad Sci U S A 1999;96:5704–9.

108. Lee H, Veazey R, Williams K, et al. Deregulation of cell growth by the K1 gene of Kaposi's sarcoma-associated herpesvirus. Nat Med 1998;4:435–40.

109. Prakash O, Tang ZY, Peng X, et al. Tumorigenesis and aberrant signaling in transgenic mice expressing the human herpesvirus-8 K1 gene. J Natl Cancer Inst 2002;94:926–35.

110. Lee BS, Connole M, Tang Z, et al. Structural analysis of the Kaposi's sarcoma-associated herpesvirus K1 protein. J Virol 2003;77:8072–86.

111. Wang L, Wakisaka N, Tomlinson CC, et al. The Kaposi's sarcoma-associated herpesvirus (KSHV/HHV-8) K1 protein induces expression of angiogenic and invasion factors. Cancer Res 2004;64:2774–81.

112. Gao SJ, Boshoff C, Jayachandra S, et al. KSHV ORF K9 (vIRF) is an oncogene which inhibits the interferon signaling pathway. Oncogene 1997;15:1979–85.

113. Jayachandra S, Low KG, Thlick AE, et al. Three unrelated viral transforming proteins (vIRF, EBNA2, and E1A) induce the MYC oncogene through the interferon-responsive PRF element by using different transcription coadaptors. Proc Natl Acad Sci USA 1999;96:11566–71.

114. Arvanitakis L, Geras-Raaka E, Varma A, et al. Human herpesvirus KSHV encodes a constitutively active G-protein-coupled receptor linked to cell proliferation. Nature 1997;385:347–50.

115. Bais C, Santomasso B, Coso O, et al. G-protein-coupled receptor of Kaposi's sarcoma-associated herpesvirus is a viral oncogene and angiogenesis activator. Nature 1998;391:86–9.

116. Cesarman E, Mesri EA, Gershengorn MC. Viral G protein-coupled receptor and Kaposi's sarcoma: a model of paracrine neoplasia? J Exp Med 2000;191:417–22.

117. Yang TY, Chen SC, Leach MW, et al. Transgenic expression of the chemokine receptor encoded by human herpesvirus 8 induces an angioproliferative disease resembling Kaposi's sarcoma. J Exp Med 2000;191:445–54.

118. Montaner S, Sodhi A, Molinolo A, et al. Endothelial infection with KSHV genes in vivo reveals that vGPCR initiates Kaposi's sarcomagenesis and can promote the tumorigenic potential of viral latent genes. Cancer Cell 2003;3:23–36.

119. Bais C, et al. Kaposi's sarcoma associated herpesvirus G protein-coupled receptor immortalizes human endothelial cells by activation of the VEGF receptor-2/ KDR. Cancer Cell 2003;3:131–43.

120. Burger M, Hartmann T, Burger JA, Schraufstatter I. KSHV-GPCR and CXCR2 transforming capacity and angiogenic responses are mediated through a JAK2-STAT3-dependent pathway. Oncogene 2005;24:2067–75.

121. Sadler R, Wu L, Forghani B, et al. A complex translational program generates multiple novel proteins from the latently expressed kaposin (K12) locus of Kaposi's sarcoma-associated herpesvirus. J Virol 1999;73:5722–30.

122. Muralidhar S, Purnfey AM, Hassani M, et al. Identification of kaposin (open reading frame K12) as a human herpesvirus 8 (Kaposi's sarcoma-associated herpesvirus) transforming gene. J Virol 1998;72:4980–8.

123. Kliche S, Nagel W, Kremmer E, et al. Signaling by human herpesvirus 8 kaposin A through direct membrane recruitment of cytohesin-1. Mol Cell 2001;7:833–43.

124. Tomkowicz B, Singh SP, Cartas M, Srinivasan A. Human herpesvirus-8 encoded kaposin: subcellular localization using immunofluorescence and biochemical approaches. DNA Cell Biol 2002;21:151–62.

125. Muralidhar S, Veytsmann G, Chandran B, et al. Characterization of the human herpesvirus 8 (Kaposi's sarcoma-associated herpesvirus) oncogene, kaposin (ORF K12). J Clin Virol 2000;16:203–13.

126. Li H, Komatsu T, Dezube BJ, Kaye KM. The Kaposi's sarcoma-associated herpesvirus K12 transcript from a primary effusion lymphoma contains complex repeat elements, is spliced, and initiates from a novel promoter. J Virol 2002;76:11880–8.

127. McCormick C, Ganem D. The kaposin B protein of KSHV activates the p38/MK2 pathway and stabilizes cytokine mRNAs. Science 2005;307:739–41.

128. Krithivas A, Young DB, Liao G, et al. Human herpesvirus 8 LANA interacts with proteins of the mSin3 corepressor complex and negatively regulates Epstein-Barr virus gene expression in dually infected PEL cells. J Virol 2000; 74:9637–45.

129. Friborg J Jr, Kong W, Hottiger MO, Nabel GJ. p53 inhibition by the LANA protein of KSHV protects against cell death. Nature 1999;402:889–94.

130. Watanabe T, Sugaya M, Atkins AM, et al. Kaposi's sarcoma-associated herpesvirus latency-associated nuclear antigen prolongs the life span of primary human umbilical vein endothelial cells. J Virol 2003;77:6188–96.

131. Knight JS, Cotter MA, Robertson ES. The latency-associated nuclear antigen of Kaposi's sarcoma-associated herpesvirus transactivates the telomerase reverse transcriptase promoter. J Biol Chem 2001;276:22971–8.

132. Verma SC, Borah S, Robertson ES. Latency-associated nuclear antigen of Kaposi's sarcoma-associated herpesvirus up-regulates transcription of human telomerase reverse transcriptase promoter through interaction with transcription factor Sp1. J Virol 2004;78:10348–59.

133. Sun Q, Zachariah S, Chaudhary PM. The human herpes virus 8-encoded viral FLICE-inhibitory protein induces cellular transformation via NF-kappaB activation. J Biol Chem 2003;278:52437–45.

134. Djerbi M, Screpanti V, Catrina AI, et al. The inhibitor of death receptor signaling, FLICE-inhibitory protein defines a new class of tumor progression factors. J Exp Med 1999;190:1025–32.

135. Verschuren EW, Jones N, Evan GI. The cell cycle and how it is steered by Kaposi's sarcoma-associated herpesvirus cyclin. J Gen Virol 2004;85:1347–61.

136. Chang Y, Moore PS, Talbot SJ, et al. Cyclin encoded by KS herpesvirus. Nature 1996;382:410.

137. Godden-Kent D, Talbot SJ, Boshoff C, et al. The cyclin encoded by Kaposi's sarcoma-associated herpesvirus stimulates cdk6 to phosphorylate the retinoblastoma protein and histone H1. J Virol 1997;71:4193–8.

138. Li M, Lee H, Yoon DW, et al. Kaposi's sarcoma-associated herpesvirus encodes a functional cyclin. J Virol 1997; 71:1984–91.

139. Swanton C, Mann DJ, Fleckenstein B, et al. Herpes viral cyclin/Cdk6 complexes evade inhibition by CDK inhibitor proteins. Nature 1997;390:184–7.

140. Ellis M, Chew YP, Fallis L, et al. Degradation of p27(Kip) cdk inhibitor triggered by Kaposi's sarcoma virus cyclin-cdk6 complex. EMBO J 1999;18:644–53.

141. Helt AM, Galloway DA. Mechanisms by which DNA tumor virus oncoproteins target the Rb family of pocket proteins. Carcinogenesis 2003;24:159–69.

142. Platt G, Carbone A, Mittnacht S. p16INK4a loss and sensitivity in KSHV associated primary effusion lymphoma. Oncogene 2002;21:1823–31.

143. Lundquist A, Barre B, Bienvenu F, et al. Kaposi sarcoma-associated viral cyclin K overrides cell growth inhibition mediated by oncostatin M through STAT3 inhibition. Blood 2003;101:4070–7.

144. Duro D, Schulze A, Vogt B, et al. Activation of cyclin A gene expression by the cyclin encoded by human herpesvirus-8. J Gen Virol 1999;80(Pt 3):549–55.

145. Mann DJ, Child ES, Swanton C, et al. Modulation of p27(Kip1) levels by the cyclin encoded by Kaposi's sarcoma-associated herpesvirus. EMBO J 1999;18:654–63.

146. Ojala PM, Tiainen M, Salven P, et al. Kaposi's sarcoma-associated herpesvirus-encoded v-cyclin triggers apoptosis in cells with high levels of cyclin-dependent kinase 6. Cancer Res 1999;59:4984–9.

147. Ojala PM, Yamamoto K, Castanos-Velez E, et al. The apoptotic v-cyclin-CDK6 complex phosphorylates and inactivates Bcl-2. Nat Cell Biol 2000;2:819–25.

148. Child ES, Mann DJ. Novel properties of the cyclin encoded by human herpesvirus 8 that facilitate exit from quiescence. Oncogene 2001;20:3311–22.

149. Kaldis P, Ojala PM, Tong L, et al. CAK-independent activation of CDK6 by a viral cyclin. Mol Biol Cell 2001;12:3987–99.

150. Verschuren EW, Klefstrom J, Evan GI, Jones N. The oncogenic potential of Kaposi's sarcoma-associated herpesvirus cyclin is exposed by *p53* loss in vitro and in vivo. Cancer Cell 2002;2:229–41.

151. Stewart ZA, Pietenpol JA. *p53* signaling and cell cycle checkpoints. Chem Res Toxicol 2001;14:243–63.

152. Verschuren EW, Hodgson JG, Gray JW, et al. The role of *p53* in suppression of KSHV cyclin-induced lymphomagenesis. Cancer Res 2004;64:581–9.

153. Wu FY, Wang SE, Tang QQ, et al. Cell cycle arrest by Kaposi's sarcoma-associated herpesvirus replication-associated protein is mediated at both the transcriptional and posttranslational levels by binding to CCAAT/enhancer-binding protein alpha and p21(CIP-1). J Virol 2003;77:8893–914.

154. Wu FY, Tang QQ, Chen H, et al. Lytic replication-associated protein (RAP) encoded by Kaposi sarcoma-associated herpesvirus causes p21CIP-1-mediated G1 cell cycle arrest through CCAAT/enhancer-binding protein-alpha. Proc Natl Acad Sci U S A 2002;99:10683–8.

155. Wang XP, Gao SJ. Auto-activation of the transforming viral interferon regulatory factor encoded by Kaposi's sarcoma-associated herpesvirus (human herpesvirus-8). J Gen Virol 2003;84:329–36.

156. Izumiya Y, Lin SF, Ellison TJ, et al. Cell cycle regulation by Kaposi's sarcoma-associated herpesvirus K-bZIP: direct interaction with cyclin-CDK2 and induction of G1 growth arrest. J Virol 2003;77:9652–61.

157. Fujimuro M, Hayward SD. The latency-associated nuclear antigen of Kaposi's sarcoma-associated herpesvirus manipulates the activity of glycogen synthase kinase-3beta. J Virol 2003;77:8019–30.

158. Fujimuro M, Wu FY, ApRhys C, et al. A novel viral mechanism for dysregulation of beta-catenin in Kaposi's sarcoma-associated herpesvirus latency. Nat Med 2003;9:300–6.

159. An FQ, Compitello N, Horwitz E, et al. The latency-associated nuclear antigen of Kaposi's sarcoma-associated herpesvirus modulates cellular gene expression and protects lymphoid cells from P16INK4A-induced cell cycle arrest. J Biol Chem 2004.,280:3862-74

160. Hayward GS. Initiation of angiogenic Kaposi's sarcoma lesions. Cancer Cell 2003;3:1–3.

161. Cornali E, Zietz C, Benelli R, et al. Vascular endothelial growth factor regulates angiogenesis and vascular permeability in Kaposi's sarcoma. Am J Pathol 1996;149:1851–69.

162. Aoki Y, Jaffe ES, Change Y, et al. Angiogenesis and hematopoiesis induced by Kaposi's sarcoma-associated herpesvirus-encoded interleukin-6. Blood 1999;93:4034–43.

163. Aoki Y, Tosato G. Role of vascular endothelial growth factor/vascular permeability factor in the pathogenesis of Kaposi's sarcoma-associated herpesvirus-infected primary effusion lymphomas. Blood 1999;94:4247–54.

164. Means RE, Choi JK, Nakamura H, et al. Immune evasion strategies of Kaposi's sarcoma-associated herpesvirus. Curr Top Microbiol Immunol 2002;269:187–201.

165. Molden J, Chang Y, You Y, et al. A Kaposi's sarcoma-associated herpesvirus-encoded cytokine homolog (vIL-6) activates signaling through the shared gp130 receptor subunit. J Biol Chem 1997;272:19625–31.

166. Osborne J, Moore PS, Chang Y. KSHV-encoded viral IL-6 activates multiple human IL-6 signaling pathways. Hum Immunol 1999;60:921–7.

167. Hideshima T, Chauhan D, Teoh G, et al. Characterization of signaling cascades triggered by human interleukin-6 versus Kaposi's sarcoma-associated herpes virus-encoded viral interleukin 6. Clin Cancer Res 2000;6:1180–9.

168. Klouche M, Brockmeyer N, Knabbe C, Rose-John S. Human herpesvirus 8-derived viral IL-6 induces PTX3 expression in Kaposi's sarcoma cells. AIDS 2002;16:F9–18.

169. Taga T. The signal transducer gp130 is shared by interleukin-6 family of haematopoietic and neurotrophic cytokines. Ann Med 1997;29:63–72.

170. Dela Cruz CS, Lee Y, Viswanathan SR, et al. N-linked glycosylation is required for optimal function of Kaposi's sarcoma herpesvirus-encoded, but not cellular, interleukin 6. J Exp Med 2004;199:503–14.

171. An J, Lichtenstein AK, Brent G, Rettig MB. The Kaposi sarcoma-associated herpesvirus (KSHV) induces cellular interleukin 6 expression: role of the KSHV latency-associated nuclear antigen and the AP1 response element. Blood 2002;99:649–54.

172. An J, Sun Y, Rettig MB. Transcriptional coactivation of c-Jun by the KSHV-encoded LANA. Blood 2004;103:222–8.

173. Hoischen SH, Vollmer P, Marz P, et al. Human herpes virus 8 interleukin-6 homologue triggers gp130 on neuronal and hematopoietic cells. Eur J Biochem 2000;267:3604–12.

174. Schulz TF. KSHV/HHV8-associated lymphoproliferations in the AIDS setting. Eur J Cancer 2001;37:1217–26.

175. Moore PS, Boshoff C, Weiss RA, Chang Y. Molecular mimicry of human cytokine and cytokine response pathway genes by KSHV. Science 1996;274:1739–44.

176. Foussat A, Wijdenes J, Bouchet L, et al. Human interleukin-6 is in vivo an autocrine growth factor for human herpesvirus-8-infected malignant B lymphocytes. Eur Cytokine Netw 1999;10:501–8.

177. Mori Y, Nishimoto N, Ohno M, et al. Human herpesvirus 8-encoded interleukin-6 homologue (viral IL-6) induces endogenous human IL-6 secretion. J Med Virol 2000;61:332–5.

178. Liu C, Okruzhnov Y, Li H, Nicholas J. Human herpesvirus 8 (HHV-8)-encoded cytokines induce expression of and autocrine signaling by vascular endothelial growth factor (VEGF) in HHV-8-infected primary-effusion lymphoma cell lines and mediate VEGF-independent antiapoptotic effects. J Virol 2001;75:10933–40.

179. Aoki Y, Tosato G, Nambu Y, et al. Detection of vascular endothelial growth factor in AIDS-related primary effusion lymphomas. Blood 2000;95:1109–10.

180. Chatterjee M, Osborne J, Bestetti G, et al. Viral IL-6-induced cell proliferation and immune evasion of interferon activity. Science 2002;298:1432–5.

181. Gazouli M, Zavos G, Papaconstantinou I, et al. The interleukin-6-174 promoter polymorphism is associated with a risk of development of Kaposi's sarcoma in renal transplant recipients. Anticancer Res 2004;24:1311–4.

182. Cesarman E, Nador RG, Bai F, et al. Kaposi's sarcoma-associated herpesvirus contains G protein-coupled recep-

tor and cyclin D homologs which are expressed in Kaposi's sarcoma and malignant lymphoma. J Virol 1996; 70:8218–23.

183. Burger M, Burger JA, Hoch RC, et al. Point mutation causing constitutive signaling of CXCR2 leads to transforming activity similar to Kaposi's sarcoma herpesvirus-G protein-coupled receptor. J Immunol 1999; 163:2017–22.

184. Munshi N, Ganju RK, Avraham S, et al. Kaposi's sarcoma-associated herpesvirus-encoded G protein-coupled receptor activation of c-jun amino-terminal kinase/stress-activated protein kinase and lyn kinase is mediated by related adhesion focal tyrosine kinase/proline-rich tyrosine kinase 2. J Biol Chem 1999;274:31863–7.

185. Couty JP, Geras-Raaka E, Weksler BB, Gershengorn MC. Kaposi's sarcoma-associated herpesvirus G protein-coupled receptor signals through multiple pathways in endothelial cells. J Biol Chem 2001;276:33805–11.

186. Montaner S, Sodhi A, Pece S, et al. The Kaposi's sarcoma-associated herpesvirus G protein-coupled receptor promotes endothelial cell survival through the activation of Akt/protein kinase B. Cancer Res 2001;61:2641–8.

187. Pati S, Cavrois M, Guo HG, et al. Activation of NF-kappaB by the human herpesvirus 8 chemokine receptor ORF74: evidence for a paracrine model of Kaposi's sarcoma pathogenesis. J Virol 2001;75:8660–73.

188. Schwarz M, Murphy PM. Kaposi's sarcoma-associated herpesvirus G protein-coupled receptor constitutively activates NF-kappa B and induces proinflammatory cytokine and chemokine production via a C-terminal signaling determinant. J Immunol 2001;167:505–13.

189. Smit MJ, Verzijl D, Casarosa P, et al. Kaposi's sarcoma-associated herpesvirus-encoded G protein-coupled receptor ORF74 constitutively activates p44/p42 MAPK and Akt via G(i) and phospholipase C-dependent signaling pathways. J Virol 2002;76:1744–52.

190. Pati S, Foulke JS, Jr., Barabitskaya O, et al. Human herpesvirus 8-encoded vGPCR activates nuclear factor of activated T cells and collaborates with human immunodeficiency virus type 1 Tat. J Virol 2003;77:5759–73.

191. Cannon ML, Cesarman E. The KSHV G protein-coupled receptor signals via multiple pathways to induce transcription factor activation in primary effusion lymphoma cells. Oncogene 2004;23:514–23.

192. Montaner S, Sodhi A, Servitja JM, et al. The small GTPase Rac1 links the Kaposi sarcoma-associated herpesvirus vGPCR to cytokine secretion and paracrine neoplasia. Blood 2004;104:2903–11.

193. Cannon M, Philpott NJ, Cesarman E. The Kaposi's sarcoma-associated herpesvirus G protein-coupled receptor has broad signaling effects in primary effusion lymphoma cells. J Virol 2003;77:57–67.

194. Boshoff C, Endo Y, Collins PD, et al. Angiogenic and HIV-inhibitory functions of KSHV-encoded chemokines. Science 1997;278:290–4.

195. Stine JT, Wood C, Hill M, et al. KSHV-encoded CC chemokine vMIP-III is a CCR4 agonist, stimulates angiogenesis, and selectively chemoattracts TH2 cells. Blood 2000;95:1151–7.

196. MacDonald MR, Li XY, Virgin HW. Late expression of a beta chemokine homolog by murine cytomegalovirus. J Virol 1997;71:1671–8.

197. Penfold ME, Dairaghi DJ, Duke GM, et al. Cytomegalovirus encodes a potent alpha chemokine. Proc Natl Acad Sci U S A 1999;96:9839–44.

198. Alcami A. Viral mimicry of cytokines, chemokines and their receptors. Nat Rev Immunol 2003;3:36–50.

199. Glenn M, Rainbow L, Aurade F, et al. Identification of a spliced gene from Kaposi's sarcoma-associated herpesvirus encoding a protein with similarities to latent membrane proteins 1 and 2A of Epstein-Barr virus. J Virol 1999;73:6953–63.

200. Choi JK, Lee BS, Shim SN, et al. Identification of the novel K15 gene at the rightmost end of the Kaposi's sarcoma-associated herpesvirus genome. J Virol 2000;74:436–46.

201. Brinkmann MM, et al. Activation of mitogen-activated protein kinase and NF-kappaB pathways by a Kaposi's sarcoma-associated herpesvirus K15 membrane protein. J Virol 2003;77:9346–58.

202. Sharp TV, Wang H, Koumi A, et al. K15 protein of Kaposi's sarcoma-associated herpesvirus is latently expressed and binds to HAX-1, a protein with antiapoptotic function. J Virol 2002;76:802–16.

203. LaCasse EC, Baird S, Korneluk RG, MacKenzie AE. The inhibitors of apoptosis (IAPs) and their emerging role in cancer. Oncogene 1998;17:3247–59.

204. Teodoro JG, Branton PE. Regulation of p53-dependent apoptosis, transcriptional repression, and cell transformation by phosphorylation of the 55-kilodalton E1B protein of human adenovirus type 5. J Virol 1997;71:3620–7.

205. Thornberry NA, Lazebnik Y. Caspases: enemies within. Science 1998;281:1312–6.

206. Ashkenazi A, Dixit VM. Death receptors: signaling and modulation. Science 1998;281:1305–8.

207. Bertin J, Armstrong RC, Ottilie S, et al. Death effector domain-containing herpesvirus and poxvirus proteins inhibit both Fas- and TNFR1-induced apoptosis. Proc Natl Acad Sci U S A 1997;94:1172–6.

208. Thome M, Schneider P, Hofmann K, et al. Viral FLICE-inhibitory proteins (FLIPs) prevent apoptosis induced by death receptors. Nature 1997;386:517–21.

209. Belanger C, Gravel A, Tomoui A, et al. Human herpesvirus 8 viral FLICE-inhibitory protein inhibits Fas-mediated apoptosis through binding and prevention of procaspase-8 maturation. J Hum Virol 2001;4:62–73.

210. Liu L, Eby MT, Rathore N, et al. The human herpes virus 8-encoded viral FLICE inhibitory protein physically associates with and persistently activates the Ikappa B kinase complex. J Biol Chem 2002;277:13745–51.

211. Sun Q, Matta H, Chaudhary PM. The human herpes virus 8-encoded viral FLICE inhibitory protein protects against growth factor withdrawal-induced apoptosis via NF-kappa B activation. Blood 2003;101:1956–61.

212. Wang HW, Sharp TV, Koumi A, et al. Characterization of an anti-apoptotic glycoprotein encoded by Kaposi's sarcoma-associated herpesvirus which resembles a spliced variant of human survivin. EMBO J 2002;21:2602–15.

213. Wang Z, Fukuda S, Pelus LM. Survivin regulates the p53 tumor suppressor gene family. Oncogene 2004;23:8146–53.

214. Dohi T, Beltrami E, Wall NR, et al. Mitochondrial survivin

inhibits apoptosis and promotes tumorigenesis. J Clin Invest 2004;114:1117–27.

215. Dohi T, Okada K, Xia F, et al. An IAP-IAP complex inhibits apoptosis. J Biol Chem 2004;279:34087–90.

216. Feng P, Park J, Lee BS, et al. Kaposi's sarcoma-associated herpesvirus mitochondrial K7 protein targets a cellular calcium-modulating cyclophilin ligand to modulate intracellular calcium concentration and inhibit apoptosis. J Virol 2002;76:11491–504.

217. Cory S, Adams JM. The Bcl2 family: regulators of the cellular life-or-death switch. Nat Rev Cancer 2002;2:647–56.

218. Cheng EH, Nicholas J, Bellows DS, et al. A Bcl-2 homolog encoded by Kaposi sarcoma-associated virus, human herpesvirus 8, inhibits apoptosis but does not heterodimerize with Bax or Bak. Proc Natl Acad Sci U S A 1997;94:690–4.

219. Widmer I, Wernli M, Bachmann F, et al. Differential expression of viral Bcl-2 encoded by Kaposi's sarcoma-associated herpesvirus and human Bcl-2 in primary effusion lymphoma cells and Kaposi's sarcoma lesions. J Virol 2002;76:2551–6.

220. Sarid R, Sato T, Bohenzky RA, et al. Kaposi's sarcoma-associated herpesvirus encodes a functional bcl-2 homologue. Nat Med 1997;3:293–8.

221. Bellows DS, Chau BN, Lee P, et al. Antiapoptotic herpesvirus Bcl-2 homologs escape caspase-mediated conversion to proapoptotic proteins. J Virol 2000;74:5024–31.

222. Hardwick JM, Bellows DS. Viral versus cellular BCL-2 proteins. Cell Death Differ 2003;10 Suppl 1:S68–76.

223. Huang Q, Petros AM, Virgin HW, et al. Solution structure of a Bcl-2 homolog from Kaposi sarcoma virus. Proc Natl Acad Sci U S A 2002;99:3428–33.

224. Inohara N, Gourley TS, Carrio R, et al. Diva, a Bcl-2 homologue that binds directly to Apaf-1 and induces BH3-independent cell death. J Biol Chem 1998;273:32479–86.

225. Stark GR, Kerr IM, Williams BR, et al. How cells respond to interferons. Annu Rev Biochem 1998;67:227–64.

226. Moore PS, Chang Y. Kaposi's sarcoma-associated herpesvirus-encoded oncogenes and oncogenesis. J Natl Cancer Inst Monogr 1998;65–71.

227. Kirchhoff S, Sebens T, Baumann S, et al. Viral IFN-regulatory factors inhibit activation-induced cell death via two positive regulatory IFN-regulatory factor 1-dependent domains in the CD95 ligand promoter. J Immunol 2002;168:1226–34.

228. Zimring JC, Goodbourn S, Offermann MK. Human herpesvirus 8 encodes an interferon regulatory factor (IRF) homolog that represses IRF-1-mediated transcription. J Virol 1998;72:701–7.

229. Nakamura H, Li M, Zarycki J, Jung JU. Inhibition of *p53* tumor suppressor by viral interferon regulatory factor. J Virol 2001;75:7572–82.

230. Seo T, Park J, Lee D, et al. Viral interferon regulatory factor 1 of Kaposi's sarcoma-associated herpesvirus binds to *p53* and represses *p53*-dependent transcription and apoptosis. J Virol 2001;75:6193–8.

231. Seo T, Shim YS, Angell JE, et al. Viral interferon regulatory factor 1 of Kaposi's sarcoma-associated herpesvirus interacts with a cell death regulator, GRIM19, and inhibits interferon/retinoic acid-induced cell death. J Virol 2002;76:8797–807.

232. Burysek L, Yeow WS, Pitha PM. Unique properties of a second human herpesvirus 8-encoded interferon regulatory factor (vIRF-2). J Hum Virol 1999;2:19–32.

233. Lubyova B, Pitha PM. Characterization of a novel human herpesvirus 8-encoded protein, vIRF-3, that shows homology to viral and cellular interferon regulatory factors. J Virol 2000;74:8194–201.

234. Esteban M, Garcia MA, Domingo-Gil E, et al. The latency protein LANA2 from Kaposi's sarcoma-associated herpesvirus inhibits apoptosis induced by dsRNA-activated protein kinase but not RNase L activation. J Gen Virol 2003;84:1463–70.

235. Nicholas J. Human herpesvirus-8-encoded signalling ligands and receptors. J Biomed Sci 2003;10:475–89.

236. Tomlinson CC, Damania B. The K1 protein of Kaposi's sarcoma-associated herpesvirus activates the Akt signaling pathway. J Virol 2004;78:1918–27.

237. Gwack Y, Hwang S, Lee D, et al. Kaposi's sarcoma-associated herpesvirus open reading frame 50 represses *p53*-induced transcriptional activity and apoptosis. J Virol 2001;75:6245–8.

238. Park J, Seo T, Hwang S, et al. The K-bZIP protein from Kaposi's sarcoma-associated herpesvirus interacts with *p53* and represses its transcriptional activity. J Virol 2000; 74:11977–82.

239. Rimessi P, Bonaccorsi A, Sturzl M, et al. Transcription pattern of human herpesvirus 8 open reading frame K3 in primary effusion lymphoma and Kaposi's sarcoma. J Virol 2001; 75:7161–74.

240. Coscoy L, Ganem D. Kaposi's sarcoma-associated herpesvirus encodes two proteins that block cell surface display of MHC class I chains by enhancing their endocytosis. Proc Natl Acad Sci U S A 2000;97:8051–6.

241. Ishido S, Choi JK, Lee BS, et al. Inhibition of natural killer cell-mediated cytotoxicity by Kaposi's sarcoma-associated herpesvirus K5 protein. Immunity 2000;13:365–74.

242. Haque M, Ueda K, Nakano K, et al. Major histocompatibility complex class I molecules are down-regulated at the cell surface by the K5 protein encoded by Kaposi's sarcoma-associated herpesvirus/human herpesvirus-8. J Gen Virol 2001;82:1175–80.

243. Ishido S, Wang C, Lee BS, et al. Downregulation of major histocompatibility complex class I molecules by Kaposi's sarcoma-associated herpesvirus K3 and K5 proteins. J Virol 2000;74:5300–9.

244. Lorenzo ME, Jung JU, Ploegh HL. Kaposi's sarcoma-associated herpesvirus K3 utilizes the ubiquitin-proteasome system in routing class major histocompatibility complexes to late endocytic compartments. J Virol 2002; 76:5522–31.

245. Means RE, Ishido S, Alvarez X, Jung JU. Multiple endocytic trafficking pathways of MHC class I molecules induced by a herpesvirus protein. EMBO J 2002;21:1638–49.

246. Coscoy L, Sanchez DJ, Ganem D. A novel class of herpesvirus-encoded membrane-bound E3 ubiquitin ligases regulates endocytosis of proteins involved in immune recognition. J Cell Biol 2001;155:1265–73.

247. Sanchez DJ, Coscoy L, Ganem D. Functional organization of MIR2, a novel viral regulator of selective endocytosis. J Biol Chem 2002;277:6124–30.

248. Coscoy L, Ganem D. A viral protein that selectively down-regulates ICAM-1 and B7-2 and modulates T cell costimulation. J Clin Invest 2001;107:1599–606.

249. Burysek L, Yeow WS, Lubyova B, et al. Functional analysis of human herpesvirus 8-encoded viral interferon regulatory factor 1 and its association with cellular interferon regulatory factors and p300. J Virol 1999;73:7334–42.

250. Li M, Dmania B, Alvarez X, et al. Inhibition of p300 histone acetyltransferase by viral interferon regulatory factor. Mol Cell Biol 2000;20:8254–63.

251. Seo T, Lee D, Lee B, et al. Viral interferon regulatory factor 1 of Kaposi's sarcoma-associated herpesvirus (human herpesvirus 8) binds to, and inhibits transactivation of, CREB-binding protein. Biochem Biophys Res Commun 2000;270:23–7.

252. Lin R, Genin P, Mamane Y, et al. HHV-8 encoded vIRF-1 represses the interferon antiviral response by blocking IRF-3 recruitment of the CBP/p300 coactivators. Oncogene 2001;20:800–11.

253. Dourmishev LA, Dourmishev AL, Palmeri D, et al. Molecular genetics of Kaposi's sarcoma-associated herpesvirus (human herpesvirus 8) epidemiology and pathogenesis. Microbiol Mol Biol Rev 2003;67:175–212, table.

254. Pozharskaya VP, Weakland LL, Zimring JC, et al. Short duration of elevated vIRF-1 expression during lytic replication of human herpesvirus 8 limits its ability to block antiviral responses induced by alpha interferon in BCBL-1 cells. J Virol 2004;78:6621–35.

255. Burysek L, Pitha PM. Latently expressed human herpesvirus 8-encoded interferon regulatory factor 2 inhibits double-stranded RNA-activated protein kinase. J Virol 2001;75:2345–52.

256. Levy DE, Garcia-Sastre A. The virus battles: IFN induction of the antiviral state and mechanisms of viral evasion. Cytokine Growth Factor Rev 2001;12:143–56.

257. Lubyova B, Kellum MJ, Frisancho AJ, Pitha PM. Kaposi's sarcoma-associated herpesvirus-encoded vIRF-3 stimulates the transcriptional activity of cellular IRF-3 and IRF-7. J Biol Chem 2004;279:7643–54.

258. Zhu FX, King SM, Smith EJ, et al. A Kaposi's sarcoma-associated herpesviral protein inhibits virus-mediated induction of type I interferon by blocking IRF-7 phosphorylation and nuclear accumulation. Proc Natl Acad Sci U S A 2002;99:5573–8.

259. Yu Y, Wang SE, Hayward GS. The KSHV immediate-early transcription factor RTA encodes ubiquitin E3 ligase activity that targets IRF7 for proteosome-mediated degradation. Immunity 2005;22:59–70.

260. Kledal TN, Rosenkilde MM, Coulin F, et al. A broad-spectrum chemokine antagonist encoded by Kaposi's sarcoma-associated herpesvirus. Science 1997;277:1656–9.

261. Dairaghi DJ, Fan RA, McMaster BE, et al. HHV8-encoded vMIP-I selectively engages chemokine receptor CCR8. Agonist and antagonist profiles of viral chemokines. J Biol Chem 1999;274:21569–74.

262. Endres MJ, Garlisi CG, Xiao H, et al. The Kaposi's sarcoma-related herpesvirus (KSHV)-encoded chemokine vMIP-I is a specific agonist for the CC chemokine receptor (CCR)8. J Exp Med 1999;189:1993–8.

263. Chen S, Bacon KB, Li L, et al. In vivo inhibition of CC and CX3C chemokine-induced leukocyte infiltration and attenuation of glomerulonephritis in Wistar-Kyoto (WKY) rats by vMIP-II. J Exp Med 1998;188:193–8.

264. Sozzani S, Luini W, Bianchi G, et al. The viral chemokine macrophage inflammatory protein-II is a selective Th2 chemoattractant. Blood 1998;92:4036–9.

265. Weber KS, Grone HJ, Rocken M, et al. Selective recruitment of Th2-type cells and evasion from a cytotoxic immune response mediated by viral macrophage inhibitory protein-II. Eur J Immunol 2001;31:2458–66.

266. Sarid R, Flore O, Bohenzky RA, et al. Transcription mapping of the Kaposi's sarcoma-associated herpesvirus (human herpesvirus 8) genome in a body cavity-based lymphoma cell line (BC-1). J Virol 1998;72:1005–12.

267. Spiller OB, Blackbourn DJ, Mark L, et al. Functional activity of the complement regulator encoded by Kaposi's sarcoma-associated herpesvirus. J Biol Chem 2003;278:9283–9.

268. Mark L, Lee WH, Spiller OB, et al. The Kaposi's sarcoma-associated herpesvirus complement control protein mimics human molecular mechanisms for inhibition of the complement system. J Biol Chem 2004;279:45093–101.

269. Chung YH, Means RE, Choi JK, et al. Kaposi's sarcoma-associated herpesvirus OX2 glycoprotein activates myeloid-lineage cells to induce inflammatory cytokine production. J Virol 2002;76:4688–98.

270. Lee BS, Alvarez X, Ishido S, et al. Inhibition of intracellular transport of B cell antigen receptor complexes by Kaposi's sarcoma-associated herpesvirus K1. J Exp Med 2000;192:11–21.

271. Zhou FC, Zhang YJ, Deng JH, et al. Efficient infection by a recombinant Kaposi's sarcoma-associated herpesvirus cloned in a bacterial artificial chromosome: application for genetic analysis. J Virol 2002;76:6185–96.

4

Epidemiology of Kaposi's Sarcoma–Associated Herpesvirus Infection

JEFFREY N. MARTIN

In 1872, Moritz Kaposi, a Hungarian dermatologist, described six patients with multifocal brown-red or blue-red nodules or plaques on the feet and hands.[1] Initially called "idiopathisches multiples pigmentsarcoma der haut" (multiple idiopathic sarcoma of the skin) by Kaposi, the condition later became known as Kaposi's sarcoma (KS). Decades later, after the epidemiology of KS began to be investigated, its uneven geographic distribution suggested that exogenous factors were etiologically important. Subsequently, as the acquired immune deficiency syndrome (AIDS) epidemic unfolded in the early 1980s, homosexual men were found to be up to 20 times more likely than other risk groups to develop KS, a markedly disproportionate risk that led to the hypothesis that the exogenous factor was a sexually transmitted infectious agent.[2] Numerous microbial candidates were proposed, but for none was convincing evidence demonstrated until Kaposi's sarcoma–associated herpesvirus (KSHV), or human herpesvirus 8 (HHV-8), was discovered in 1994.[3] In a short period following the discovery of KSHV, consensus rapidly developed that it is a necessary, albeit not sufficient, causal agent of KS.[4–8] This discovery was more than academic, in that because of the AIDS epidemic, KS is now worldwide the fourth most common cancer caused by an infectious agent, following gastric, cervical, and hepatic cancers. Now that the clinical importance of KSHV has been established, attention has turned toward the unraveling of what is proving to be a complicated epidemiologic profile for the virus.

DIAGNOSIS OF KSHV INFECTION

While nucleic acid amplification techniques were originally used to identify the presence of KSHV DNA in KS tissue, when applied to peripheral blood, these techniques are much less sensitive as compared with detection of KSHV-specific antibodies. For this reason, there is currently little role for nucleic acid–based testing of peripheral blood in the diagnosis of KSHV infection.[9] Instead, the primary means of KSHV diagnosis is antibody testing, and what follows is an overview of serologic testing that provides the requisite perspective for which to interpret epidemiologic studies of the distribution and transmission of KSHV.

Initial Serologic Assays for KSHV Antibodies

After the finding that DNA from primary effusion lymphoma (PEL) biopsy specimens contained KSHV sequences, the original assays for KSHV antibodies were developed using cell lines obtained from patients with PEL.[10–14] One of the first platforms were indirect immunofluorescence assays (IFAs) that used the cell lines in an uninduced state, where KSHV is primarily in its latent phase. These assays detect antibodies to KSHV latency-associated nuclear antigen (LANA or LANA-1), the product of open reading frame (ORF) 73.[15,16] Extensive evaluation of these assays determined that anti-LANA seropositivity is found in approximately 80% of persons with KS and < 5% of female homosexual adults in the United States or Northern Europe (ie, specificity of at least 95%).[12–14] Subsequently, it was determined that induction, using phorbol ester, of KSHV into a lytic phase resulted in IFAs with greater, albeit not complete, sensitivity (approximately 95%) in terms of identifying KS patients, while maintaining seropositivity of < 10% in nonhomosexual adults in the United States.[17] In an attempt to improve throughput and eliminate the subjective interpretation inherent in IFAs, a variety of other first-generation assays with comparable performance characteristics were developed. These include enzyme immunoassays (EIA) detecting antibodies against (1) bacterially derived recombinant portions of a minor capsid protein (ORF65), LANA, and glycoprotein K8.1[7,14,18,19]; (2) synthetic peptides of *K8.1* and ORF65[9,20]; and (3) whole virus.[21,22]

Methodologic Challenges in Serologic Assay Development

Although first-generation antibody assays, particularly those detecting anti-LANA antibodies, have been useful in epidemiologic work, no single first-generation serologic assay has demonstrated extremely high sensitivity and specificity, and agreement between assays has been suboptimal. In a study of seven first-generation antibody assays examining 143 serum specimens, the percentage of KSHV-seropositive specimens determined by the different assays ranged from 0 to 54% for the subset of specimens from blood donors, 27 to 60% for HIV-infected persons without KS, and 49 to 93% for KS patients.[23] More recently, a comparison of KSHV antibody testing from six laboratories, using newly developed assays or second generations of previously examined assays, found improved agreement when testing serum specimens from persons with KS (all six laboratories found all 21 specimens to be positive) but only modest agreement when evaluating 1,000 specimens from blood donors (a low-risk group for KSHV infection).[24] In part, this interassay disagreement may be because certain assays target different antibodies for which inherent sensitivity and specificity for KSHV infection may differ (eg, antibodies against lytic-phase versus latent-phase antigens). In other instances, however, assay calibration (ie, differentiating positive from negative results) has not been done in a standardized fashion across assays with reference to a wide spectrum of "gold standard" KSHV-infected (true positive) and KSHV-uninfected (true negative) subjects. Determining assay sensitivity by limiting the true-positive reference group to persons with KS, as has been typically done in the initially described assays, may result in estimates of sensitivity that are unrealistically inflated. This is because it is now recognized that among KSHV-infected persons, antibody titer is highest and therefore easier to detect in KS patients.[13] One attempt to reduce this "spectrum bias" was by Engels and colleagues, who used diluted serum from KS patients in an attempt to mimic KSHV-infected persons without KS and found rapidly diminishing sensitivity with only minimal dilution.[19,25] However, the amount of dilution needed to mimic infected but nondiseased persons is not known. Another attempt was the use of homosexual men without KS but who had detectable KSHV in their saliva.[26] These persons, however, may be enriched for antibody positivity if the presence of KSHV antigen drives antibody production. Therefore, more work is needed in identifying gold standard KSHV-infected reference subjects without KS for the evaluation of assay sensitivity.

Whereas early serologic investigators at a minimum had the presence of KS as a basis for forming a true-positive reference group, assembling a true-negative (KSHV-uninfected) reference group has been particularly vexing because of the lack of any analogous gold standard certifying absence of infection. For example, the use of blood donors is problematic, because they may include men with undisclosed homosexual activity, the primary risk factor for KSHV infection in developed countries (described below).[14,20,23,27] Approaches used in more recent work to optimize the assembly of a true-negative reference group have capitalized on what is now known about the epidemiology of KSHV infection and of KS per se. In the United States, for example, this includes the use of virginal women and of young children who are just past the age of harboring maternal antibodies[22]; HIV-infected hemophiliacs and their female sexual partners, both of whom were known not to subsequently develop KS after a substantial period of observation[19]; and homosexual women.[26]

Seroreversion

Further complicating the interpretation of serologic testing is the phenomenon of a negative result following a positive result, termed seroreversion, noted in longitudinal observation of individual subjects. For example, Quinlivan and colleagues found that 27 of 33 (82%) subjects, who had at least one time point been seropositive for antibodies to LANA, had at least one subsequent time point exhibiting seroreversion.[28] This has also been reported by others.[29] Whether seroreversion is the result of assay measurement error (ie, inadequate reproducibility) or whether it reflects true biologic diminution or loss of antibody is not known. In any case, its presence clouds the interpretation of a single seronegative serologic test result in a cross-sectional study.

Use of Currently Available Serologic Assays

For epidemiologic work where between-group comparisons are the primary focus, even using first-generation serologic assays, despite their poor interlaboratory agreement, has resulted in reproducible and plausible inferences (described below). Use of currently available serologic assays for individual-level diagnosis, however, be it in an epidemiologic study in the determination of seroconversion among individual subjects, or in the clinical setting, requires greater caution. The lack of gold standards in the development of assays, the apparent lack of concurrent high-level sensitivity and specificity among those first-generation assays that have been evaluated most extensively, and the phenomenon of seroreversion make definitive diagnosis of the presence or absence of KSHV infection problematic at an individual level. The only exception is persons who test positive on a very specific assay, such as the anti-LANA IFA (at least as performed in experienced laboratories). Currently, there is no Food and Drug Administration–licensed assay for KSHV antibodies; testing is limited to research laboratories.

EPIDEMIOLOGY OF KSHV INFECTION

Prevalence of Infection

Geographic Distribution

Extensive worldwide surveys of KSHV seroprevalence using the same serologic assay and same method of sampling of subjects (eg, similar age groups) have not been performed. Even with this limitation, three major patterns of seroprevalence have reproducibly emerged: high-level endemic, intermediate-level endemic, and non-endemic. High-level endemic areas are defined by those with seroprevalences of between 30 and 70% among general adult populations, and are found throughout Africa and many parts of the Middle East (eg, Egypt).[30–33] As is discussed below, it is the catastrophic intersection between the KSHV endemic and the human immunodeficiency virus (HIV) epidemic in sub-Saharan Africa that has resulted in KS becoming the most common adult malignancy in many areas there.[34,35] Intermediate-level endemic areas feature KSHV seroprevalences of between 10 and 25% in the general population and are found primarily in the Mediterranean area.[36–38] Non-endemic areas are those with seroprevalences < 10% in the general population. These include North America, Central America, South America, Northern Europe, and Asia. In these non-endemic areas, however, certain population groups have seroprevalences that rival those in high and intermediate-level prevalence regions. In particular, it is homosexual men across these non-endemic areas that have consistently been shown to have the highest seroprevalence; between 30 to 60% of HIV-infected homosexual men in these areas and 20 to 30% of HIV-uninfected homosexual men are KSHV-infected.[6,8,12,17,39,40] This contrasts with < 10% prevalence in most reports of women and nonhomosexual men in the general population of these areas.[6,12,41,42]

Temporal Patterns

Studies of genomic strain variability have concluded that KSHV is an ancient human virus, introduced at least tens of thousands of years ago (see "Genotypic

Diversity of Infection," below).[43] Descriptions of KS in the 1800s and the finding of high KSHV sero-prevalences in geographically distinct and remote isolated populations substantiate this.[1,44–46] There is, however, debate as to its introduction in sentinel populations such as homosexual men in the United States and Northern Europe. Two initial reports hypothesized that an epidemic of KSHV infection in homosexual men took place concurrently with that of HIV infection.[8,39] This hypothesis was based upon the finding of an initial high incidence of KSHV infection in these studies at the beginning of their observation in 1981 and 1982, respectively. How-ever, a more direct examination of homosexual men in San Francisco as early as 1978, prior to the HIV epidemic, found that seroprevalence was already 24.9%.[47] An endemic state of KSHV infection in homosexual men has also been suggested in Den-mark in the 1970s, both in a study directly measur-ing KSHV seroprevalence and in a study of KS that found that never-married men (a crude surrogate for homosexual men) were significantly at risk.[48,49] Therefore, the introduction of KSHV infection appears to have substantially preceded that of HIV.

There is little information on the patterns of KSHV infection in different populations over time. In Africa, among samples collected between 1972 and 1978 in Uganda and Tanzania, the seropreva-lence of KSHV infection was similar to that found in the 1980s and 1990s, suggesting that there has been little influence from the emerging HIV epidemic.[50] In homosexual men in developed countries, there had been speculation, based upon the report of either decreased incidence of AIDS-associated KS or a decline in KS as a proportion of new AIDS cases, that the prevalence of KSHV infection had fallen in the late 1980s and early 1990s.[51–53] However, a decline in the overall KS incidence rate could have been caused by reduced HIV transmission alone, resulting in fewer immunocompromised persons available to develop KS. Similarly, a decline in KS as a proportion of new AIDS cases could be caused by a decline in the proportion of new cases occur-ring in homosexual men, since KS is uncommon in risk groups other than homosexual men. Direct examination of KSHV seroprevalence in homo-sexual men in San Francisco (including both HIV-infected and uninfected men) found a stable prevalence between 26 to 29% in the periods span-ning 1978 to 1980, 1984 to 1985, and 1995 to 1996.[47] Similarly, KSHV seroprevalence was stable at approximately 60% in the period spanning 1985 to 1995 among homosexual men in Italy who had recently acquired HIV infection.[54]

Genotypic Diversity of Infection

The entire KSHV genome was sequenced shortly after its detection, and considerable work thereafter has documented extensive genotypic heterogeneity across populations.[55,56] Initial work examining geno-typic diversity focused on segments of ORF26 and ORF75, and although there was not extensive over-all variation (only 1.5% of nucleotide positions), there was enough clustering to form three distinct but narrow subtypes in the initial 12 specimens examined.[57] Subsequently, ORF $K1$, $K12$, 73, $K14.1$, and $K15$ have also been examined in many more specimens, resulting in the finding of significantly more genotypic heterogeneity and a much more complicated interpretation. Of these regions, the far left hand (ORF $K1$) and right hand (ORF $K15$) sides of the genome are most interesting. ORF $K1$ is the most heterogeneous, with up to 44% of amino acid differences across strains, allowing for the formation of at least 5 major subtypes and at least 24 sub-groups, many of which indicate intertype recombi-nation.[44,58–62] This degree of diversity has been seen with relatively few isolates examined thus far (< 250); as more are sequenced, it is apparent that even more distinct subtypes will be identified.[46] ORF $K15$ features two highly diverged alleles, termed P (for predominant) and M (for minor), cor-responding to their prevalence in isolates examined to date, which have only 33% amino acid homology to one another.[63] The two alleles are so disparate that it has been suggested the minor form was introduced via a recombination event with a related but as yet undocumented primate virus.[63]

Nomenclature schemes for the genotypic diver-sity are still in evolution and not yet standardized between authors. Based on ORF $K1$ typing alone, at least three approaches have been proposed. Zong and colleagues proposed naming subtypes A through D, with numerical subgroups within subtypes (eg, A1 through A5).[59] Cook and colleagues proposed subtypes A through C, with two forms of subgroups, one denoted with numbers (eg, A3 and A5) and another with superscripts (eg, A').[60] Finally, Meng and colleagues proposed genotypes I through IV with subtypes (eg, I-A to I-F).[61] To each of these schemes, a fifth major subtype (termed subtype E) was subsequently described among remote, isolated South American populations.[44,46] Overall genotypic classification is even more complicated because there is not complete linkage in strain diversity across the genome. For example, diversity in ORF *K15*, although limited to the P versus M nomenclature, is largely independent of ORF *K1* genotype.[62,64] When the internal coding regions (eg, ORF26, *K12*, 73, 75) are also considered, there becomes the need to describe at least three or four segments to fully describe a strain (eg, as C3/A/A2/M).[62]

Despite the complexity in nomenclature, there do appear to be emerging patterns in the geographic distribution of the different subtypes. Following the classification scheme proposed by Zong and colleagues for ORF K1, it has been observed that B subtypes are found almost exclusively in sub-Saharan Africa, D subtypes in South Asia/Australia/Pacific, and A and C subtypes in the United States/Europe/North Asia (with a notable exception being the presence of A5 subtypes in Africa).[59,62] This has led to the speculation that KSHV was present in the origins of modern humans in Africa (B subtype), and that the separation into the three main branches (A/C, B, and D) is explained by isolation and founder effects associated with the original migrations of humans out of Africa, first to the Middle East, and then South Asia (D subtype), and later to Europe, North Asia, and the Americas (A and C subtypes).[43,62] Notable examples of this geographic association are seen in immigrants whose KSHV sequences match those of their countries of origin rather than their adopted residence.[62] The story is not entirely consistent, however, because of the unexpected finding of subtype E in isolated South American populations.[44,46] Whereas it would have been expected that novel subtypes in South America would be most closely related to subtypes A and C (or even B), subtype E is most closely related to subtype D.

Aside from tracing the spread of KSHV over time and across human populations, the other implications of the substantial genotypic diversity are not well understood. First, although it is likely that the considerable heterogeneity in ORF *K1* is providing clues regarding a powerful biologic selection process, whether this involves immune evasion or some other mechanism is not known. Second, it is not known whether genotype plays a role in the ease of transmissibility and acquisition of KSHV. For example, it has not been established whether the localization of the B subtype in Africa can explain the high KSHV seroprevalence there compared with other regions. If genotype is important in viral transmission, then a high transmissibility is likely not limited to subtype B, as E subtypes in remote South American populations are also associated with very high community seroprevalences.[44,46] Third, there has thus far been no convincing evidence for the importance of genotype in either the development of KSHV-related disease per se, the type of KSHV-related disease manifestation (KS versus PEL versus multicentric Castleman's diseases), or clinical severity once disease occurs. Of these potential questions, data are most abundant, but not yet definitive, on the issue of association with the type of disease where work to date finds no correlation.[62,65] One report found an association between single nucleotide polymorphisms (SNPs) at nucleotide positions 1032 and 1055 of ORF26, but this was among many SNPs evaluated and requires confirmation.[66]

Routes of Transmission

Current knowledge about KSHV transmission can be summarized as follows: there is definitive evidence that it is transmitted by some form of intimate contact between homosexual men; equally persuasive evidence that it is transmitted in childhood by a horizontal nonsexual route in high-level endemic areas; and strong evidence that it is transmitted by infected organs in transplantation, by sharing of equipment among injection drug users, and by transfusion of whole unprocessed blood in high-level endemic areas. What is not known are the specific sexual behaviors that transmit among homosexual men, the exact means of horizontal spread to children in endemic areas, whether KSHV is transmitted vertically, and whether transmission occurs via transfusion of blood products that have undergone modern processing techniques.

Transmission in Non-endemic Areas

Sexual transmission. Initial seroepidemiologic studies postulated that KSHV was sexually transmitted by showing that other than in KS patients, seroprevalence was highest in homosexual men and other groups at highest risk for sexually transmitted disease (STD). Reports of this type, however, describing an association between risk of STD and KSHV seroprevalence, provide only indirect evidence for sexual transmission. More definitive evidence is found in studies with direct measurement of sexual activity. For example, among a population-based sample of homosexual men in San Francisco, KSHV seroprevalence increased linearly with the number of male intercourse partners in the previous 2 years (Figure 4–1).[6] The strength of this association, confirmed by other researchers, leaves little doubt that some form of intimate contact transmits the virus among homosexual men.[8,39,67–71] However, because "sexual partner" is defined broadly in most of these reports to include a variety of practices (eg, insertive and receptive penile-anal intercourse, penile-oral intercourse, and oral-anal contact), these data alone do not pinpoint the specific route of sexual transmission.

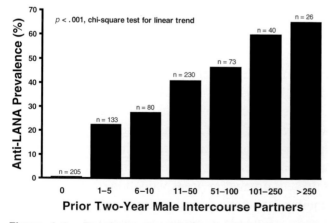

Figure 4–1. Prevalence of antibodies to Kaposi's sarcoma–associated herpesvirus latency-associated nuclear antigen (LANA) by number of prior 2-year male intercourse partners among men in San Francisco. The number atop each column signifies the number of subjects in each group. Reproduced with permission from Martin JN et al.[6]

Even prior to the discovery of KSHV, many studies had sought to identify the specific route of transmission for the putative KS agent. Some, but not all, found that insertive oral-anal sexual practices ("rimming") were a risk factor for KS and, by extension, were a risk factor for the as-yet-undiscovered KS agent.[72–78] The discovery of KSHV was hoped to bring clarity to this question, but initial studies among homosexual men have been conflicting, variously reporting the strongest association for penile-anal intercourse, penile-oral intercourse, oral-anal contact, or kissing. To date, at least eight studies have evaluated specific practices (Table 4–1).[8,39,67–71,79] For almost all of the acts, at least one study has reported an association. However, for no act have all (or nearly all) studies found an association. Receptive penile-anal intercourse, the act that has attracted the most support, is paradoxically one in which the *apparent* culprit body fluid, semen, is now known to rarely harbor KSHV.[68,80,81]

Recognition that saliva is the body fluid that most commonly harbors KSHV has naturally focused attention on transmission by kissing.[68] However, because kissing is common in all population groups, the low prevalence of KSHV in the general population argues against kissing as a dominant route of spread. Indeed, other herpesviruses transmitted by kissing (eg, Epstein-Barr Virus) are highly prevalent in the general population. One scenario where kissing could be the major route of spread but still not result in high prevalence in the general population is if KSHV was recently introduced into homosexual men and has not yet spread to others. Data from San Francisco, however, show that KSHV was not recently introduced into homosexual men. Seroprevalence among homosexual men in San Francisco in 1978 to 1980 was estimated to be 28.4% compared with 26.4% in 1995 to 1996, arguing against kissing as the dominant route of spread.[47]

The most recent US Public Health Service guidelines for the prevention of KSHV infection reflect the uncertainty in the literature about its transmission.[82] They state that the major routes of KSHV transmission appear to be "oral, (via) semen, and through blood via needle sharing" and that patients should be counseled that "kissing and sexual intercourse with persons who have high risk of

Table 4 1. STUDIES EVALUATING SPECIFIC SEXUAL PRACTICES AS ROUTES OF KAPOSI'S SARCOMA–ASSOCIATED HERPESVIRUS TRANSMISSION IN HOMOSEXUAL MEN

Study	Design	Penile-Anal Intercourse		Penile-Oral Intercourse		Oral-Anal Contact		Kissing
		Ins.*	Rec.*	Ins.	Rec.	Ins.	Rec.	
Melbye et al, 1998[39]	Cohort	NE‡	+†	NE	–†	–	–	–
O'Brien et al, 1999[8]	Cohort	+	+	–	–	+	–	NE
Grulich et al, 1999[79]	Cross-sectional	–	–	–	–	–	–	NE
Dukers et al, 2000[67]	Cohort	–	–	+	+	–	–	NE
Jacobson et al, 2000[69]	Cohort	NE	+	–	–	NE	NE	NE
Pauk et al, 2000[68]	Cross-sectional	NE	NE	NE	NE	NE	NE	+
Diamond et al, 2001[70]	Cross-sectional	–	+	NE	NE	NE	NE	NE
Casper et al, 2002[71]	Cross-sect/cohort	–	–	NE	NE	–	–	NE

*"Ins." denotes insertive practice of the act; "Rec." denotes receptive practice of the act,
†"+" indicates an association was found; "–" indicates no association was found.
‡NE denotes the act was not evaluated.

being infected with KSHV (eg, persons who have KS or who are HIV infected), might lead to acquisition of the agent that causes KS." Admittedly, this guideline is rated CIII (meaning evidence for efficacy is insufficient), but it poses a quandary for homosexual men, leaving great uncertainty about whether any form of contact is safe.

In contrast to the data for sexual transmission in homosexual men, evidence for sexual transmission in heterosexual men or women is less convincing. In a large study of 2,718 STD clinic attendees in London, KSHV seroprevalence in heterosexual men and women was 4.6% compared to 18.5% in (mostly HIV-uninfected) homosexual men.[41] Among the heterosexual men and women, there was no association between KSHV seropositivity and either the number of sexual partners or current or prior history of STDs. Several other studies have found associations between KSHV seropositivity and STD history (either HIV, genital warts, syphilis, gonorrhea, herpes simplex virus 2, or chlamydial infection) among women, but whether this truly represents sexual transmission rather than a surrogate for other types of incompletely controlled-for behavior (eg, injection drug use) is not clear.[83–88] Among the two studies that best controlled for injection drug use by restricting to those women who denied either injection drug use, or who were seronegative for hepatitis C virus infection, one study reported an association between STD history and KSHV seropositivity but the other did not.[85,88] To date, although one report found a trend toward higher seropositivity in women with earlier sexual debut, no study has revealed the same unequivocal direct relationship between KSHV seropositivity and number of sexual partners as seen in homosexual men.[89] Moreover, in what should be the most powerful evaluation of heterosexual transmission among women, a history of sex with male bisexual partners has not been associated with KSHV seropositivity.[85,86] Given the scarcity of KSHV in semen, the lack of significant heterosexual transmission of KSHV is not surprising.

Injection drug use. The paucity of KS among HIV-infected nonhomosexual injection drug users led to the prediction that the putative agent of KS would be low among injection drug users.[2] Indeed, KSHV seroprevalence in injection drug users is much lower than in homosexual men, but whether injection drug use can transmit KSHV to any extent is under active investigation.[7,14] The strongest evidence comes from Cannon and colleagues, who evaluated women in the US-based HIV Epidemiology Research Study (HERS).[85] Compared with nonusers, injection drug users were more likely to be KSHV-infected in a dose-response manner, depending on drug use frequency. Furthermore, when restricted to women with low-risk sexual behavior, those who were infected with hepatitis C virus were 20 times more likely to be KSHV-infected. The inference that KSHV can be transmitted through injection drug use has subsequently been supported in at least three other studies in women and men.[70,88,90] In contrast, no association for injection drug use was reported among women in the Women's Interagency HIV Study (WIHS), but this cross-sectional analysis evaluated only the prior 6-month injection drug use history and did not evaluate dose-response trends or an association with HCV seropositivity (a better marker of lifetime injection drug use).[86] Similarly, no association was found among injection drug users in Baltimore, but again, the study lacked accurate measurement of the lifetime magnitude of injection drug use behavior, critical in a population where everyone has practiced at least some of this behavior.[91] Finally, a study of both male and female drug users in Amsterdam also failed to show an association for injection drug use, but admittedly lacked adequate statistical power.[92] Taken together, the available data do support that injection drug use can transmit KSHV. Nonetheless, the efficiency of spread by injection drug use (defined as the probability of transmission per each contact with a KSHV-infected person where injection drug use equipment is shared) is likely very low, as evidenced by the markedly lower prevalence in injection drug users as compared with homosexual men.

Blood transfusion. The possibility of transmission by blood transfusion was raised by Blackbourn and colleagues, who recovered KSHV from peripheral blood mononuclear cells from a single blood donor and were able to propagate the virus in previously uninfected target cells.[93] Further concern was introduced with the finding, reviewed above, that injection drug use (ie, exposure to minute quantities of blood) can apparently transmit KSHV, as well as from the apparent transmission via blood transfusion in two cases following postsurgical transfusions in a retrospective report from cases in the 1980s.[94] However, two other retrospective studies of known KSHV antibody-positive blood donors and their associated recipients failed to identify KSHV transmission.[95,96] Although not excluding the possibility that transfusion transmission can occur, these retrospective studies estimated that the risk per individual transfused is likely very low (95% CI for transmission risk per individual transfused, 0–9%), and other epidemiologic data support this view. For example, for transfusion of noncellular components such as fresh frozen plasma, cryoprecipitate, or factor concentrates, that the risk from transfusion, at least in non-

endemic areas, is likely very low is substantiated by indirect data in (1) hemophiliacs where KSHV seroprevalence is very low (0 to 3%), and (2) HIV-infected hemophiliacs in the 1980s who had a very low incidence of KS.[2,12–14] For transfusion of cellular components such as red blood cells, the low incidence of KS among the initial cohort of persons in the 1980s, other than hemophiliacs, who acquired HIV via blood transfusion similarly argues for a very low risk of transmission.[2] Both the hemophiliacs and generic blood transfusion recipients were in many cases infected by blood donations from homosexual men who harbored HIV and who likely also had a high prevalence of KSHV infection. The fact that so few developed KS strongly suggests that KSHV is very inefficiently spread, if at all, via transfusion in non-endemic areas with modern blood-banking practices. Consequently, there has been to date no forceful movement in the international blood-banking community to universally screen for KSHV.

The fact that KSHV transmission by injection drug use (where only minute quantities of blood are exchanged) has been established in non-endemic areas, but transmission by transfusion (where large quantities are exchanged) has not, is seemingly inconsistent. The paradox may be explained by the composition of the material exchanged. In injection drug use, fresh whole blood is exchanged, which is replete with mononuclear cells, the host cells for KSHV when it is present in the circulation. In contrast, mononuclear cells are intentionally (albeit not completely) removed in all forms of blood transfusion in most non-endemic areas. Although elements of blood plasma are exchanged in both injection drug use and transfusion, cell-free KSHV DNA is rarely found in plasma. In addition, it has required the presence of multiply exposed injection drug users (eg, daily drug use over several decades) to delineate a risk associated with this practice. The only comparably exposed group in non-endemic areas to be examined in transfusion medicine were 19 persons from France with thalassemia or sickle cell disease, who received a mean of 326 red blood cell transfusions.[97] No instances of KSHV infection were found in these individuals, but of note, they received only white blood cell–reduced (a more complete technique of white blood cell removal than standard processing) red cells, and they were examined for the presence of KSHV only with polymerase chain reaction (PCR) techniques, not by antibody testing. In a smaller group ($n = 9$) of patients with sickle cell disease, who had over 100 red blood cell transfusions and did have KSHV antibody testing performed, two were seropositive, but the sample size was too small to ascertain whether this was significantly greater than the background seroprevalence in the population.[98]

Organ transplantation. Several studies have confirmed the ability of KSHV to be transmitted through renal transplantation.[99–101] The initial sentinel work from Switzerland found that 12% (25 of 206) of renal transplant recipients, negative for antibodies to KSHV prior to surgery, seroconverted within 1 year after transplantation.[99] Two of the 25 patients developed KS. The inference that most, if not all, of these apparent seroconversions were caused by the allograft was strengthened by the finding that serum from 5 out of 6 donors to seroconverters were positive for KSHV antibodies compared with 0 out of 8 donors to nonseroconverters. In addition, transmission through blood products was ruled out in several cases. Subsequently, elegant molecular work performed on 8 renal transplant recipients with posttransplant KS determined that among 5 patients, individual cells microdissected from KS lesions were of donor origin and were KSHV infected.[102] This finding not only substantiates the ability of KSHV to be transmitted via renal transplantation but implies that, in at least some cases, the virus is spread not as free virus but instead in a cell-associated form in KS progenitor cells. Finally, although the data are not as conclusive, transmission through liver transplantation has also been reported.[103] Now that transmission through solid organ transplantation has been confirmed, there are beginning to be calls for routine screening of organ donors and recipients.[104,105] Difficulties in the assays for KSHV antibodies will make this an imperfect process, but the idea seems most warranted in non-endemic areas where the low prevalence of KSHV infection among donors means that few organs will need to be discarded because of KSHV seropositivity, and those that are may be given to recipients who are seropositive.

Transmission in Endemic Areas

Nonsexual horizontal transmission. In high-level endemic areas, such as the Middle East and Africa, an age-dependent increase in KSHV seroprevalence during childhood provides strong evidence for some form of nonsexual horizontal transmission (Table 4–2). In intermediate-level endemic areas such as the Mediterranean, fewer comparable data exist, and although only one report is suggestive of an age-dependent increase in KSHV seroprevalence before puberty, this is substantiated by the finding of increased seroprevalence in the children of patients with KS, relative to persons without KS.[36,106,107] Indeed, the fact that prevalence at the time of puberty in some high-level endemic areas is nearly that seen in adulthood suggests that nonsexual horizontal transmission is the dominant route of spread; this, of course, assumes that seroreversion is not common and therefore not masking the occurrence of a continuing high incidence of infection in adulthood. For example, in Cameroon, Gessain and colleagues demonstrated that after loss of maternal antibody by 6 months of age, there was a monotonic increase in KSHV seroprevalence from 13% in 7- to 24-month-olds, to 39% in 12- to 14-year-olds.[32] There was a similar pattern found among Ugandan children.[31] In Egypt, prevalence was 17% in children aged 1-year-old and under, ranging up to 58% among children aged 7 to 9 years old.[33]

The fact that saliva is the body fluid that most commonly harbors KSHV lends the biologic plausibility that some form of nonsexual horizontal transmission is the dominant form of spread in endemic areas. The exact mode of spread, however, is not known. Some of the first reports from sub-Saharan Africa found that maternal KSHV seropositivity was a risk factor for seropositivity among children, leading to the conclusion that mother-to-child spread was the most significant route.[108,109] These data, however, were not controlled for the family's community of residence (and hence background prevalence of KSHV infection), and did not consider whether this association might be confounded by father-to-child, sibling-to-sibling, or extrafamilial spread. In a cross-sectional study that evaluated all family members, Plancoulaine and colleagues found evidence for both mother-to-child and sibling-to-sibling spread, but not father-to-

Table 4–2. STUDIES EVALUATING THE ASSOCIATION BETWEEN AGE AND KAPOSI'S SARCOMA–ASSOCIATED HERPESVIRUS (KSHV) SEROPREVALENCE IN PREPUBESCENT CHILDREN IN AFRICA, THE MIDDLE EAST, AND ITALY

Country/Population (reference)	Age Group	N	Percent KSHV Seropositive*	
			Antilatent Antibody	Antilytic Antibody
Uganda/Hospital outpatients (Mayama et al, 1998[31])	0–5 years	35	20[†]	28[†]
	5–9 years	48	38	42
	20–24 years	53	36	46
Cameroon/Clinic patients (Gessain et al, 1999[32])	7–12 months	32	12.5	
	13–24 months	28	-	14.3
	3–4 years	36	-	13.9
	5–8 years	34	-	23.5
	9–11 years	36	-	25.0
	12–14 years	28	-	39.2
	15–20 years	27	-	48.0
	Pregnant women	189	-	54.5
Egypt/Vaccinees (Andreoni et al, 1999[33])	< 1 year	42	7.1	16.6
	1–3 years	40	10.0	37.5
	4–6 years	40	7.5	45.0
	7–9 years	38	10.5	57.8
	10–12 years	36	5.5	52.7
Italy/Hospital inpatients (Whitby et al, 2000[107])	3–5 years	90	1.1	
	6–10 years	94	6.3	
	11–15 years	38	7.8	

*An immunofluorescence assay detecting antibodies to both lytic- and latent-phase antigens was used.
†Percentages extrapolated from Figure 4–1.

child or spouse-to-spouse.[110] This, however, was performed in French Guiana, where a seroprevalence of only 15% among persons aged 15 to 40 years was reported, even when using a more sensitive induced IFA antibody assay. Whether or not the findings apply to areas with much higher prevalence, such as Africa, is not clear. A similar cross-sectional family study from Israel, where seroprevalence among adults was also only slightly > 10%, found a role for mother-to-child spread but did not examine the role of sibling-to-sibling spread.[111] Most recently, a study of children in a high prevalence area in rural Tanzania found that having a KSHV-seropositive mother, father, or next-older sibling was associated with being KSHV seropositive and that the magnitude of the risk was about the same across these relatives.[112] Importantly, there was also an age-dependent increase in KSHV seroprevalence among children who did not have a seropositive first-degree relative, suggesting that non-familial transmission also occurs. Transmission emanating from outside of the immediate family has also been reported in initial molecular epidemiologic work performed among family members in Malawi.[113,114]

Taken together, these studies suggest that a variety of relationship types (ie, mother-to-child, father-to-child, sibling-to-child, nonfamily member–to-child) may be important in KSHV transmission. It is likely that no single relationship type has any universal significance per se in transmitting KSHV, but rather that transmission is a product of salivary shedding in the infected individual and as-of-yet undetermined sociocultural practices that promote saliva passage to either interrupted skin or mucosal surfaces in the uninfected child.

As has been the case for horizontal transmission of hepatitis B virus infection in endemic areas, identifying the precise mechanisms by which KSHV is spread to children will be a considerable challenge. The exact mode of spread notwithstanding, why nonsexual horizontal transmission in children is so common in one part of the world but so uncommon in others (eg, the United States) is not understood. An association between lower education and KSHV seropositivity in some studies in endemic areas suggests that region-specific behavioral factors may be important, but the role of region-specific differences in host-mediated response to KSHV remains largely unexplored.[115,116] Although a culprit gene has not yet been identified, segregation analysis in a French Guiana population suggests that a recessive gene controlling susceptibility to KSHV infection may explain the rapidly rising KSHV seroprevalence up to puberty in the population with a subsequent plateau thereafter.[117]

Sexual transmission. Whereas sexual transmission among homosexual men appears to occur in KSHV-endemic areas just as it does in non-endemic areas, data on heterosexual transmission in endemic areas are conflicting.[106,118] The best evidence for heterosexual transmission in intermediate-level endemic areas comes from one report from Sicily, showing an association between prostitution, STD clinic attendance, and KSHV seropositivity, although others have not confirmed this.[106,119] In high-level endemic areas, the best evidence is from two studies from Cameroon, two from Kenya, and one from Nigeria, each showing a relationship between KSHV seropositivity and prostitution and/or history of at least one STD.[120–124] The work from Kenya was also notable for associations between KSHV seropositivity and lack of condom use and lack of circumcision.[122] However, several other studies have found no role for heterosexual transmission.[31,116,118,125–129] In particular, there is marked inconsistency in high-level endemic areas between what should be a powerful marker of sexual behavior, HIV infection, and KSHV serostatus, with some studies showing an association but others not.[115,120,122,125,128,130–134] This is in contrast to the universal association seen between HIV infection and KSHV serostatus in homosexual men in low-level endemic areas.[6–8] In terms of direct information on the number of sexual partners in endemic areas, Sitas and colleagues found a very small risk associated with lifetime sexual partners, but others have not confirmed this.[115,122,123] Of particular acts examined, the one report that examined kissing did not show an association with KSHV seropositivity.[123] To date, no longitudinal studies evaluating sexual transmission of KSHV that follow initially seronegative adults have been performed. Given the high prevalence of infection that is already present by puberty in endemic areas, attempts with cross-sectional studies to assess the role of either current or past sexual behavior in determining KSHV serostatus are methodologically challenging. The expectation of these cross-sectional studies would be associations that are attenuated. Therefore, definitive evidence will likely await longitudinal study.

Vertical transmission. The occurrence of KS in young children, and in particular, a case report of KS in a 6-day-old child, has suggested that KSHV can be vertically transmitted.[135] Because of the presence of maternal antibody in infants, documentation of vertical transmission relies upon detection of KSHV DNA. Mantina and colleagues evaluated the newborns of 89 Zambian women who were KSHV-antibody positive.[136] In a blood draw taken at 24 hours of life, 2 of 89 (2.2%) had detectable KSHV DNA in peripheral blood cells by PCR. Because KSHV DNA sequences could not be detected from the mothers, it cannot be determined whether or not these 2 cases represent true vertical infection or PCR contamination. Even if they do represent true infection, it would appear that the incidence and efficiency of vertical infection is quite low.

Blood transfusion. Because of the high prevalence of KSHV infection in endemic areas, if transmission via blood transfusion occurred, even if inefficient, it could pose a significant public health concern. A study of Ugandan children with sickle cell disease found a dose-response relationship between number of transfusions received and KSHV seropositivity, even after adjustment for age.[137] The overall estimated KSHV transmission risk was 2.6% (95% CI, 1.9–3.3%) per unit transfusion. If it is assumed that the prevalence of KSHV among donors in Uganda is approximately 50%, then the risk associated with receipt of a transfusion from a KSHV-seropositive donor is 5%. Of note, however, is that in Uganda, transfusion recipients are given fresh unprocessed whole blood. Whether or not these same per-unit risks occur when fractionated blood products such as leukocyte-depleted red blood cells or plasma are used, as is the case in more developed settings, is not known. The finding of KSHV DNA in the serum of a substantial proportion of blood donors in at least one African population lends credence to the concern.[129]

DISEASE MANIFESTATIONS

Primary Infection Syndrome

Very little is known about the clinical manifestations of primary KSHV infection. A major reason for this is the absence of clinically available diagnostic tests that could be used to evaluate large numbers of symptomatic persons. Furthermore, the phenomenon of seroreversion, which occurs with the currently available research-level serologic assays, makes identification of seroconversion uncertain in the absence of long-standing and repeated documentation of seronegativity (as would only be available in a formal cohort study). Therefore, in adults, all that is known comes from three reports of what are believed to represent primary infection. In the first, an HIV-infected man developed a sudden but transient onset of angiolymphoid hyperplasia with fever, arthralgia, cervical adenopathy, and splenomegaly.[138] The second report involved two transplant recipients who each received a kidney from the same KSHV-seropositive donor; one recipient developed disseminated KS and the other had fever, splenomegaly, and pancytopenia.[139] These reports emphasize the potential severity of primary infection, but because they were identified on the basis of symptoms, they do not indicate what percentage of new infections are associated with clinical symptoms. Moreover, the reports may not represent primary infection in immunocompetent hosts. The third report described five cases of KSHV seroconversion that developed during the longitudinal observation of HIV-uninfected homosexual men.[140] Four of the five cases had one or more symptoms of lymphadenopathy, diarrhea, fatigue, or rash. Although the symptoms were self-limiting, their longevity and severity were difficult to ascertain from the retrospective study design. Furthermore, this study reported a KSHV incidence of only 3.7 cases per 1,000 person-years, which seemingly could not account for the prevalence of 9.2% observed at the beginning of the cohort's observation, raising questions about whether the seroconversions detected represented only the cases that were the most overt immunologically and perhaps clinically.

In children, a study of 1- to 4-year-olds ($n = 86$) in Egypt with fever of undetermined origin found 6 children with KSHV DNA in saliva but without KSHV antibodies, thus presumably representing primary infection.[141] Of the three children for whom a follow-up blood sample was obtained, all developed KSHV antibodies. In addition to fever, 5 of the 6 children developed a rash that first appeared on the face and gradually spread to the trunk, arms, and legs. Five of the 6 children also had upper respiratory tract infection symptoms, and 2 had lower respiratory tract infection symptoms. Although this report again demonstrates the severity of disease that can occur, its hospital-based sampling precludes an understanding of the overall frequency of symptomatic disease among children with primary infection. There has also been one report of a 1-month-old girl with DiGeorge anomaly, a primary immunodeficiency, who had widespread KSHV dissemination with virus detected in peripheral blood mononuclear cells, bone marrow, spleen, and lymph nodes as well as in endothelial and epithelial cells of the skin, lungs, esophagus, intestine, choroid plexus, and heart.[142] She died of multiorgan failure. Of interest from a transmission viewpoint is that there was no evidence of KSHV infection in her mother.

Kaposi's Sarcoma

There are four forms of KS, defined on the basis of their epidemiologic context. "Classic" KS is the syndrome originally described by Kaposi, and it has recently been thoroughly reviewed.[1,143] It is found most frequently in older men (> 50 years) of Mediterranean or Eastern European heritage and is characterized initially by bluish-red painless spots on the feet and lower legs that subsequently, if untreated, progress to form raised nodular growths that may ulcerate and bleed. In the latter stages of disease, the entire lower extremities as well as the hands and arms may become involved. Although the disease course is typically indolent, internal involvement does occur in approximately 10% of cases. African or "endemic" KS is most common in sub-Saharan Africa. Even before the AIDS epidemic, portions of sub-Saharan Africa, particularly the Nile-Congo watershed, had among the highest incidences of KS in the world.[144,145] In these areas, KS represented 4 to 10% of all adult cancers and was mainly a disease of men aged 30 to 50 years old. Like classic KS, endemic KS manifests primarily as localized plaques and nodules on the feet and lower legs, but visceral involvement is more common than in the classic form. The third form of KS was described shortly after the advent of solid organ transplantation, and foreshadowed the powerful influence of immunosuppression on KS development.[146,147] In this form, called "posttransplant" or "iatrogenic" KS, both disseminated cutaneous involvement and visceral disease are common. As noted earlier, recent work has shown that among cases that develop because of de novo transmission of KSHV, cells within the KS lesions are often of donor origin.[102] This implies that either circulating KSHV-infected spindle-like cells or lymphoid cells trapped in the allograft or endothelial cells (or their precursors) residing in the allograft are the critical transplanted element that leads to KS lesion formation. Interestingly, lesions often diminish with lessening of the immunosuppressive regimen, but because this reduction is often accompanied by organ rejection, KS is a feared posttransplant complication.[147] The finding that KS lesions are sometimes of donor cellular origin implies that donor-derived KSHV-specific cytotoxic T cells could be a useful form of therapy that could obviate the need to lessen immunosuppression.

The fourth form of KS, originally described in young homosexual men, heralded the beginning of the HIV epidemic in 1981 (Figure 4–2).[148,149] "Epidemic" or "AIDS-associated" KS became the most common HIV-associated malignancy, particularly affecting persons who acquired HIV via male homosexual behavior.[2] Prior to the introduction of effective anti-HIV therapy, HIV-infected homosexual men were estimated to have a 20-fold higher risk of KS development than other HIV transmission risk groups and a lifetime cumulative incidence of 37%.[2,150] Cutaneous AIDS-related KS, typically the earliest presentation, is often disseminated, cosmetically disfiguring, and complicated by bulky lesions, lymphatic obstruction, and extremity or facial swelling (Figure 4–3).[151] Subsequent visceral manifestations, especially pulmonary and gastrointestinal involvement, are common and convey a poor prognosis.[152,153] Prior to 1996 (ie, prior to the era of highly active antiretroviral therapy for HIV and improved chemotherapy for KS), the median survival for HIV-infected persons with visceral involvement was 15 months.[154] However, even persons with KS confined to the skin and/or lymph nodes also had significant mortality, with a median survival of 27 months.[154] As it has with

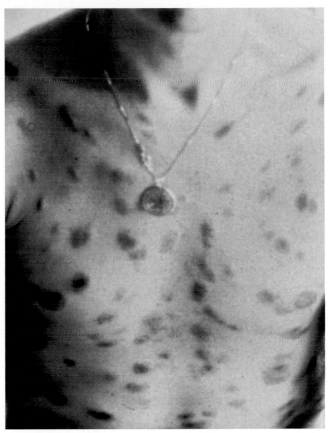

Figure 4–2. Diffuse cutaneous Kaposi's sarcoma in a homosexual man.

other complications of HIV infection, the advent of highly active antiretroviral therapy has dramatically altered the prognosis of AIDS-associated KS. In a study of 287 patients with KS from 1990 to 1999, use of highly active antiretroviral therapy was associated with an 81% reduction in mortality.[155]

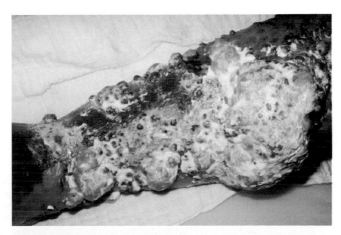

Figure 4–3. Fulminant nodular Kaposi's sarcoma of the lower extremity in a patient with acquired immunodeficiency syndrome.

The introduction of potent anti-retroviral therapy for HIV infection in the mid-1990s has also led to a dramatic reduction in the incidence of AIDS-associated KS in resource-rich settings.[156,157] In contrast, in portions of sub-Saharan Africa, where KSHV is endemic and antiretroviral therapy is not widely available, KS is now the most common adult malignancy. For example, in Uganda, the incidence of KS between 1964 to 1968 and 1989 to 1991 has increased more than 20-fold in men.[158] A similar situation exists in Zimbabwe, where the HIV epidemic is largely unchecked and where KS is now the most common cancer overall in adults, most common in men (40% of all cancers), and the second most common in women (18% of all cancers) and children (10% of all cancers).[34] As is seen in AIDS-associated KS in resource-rich settings, the clinical manifestations of KS in sub-Saharan Africa have also changed. The most common presentations are now more aggressive forms, such as lymphadenopathic or visceral KS, for which effective and affordable treatment is generally unavailable.[158,159]

The disproportionate risk of KS among HIV-infected homosexual men led to the hypothesis that a sexually transmitted infectious agent, other than HIV, was etiologically important.[2] This epidemiologically driven hypothesis reinvigorated an intense laboratory investigation for the causative agent that ultimately resulted in the identification of KSHV.[3] In a relatively short period of time since the discovery of KSHV, there have been a large number of epidemiologic studies evaluating its causal role in KS (Table 4–3). In the absence of experimental evidence (eg, Koch's postulates), epidemiologists assess causality using Hill's criteria.[160] These criteria are discussed in Table 4–4 in order of their importance. The overwhelming assessment of these criteria, coupled with the finding that KSHV is invariably present in KS tumor specimens from all forms of KS throughout the world, is that KSHV is a necessary causal agent of KS.[161] However, because only a small fraction of persons infected with KSHV develop KS, it is concluded that KSHV is a necessary, but not sufficient, causal agent of KS.

Of other potential cofactors operating along with KSHV infection in the etiology of KS, immunosuppression in general, and HIV infection in particular,

Table 4–3. STUDIES ESTIMATING THE ASSOCIATION BETWEEN KAPOSI'S SARCOMA–ASSOCIATED HERPESVIRUS (KSHV) INFECTION AND ACQUIRED IMMUNE DEFICIENCY SYNDROME (AIDS)-RELATED KAPOSI'S SARCOMA*

Reference	KSHV Antigen Targeted	Antibody Assay Format	Association Between KSHV and AIDS-KS, Point Estimate[†] (95% CI)
Case-Control Studies			
Miller et al, 1996[11]	p40	Immunoblot	13.4 (4.5–42)
Miller et al, 1996[11]	Lytic cycle	IFA	12.2 (4.1–38)
Gao et al, 1996[5]	LNA	Immunoblot	18.9 (5.4–70)
Kedes et al, 1996[12]	LNA	IFA	8.5 (3.1–23)
Gao et al, 1996[13]	LNA	IFA	16.3 (5.3–50)
Simpson et al, 1996[14]	LNA	IFA	10.2 (4.2–25)
Simpson et al, 1996[14]	ORF65	EIA	9.2 (2.7–31)
Lennette et al, 1996[184]	Lytic cycle	IFA	1.8 (0.53–5.8)
Lennette et al, 1996[184]	LNA	IFA	4.2 (2.2–8.0)
Longitudinal Studies			
Martin et al, 1998[6]	LNA	IFA	2.5 (1.7–3.8)
Renwick et al, 1998[7]	ORF65.2; ORF73	EIA	3.3[‡] (1.9–5.8)
Renwick et al, 1998[7]	ORF65.2; ORF73	EIA	5.2[§] (2.9–9.3)
O'Brien et al, 1999[8]	LNA	IFA	3.6 (1.7–9.5)

EIA = enzyme immunoassay; IFA = immunofluorescence assay; LNA = latent nuclear antigen; ORF = open reading frame.
*Limited to studies that measure KSHV infection by antibody response and either directly control for number of sexual partners or restrict analyses to human immunodeficiency virus–infected homosexual men.
[†]Odds ratios are reported for case-control studies and hazard ratios for longitudinal studies.
[‡]Hazard ratio shown is for KSHV-prevalent infection.
[§]Hazard ratio shown is for KSHV seroconverters.

Table 4–4. ASSESSMENT OF THE HILL CRITERIA FOR THE ROLE OF KAPOSI'S SARCOMA–ASSOCIATED HERPESVIRUS (KSHV) INFECTION IN THE ETIOLOGY OF KAPOSI'S SARCOMA (KS)

Criterion	Comment
Temporality	Demonstrating that KSHV infection precedes KS is the sine qua non for causality. KSHV infection has been shown to precede KS in several studies, thus dispelling notions that KS tumors, by being hospitable breeding grounds, result in the subsequent presence of KSHV.[4–8,185,100] Importantly, KSHV infection is temporally associated with KS, independent of degree of sexual exposure (excluding the possibility that KSHV is just a marker for another as-yet-undiscovered sexually transmitted pathogen) and immunocompromise.[4–8]
Strength of association	After adjusting for all known potential confounding factors, statistical associations between a putative cause and disease that maintain a large magnitude are less likely to be explained by unaccounted for confounding factors and hence more likely to be valid associations. In longitudinal studies of KSHV and KS, the relevant association to be evaluated is KS incidence in KSHV-infected persons compared with KSHV-uninfected persons. If it is accepted that KS per se does not cause KSHV infection to be detected, then associations from case-control studies are also relevant. Of the studies of AIDS-related KS that measured KSHV infection by serologic means and directly controlled for number of sexual partners or restricted analyses to homosexual men, the magnitude of association between KSHV and KS ranges from 2.5 to 5.2 (hazard ratios) in longitudinal studies and 1.8 to 18.9 (odds ratios) in case-control studies.[5–8,11–14,184]
Consistency	All published epidemiologic reports addressing a possible association between KSHV and KS, with the exception of one, have found a direct association. Although it is formally possible that an unrecognized bias in either subject selection or variable measurement could account for the association between KSHV and KS seen in all studies to date, this is improbable because such a bias is unlikely to be consistently present in such a wide array of studies that vary by design, participant selection, and assay formats. Furthermore, the remarkable consistency in results makes chance a very unlikely explanation.
Biologic plausibility	There are several potential biologic mechanisms by which KSHV may cause KS.
Dose-response relationship	Among human immunodeficiency virus and KSHV co-infected homosexual men, this criterion has been satisfied by the finding that detectable peripheral blood mononuclear cell-associated KSHV is associated with the subsequent development of KS.[187]
Coherence	This criterion implies that a cause-and-effect interpretation for the association in question does not conflict with what is otherwise known about either the disease or the putative causal agent. A causal role for KSHV in KS is compatible with existing knowledge, in that the epidemiology of KSHV per se matches that long predicted for the agent of KS (eg, highest prevalences in groups at greatest risk for KS and, in developed settings, sexually transmitted).
Analogy	Although a weak criterion, there is analogous evidence for a causal role of KSHV in KS. Two herpesviruses closely related to KSHV, herpesvirus saimiri and Epstein-Barr virus, are oncogenic.
Specificity	That a single cause must cause a single disease is clearly outdated and likely violated by KSHV, which has also at least been associated with primary effusion lymphoma and multicentric Castleman's disease.[10,173,188]
Experimental evidence	In SCID mice, injection of KSHV into transplanted human skin results in the formation of lesions that are morphologically and phenotypically consistent with KS.[189]

SCID = severe combined immunodeficiency.

confer the greatest risk. Among HIV-infected persons, the magnitude of immunosuppression, as evidenced by CD4 T-cell count, is predictive of development of KS.[7,162] Timing of KSHV infection relative to HIV infection may be important as well (the risk of developing KS was significantly greater in one study, and of similar magnitude but not statistically significant in a second study) in persons who acquire KSHV after, as compared with before, HIV infection.[7,162] Studies of this nature have potential methodologic pitfalls, however, and what appears to be KSHV seroconversion could conceivably be KSHV reactivation and reappearance of antibody positivity.[163] Two potential genetic risk factors have also been described and await confirmation. The FF genotype of the low-affinity Fc gamma receptor IIIA is underrepresented in patients with KS, whereas the VF genotype confers greater risk.[164] Homozygosity for allele G at amino acid 174 of the interleukin-6 (IL-6) promoter, associated with increased IL-6 production, has been related to the development of KS whereas homozygosity of allele C appears protective.[165] However, it is not known whether these genetic factors influence development of KS via pathogenic acceleration among

KSHV-infected persons or via enhancement of the acquisition of KSHV per se.

Despite substantial investigation, the identification of cofactors, in addition to KSHV, for development of KS among immunocompetent individuals is largely incomplete. The role of cofactors is particularly evident in Africa, where prior to the AIDS epidemic, there was tremendous heterogeneity in KS incidence; this heterogeneity is not fully explained by underlying geographic differences in KSHV prevalence.[166] The absence of KS among Ethiopian immigrants to Israel compared with Israeli-born residents, despite higher KSHV seroprevalence in the Ethiopians, is a well-documented example of some heretofore undiscovered protective factor.[167] Studies that have evaluated factors associated with KS, which were performed prior to the identification of KSHV, have had their interpretations clouded by the possibility that these factors are associated with acquisition of KSHV. This pertains to, for example, genetic studies where, in at least some reports, an increased risk for classic KS has been observed in persons with human leukocyte antigen (HLA)-DR5 and a protective effect observed for HLA-DR3.[168] Both male gender and older age have long been identified as significant risk factors for KS, and neither can be fully explained by an increased risk for acquisition of KSHV infection. However, mechanistic explanation for these factors is unknown. Higher levels of immune activation, measured by circulating neopterin and β-2-microglobulin, have also been associated with classic KS, but it has not been determined whether this is a cause or a consequence of KS.[169] More recent studies that were either limited to participants with KSHV infection or adjusted for KSHV infection are most notable for the absence of demonstrable associations. Nonetheless, two new potential behavioral factors have been identified that require further investigation. In classic KS, smoking was found to be protective; the effect of smoking on inflammatory cytokines was the speculated mechanism.[170] In endemic KS, going barefoot more than half the time was a risk factor.[171] It has been suggested that fine soil particles might pass through the skin of barefooted individuals and block the lymphatic system, causing local immunosuppression in the lower limbs and predisposing to the development of KS.[172]

Other Diseases

KSHV also has been associated with PEL, multicentric Castleman's disease, and hemophagocytic lymphohistiocytosis.[10,173,174] Among other diseases that have been hypothesized to be caused by KSHV, multiple myeloma has generated the most interest because of its frequency and clinical severity.[175] From an ecologic viewpoint, the association lacks plausibility given that multiple myeloma is not more common in populations in which KSHV prevalence is high. In addition, numerous individual subject-level studies have failed to confirm the initial claim.[176–180] Most recently, claims have also been made for an association between KSHV infection and pulmonary hypertension, prostate cancer, and amyotrophic lateral sclerosis.[181–183] The clinical impact of these conditions, especially prostate cancer, is sure to prompt much additional work in the next several years seeking to confirm these associations.

REFERENCES

1. Kaposi M. Idiopathisches multiples Pigmentsarcom der Haut. Arch Dermatol Syph (Prague) 1872;4:265–78.
2. Beral V, Peterman TA, Berkelman RL, Jaffe HW. Kaposi's sarcoma among persons with AIDS: a sexually transmitted infection? Lancet 1990;335:123–8.
3. Chang Y, Cesarman E, Pessin MS, et al. Identification of herpesvirus-like DNA sequences in AIDS-associated Kaposi's sarcoma. Science 1994;266:1865–9.
4. Whitby D, Howard MR, Tenant-Flowers M, et al. Detection of Kaposi sarcoma associated herpesvirus in peripheral blood HIV-infected individuals and progression to Kaposi's sarcoma. Lancet 1995;346:799–802.
5. Gao SJ, Kingsley L, Hoover DR, et al. Seroconversion to antibodies against Kaposi's sarcoma-associated herpesvirus-related latent nuclear antigens before the development of Kaposi's sarcoma. N Engl J Med 1996;335:233–41.
6. Martin JN, Ganem DE, Osmond DH, et al. Sexual transmission and the natural history of human herpesvirus 8 infection. N Engl J Med 1998;338:948–54.
7. Renwick N, Halaby T, Weverling GJ, et al. Seroconversion for human herpesvirus 8 during HIV infection is highly predictive of Kaposi's sarcoma. AIDS 1998;12:2481–8.
8. O'Brien T, Kedes D, Ganem D, et al. Evidence for concurrent epidemics of human herpesvirus 8 and human immunodeficiency virus type 1 in US homosexual men: rates, risk factors, and relationship to Kaposi's sarcoma. J Infect Dis 1999;180:1010–7.
9. Spira TJ, Lam L, Dollard SC, et al. Comparison of serologic assays and PCR for diagnosis of human herpesvirus 8 infection. J Clin Microbiol 2000;38:2174–80.
10. Cesarman E, Chang Y, Moore PS, et al. Kaposi's sarcoma-

associated herpesvirus-like DNA sequences in AIDS-related body-cavity-based lymphomas. N Engl J Med 1995;332:1186–91.

11. Miller G, Rigsby MO, Heston L, et al. Antibodies to butyrate-inducible antigens of Kaposi's sarcoma-associated herpesvirus in patients with HIV-1 infection. N Engl J Med 1996;334:1292–7.

12. Kedes DH, Operskalski E, Busch M, et al. The seroepidemiology of human herpesvirus 8 (Kaposi's sarcoma-associated herpesvirus): distribution of infection in KS risk groups and evidence for sexual transmission. Nat Med 1996;2:918–24.

13. Gao SJ, Kingsley L, Li M, et al. KSHV antibodies among Americans, Italians and Ugandans with and without Kaposi's sarcoma. Nat Med 1996;2:925 8.

14. Simpson GR, Schulz TF, Whitby D, et al. Prevalence of Kaposi's sarcoma associated herpesvirus infection by antibodies to recombinant capsid protein and latent antigen. Lancet 1996;348:1133–8.

15. Rainbow L, Platt GM, Simpson GR, et al. The 222- to 234-kilodalton latent nuclear protein (LNA) of Kaposi's sarcoma-associated herpesvirus (human herpesvirus 8) is encoded by orf73 and is a component of the latency-associated nuclear antigen. J Virol 1997;71:5915–21.

16. Kedes DH, Lagunoff M, Renne R, Ganem D. Identification of the gene encoding the major latency-associated nuclear antigen of the Kaposi's sarcoma-associated herpesvirus. J Clin Invest 1997;100:2606–10.

17. Chandran B, Smith MS, Koelle DM, et al. Reactivities of human sera with human herpesvirus-8-infected BCBL-1 cells and identification of HHV-8-specific proteins and glycoproteins and the encoding cDNAs. Virology 1998;243:208–17.

18. Raab MS, Albrecht JC, Birkmann A, et al. The immunogenic glycoprotein gp35-37 of human herpesvirus 8 is encoded by open reading frame K8.1. J Virol 1998;72:6725–31.

19. Engels EA, Whitby D, Goebel PB, et al. Identifying human herpesvirus 8 infection: performance characteristics of serologic assays. J Acquir Immune Defic Syndr 2000;23:346–54.

20. Pau CP, Lam LL, Spira TJ, et al. Mapping and serodiagnostic application of a dominant epitope within the human herpesvirus 8 ORF 65-encoded protein. J Clin Microbiol 1998;36:1574–7.

21. Chatlynne LG, Lapps W, Handy M, et al. Detection and titration of human herpesvirus-8-specific antibodies in sera from blood donors, acquired immunodeficiency syndrome patients, and Kaposi's sarcoma patients using a whole virus enzyme-linked immunosorbent assay. Blood 1998;92:53–8.

22. Martin JN, Amad Z, Cossen C, et al. Use of epidemiologically well-defined subjects and existing immunofluorescence assays to calibrate a new enzyme immunoassay for human herpesvirus 8 antibodies. J Clin Microbiol 2000;38:696–701.

23. Rabkin CS, Schulz TF, Whitby D, et al. Interassay correlation of human herpesvirus 8 serologic tests. HHV-8 Interlaboratory Collaborative Group. J Infect Dis 1998;178:304–9.

24. Pellett PE, Wright DJ, Engels EA, et al. Multicenter comparison of serologic assays and estimation of human her-pesvirus 8 seroprevalence among US blood donors. Transfusion 2003;43.1260–8.

25. Ransohoff DF, Feinstein AR. Problems of spectrum and bias in evaluating the efficacy of diagnostic tests. N Engl J Med 1978;299:926–30.

26. Casper C, Krantz E, Taylor II, et al. Assessment of a combined testing strategy for detection of antibodies to human herpesvirus 8 (HHV-8) in persons with Kaposi's sarcoma, persons with asymptomatic HHV-8 infection, and persons at low risk for HHV-8 infection. J Clin Microbiol 2002;40:3822–5.

27. Tedeschi R, De Paoli P, Schulz TF, Dillner J. Human serum antibodies to a major defined epitope of human herpesvirus 8 small viral capsid antigen. J Infect Dis 1999;179:1016–20.

28. Quinlivan EB, Wang RX, Stewart PW, et al. Longitudinal sero-reactivity to human herpesvirus 8 (KSHV) in the Swiss HIV cohort 4.7 years before KS. Swiss HIV Cohort Study. J Med Virol 2001;64:157–66.

29. Chohan BH, Taylor H, Obrigewitch R, et al. Human herpesvirus 8 seroconversion in Kenyan women by enzyme-linked immunosorbent assay and immunofluorescence assay. J Clin Virol 2004;30:137–44.

30. Olsen SJ, Chang Y, Moore PS, et al. Increasing Kaposi's sarcoma-associated herpesvirus seroprevalence with age in a highly Kaposi's sarcoma endemic region, Zambia in 1985. AIDS 1998;12:1921–5.

31. Mayama S, Cuevas LE, Sheldon J, et al. Prevalence and transmission of Kaposi's sarcoma-associated herpesvirus (human herpesvirus 8) in Ugandan children and adolescents. Int J Cancer 1998;77:817–20.

32. Gessain A, Mauclere P, van Beveren M, et al. Human herpesvirus 8 primary infection occurs during childhood in Cameroon, Central Africa. Int J Cancer 1999;81:189–92.

33. Andreoni M, El-Sawaf G, Rezza G, et al. High seroprevalence of antibodies to human herpesvirus-8 in Egyptian children: evidence of nonsexual transmission. J Natl Cancer Inst 1999;91:465–9.

34. Chokunonga E, Levy LM, Bassett MT, et al. Cancer incidence in the African population of Harare, Zimbabwe: second results from the cancer registry 1993–1995. Int J Cancer 2000;85:54–9.

35. Wabinga HR, Parkin DM, Wabwire-Mangen F, Nambooze S. Trends in cancer incidence in Kyadondo County, Uganda, 1960–1997. Br J Cancer 2000;82:1585–92.

36. Angeloni A, Heston L, Uccini S, et al. High prevalence of antibodies to human herpesvirus 8 in relatives of patients with classic Kaposi's sarcoma from Sardinia. J Infect Dis 1998;177:1715–8.

37. Whitby D, Luppi M, Barozzi P, et al. Human herpesvirus 8 seroprevalence in blood donors and lymphoma patients from different regions of Italy. J Natl Cancer Inst 1998;90:395–7.

38. Cattani P, Cerimele F, Porta D, et al. Age-specific seroprevalence of human herpesvirus 8 in Mediterranean regions. Clin Microbiol Infect 2003;9:274–9.

39. Melbye M, Cook PM, Hjalgrim H, et al. Risk factors for Kaposi's-sarcoma-associated herpesvirus (KSHV/HHV-8) seropositivity in a cohort of homosexual men, 1981–1996. Int J Cancer 1998;77:543–8.

40. Dukers NH, Renwick N, Prins M, et al. Risk factors for human herpesvirus 8 seropositivity and seroconversion in a cohort of homosexual men. Am J Epidemiol 2000;151: 213–24.

41. Smith NA, Sabin CA, Gopal R, et al. Serologic evidence of human herpesvirus 8 transmission by homosexual but not heterosexual sex. J Infect Dis 1999;180:600–6.

42. Kedes DH, Ganem D, Ameli N, et al. The prevalence of serum antibody to human herpesvirus 8 (Kaposi sarcoma-associated herpesvirus) among HIV-seropositive and high-risk HIV-seronegative women. JAMA 1997;277:478–81.

43. Hayward GS. KSHV strains: the origins and global spread of the virus. Semin Cancer Biol 1999;9:187–99.

44. Biggar RJ, Whitby D, Marshall V, et al. Human herpesvirus 8 in Brazilian Amerindians: a hyperendemic population with a new subtype. J Infect Dis 2000;181:1562–8.

45. Rezza G, Danaya RT, Wagner TM, et al. Human herpesvirus-8 and other viral infections, Papua New Guinea. Emerg Infect Dis 2001;7:893–5.

46. Whitby D, Marshall VA, Bagni RK, et al. Genotypic characterization of Kaposi's sarcoma-associated herpesvirus in asymptomatic infected subjects from isolated populations. J Gen Virol 2004;85:155–63.

47. Osmond DH, Buchbinder S, Cheng A, et al. Prevalence of Kaposi sarcoma-associated herpesvirus infection in homosexual men at beginning of and during the HIV epidemic. JAMA 2002;287:221–5.

48. Hjalgrim H, Lind I, Rostgaard K, et al. Prevalence of human herpesvirus 8 antibodies in young adults in Denmark (1976–1977). J Natl Cancer Inst 2001;93:1569–71.

49. Hjalgrim H, Melbye M, Lecker S, et al. Epidemiology of classic Kaposi's sarcoma in Denmark between 1970 and 1992. Cancer 1996;77:1373–8.

50. de-Thé G, Bestetti G, van Beveren M, Gessain A. Prevalence of human herpesvirus 8 infection before the acquired immunodeficiency disease syndrome-related epidemic of Kaposi's sarcoma in East Africa. J Natl Cancer Inst 1999;91:1888–9.

51. Rutherford GW, Payne SF, Lemp GF. The epidemiology of AIDS-related Kaposi's sarcoma in San Francisco. J Acquir Immune Defic Syndr 1990;3 Suppl 1:S4–7.

52. Dore GJ, Li Y, Grulich AE, et al. Declining incidence and later occurrence of Kaposi's sarcoma among persons with AIDS in Australia: the Australian AIDS cohort. AIDS 1996;10:1401–6.

53. Jones JL, Hanson DL, Dworkin MS, et al. Effect of anti-retroviral therapy on recent trends in selected cancers among HIV-infected persons. Adult/Adolescent Spectrum of HIV Disease Project Group. J Acquir Immune Defic Syndr 1999;21 Suppl 1:S11–7.

54. Rezza G, Dorrucci M, Serraino D, et al. Incidence of Kaposi's sarcoma and HHV-8 seroprevalence among homosexual men with known dates of HIV seroconversion. Italian Seroconversion Study. AIDS 2000;14:1647–53.

55. Russo JJ, Bohenzky RA, Chien MC, et al. Nucleotide sequence of the Kaposi sarcoma-associated herpesvirus (HHV8). Proc Natl Acad Sci U S A 1996;93:14862–7.

56. Neipel F, Albrecht JC, Fleckenstein B. Cell-homologous genes in the Kaposi's sarcoma-associated rhadinovirus human herpesvirus 8: determinants of its pathogenicity? J Virol 1997;71:4187–92.

57. Zong JC, Metroka C, Reitz MS, et al. Strain variability among Kaposi sarcoma-associated herpesvirus (human herpesvirus 8) genomes: evidence that a large cohort of United States AIDS patients may have been infected by a single common isolate. J Virol 1997;71:2505–11.

58. Nicholas J, Zong JC, Alcendor DJ, et al. Novel organizational features, captured cellular genes, and strain variability within the genome of KSHV/HHV8. J Natl Cancer Inst Monogr 1998:79–88.

59. Zong JC, Ciufo DM, Alcendor DJ, et al. High-level variability in the ORF-K1 membrane protein gene at the left end of the Kaposi's sarcoma-associated herpesvirus genome defines four major virus subtypes and multiple variants or clades in different human populations. J Virol 1999;73:4156–70.

60. Cook PM, Whitby D, Calabro ML, et al. Variability and evolution of Kaposi's sarcoma-associated herpesvirus in Europe and Africa. International Collaborative Group. AIDS 1999;13:1165–76.

61. Meng YX, Spira TJ, Bhat GJ, et al. Individuals from North America, Australasia, and Africa are infected with four different genotypes of human herpesvirus 8. Virology 1999;261:106–19.

62. Zong J, Ciufo DM, Viscidi R, et al. Genotypic analysis at multiple loci across Kaposi's sarcoma herpesvirus (KSHV) DNA molecules: clustering patterns, novel variants and chimerism. J Clin Virol 2002;23:119–48.

63. Poole LJ, Zong JC, Ciufo DM, et al. Comparison of genetic variability at multiple loci across the genomes of the major subtypes of Kaposi's sarcoma-associated herpesvirus reveals evidence for recombination and for two distinct types of open reading frame K15 alleles at the right-hand end. J Virol 1999;73:6646–60.

64. Lacoste V, Kadyrova E, Chistiakova I, et al. Molecular characterization of Kaposi's sarcoma-associated herpesvirus/human herpesvirus-8 strains from Russia. J Gen Virol 2000;81(Pt 5):1217–22.

65. Lacoste V, Judde JG, Briere J, et al. Molecular epidemiology of human herpesvirus 8 in Africa: both B and A5 K1 genotypes, as well as the M and P genotypes of K14.1/K15 loci, are frequent and widespread. Virology 2000;278:60–74.

66. Endo T, Miura T, Koibuchi T, et al. Molecular analysis of human herpesvirus 8 by using single nucleotide polymorphisms in open reading frame 26. J Clin Microbiol 2003; 41:2492–7.

67. Dukers NHTM, Renwick N, Prins M, et al. Risk factors for human herpesvirus 8 seropositivity and seroconversion in a cohort of homosexual men. Am J Epidemiol 2000;151: 213–24.

68. Pauk J, Huang ML, Brodie SJ, et al. Mucosal shedding of human herpesvirus 8 in men. N Engl J Med 2000;343:1369–77.

69. Jacobson LP, Springer G, Jenkins FJ, et al. HHV-8 infection: incidence and risk factors in the Multicenter AIDS Cohort Study (MACS), 3rd International Workshop on Kaposi Sarcoma-Associated Herpesviruses and Related Agents. 2002. Amherst, Massachusetts.

70. Diamond C, Thiede H, Perdue T, et al. Seroepidemiology of human herpesvirus 8 among young men who have sex with men. The Seattle Young Men's Survey Team. Sex Transm Dis 2001;28:176–83.

71. Casper C, Wald A, Pauk J, et al. Correlates of prevalent and

incident Kaposi's sarcoma-associated herpesvirus infection in men who have sex with men. J Infect Dis 2002; 185:990–3.

72. Jacobson LP, Munoz A, Fox R, et al. Incidence of Kaposi's sarcoma in a cohort of homosexual men infected with the human immunodeficiency virus type 1. The Multicenter AIDS Cohort Study Group. J Acquir Immune Defic Syndr 1990;3 Suppl 1:S24–31.

73. Beral V, Bull D, Darby S, et al. Risk of Kaposi's sarcoma and sexual practices associated with faecal contact in homosexual or bisexual men with AIDS. Lancet 1992;339:632–5.

74. Grulich AE, Kaldor JM, Hendry O, et al. Risk of Kaposi's sarcoma and oroanal sexual contact. Am J Epidemiol 1997;145:673–9.

75. Archibald CP, Schechter MT, Craib KJ, et al. Risk factors for Kaposi's sarcoma in the Vancouver Lymphadenopathy-AIDS Study. J Acquir Immune Defic Syndr 1990;3 Suppl 1:S18–23.

76. Lifson AR, Darrow WW, Hessol NA, et al. Kaposi's sarcoma in a cohort of homosexual and bisexual men. Epidemiology and analysis for cofactors. Am J Epidemiol 1990;131: 221–31.

77. Page-Bodkin K, Tappero J, Samuel M, Winkelstein W. Kaposi's sarcoma and faecal-oral exposure [letter]. Lancet 1992;339:1490.

78. Elford J, Tindall B, Sharkey T. Kaposi's sarcoma and insertive rimming [letter]. Lancet 1992;339:938.

79. Grulich AE, Olsen SJ, Luo K, et al. Kaposi's sarcoma-associated herpesvirus: a sexually transmissible infection? J Acquir Immune Defic Syndr Hum Retrovirol 1999; 20:387–93.

80. Diamond C, Huang ML, Kedes DH, et al. Absence of detectable human herpesvirus 8 in the semen of human immunodeficiency virus-infected men without Kaposi's sarcoma. J Infect Dis 1997;176:775–7.

81. Koelle DM, Huang ML, Chandran B, et al. Frequent detection of Kaposi's sarcoma-associated herpesvirus (human herpesvirus 8) DNA in saliva of human immunodeficiency virus-infected men: clinical and immunologic correlates. J Infect Dis 1997;176:94–102.

82. U.S. Public Health Service and Infectious Diseases Society of America. Guidelines for Preventing Opportunistic Infections Among HIV-infected Persons. MMWR Morb Mortal Wkly Rep 2002;51:1–46.

83. Sosa C, Klaskala W, Chandran B, et al. Human herpesvirus 8 as a potential sexually transmitted agent in Honduras. J Infect Dis 1998;178:547–51.

84. Tedeschi R, Caggiari L, Silins I, et al. Seropositivity to human herpesvirus 8 in relation to sexual history and risk of sexually transmitted infections among women. Int J Cancer 2000;87:232–5.

85. Cannon MJ, Dollard SC, Smith DK, et al. Blood-borne and sexual transmission of human herpesvirus 8 in women with or at risk for human immunodeficiency virus infection. HIV Epidemiology Research Study Group. N Engl J Med 2001;344:637–43.

86. Greenblatt RM, Jacobson LP, Levine AM, et al. Human herpesvirus 8 infection and Kaposi's sarcoma among human immunodeficiency virus-infected and -uninfected women. J Infect Dis 2001;183:1130–4.

87. Janier M, Agbalika F, de La Salmoniere P, et al. Human herpesvirus 8 seroprevalence in an STD clinic in Paris: a study of 512 patients. Sex Transm Dis 2002;29:698–702.

88. Goedert JJ, Charurat M, Blattner WA, et al. Risk factors for Kaposi's sarcoma-associated herpesvirus infection among HIV-1-infected pregnant women in the USA. AIDS 2003; 17:425–33.

89. de Sanjose S, Marshall V, Sola J, et al. Prevalence of Kaposi's sarcoma-associated herpesvirus infection in sex workers and women from the general population in Spain. Int J Cancer 2002;98:155–8.

90. Atkinson J, Edlin BR, Engels EA, et al. Seroprevalence of human herpesvirus 8 among injection drug users in San Francisco. J Infect Dis 2003;187:974–81.

91. Bernstein KT, Jacobson LP, Jenkins FJ, et al. Factors associated with human herpesvirus type 8 infection in an injecting drug user cohort. Sex Transm Dis 2003;30:199–204.

92. Renwick N, Dukers NH, Weverling GJ, et al. Risk factors for human herpesvirus 8 infection in a cohort of drug users in the Netherlands, 1985–1996. J Infect Dis 2002;185: 1808–12.

93. Blackbourn DJ, Ambroziak J, Lennette E, et al. Infectious human herpesvirus 8 in a healthy North American blood donor. Lancet 1997;349:609–11.

94. Dollard SC, Nelson KE, Ness PM, et al. Possible transmission of human herpesvirus-8 by blood transfusion in a historical United States cohort. Transfusion 2005;45:500–3.

95. Operskalski EA, Busch MP, Mosley JW, Kedes DH. Blood donations and viruses. Lancet 1997;349:1327.

96. Engels EA, Eastman H, Ablashi DV, et al. Risk of transfusion-associated transmission of human herpesvirus 8. J Natl Cancer Inst 1999;91:1773–5.

97. Lefrere JJ, Mariotti M, Girot R, et al. Transfusional risk of HHV-8 infection. Lancet 1997;350:217.

98. Challine D, Roudot-Thoraval F, Sarah T, et al. Seroprevalence of human herpes virus 8 antibody in populations at high or low risk of transfusion, graft, or sexual transmission of viruses. Transfusion 2001;41:1120–5.

99. Regamey N, Tamm M, Wernli M, et al. Transmission of human herpesvirus 8 infection from renal-transplant donors to recipients. N Engl J Med 1998;339:1358–63.

100. Diociaiuti A, Nanni G, Cattani P, et al. HHV8 in renal transplant recipients. Transplant Int 2000;13 Suppl 1:S410–2.

101. Luppi M, Barozzi P, Santagostino G, et al. Molecular evidence of organ-related transmission of Kaposi sarcoma-associated herpesvirus or human herpesvirus-8 in transplant patients. Blood 2000;96:3279–81.

102. Barozzi P, Luppi M, Facchetti F, et al. Post-transplant Kaposi sarcoma originates from the seeding of donor-derived progenitors. Nat Med 2003;9:554–61.

103. Andreoni M, Goletti D, Pezzotti P, et al. Prevalence, incidence and correlates of HHV-8/KSHV infection and Kaposi's sarcoma in renal and liver transplant recipients. J Infect 2001;43:195–9.

104. Moore PS. Transplanting cancer: donor-cell transmission of Kaposi sarcoma. Nat Med 2003;9:506–8.

105. Michaels MG, Jenkins FJ. Human herpesvirus 8: is it time for routine surveillance in pediatric solid organ transplant recipients to prevent the development of Kaposi's sarcoma? Pediatr Transplant 2003;7:1–3.

106. Perna AM, Bonura F, Vitale F, et al. Antibodies to human herpes virus type 8 (HHV8) in general population and in individuals at risk for sexually transmitted diseases in Western Sicily. Int J Epidemiol 2000;29:175–9.

107. Whitby D, Luppi M, Sabin C, et al. Detection of antibodies to human herpesvirus 8 in Italian children: evidence for horizontal transmission. Br J Cancer 2000;82:702–4.

108. Bourboulia D, Whitby D, Boshoff C, et al. Serologic evidence for mother-to-child transmission of Kaposi sarcoma-associated herpesvirus infection [letter]. JAMA 1998;280:31–2.

109. Sitas F, Newton R, Boshoff C. Increasing probability of mother-to-child transmission of HHV-8 with increasing maternal antibody titer for HHV-8 [letter]. N Engl J Med 1999;340:1923.

110. Plancoulaine S, Abel L, van Beveren M, et al. Human herpesvirus 8 transmission from mother to child and between siblings in an endemic population. Lancet 2000;356: 1062–5.

111. Davidovici B, Karakis I, Bourboulia D, et al. Seroepidemiology and molecular epidemiology of Kaposi's sarcoma-associated herpesvirus among Jewish population groups in Israel. J Natl Cancer Inst 2001;93:194–202.

112. Mbulaiteye SM, Pfeiffer RM, Whitby D, et al. Human herpesvirus 8 infection within families in rural Tanzania. J Infect Dis 2003;187:1780–5.

113. Cook RD, Hodgson TA, Molyneux EM, et al. Tracking familial transmission of Kaposi's sarcoma-associated herpesvirus using restriction fragment length polymorphism analysis of latent nuclear antigen. J Virol Methods 2002;105:297–303.

114. Cook RD, Hodgson TA, Waugh AC, et al. Mixed patterns of transmission of human herpesvirus-8 (Kaposi's sarcoma-associated herpesvirus) in Malawian families. J Gen Virol 2002;83:1613–9.

115. Sitas F, Carrara H, Beral V, et al. Antibodies against human herpesvirus 8 in black South African patients with cancer. N Engl J Med 1999;340:1863–71.

116. Newton R, Ziegler J, Bourboulia D, et al. The sero-epidemiology of Kaposi's sarcoma-associated herpesvirus (KSHV/HHV-8) in adults with cancer in Uganda. Int J Cancer 2003;103:226–32.

117. Plancoulaine S, Gessain A, van Beveren M, et al. Evidence for a recessive major gene predisposing to human herpesvirus 8 (HHV-8) infection in a population in which HHV-8 is endemic. J Infect Dis 2003;187:1944–50.

118. Rezza G, Lennette ET, Giuliani M, et al. Prevalence and determinants of anti-lytic and anti-latent antibodies to human herpesvirus-8 among Italian individuals at risk of sexually and parenterally transmitted infections. Int J Cancer 1998;77:361–5.

119. Masini C, Abeni DD, Cattaruzza MS, et al. Antibodies against human herpesvirus 8 in subjects with non-venereal dermatological conditions. Br J Dermatol 2000;143:484–90.

120. Bestetti G, Renon G, Mauclere P, et al. High seroprevalence of human herpesvirus-8 in pregnant women and prostitutes from Cameroon [letter]. AIDS 1998;12:541–3.

121. Rezza G, Tchangmena OB, Andreoni M, et al. Prevalence and risk factors for human herpesvirus 8 infection in northern Cameroon. Sex Transm Dis 2000;27:159–64.

122. Baeten JM, Chohan BH, Lavreys L, et al. Correlates of human herpesvirus 8 seropositivity among heterosexual men in Kenya. AIDS 2002;16:2073–8.

123. Lavreys L, Chohan B, Ashley R, et al. Human herpesvirus 8: seroprevalence and correlates in prostitutes in Mombasa, Kenya. J Infect Dis 2003;187:359–63.

124. Eltom MA, Mbulaiteye SM, Dada AJ, et al. Transmission of human herpesvirus 8 by sexual activity among adults in Lagos, Nigeria. AIDS 2002;16:2473–8.

125. Enbom M, Tolfvenstam T, Ghebrekidan H, et al. Seroprevalence of human herpes virus 8 in different Eritrean population groups. J Clin Virol 1999;14:167–72.

126. Wawer MJ, Eng SM, Serwadda D, et al. Prevalence of Kaposi sarcoma-associated herpesvirus compared with selected sexually transmitted diseases in adolescents and young adults in rural Rakai District, Uganda. Sex Transm Dis 2001;28:77–81.

127. Vitale F, Viviano E, Perna AM, et al. Serological and virological evidence of non-sexual transmission of human herpesvirus type 8 (HHV8). Epidemiol Infect 2000;125: 671–5.

128. Marcelin AG, Grandadam M, Flandre P, et al. Kaposi's sarcoma herpesvirus and HIV-1 seroprevalences in prostitutes in Djibouti. J Med Virol 2002;68:164–7.

129. Enbom M, Urassa W, Massambu C, et al. Detection of human herpesvirus 8 DNA in serum from blood donors with HHV-8 antibodies indicates possible bloodborne virus transmission. J Med Virol 2002;68:264–7.

130. Nuvor SV, Katano H, Ampofo WK, et al. Higher prevalence of antibodies to human herpesvirus 8 in HIV-infected individuals than in the general population in Ghana, West Africa. Eur J Clin Microbiol Infect Dis 2001;20:362–4.

131. Hladik W, Dollard SC, Downing RG, et al. Kaposi's sarcoma in Uganda: risk factors for human herpesvirus 8 infection among blood donors. J Acquir Immune Defic Syndr 2003;33:206–10.

132. He J, Bhat G, Kankasa C, et al. Seroprevalence of human herpesvirus 8 among Zambian women of childbearing age without Kaposi's sarcoma (KS) and mother-child pairs with KS. J Infect Dis 1998;178:1787–90.

133. Lampinen TM, Kulasingam S, Min J, et al. Detection of Kaposi's sarcoma-associated herpesvirus in oral and genital secretions of Zimbabwean women. J Infect Dis 2000;181:1785–90.

134. DeSantis SM, Pau CP, Archibald LK, et al. Demographic and immune correlates of human herpesvirus 8 seropositivity in Malawi, Africa. Int J Infect Dis 2002;6:266–9.

135. Gutierrez-Ortega P, Hierro-Orozco S, Sanchez-Cisneros R, Montano LF. Kaposi's sarcoma in a 6-day-old infant with human immunodeficiency virus. Arch Dermatol 1989; 125:432–3.

136. Mantina H, Kankasa C, Klaskala W, et al. Vertical transmission of Kaposi's sarcoma-associated herpesvirus. Int J Cancer 2001;94:749–52.

137. Mbulaiteye SM, Biggar RJ, Bakaki PM, et al. Human herpesvirus 8 infection and transfusion history in children with sickle-cell disease in Uganda. J Natl Cancer Inst 2003;95:1330–5.

138. Oksenhendler E, Cazals-Hatem D, Schulz TF, et al. Transient angiolymphoid hyperplasia and Kaposi's sarcoma after primary infection with human herpesvirus 8 in a patient

with human immunodeficiency virus infection. N Engl J Med 1998;338:1585–90.

139. Luppi M, Barozzi P, Schulz TF, et al. Bone marrow failure associated with human herpesvirus 8 infection after transplantation. N Engl J Med 2000;343:1378–85.

140. Wang QJ, Jenkins FJ, Jacobson LP, et al. Primary human herpesvirus 8 infection generates a broadly specific CD8(+) T-cell response to viral lytic cycle proteins. Blood 2001;97:2366–73.

141. Andreoni M, Sarmati L, Nicastri E, et al. Primary human herpesvirus 8 infection in immunocompetent children. JAMA 2002;287:1295–300.

142. Sanchez-Velasco P, Ocejo-Vinyals JG, Flores R, et al. Simultaneous multiorgan presence of human herpesvirus 8 and restricted lymphotropism of Epstein-Barr virus DNA sequences in a human immunodeficiency virus-negative immunodeficient infant. J Infect Dis 2001;183:338–42.

143. Iscovich J, Boffetta P, Franceschi S, et al. Classic Kaposi sarcoma: epidemiology and risk factors. Cancer 2000;88: 500–17.

144. Davies JNP, Elmes S, Hutt MSR. Cancer in an African community, 1897–1956. An analysis of the records of Mengo Hospital, Kampala, Uganda: Part 1. BMJ 1964;1:259–64.

145. Hutt MSR, Burkitt D. Geographical distribution of cancer in East Africa: a new clinicopathological approach. BMJ 1965;2:719–22.

146. Siegel JH, Janis R, Alper JC, et al. Disseminated visceral Kaposi's sarcoma. Appearance after human renal homograft operation. JAMA 1969;207:1493–6.

147. Penn I. Kaposi's sarcoma in organ transplant recipients: report of 20 cases. Transplantation 1979;27:8–11.

148. Friedman-Kien AE. Disseminated Kaposi's sarcoma syndrome in young homosexual men. J Am Acad Dermatol 1981;5:468–71.

149. Hymes KB, Cheung T, Greene JB, et al. Kaposi's sarcoma in homosexual men: a report of eight cases. Lancet 1981;2:598–600.

150. Hoover DR, Black C, Jacobson LP, et al. Epidemiologic analysis of Kaposi's sarcoma as an early and later AIDS outcome in homosexual men. Am J Epidemiol 1993;138:266–78.

151. Kaplan LD, Northfelt DW. Malignancies associated with AIDS. In: Sande MA, Volberding PA, editors. The medical management of AIDS. Philadelphia: W.B. Saunders; 1997. p. 413–22.

152. Friedman SL, Wright TL, Altman DF. Gastrointestinal Kaposi's sarcoma in patients with acquired immunodeficiency syndrome. Endoscopic and autopsy findings. Gastroenterology 1985;89:102–8.

153. Mitchell DM, McCarty M, Fleming J, Moss FM. Bronchopulmonary Kaposi's sarcoma in patients with AIDS. Thorax 1992;47:726–9.

154. Krown SE, Testa MA, Huang J. AIDS-related Kaposi's sarcoma: prospective validation of the AIDS Clinical Trials Group staging classification. AIDS Clinical Trials Group Oncology Committee. J Clin Oncol 1997;15:3085–92.

155. Tam HK, Zhang ZF, Jacobson LP, et al. Effect of highly active antiretroviral therapy on survival among HIV-infected men with Kaposi sarcoma or non-Hodgkin lymphoma. Int J Cancer 2002;98:916–22.

156. Eltom MA, Jemal A, Mbulaiteye SM, et al. Trends in Kaposi's sarcoma and non-Hodgkin's lymphoma incidence in the United States from 1973 through 1998. J Natl Cancer Inst 2002;94:1204–10.

157. Portsmouth S, Stebbing J, Gill J, et al. A comparison of regimens based on non-nucleoside reverse transcriptase inhibitors or protease inhibitors in preventing Kaposi's sarcoma. AIDS 2003;17:F17–22.

158. Wabinga HR, Parkin DM, Wabwire-Mangen F, Mugerwa JW. Cancer in Kampala, Uganda, in 1989–91: changes in incidence in the era of AIDS. Int J Cancer 1993;54:26–36.

159. Desmond-Hellmann SD, Mbidde EK, Kizito A, et al. The value of a clinical definition for epidemic KS in predicting HIV seropositivity in Africa. J Acquir Immune Defic Syndr 1991;4:647–51.

160. Hill AB. The environment and disease: association or causation? Proc R Soc Med 1965;58:295–300.

161. IARC Working Group. Kaposi's sarcoma herpesvirus/human herpesvirus 8. IARC Monogr Eval Carcinog Risks Hum 1997;70:375–492.

162. Jacobson LP, Jenkins FJ, Springer G, et al. Interaction of human immunodeficiency virus type 1 and human herpesvirus type 8 infections on the incidence of Kaposi's sarcoma. J Infect Dis 2000;181:1940–9.

163. Cannon MJ, Pellett PE. Effect of order of infection with human immunodeficiency virus and human herpesvirus 8 on the incidence of Kaposi's sarcoma. [Comment on: J Infect Dis 2000;181:1940–9 UI: 20298916]. J Infect Dis 2001;183:1304–5.

164. Lehrnbecher TL, Foster CB, Zhu S, et al. Variant genotypes of FcgammaRIIIA influence the development of Kaposi's sarcoma in HIV-infected men. Blood 2000;95:2386–90.

165. Foster CB, Lehrnbecher T, Samuels S, et al. An IL6 promoter polymorphism is associated with a lifetime risk of development of Kaposi sarcoma in men infected with human immunodeficiency virus. Blood 2000;96:2562–7.

166. Dedicoat M, Newton R. Review of the distribution of Kaposi's sarcoma-associated herpesvirus (KSHV) in Africa in relation to the incidence of Kaposi's sarcoma. Br J Cancer 2003;88:1–3.

167. Grossman Z, Iscovich J, Schwartz F, et al. Absence of Kaposi sarcoma among Ethiopian immigrants to Israel despite high seroprevalence of human herpesvirus 8. Mayo Clin Proc 2002;77:905–9.

168. Contu L, Cerimele D, Pintus A, et al. HLA and Kaposi's sarcoma in Sardinia. Tissue Antigens 1984;23:240–5.

169. Touloumi G, Hatzakis A, Potouridou I, et al. The role of immunosuppression and immune-activation in classic Kaposi's sarcoma. Int J Cancer 1999;82:817–21.

170. Goedert JJ, Vitale F, Lauria C, et al. Risk factors for classical Kaposi's sarcoma. J Natl Cancer Inst 2002;94:1712–8.

171. Ziegler J, Newton R, Bourboulia D, et al. Risk factors for Kaposi's sarcoma: a case-control study of HIV-seronegative people in Uganda. Int J Cancer 2003;103:233–40.

172. Ziegler JL. Endemic Kaposi's sarcoma in Africa and local volcanic soils. Lancet 1993;342:1348–51.

173. Soulier J, Grollet L, Oksenhendler E, et al. Kaposi's sarcoma-associated herpesvirus-like DNA sequences in multicentric Castleman's disease. Blood 1995;86:1276–80.

174. Fardet L, Blum L, Kerob D, et al. Human herpesvirus 8-associated hemophagocytic lymphohistiocytosis in human

immunodeficiency virus-infected patients. Clin Infect Dis 2003;37:285–91.

175. Rettig MB, Ma HJ, Vescio RA, et al. Kaposi's sarcoma-associated herpesvirus infection of bone marrow dendritic cells from multiple myeloma patients. Science 1997; 276:1851–4.

176. Parravicini C, Lauri E, Baldini L, Neri A. Kaposi's sarcoma-associated herpesvirus infection and multiple myeloma. Science 1997;278:1969–79.

177. Masood R, Zheng T, Tulpule A, Arora N. Kaposi's sarcoma-associated herpesvirus infection and multiple myeloma. Science 1997;278:1970–71.

178. Whitby D, Boshoff C, Luppi M, Torelli G. Kaposi's sarcoma-associated herpesvirus infection and multiple myeloma. Science 1997;278:1971–2.

179. Ablashi DV, Chatlynne L, Thomas D, et al. Lack of serologic association of human herpesvirus-8 (KSHV) in patients with monoclonal gammopathy of undetermined significance with and without progression to multiple myeloma. Blood 2000;96:2304–6.

180. Brander C, Raje N, O'Connor PG, et al. Absence of biologically important Kaposi sarcoma-associated herpesvirus gene products and virus-specific cellular immune responses in multiple myeloma. Blood 2002;100:698–700.

181. Cool CD, Rai PR, Yeager ME, et al. Expression of human herpesvirus 8 in primary pulmonary hypertension. N Engl J Med 2003;349:1113–22.

182. Hoffman LJ, Bunker CH, Pellett PE, et al. Elevated sero-prevalence of human herpesvirus 8 among men with prostate cancer. J Infect Dis 2004;189:15–20.

183. Cermelli C, Vinceti M, Beretti F, et al. Risk of sporadic amyotrophic lateral sclerosis associated with seropositivity for herpesviruses and echovirus-7. Eur J Epidemiol 2003; 18:123–7.

184. Lennette ET, Blackbourn DJ, Levy JA. Antibodies to human herpesvirus type 8 in the general population and in Kaposi's sarcoma patients. Lancet 1996;348:858–61.

185. Moore PS, Kingsley LA, Holmberg SD, et al. Kaposi's sarcoma-associated herpesvirus infection prior to onset of Kaposi's sarcoma. AIDS 1996;10:175–80.

186. Lefrere JJ, Meyohas MC, Mariotti M, et al. Detection of human herpesvirus 8 DNA sequences before the appearance of Kaposi's sarcoma in human immunodeficiency virus (HIV)-positive subjects with a known date of HIV seroconversion. J Infect Dis 1996;174:283–7.

187. Engels EA, Biggar RJ, Marshall VA, et al. Detection and quantification of Kaposi's sarcoma-associated herpesvirus to predict AIDS-associated Kaposi's sarcoma. AIDS 2003;17:1847–51.

188. Rothman KJ, Greenland S. Causation and causal inference. In: Modern epidemiology. Philadelphia (PA): Lippincott-Raven; 1998. p. 7–28.

189. Foreman KE, Friborg J, Chandran B, et al. Injection of human herpesvirus-8 in human skin engrafted on SCID mice induces Kaposi's sarcoma-like lesions. J Dermatol Sci 2001;26:182–93.

5

Clinical Features and Management of Kaposi's Sarcoma

ROBERTA CINELLI
EMANUELA VACCHER
UMBERTO TIRELLI

Acquired immune deficiency syndrome (AIDS)–related Kaposi's sarcoma (KS) is a mesenchymal tumor involving blood and lymphatic vessels of multifactorial origin and is usually seen in men who have sex with men. Its clinical course is highly variable, ranging from minimal stable disease (presenting as an incidental finding) to explosive growth resulting in significant morbidity and mortality.[1] KS can be diagnosed at any stage of human immunodeficiency virus (HIV) infection although it more commonly occurs in severely immunocompromised patients.[2,3]

CLINICAL FEATURES

KS commonly presents as cutaneous lesions that may occur at any site but usually begin in the head and neck area, upper torso, extremities, oral mucosa, and genitalia. The lesions are often elliptical, are quite symmetric, and may be arranged in a linear fashion along skin tension lines. These lesions are pigmented, their colors including many hues of pink, red, purple, and brown; yellow perilesional halos may occasionally be seen (Figures 5–1 to 5–4). Lesions may arise quickly in a few days, vary in size and shape, and are generally nonpruritic and painless. They can be flat, plaquelike (especially on the soles of the feet and on the thigh), nodular or exophytic, and fungating, with breakdown of overlying skin. Moreover, they can coalesce to form large areas of tumorous involvement (Figure 5–5). These

large lesions are often associated with edema (particularly in the face, genitalia, and lower extremities) that responds poorly to therapy.[1,2,4,5] Lymphedema may also be out of the extent of cutaneous disease and may be related both to vascular obstruction caused by lymphadenopathy and to the cytokines involved in the pathogenesis of KS[1] (Figure 5–6 A and B). Other variants of KS include telangiectatic KS (translucent nodules with prominent telangiectasia), ecchymotic KS (appearing as periorbital ecchymoses with a large number of extravasated red blood cells), keloidal KS (brown-violaceous nodules with a keloidal component), cavernous KS (a rare type of

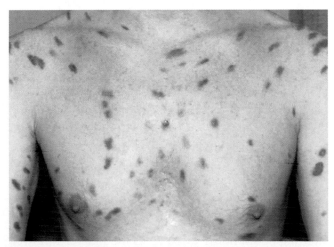

Figure 5–1. Pink KS lesions, mostly macules, on a fair-skinned patient. Courtesy of Susan E. Krown, MD, Memorial Sloan-Kettering Cancer Center.

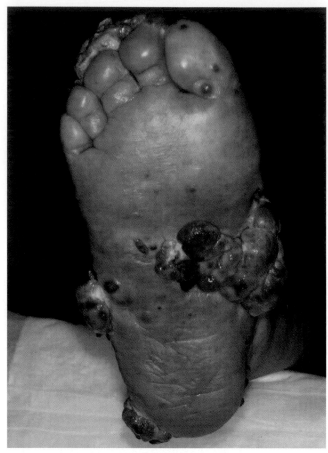

Figure 5–2. Red, nodular KS lesions on the foot of a patient. Courtesy of Susan E. Krown, MD, Memorial Sloan-Kettering Cancer Center.

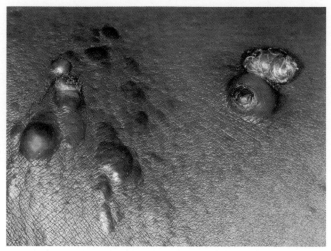

Figure 5–3. Dark brown, nodular KS lesions on the skin of an African American patient. Courtesy of Susan E. Krown, MD, Memorial Sloan-Kettering Cancer Center.

locally aggressive KS that histologically resembles cavernous hemangiomas), and lymphangioma-like KS (a rare variant in which dilated vascular spaces produce a bullous-appearing eruption, typically on the lower legs; the lesions are easily compressible and appear clinically to be fluid filled).[4]

Visible lesions carry a social stigmatization (and an associated psychosocial burden) that can result in emotional distress, guilt, anger, ostracism, and loss of employment.[1,4–6] Moreover, dermal and lymphatic infiltration with KS may result in debilitating and cosmetically unacceptable edema in the periorbital areas, genitals, or extremities, causing difficulty in walking.[4]

Extracutaneous spread of KS is common. The oral cavity is involved in approximately 20% of patients at the time of initial diagnosis[4]; the intraoral site most commonly affected is the palate, followed by the gingiva (Figures 5–7 and 5–8). Although usually asymptomatic, these lesions can cause pain and

discomfort; may become easily traumatized during normal chewing, causing bleeding, ulceration, and secondary infection; and may interfere with nutrition and speech (Figure 5–9).[1,2,4,5,7] Involvement of the oral cavity has been associated with KS in other areas of the gastrointestinal tract.[7] Macular lesions of the conjunctiva may occur, but they are relatively benign.[4] Although a trained observer can often make a presumptive diagnosis of KS quite easily, it is important to confirm the suspicion by a simple skin biopsy because early lesions can be mistaken for purpura, hematomas, angiomas, dermatofibromas, or nevi.[2,5] It is especially important to perform biopsies of lesions that are less typical of KS or that appear or progress rapidly, to rule out bacillary

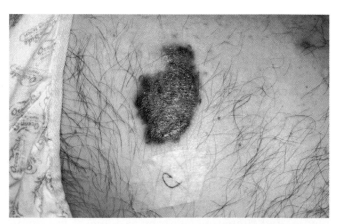

Figure 5–4. Violaceous KS lesion with surrounding yellow-green halo. Courtesy of Susan E. Krown, MD, Memorial Sloan-Kettering Cancer Center.

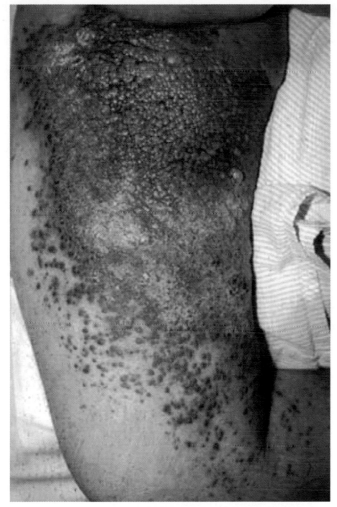

Figure 5–5. Coalesced KS lesions on leg. Courtesy of Susan E. Kraun, MD, Memorial Sloan-Kettering Cancer Center.

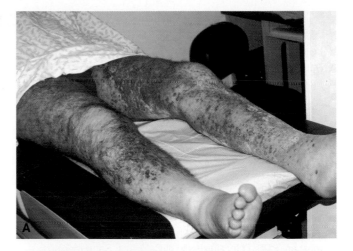

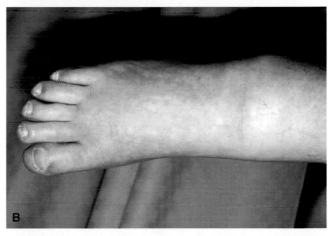

Figure 5–6. *A*, Extensive bilateral lymphedema of the lower extremities with confluent flat plaque-like KS lesions. *B*, Lymphedema of the foot in the same patient as *A*. Courtesy of Susan E. Krown, MD, Memorial Sloan-Kettering Cancer Center.

angiomatosis (BA) (Figures 5–10 A and B). BA is the most important differential diagnosis of KS although KS and BA can occur simultaneously.[5]

Although dermatologic manifestations of KS can be alarming, the involvement of visceral organs is more commonly life threatening because KS causes significant morbidity with organ dysfunction such as lymphatic obstruction, gastrointestinal bleeding, or rapidly progressive pulmonary failure. Other areas such as the pharynx, heart, bone marrow, prostate, testis, bladder, penis, and kidney are less commonly affected.[4]

Visceral involvement in KS occurs in more than 50% of cases although only a subset of patients becomes symptomatic. The gastrointestinal (GI) tract is the most common site of extracutaneous KS[3] and may be found in 40% of cases at initial diagno-

sis and up to 80% of cases at autopsy; involvement can occur in the absence of cutaneous disease.[5] The stomach, colon, or small bowel may all be affected; KS in the liver, spleen, pancreas, and omentum has also been described. When symptomatic, GI KS may present as weight loss, abdominal pain, nausea, vomiting, upper or lower GI tract bleeding, or diarrhea.[1,2,5,8] Testing the stool for occult blood is an excellent way to screen for GI involvement. For patients with occult blood or GI symptoms, further studies are often recommended. Lesions in the GI tract may be recognized quite easily by the endoscopist; they typically appear as hemorrhagic nodules that are either isolated or confluent, and they can be located in any portion of the tract. Since they tend to be submucosal, biopsy specimens may not demonstrate KS.[1,4,5,9]

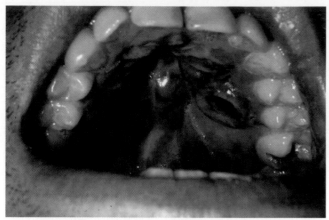

Figure 5–7. KS lesion on the palate. Courtesy of Deborah Greenspan, BDS, DSc, University of California, San Francisco.

Lymph node involvement is not uncommon in KS and may be present in patients without evidence of mucocutaneous disease.[5]

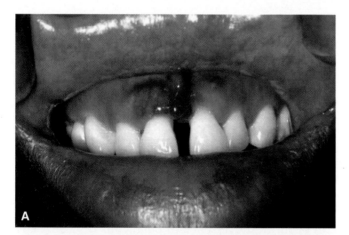

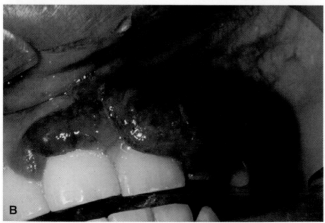

Figure 5–8. *A*, KS lesion of the gingiva. Courtesy of Susan E. Krown, MD, Memorial Sloan-Kettering Cancer Center. *B*, Large KS lesion of the gingiva. Courtesy of Deborah Greenspan, BDS, DSc, University of California, San Francisco.

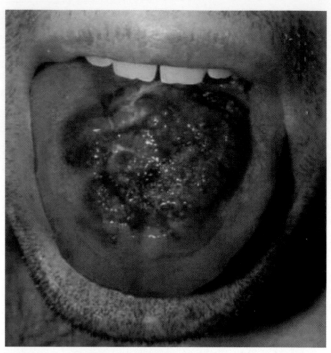

Figure 5–9. KS lesion of the tongue. Courtesy of Susan E. Krown, MD, Memorial Sloan-Kettering Cancer Center.

The pulmonary area is the second most common site of extracutaneous involvement, and pulmonary KS is the most life-threatening form of the disease.[2,10] Pulmonary KS may be difficult to differentiate from other infectious or neoplastic conditions, yet the distinction is essential for without treatment, patients with pulmonary KS have a median survival of only a few months.[11] Even before the introduction of highly active anti-retroviral therapy (HAART), the prevalence of pulmonary KS was uncertain because radiographic changes due to the tumor were often attributed to pulmonary infections.[12] When postmortem examinations have been conducted on HIV-infected patients already known to have cutaneous disease, the prevalence of pulmonary involvement has ranged from 47 to 75%.[13,14] Pulmonary KS in the absence of mucocutaneous disease is generally considered a rare event.[15] The frequency of isolated pulmonary KS has ranged from 0.0 to 15.3%.[13,14,16] The clinical presentation of pulmonary KS is nonspecific and may be indistinguishable from that of pneumonia. Dyspnea and cough are the most common presenting symptoms, but fever, night sweats, hemoptysis, and chest pain may also occur.[1,2,4,5,10] When bleeding occurs, its origin is not

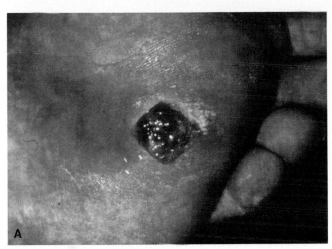 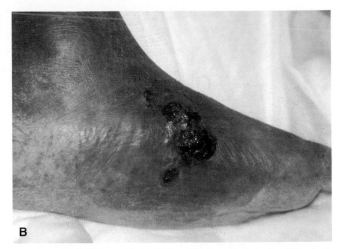

Figure 5–10. Images demonstrating the similarity of KS and bacillary angiomatosis (BA) in the feet. *A,* Bacillary angiomatosis of the foot. *B,* Kaposi's sarcoma lesions of the foot. Reproduced with permission from JW Tappero, JE Koeler. Images in clinical medicine. Bacillary angiomatosis or Kaposi's sarcoma? N Engl J Med 1997;337:1888. Copyright 1997 Massachusetts Medical Society.

always obvious.[8] Hoarseness and stridor are relatively infrequent; when present, they usually connote tumor involvement of the trachea or larynx.[10] Isolated pulmonary KS may present in a variety of fashions ranging from a slow-growing and asymptomatic peripheral nodule without accompanying adenopathy or pleural effusion[17] to a rapidly progressive interstitial infiltrate culminating in acute respiratory failure[18]; it may also be the only cause of persistent fever in a patient with HIV infection.[19] Usually, plain chest radiography reveals thickening along bronchovascular bundles, often emanating from a perihilar origin; as the tumor grows, a reticulonodular infiltrate appears, mainly in the lower lobes. With continued growth, nodules become irregular and confluent, and this, along with interstitial infiltrates, leads to dense airspace consolidation (Figure 5–11). Pleural effusions are present in as many as 50% of cases, and hilar or mediastinal lymphadenopathy is evident in 10 to 60%. The degree of radiographic abnormalities usually correlates with findings on endoscopy.[20] Computed tomography (CT) offers additional benefits over conventional radiography, not only in terms of identifying KS but also in terms of providing greater details regarding other lung diseases. However, these differences are usually modest, and in most patients, conventional radiography can provide adequate information.[10] Gallium-thallium radionuclide imaging is also used to distinguish KS from other pulmonary diseases in

patients with HIV infection; KS is thallium avid but, unlike other infectious or neoplastic disorders, does not take gallium.[21] Direct bronchoscopic inspection of lesions may be the most sensitive technique available to establish a diagnosis of pulmonary KS, but parenchymal lesions may occur in the absence of tracheobronchial lesions. Pleural effusions may be bloody or serosanguineous transudates or exudates. Pleural involvement occurs in the presence of pulmonary lesions; thoracentesis rarely leads to a diagnosis of KS, but it should be performed to rule out the presence of malignancy or infections.[10]

KS is more aggressive and life threatening in women than in men; women have an increased incidence of lymphedema, lymph node disease, and visceral disease, and their overall survival is shorter than that of men.[22] In a series of 54 women and 108 men with AIDS-related KS, Nasti and colleagues found that KS occurred at an earlier age, was associated with a more severe immunodeficiency and more advanced stages of HIV disease, and had a more aggressive presentation in women than in men. At KS diagnosis, women had a significantly increased proportion of visceral disease (particularly pulmonary involvement) and an increase in atypical sites of involvement. The number of deaths due to KS was significantly higher among female patients. In addition, women showed a decreased overall survival rate compared with that of men, and the CD4 cell count at diagnosis significantly influenced their

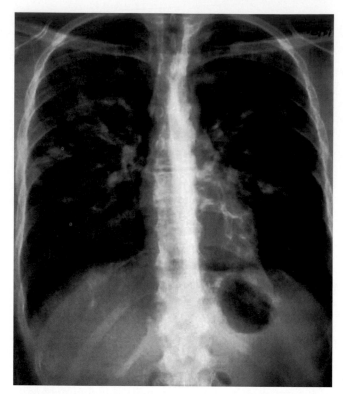

Figure 5–11. Bilateral, patchy lung infiltrates showing pulmonary KS. Courtesy of Susan E. Krown, MD, Memorial Sloan-Kettering Cancer Center.

survival. It remains unclear whether the more aggressive course of KS in women is an intrinsic characteristic of the disease in female patients or whether it is due to other factors, such as hormonal status.[23]

MANAGEMENT

Care for patients with KS has to take into account (1) the type of KS, (2) the extent of the tumor, (3) the organs involved, (4) the potential effect on the patient's overall clinical condition, and (5) virologic, immunologic, and hematologic status.[4]

The initial evaluation of a patient with KS consists of a thorough physical examination with special attention paid to those areas typically affected by the disease. Testing the stool for occult blood is an optimal way to screen for GI involvement; endoscopy can be reserved for those patients with occult blood or with GI symptoms. Similarly, chest radiography is an excellent screening test for pulmonary lesions; bronchoscopy should be reserved for patients with an abnormal film or persistent respiratory symptoms when no other cause has been found. A CD4 cell count and an assessment of HIV viral load are important for staging and initial treatment decisions.[5]

Early trials of various therapeutic agents for KS were impaired by the lack of a uniform staging system. Furthermore, prognosis is related to factors other than the tumor burden itself, such as the patient's underlying immunologic status and the presence of other HIV-related diseases. For this reason, the AIDS Clinical Trials Group devised a staging system in which patients are divided into good-risk and poor-risk categories according to three parameters: extent of tumor (T), immune status (I), and severity of systemic illness (S).[24] This classification has been shown to predict survival: when comparing good-risk patients with poor-risk patients for each of three parameters, respective median survival was 27 versus 15 months according to T, 40 versus 13 months according to I, and 22 versus 16 months according to S.[25]

AIDS-related KS is not currently curable. Moreover, the disease is quite variable, ranging from a very indolent process, requiring close observation and little if any therapy, to a rapidly progressive life-threatening disease. Numerous therapeutic options do exist and must be evaluated to respond to each patient's need. As no curative therapy exists, the primary goal of therapy must be to provide safe and effective palliation. Treatment options depend greatly on the tumor (extent of the disease, rate of growth), the HIV viral load, and the host (CD4 cell count, overall medical conditions). In terms of the host, it is important to assess any impairment in organ function and the potential for drug interactions that may increase overall toxicities. Thus, considering the palliative role of KS therapy, the potential benefits of therapy must be weighed against the high risk of adverse effects. Therefore, quality-of-life assessment becomes an integral component of therapeutic decisions.

Highly Active Anti-retroviral Therapy

The diagnosis of KS should not prompt a reflexive move to treat; for all patients, a critical aspect of tumor control is the optimizing of anti-HIV therapy.[26]

Highly active anti-retroviral therapy (HAART) has profoundly influenced the natural history of

AIDS-related KS. Not only has the incidence of the disease declined sharply since HAART became widely available,[27–37] but HAART has also been associated with a lengthening of the time to treatment failure[38] as well as with a longer survival among patients with pulmonary KS who have undergone chemotherapy.[39] Response of preexisting KS to HAART alone has been documented in up to 86% of patients, a rate exceeding that of most cytotoxic chemotherapy studies.[40] This response is generally durable and gradually increases over time.[26] The underlying mechanisms behind the significant decline in incidence of AIDS-related KS that has resulted from the widespread use of HAART have yet to be elucidated,[27–37] but restored immunity to human herpesvirus 8 (HHV-8), decreased levels of angiogenic factors that stimulate KS proliferation, and direct angiogenesis-inhibiting effects of HIV protease inhibitors may be all involved. Such a direct anti-KS effect has recently been suggested in a study by Sgadari and colleagues, who administrated indinavir or saquinavir (both protease inhibitors) to nude mice, achieving the blocked development and regression of angioproliferative KS-like lesions promoted by primary human KS cells.[41] The effects were mediated by the inhibition of endothelial- and KS-cell invasion and the inhibition of matrix metalloproteinase 2 (MMP-2) proteolytic activation by protease inhibitors at the concentration present in the plasma of treated individuals.[41]

There are a few recent reports about the regression of AIDS-related KS after treatment with HAART using either protease inhibitors (PIs) or nonnucleoside reverse transcriptase inhibitors (NNRTIs).[42–60] Particularly, Cattelan and colleagues[42] found that the clinical response to PI-containing HAART regimens correlated with a decrease in plasma HIV ribonucleic acid levels, an increase in CD4 cell counts, and a decrease in antibodies to ORF65 HHV-8 protein. Nasti and colleagues[61] conducted a retrospective cohort study comparing epidemiologic, clinical, and outcomes data from 160 patients who were naive for HAART at the time of KS diagnosis with the corresponding data from 51 patients who were already undergoing HAART at the time of KS diagnosis; the authors found that immunologic and virologic parameters at the time of

KS diagnosis were significantly more favorable in patients who were already undergoing HAART than in naive patients. The frequency of cutaneous involvement was similar in both groups, but cutaneous disease was more indolent among patients who were already undergoing HAART at the time of KS occurrence. Moreover, a smaller proportion of them presented visceral involvement. In particular, GI involvement was significantly less frequent among patients who were already undergoing HAART at the time of KS diagnosis although the 3-year survival rates of patients already undergoing HAART at the time of KS diagnosis were not significantly different from those of patients who were HAART naive at the time of KS diagnosis. The authors concluded that KS has a less aggressive presentation in patients who are already undergoing HAART when compared with patients who are naive for HAART at KS diagnosis whereas natural history and outcome do not appear to be influenced by the initiation of HAART before the development of KS.

In another study, Tam and colleagues[29] concluded that HAART is associated with improved overall survival even when initiated after the diagnosis of KS and that HAART appears to be effective at prolonging survival independently from the baseline CD4 cell count and other prognostic factors among men with KS.

Immune reconstitution due to HAART may be a reasonable explanation for the observed improvement in survival after HAART treatment. HAART may also lead to an increase in host T-cell immunity to HHV8, which could result in enhanced control of the virus and its oncogenic properties.[62] The evidence that CD8 cytotoxic T-cell response to HHV-8 is lower in HIV-infected people supports this hypothesis.[63–65] Furthermore, Jung and colleagues[66] found that HAART is also effective in enhancing the efficiency of KS cancer treatment. For example, patients on HAART were able to sustain longer courses of chemotherapy without experiencing relapse at its discontinuation.

Although HAART plays an important role, it is often insufficient for patients with aggressive disease; given the potential for aggressive or symptomatic KS to worsen prognosis, tumor-specific therapy may be indicated. There are insufficient data on which to base conclusions about the activity of

HAART in patients with advanced symptomatic disease. In most prospective studies, patients with advanced KS either received chemotherapy from the outset of HAART or had chemotherapy added after the KS failed to respond to HAART alone. The KS lesions of such patients regressed less often and more slowly than did the lesions of patients with less severe KS who received only HAART. Once KS regression is achieved with a combination of HAART and systemic KS therapy, however, chemotherapy can be withdrawn.[67] Vaccher and colleagues described the case of a patient whose stage T1 KS progressed during initial HAART despite the suppression of HIV viral load and an increase in the CD4 cell count. Chemotherapy was then added, and a partial remission was achieved. On the discontinuation of tumor-specific therapy, residual lesions regressed completely with the only use of HAART during the subsequent 5 months.[68]

Although HAART is an important component of KS treatment, evidence that HAART induces regression of advanced symptomatic KS without concomitant specific tumor treatment is scant. Nevertheless, for patients with limited KS and who have not undergone HAART previously, it is appropriate to require an extended period of stable HAART before initiating new KS treatments.[67]

Local Treatment

Tumor treatment may be locally applied to patients with limited and accessible lesions. Such treatment includes surgical excision; cryotherapy with liquid nitrogen; laser therapy; radiotherapy; local injection with vinblastine, vincristine, or bleomycin; and the use of alitretinoin gel 0.1% (9-cis-retinoic acid). With any local modality, there is generally residual evidence of the disease process. The chosen modality depends mainly on the expected adverse effects of the intervention. Alitretinoin gel 0.1% is the only topical patient-administered therapy approved for KS treatment. It is a naturally occurring retinoid that binds to both retinoic acid receptors and to retinoid-X receptors. In a phase III study, alitretinoin, when compared with vehicle gel, was associated with a shorter time to tumor response, a more prolonged duration of response, and a more prolonged time to

disease progression. Most patients required 4 to 8 weeks of treatment before response was seen, and response appeared in patients with a wide range of baseline CD4 cell counts. Dermal irritation, generally mild or moderate, was a common side effect. Dark-skinned patients may occasionally experience fastidious skin lightening.[69]

Radiotherapy is an important treatment in the local management of KS. Whole-body electron beam therapy, fractionated focal radiation therapy in doses of up to 4,500 cGy, and single-dose treatments of 800 cGy produced complete remissions in 50 to 80% of patients. However, postradiation hyperpigmentation remained in 20% of lesions, and 10% of patients had local recurrences. Treatment of the oral cavity and pharynx has resulted in unexpectedly severe mucositis in some HIV-positive patients, and treatment of large volumes of the skin has led to the development of lymphedema.[70–73] Late complications of radiation therapy include fibrosis, ulceration, and superinfections. Large-field irradiation must be used cautiously, especially in the lower extremities; even with low doses, considerable brawny induration may develop in the treatment fields within months. This phenomenon occurs at a much lower dose than would be expected in the setting of HIV-negative patients.[74] Complications of radiation therapy may take many months to appear and may be aggravated by subsequent therapies such as doxorubicin-containing regimens.[75] To find the best dosage regimen, Stelzer and Griffin, in a prospective randomized trial, treated patients' KS lesions with one of three regimens: 800 cGy in a single fraction, 20 Gy in 10 fractions, or 40 Gy in 20 fractions. Complete-response rates and duration of disease control were superior in the two higher-dose arms. Lesions treated with the highest doses showed a complete-remission rate of 79 to 83% whereas the complete-remission rate for the 800 cGy arm was only 50%. No differences in acute toxicity were seen between the three arms, and late toxicity was reported only in the high-dose arm.[76] In general, a single dose of 800 cGy is effective in reducing symptoms associated with KS in patients with advanced disease whereas a fractionated course is more suitable for patients with more extensive disease and a longer life expectancy.

Intralesional injections of vinblastine, vincristine, bleomycin, and interferon-α (IFN-α) have been reported to be effective local treatments of KS.[77–79] Vinblastine is probably the most widely used intralesional agent and yields a response rate of 70%[80]; the only adverse effects are local pain and skin irritation. Intralesional injection of β human chorionic gonadotropin (β-hCG) has been shown to be useful in the local treatment of small lesions in a dose-dependent manner. In a phase I-to-II trial, 24 patients received intralesional injections of β-hCG three times per week for 2 weeks at doses of 250, 500, 1,000, and 2,000 IU (six patients each). There was complete resolution of KS lesions in 10 of 12 patients receiving the higher-dosage regimens. Treatment was well tolerated at all dosages.[81]

Interferon

IFN-α is a biologic response modifier that can produce clinically significant responses in KS patients, especially those patients with disease limited to the skin and with relatively modest degrees of immunosuppression.[82] IFN-α has multiple effects on cell proliferation, angiogenesis, immune function, and gene expression, as well as antiviral effects that are important in the control of KS. Recently, IFN-α was also shown to inhibit HHV-8 lytic viral reactivation in latently infected cultured peripheral-blood mononuclear cells and to reduce HHV-8 viral load in cultured peripheral-blood mononuclear cells from KS patients.[83] IFN-α inhibits endothelial cell proliferation and has been shown to inhibit the proliferation of KS-derived spindle cells by down-regulation of c-*myc* expression.[84]

Many trials of IFN-α in KS treatment have been conducted in the past 20 years. Tumor regression has been documented in many trials that used either recombinant or lymphoblastoid IFN-α administered daily or three times a week.[85–94] These studies also demonstrated that high doses of IFN-α ($\geq$ 20 million U/m^2 of body surface) were superior to lower doses; objective tumor response rates ranging from 18 to 46% were observed for patients treated with higher doses of IFN-α whereas response rates of < 10% were observed for patients treated with doses ranging from 1.0 to 7.5 million U/m^2.[85–94]

The first sign of tumor regression is usually noted within 4 to 8 weeks, but maximal responses generally require 6 or more months of treatment. The optimal duration of IFN-α treatment is unknown. Factors associated with a poor response to IFN-α therapy include prior opportunistic infections, the presence of systemic symptoms, and a CD4 cell count of < 200 cells/mm^3.[74]

Adverse events usually consist of myelosuppression, hepatic abnormalities, flulike symptoms (fever, chills, myalgias, anorexia, fatigue), psychiatric disorders, and moderate hair loss.

For some patients with asymptomatic but relatively disseminated disease, IFN-α in combination with anti-retroviral agents may be a reasonable option before starting other more toxic treatments such as chemotherapy.

Chemotherapy

For patients with edema, extensive mucocutaneous disease, or symptomatic pulmonary or GI involvement, systemic chemotherapy is appropriate and is generally well tolerated.

Several single agents have been reported to be active in AIDS-related KS; these include the vinca alkaloids vincristine and vinblastine, the anthracyclines doxorubicin and epirubicin, the epipodophyllotoxins etoposide and teniposide, and bleomycin.[95] Although many of these older chemotherapeutic agents have been found to be active against KS both as single agents and in combination, the current chemotherapy for KS revolves around the newer liposomal anthracyclines and paclitaxel. A randomized phase III trial was conducted to compare the safety and efficacy of liposomal daunorubicin at 40 mg/m^2 with that of the Adriamycin (doxorubicin)/bleomycin/vincristine (ABV) regimen (doxorubicin, 10 mg/m^2; bleomycin, 15 U; and vincristine, 1 mg), administered intravenously every 2 weeks. Concomitant HAART was permitted. Overall response rates (25% for liposomal daunorubicin and 28% for ABV), time to treatment failure, and overall survival were similar for both groups. This trial's results confirm that liposomal daunorubicin is effective in the treatment of AIDS-related KS (as is the ABV regimen) but is associated with significantly less alopecia and neuropathy and produces no evidence of cardiac adverse events.[96]

Polyethylene glycol (PEG)/liposomal doxorubicin is a formulation in which doxorubicin is encapsulated in PEG-coated liposomes. This alters the drug's pharmacokinetic properties, prolonging circulation time and enhancing its localization to tumors.[97] This selective increased drug delivery to the tumors was shown to result in a significant improvement in therapeutic efficacy, with no increase in adverse effects. Whereas liposomal daunorubicin has a half-life of approximately 8 hours, the liposome in liposomal doxorubicin is additionally modified with the addition of PEG, which reduces uptake by the reticuloendothelial system and results in a half-life of approximately 30 hours.[98]

PEG/liposomal doxorubicin (20 mg/m^2) administered as monotherapy every 2 or 3 weeks for up to 6 cycles produced overall response rates ranging from 46 to 88% in studies involving 79 to 258 patients.[99,100] The reported duration of response was 90 to 142 days. PEG/liposomal doxorubicin is at least as effective as bleomycin plus vincristine (BV regimen) at producing a response,[100] and it produced a significantly higher overall response rate than did the standard ABV regimen).[99] In one study, involving 241 patients, Stewart and colleagues found that PEG/liposomal doxorubicin (20 mg/m^2) as monotherapy every 2 or 3 weeks produced a significantly higher overall response than that produced by the BV regimen (59% versus 23%).[100]

High peak plasma concentrations and lifetime cumulative doses of standard doxorubicin are thought to be important factors contributing to the cardiotoxicity of the drug. The risk of developing impaired myocardial function is estimated to be 5 to 8% at a total cumulative dose of 450 mg/m^2; above this level, the incidence of congestive heart failure increases. PEG/liposomal doxorubicin is less cardiotoxic than standard doxorubicin because after PEG/liposomal doxorubicin administration, very little drug circulates freely in plasma, and this formulation does not as readily traverse the continuous capillaries in myocardial tissue.[97]

In randomized trials, the percentage of patients experiencing a reduction of left ventricular ejection fraction greater than 20% appeared to be lower with PEG/liposomal doxorubicin than with the ABV regimen (4.3% versus 9.1%); however, cardiotoxicity appeared to be more common with PEG/liposomal doxorubicin than with the BV regimen (1.7% versus 0.8%).[100] Quite recently, some investigators used cardiac biopsies to evaluate doxorubicin-induced cardiac damage in KS patients treated with PEG/liposomal doxorubicin. PEG/liposomal doxorubicin produced significantly lower cardiac histopathologic changes than did standard doxorubicin; the median endomyocardial biopsy score from 10 patients who had received a mean cumulative dose of PEG/liposomal doxorubicin of 623 mg/m^2 was significantly lower than the median biopsy score from 10 historical patients with various types of cancer who were matched by cumulative standard doxorubicin dose (mean, 565 mg/m^2) (0.3% versus 3.0%).[101]

The overall incidences of adverse events associated with PEG/liposomal doxorubicin and BV or ABV do not appear to differ. However, fewer early withdrawals because of adverse events occurred with PEG/liposomal doxorubicin than with BV (10.7% versus 26.7%), and there were differences between regimens with regard to specific events. PEG/liposomal doxorubicin was associated with significantly less constipation and paresthesia than was BV and with significantly less grade 3 or 4 nausea and vomiting, alopecia, and peripheral neuropathy than was ABV. Instead, PEG/liposomal doxorubicin was associated with significantly more opportunistic infections, and grade 3 or 4 mucositis and stomatitis than was BV, and it produced a significantly higher incidence of leukopenia than did BV and ABV.[99,100]

PEG/liposomal doxorubicin has been shown to be better than ABV and BV at improving some aspects of quality of life and at producing clinical benefits for KS patients. The effect of PEG/liposomal doxorubicin, as compared with ABV, on health-related quality of life was assessed in a randomized study, and the results were published separately.[99,102] From baseline to the end of treatment, KS patients treated with PEG/liposomal doxorubicin improved significantly in the domains of pain, cognitive functioning, social functioning, and health distress whereas KS patients treated with ABV deteriorated significantly in the fatigue domain. The duration of response was longer in KS patients treated with PEG/liposomal doxorubicin than in patients treated with ABV; nearly 40% of those treated with PEG/liposomal doxorubicin who achieved a clinically significant change in overall score for quality of life maintained this response for 70 days, compared with none of the patients treated with ABV.[102]

A combination of HAART and liposomal anthracycline chemotherapy thus represents the standard of care for advanced AIDS-related KS despite concerns that chemotherapy could adversely affect lymphocyte subset and HIV viral load. Esdaile and colleagues demonstrated that liposomal anthracyclines together with HAART did not lead to a significant loss of CD4 or CD8 cells or to an increase in HIV-1 viremia during chemotherapy or up to 12 months after chemotherapy.[103]

Paclitaxel is a cytotoxic agent for which there is evidence of antitumor efficacy in KS patients; it exerts its antitumor activity by several mechanisms, most prominently by polymerizing microtubules, inhibiting cell division and inducing cell death.[104] Paclitaxel has also been shown to inhibit angiogenesis in preclinical models.[105,106] Some studies have shown that paclitaxel concentrations that are lower than those used for other tumor types may induce tumor cell death in KS models.[107]

Neutropenia is the primary dose-limiting adverse event during chemotherapy with paclitaxel; a reduction in the neutrophil count is usually observed by day 8, the nadir occurring on days 8 to 11. Neutropenia is not cumulative in most patients. Neutrophil count nadirs usually remain unchanged during subsequent courses of chemotherapy, suggesting that paclitaxel does not produce irreversible stem cell toxicity. Recovery generally occurs by days 15 to 21. Peripheral neuropathy may also be severe and occasionally dose limiting. Hypersensitivity reactions, dyspnea, hypotension, and angioedema have also occurred, so that patients have to receive premedication with steroids and antihistamines. Other adverse events include alopecia, arthralgia, myalgia, GI disturbances, mucositis, bradycardia and cardiac conduction irregularities, rashes, and elevated liver enzyme levels.[74] Paclitaxel is quite well tolerated, but the higher prevalence of alopecia, myalgias, arthralgias and bone marrow suppression, together with the need for a 3-hour infusion, make it less attractive than liposomal anthracyclines as initial therapy for disseminated disease.

Recommended dosing schedules for paclitaxel are 100 mg/m^2 over 3 hours every 2 weeks or 135 mg/m^2 over 3 hours every 3 weeks.[108–111] The usual regimens of premedication include diphenydramine and ranitidine plus dexamethasone.

Objective response rates to paclitaxel range from 56 to 71% in some trials involving pretreated patients with disseminated disease, and the median duration of response ranges from 7.4 to 10.4 months.[108–111] Neither TIS stage nor site of disease affected response to therapy, and major response rates were similar when patients who were not on a PI at the time of response were compared with patients who were on a PI at the time of response. Conversely, PI use had an impact on time to disease progression, on time to treatment failure, and on survival.[110] Response to paclitaxel therapy correlates with a fall in plasma levels of interleukin (IL)-6 but correlates poorly with known angiogenic cytokines.[111] These studies lead us to conclude that paclitaxel is effective and quite well tolerated in the treatment of advanced and previously treated patients with AIDS-related KS.

Drug metabolism of many of the approved antiretroviral agents, particularly PIs and NNRTIs, involves cytochrome P-450 metabolic pathways. Taxanes are oxidized to less active metabolites by hepatic cytochrome P-450 enzymes. Toxicities noted in some patients receiving paclitaxel have been ascribed to a toxic interaction between this drug and HAART, so that caution is urged when agents that use the same metabolic pathways are coadministered.

Although liposomal anthracyclines and paclitaxel induce high response rates, responding subjects often relapse and some patients fail to respond; thus, new therapeutic interventions are needed. Etoposide was one of the first drugs shown to be active against AIDS-related KS, and Evans and colleagues treated 36 high-risk KS patients with oral etoposide (50 mg per day) for 7 consecutive days every 2 weeks. All patients' disease had relapsed or progressed after previous combination chemotherapy or anthracycline therapy. For patients without a complete or partial response after two cycles of therapy and no toxicities greater than grade 2, the dose of etoposide was raised to 100 mg per day orally on days 1 to 7 of each 14-day cycle. The overall objective response rate was 36.1%, and the median time to response was 17.7 weeks. Toxicities were mild to moderate and consisted of fever, agitation, irregular cardiac rhythm, difficulty with concentration, paresthesias, diarrhea, nausea, and mucositis. Both treatment response and toxicities were linked to changes in specific areas of quality of life; except for appearance, all scales worsened for nonresponders. Only symptoms of distress worsened for responders, and all changes were more favorable for responders than for nonresponders. The authors concluded that low-dose chronic administration of etoposide may be a useful option for patients with progressive or refractory KS after chemotherapy with liposomal anthracyclines or paclitaxel and that oral etoposide may be of greater value in underdeveloped areas of the world, in which an effective, minimally toxic, and easily administered therapeutic agent may be of particular importance.[112]

Other Agents

Because chemotherapeutic approaches are not curative and because all are associated with toxicity, there is an interest in pathogenesis-based approaches that may be more selective for the tumor.

Thalidomide shows a range of activities that could influence the growth of KS lesions. It has been shown to inhibit both basic fibroblast growth factor–induced and vascular endothelial growth factor (VEGF)–induced angiogenesis in models of corneal vascularization,[113] an effect that requires species-dependent metabolic activation.[114] The inhibition of vascular endothelial cell proliferation induced by thalidomide occurs in association with a marked decrease in the activity of nuclear factor-SP1, a transcription factor involved in the expression of extracellular matrix genes, and moderate inhibition of nuclear factor-κB activation in nuclear extracts.[115] The blockade of nuclear factor-κB activation involves inhibition of the activity of the IκB kinase and is associated with inhibition of the cytokine-induced expression of nuclear factor-κB–regulated genes.[116]

Thalidomide-induced regression of KS has been documented in some studies.[117–119] The first report was about a single patient whose KS was shown to regress during thalidomide treatment for aphthous stomatitis and who had a clearance of HHV-8 deoxyribonucleic acid from blood.[117] In the second study, the authors treated 17 patients with a once-nightly dose of thalidomide (100 mg) for 8 weeks and observed a partial remission in 35% of patients.[118] The last study used escalating daily doses of thalidomide, beginning with a nightly dose of 200 mg and increasing the dose at 2-week intervals to a maximum of 1,000 mg, according to patients' tolerance; 47% of patients achieved a partial response, which lasted a median of 7.1 months.[119] Toxicities included depression, fever, rash, and neurologic toxicity. The results of these small studies suggest that there may be a role for thalidomide in KS treatment.

Several retinoids have activity in AIDS-related KS. As discussed above, alitretinoin gel 0.1% (9-*cis*-retinoic acid) is the only topical patient-administered therapy approved for KS treatment. In an attempt to discover new effective drugs against KS, Miles and colleagues treated 66 KS patients with once-daily oral 9-*cis*-retinoic acid at doses up to 140 mg/m^2 (most patients received a maximum dose of 100 mg/m^2). They achieved a tumor response rate of 37%, and it was associated with an improvement in quality-of-life measures. The median time to response was 9 weeks. The main adverse events were headache and skin toxicity.[120]

Bernstein and colleagues treated 76 AIDS-related KS patients with escalating doses of liposomal tretinoin (all-*trans*-retinoic acid) administered once or three times weekly. Patients were randomized to receive the study drug once or three times weekly. The starting dose was 60 mg/m^2; this was raised to 90 mg/m^2 and then to 120 mg/m^2 if the drug was well tolerated (≤ grade II toxicity). Four weeks of therapy constituted one cycle, and patients could receive up to eight cycles. Those who completed the eight cycles were given the option to receive extended therapy; 28.9% of patients responded (no complete remissions). Concomitant or prior use of HAART containing PIs did not appear to affect patients' response to treatment.[121]

The biologic effects of retinoids in KS are mediated by retinoic acid receptors and retinoid-X receptors, which belong to the superfamily of steroid/thyroid hormone nuclear receptors. The nuclear receptor for 1-α,25-dihydroxyvitamin D$_3$ (the active form of vitamin D$_3$), or the vitamin D$_3$ receptor (VDR), also belongs to the steroid/thyroid hormone nuclear receptor superfamily. 1-α,25-dihydroxyvitamin D$_3$ is an important regulator of cell growth and differentiation of various cell types,[122,123] and it inhibits the production of IL-6 and IL-8 in cultured keratinocytes.[124–126] Because IL-6 and IL-8 are autocrine growth factors for KS cells,[127] Masood and colleagues sought to determine whether a VDR agonist would inhibit the growth of KS cells in vitro and in vivo. They determined that 1-α,25-dihydroxyvitamin D$_3$ inhibits the growth of KS cells in vitro by inhibiting the production of both IL-6 and IL-8. They also showed that a synthetic VDR agonist, calcipotriol, has antitumor effects in patients with KS.[128] 1-α,25-dihydroxyvitamin D$_3$ and its analogues may thus be candidates for clinical development in KS patients.

A phase I clinical study was conducted to evaluate toxicity, pharmacokinetics, and tumor response of the angiogenesis inhibitor TNP-470 among patients with early AIDS-related KS. Thirty-eight patients received TNP-470 by weekly intravenous infusion over 1 hour at one of six dose levels for up to 24 weeks. The dose levels tested included 10, 20, 30, 40, 50, and 70 mg/m^2. Eighteen percent of patients achieved a partial response; the median time to response was 4 weeks, and the median duration of response was 11 weeks. Tumor response was observed in a substantial number of cases and occurred at various dose levels. Adverse events included neutropenia, hemorrhage, and urticaria.[129] Thus, TNP-470 should be evaluated further for patients with AIDS-related KS, both as a single agent and in combination with other biologic response modifiers in early disease or after an initial response to chemotherapy.

IM-862 is a dipeptide of L-glutamyl-L-tryptophan that was initially isolated from the thymus. It has been produced synthetically, and preclinical studies have shown that the dipeptide inhibits angiogenesis in chorioallantoic membrane assays. IM-862 mediates these effects by inhibiting the production of VEGF and by activating natural killer cell function. In animal studies using IM-862 and in which intranasal, subcutaneous, intravenous, and intramuscular administration routes were investigated, no difference in antitumor activity was observed among these routes of administration.[130] Intranasal administration allowed a bioavailability of 71%, so it has been chosen for human trials. Tulpule and colleagues treated 44 patients with advanced AIDS-related KS, using IM-862 as intranasal drops at a dose of 5 mg. Patients were randomized to two dosing schedules given in repeated cycles until disease progression or toxicity: (1) 5 days of therapy followed by 5 days off and (2) daily dosing. Major responses, occurring after a median of 6 weeks, were documented in 36% of patients. Adverse events were limited to mild and transient headache, fatigue, tingling, and nausea, without any hematologic adverse events.[131]

Matrix metalloproteinases (MMPs) are a family of zinc-dependent endopeptidases that are involved in the destruction of extracellular matrix proteins.[132] MMPs may be divided into three classes, based on their substrate specificity: collagenases, gelatinases, and stromelysins. MMP-2 (gelatinase A) and MMP-9 (collagenase B) degrade collagen type IV, which is the major component of basement membranes and is involved in tumor invasion and metastases.[133–135] MMP-2 and MMP-9 are constitutively overexpressed in KS cells.[136] Naturally occurring tissue matrix metalloproteinase inhibitors (MMPIs) have been shown to inhibit tumor cell invasion and angiogenesis.[137] 6-Demethyl-6-deoxy-4-dedimethylaminotetracycline (COL-3) is a chemically modified tetracycline; it inhibits the in vitro activity of activated neutrophil gelatinase and the expression of MMPs in human colon and breast carcinoma cell lines in a dose-dependent manner. Moreover, it inhibits the invasion of multiple carcinoma cell lines into Matrigel and the invasiveness of a human melanoma cell line through basement membrane matrix. The potential of COL-3 to inhibit the activity, activation, and production of MMPs distinguishes it from other MMPIs, which target only the active enzyme.[138] Cianfrocca and colleagues[139] used a daily oral schedule of COL-3 to assess its safety and antitumor activity in patients with AIDS-related KS. They treated 18 patients, using COL-3 in dosing cohorts of 25, 50, and 70 mg/m^2/d. Almost all of the patients had received previous KS therapy. The overall response rate was 44%, and the median duration of response was 25 weeks. There was a significant difference between responders and nonresponders with respect to the change in MMP-2 serum levels from baseline to minimum value on treatment. Adverse events included photosensitivity, rash, and headache. Photosensitivity was dose related.[139] This study supports further evaluation of COL-3 as a single agent for patients with early KS and in combination with other agents for patients with more advanced disease.

The positive activity of β human chorionic gonadotropin (β-hCG) on tumorigenesis and metastasis of the KS cell line in immunodeficient mice has been described.[140] Since that trial, some small clinical studies have been performed to test the antitumor activity of β-hCG; the results of these trials conflict.

Harris and colleagues first achieved marked tumor regression by treating six patients with escalating doses of human chorionic gonadotropin (between 150,000 and 700,000 IU for intramuscular administration) thrice weekly.[141] Conversely, Tirelli and colleagues did not find any evidence of activity when treating 13 patients with human chorionic gonadotropin in doses ranging from 4,000 to 32,000 IU thrice weekly for 4 months and from 100,000 to 300,000 IU thrice weekly for 3 months.[142] Major adverse events were malaise, fatigue, ascites, impaired renal function, and anemia. At present, β-hCG has shown limited efficacy in KS patients and also the potential to produce serious adverse events, so it should not be recommended outside of investigational trials.

Anti-HHV-8 Therapy

The discovery of HHV-8 as the etiologic agent for KS has raised the hypothesis of using antiviral agents as treatment or prophylaxis of AIDS-related KS. Sensitivity studies have shown HHV-8 to be resistant to acyclovir and penciclovir and susceptible to ganciclovir, cidofovir, adefovir, and foscarnet.[143,144] On the basis of these in vitro results, patients with KS who are treated for cytomegalovirus disease had a significantly longer time to progression of the existing KS if they received foscarnet instead of ganciclovir.[145] Conversely, patients with cytomegalovirus disease who received oral ganciclovir had a decreased risk of developing KS, suggesting a prophylactic effect.[146] In this trial, patients were randomized to receive either a ganciclovir retinal implant alone or the implant with additional systemic ganciclovir. Patients randomized to receive systemic ganciclovir had a statistically decreased risk of developing KS over time. The hypothesis that lytic HHV-8 infection could be treated with ganciclovir and that such treatment could have a positive effect on the development of KS is very interesting, and further work is expected.

Risks and Benefits

In AIDS-related KS, for which only palliative treatments are available, knowledge of the adverse effects of drugs and their impact on quality of life is of particular importance in assessing the role of drugs in disease management.

Treatment of KS presents several problems, such as the presence of widespread aggressive disease in some patients, the presence of opportunistic infections that complicate the administration of chemotherapy, and the presence of a HIV-related myelodysplastic disease that makes the administration of immunosuppressive drugs difficult. Moreover, in regard to KS therapy, the integration of antiviral therapy with other kinds of therapy can be foreseen.

To obtain the highest benefit-risk ratio, KS treatment has to be individualized on the basis of the patient's overall clinical and immunologic status as well as the toxic profile of concomitant HAART therapy.

All patients who are not receiving HAART and who develop mild, moderate, or asymptomatic KS should be treated with HAART as a first option.

Immediate therapeutic intervention is unnecessary for a patient with stable or slowly progressive cutaneous disease and no cosmetic complications.

Local therapy is suitable for patients with few lesions, particularly if they are causing emotional or physical distress. The modality chosen depends mainly on the expected adverse effects of intervention. When radiation therapy is used, the clinicians have to consider that no single dosage schedule is appropriate for all patients, and so doses and schedules of treatment depend on life expectancies and the extent of the lesions. Prolonged follow-up after irradiation is mandatory because complications may occur after some months and can be worsened by subsequent systemic chemotherapies.

For patients with moderately extensive cutaneous or mucosal disease and a CD4 cell count > 200 cells/mm^3, immunotherapy with IFN-α and HAART is indicated.

Systemic chemotherapy is necessary for patients with aggressive, extensive, and rapidly progressive mucocutaneous disease or with symptomatic visceral involvement. Liposomal anthracyclines are the first-line drugs for treating KS; liposomal daunorubicin has shown the best benefit-risk ratio at a dosage of 40 mg/m^2 every 2 weeks whereas liposomal doxorubicin has shown the best benefit-risk ratio at a dosage of 20 mg/m^2 every 2 or 3 weeks.

Paclitaxel at dosages of 100 mg/m^2 every 2 weeks or 135 mg/m^2 every 3 weeks is another suitable option for KS treatment. Institution or continuation of effective HAART and prophylaxis of opportunistic infections should be recommended for all patients receiving chemotherapy. In choosing an effective HAART regimen, clinicians must give attention to potential drug interactions and agents that do not alter the metabolism of cytotoxic agents.

KS is a multifactorial disorder, resulting from the interaction of various factors such as HHV-8 infection and underlying immunosuppression, occurring within the setting of an abnormal cytokine milieu and angiogenic peptides. Whereas traditional chemotherapeutic approaches may be effective for patients with disseminated or aggressive disease, newer concepts of therapy target factors associated with the pathogenesis of the disease, which may be better in terms of benefit-risk ratio.

REFERENCES

1. Dezube BJ. Acquired immunodeficiency syndrome–related Kaposi's sarcoma: clinical features, staging and treatment. Semin Oncol 2000;27:424–30.
2. Levine AM, Tulpule A. clinical aspects and management of AIDS-related Kaposi's sarcoma. Eur J Can 2001;37:1288–95.
3. Tappero JW, Conant MA, Wolfe SF, et al. Kaposi's sarcoma: epidemiology, pathogenesis, histology, clinical spectrum, staging criteria and therapy. J Am Acad Dermatol 1993;28:371–95.
4. Hengge UR, Ruzicka T, Tyring SK, et al. Update on Kaposi's sarcoma and other HHV8 associated diseases. Part 1: epidemiology, environmental predispositions, clinical manifestations and therapy. Lancet Infect Dis 2002;2:281–92.
5. Dezube BJ. Management of AIDS-related Kaposi's sarcoma:
advances in target discovery and treatment. Expert Rev Anticancer Ther 2002;2:89–96.
6. Holland JC, Tross S. Psychosocial considerations in the therapy of epidemic Kaposi's sarcoma. Semin Oncol 1987;14(2 Suppl 3):48–53.
7. Ficarra G, Berson AM, Silverman SJ, et al. Kaposi's sarcoma of the oral cavity: a study of 134 patients with a review of the pathogenesis, epidemiology, clinical aspects and treatment. Oral Surg Oral Med Oral Pathol 1998;66:543–50.
8. Danzig JB, Brandt LJ, Reinus JF, Klein RS. Gastrointestinal malignancy in patients with AIDS. Am J Gastroenterol 1991;86:715–8.
9. Ioachim HL, Adsay V, Giancotti FR, et al. Kaposi's sarcoma of internal organs. A multiparameter study of 86 cases. Cancer 1995;75:1376–85.
10. Aboulafia DM. The epidemiologic, pathologic and clinical features of AIDS-associated pulmonary Kaposi's sarcoma. Chest 2000;117:1128–45.
11. Garay SM, Belenko M, Fazzini E, et al. Pulmonary manifestations of Kaposi's sarcoma. Chest 1987;91:39–43.
12. Pothoff G, Pohler E, Diekmann M, et al. Difficulties in the diagnosis of AIDS-associated intrapulmonary Kaposi's sarcoma. Pneumologie 1990;44:74–7.
13. Lemlich G, Schwam L, Lebwhol M. Kaposi's sarcoma in acquired immunodeficiency syndrome: postmortem findings in twenty-four cases. J Am Acad Dermatol 1987;16:319–25.
14. Miller RF, Tomlinson NC, Cottril CP, et al. Bronchopulmonary Kaposi's sarcoma in patients with AIDS. Thorax 1992;47:721–5.
15. Fouret PJ, Touboul JL, Maynaoud CM, et al. Pulmonary Kaposi's sarcoma in patients with acquired immunodeficiency syndrome: a clinicopathological study. Thorax 1987;42:262–8.
16. Huang L, Schnapp LM, Gruden JF, et al. Presentation of AIDS-related pulmonary Kaposi's sarcoma diagnosed by bronchoscopy. Am J Respir Crit Care Med 1996;153:1385–90.
17. Gruden JF, Huang L, Webb WR, et al. AIDS-related Kaposi's sarcoma of the lung: radiographic findings and staging system with bronchoscopy correlation. Radiology 1995;195:545–52.
18. Roux FJ, Bancal C, Dombret MC, et al. Pulmonary Kaposi's sarcoma revealed by a solitary nodule in a patient with acquired immunodeficiency syndrome. Am J Respir Crit Care Med 1994;149:1041–3.
19. Sadaghdar H, Eden E. Pulmonary Kaposi's sarcoma presenting as fulminant respiratory failure. Chest 1991;100:858–60.
20. Bach MC, Bagwell SP, Fanning JP. Primary pulmonary Kaposi's sarcoma in the acquired immunodeficiency syndrome: a cause of persistent pyrexia. Am J Med 1988;85:274–5.
21. Lee VW, Fuller JD, O'Brien MJ, et al. Pulmonary Kaposi's sarcoma in patients with AIDS: scintigraphic diagnosis with sequential thallium and gallium scanning. Radiology 1991;180:409–12.
22. Cooley TP, Hirschhorn LR, O'Keane JC. Kaposi's sarcoma in women with AIDS. AIDS 1996;10:1221–5.
23. Nasti G, Serraino D, Ridolfo A, et al. AIDS-associated Kaposi's sarcoma is more aggressive in women: a study of

54 patients. J Acquir Immune Defic Syndr Hum Retrovirol 1999;20:337–41.

24. Krown SE, Metroka C, Wernz JC. Kaposi's sarcoma in the acquired immunodeficiency syndrome: a proposal for evaluation, response and staging criteria. AIDS Clinical Trials Group Oncology Committee. J Clin Oncol 1989;7:1201–7.

25. Krown SE, Testa MA, Huang J. AIDS-related Kaposi's sarcoma: perspective validation of the AIDS Clinical Trials Group staging classification. AIDS Clinical Trials Group Oncology Committee. J Clin Oncol 1997;15:3085–92.

26. Scadden DT. AIDS-related malignancies. Ann Rev Med 2003;54:285–03.

27. Ledergerber B, Talenti A, Egger M. Risk of HIV related Kaposi's sarcoma and non-Hodgkin's lymphoma with potent antiretroviral therapy: prospective cohort study. BMJ 1999;319:23–4.

28. Jacobson LP, Yamashita TE, Detels R, et al. Impact of potent antiretroviral therapy on the incidence of Kaposi's sarcoma and non-Hodgkin's lymphomas among HIV-infected individuals: multicenter AIDS cohort study. J Acquir Immune Defic Syndr 1999;21 Suppl 1:S34–41.

29. Tam HK, Zhang Z-F, Jacobson LP, et al. Effect of highly active antiretroviral therapy on survival among HIV-infected men with Kaposi sarcoma or non-Hodgkin lymphoma. Int J Cancer 2002;98:916–22.

30. Jones JL, Hanson DL, Dworking MS, et al. Incidence and trends in Kaposi's sarcoma in the era of effective antiretroviral therapy. J Acquir Immune Defic Syndr 2000;24: 270–4.

31. Ives NJ, Gazzard BG, Easterbrook PJ. The changing pattern of AIDS-defining illnesses with the introduction of highly active antiretroviral therapy (HAART) in a London clinic. J Infect 2001;42:134–9.

32. Buchbinder SP, Homberg SD, Scheer S, et al. Combination antiretroviral therapy and incidence of AIDS-related malignancies. J Acquir Immune Defic Syndr 1999;21 Suppl 1:S23–6.

33. Rabkin CS, Testa M, Huang J, et al. Kaposi's sarcoma and non-Hodgkin's lymphoma incidence in AIDS Clinical Trials Group study participants. J Acquir Immune Defic Syndr 1999;21 Suppl 1:S31–3.

34. Appleby P, Beral V, Newton R, et al. Imperial Cancer Research Fund Cancer Epidemiology Unit: highly active antiretroviral therapy and incidence of cancer in human immunodeficiency virus infected adults. J Natl Cancer Inst 2000;92:1823–30.

35. Sparano JA, Anand K, Desai J, et al. Effect of highly active antiretroviral therapy on the incidence of HIV associated malignancies at an urban medical center. J Acquir Immune Defic Syndr 1999;21 Suppl 1:S18–22.

36. Carrieri MP, Pradier C, Piselli P, et al. Reduced incidence of Kaposi's sarcoma and of systemic non-Hodgkin's lymphoma in HIV-infected individuals treated with highly active antiretroviral therapy. Int J Cancer 2003;103:142–4.

37. Mocroft A, Kirk O, Clumeck N, et al. The changing pattern of Kaposi's sarcoma in patients with HIV, 1994-2003. Cancer 2004;100:2644–54.

38. Bower M, Fox P, Fife K, et al. Highly active anti-retroviral therapy (HAART) prolongs time to treatment failure in Kaposi's sarcoma. AIDS 1999;13:2105–11.

39. Holkova B, Takeshita K, Cheng DM, et al. Effect of highly active antiretroviral therapy on survival in patients with AIDS associated Kaposi's sarcoma treated with chemotherapy. J Clin Oncol 2001;19:3848–51.

40. Cattelan A, Calabrò M, Gasperini P, et al. Acquired immunodeficiency syndrome-related Kaposi's sarcoma regression after highly active antiretroviral therapy: biologic correlates of clinical outcome. J Natl Cancer Inst Monogr 2001;28:44–9.

41. Sgadari C, Barillari G, Toschi E, et al. HIV protease inhibitors are potent anti-angiogenic molecules and promote regression of Kaposi's sarcoma. Nat Med 2002;8: 225–32.

42. Cattelan AM, Calabrò ML, Aversa SML, et al. Regression of AIDS-related Kaposi's sarcoma following antiretroviral therapy with protease inhibitors: biological correlates of clinical outcome. Eur J Cancer 1999;35:1809–15.

43. Dupont C, Vasseur E, Beauchet A, et al. Long-term efficacy on Kaposi's sarcoma of highly active antiretroviral therapy in a cohort of HIV-positive patients. AIDS 2000;14:987–93.

44. Shaw A, McLean K. Kaposi's sarcoma regression following treatment with a triple antiretroviral regimen containing nevirapine. Int J STD AIDS 1999;10:417–8.

45. Murphy M, Armstrong D, Sepkowitz KA, et al. Regression of AIDS-related Kaposi's sarcoma following treatment with an HIV-1 protease inhibitor. AIDS 1997;11:261–2.

46. Blum L, Pellet C, Agbalika F, et al. Complete regression af AIDS-related Kaposi's sarcoma associated with undetectable human herpesvirus-8 sequences during anti-HIV protease therapy. AIDS 1997;11:1653–5.

47. Benfield T, Kirk O, Elbrong B, et al. Complete histological regression of Kaposi's sarcoma following treatment with protease inhibitors despite persistence of HHV-8 in lesions. Scand J Infect Dis 1998;30:613–5.

48. Martinelli C, Zazzi M, Ambu S, et al. Complete regression of AIDS-related Kaposi's sarcoma-associated human herpesvirus-8 during therapy with indinavir. AIDS 1998;12: 1717–9.

49. Murdaca G, Campelli A, Sett M, et al. Complete remission of AIDS/Kaposi's sarcoma after treatment with a combination of two nucleoside reverse transcriptase inhibitors and one non-nucleoside reverse transcriptase inhibitor. AIDS 2002;16:304–5.

50, Niehues T, Horneff G, Megahed M, et al. Complete regression of AIDS-related Kaposi's sarcoma in AIDS. AIDS 1999;13:1148–9.

51. Aboulafia DM. Regression of acquired immunodeficiency syndrome-related pulmonary Kaposi's sarcoma after highly active antiretroviral therapy. Mayo Clin Proc 1998;73:439–43.

52. Burdick AE, Carmichael C, Rady PL, et al. Resolution of Kaposi's sarcoma associated with undetectable level of human herpesvirus 8 DNA in a patient with AIDS after protease inhibitor therapy. J Am Acad Dermatol 1997;37: 648–9.

53. Parra R. Leal M, Delgado J, et al. Regression of invasive AIDS-related Kaposi's sarcoma following antiretroviral therapy. Clin Infect Dis 1998;26:218–9.

54. Genka I, Yasuoka A, Saitoh K, Oka S. Highly active antiretroviral therapy for the treatment of Kaposi's sarcoma

associated with primary human immunodeficiency virus type-1 infection. Jpn J Infect Dis 2000;53:166–7.

55. Diz Dios P, Ocampo Hermida A, Miralles Alvarez C, et al. Regression of AIDS-related Kaposi's sarcoma following ritonavir therapy. Oral Oncol 1998;34:236–8.

56. Conant MA, Opp KM, Poretz D, et al. Reduction of Kaposi's sarcoma lesions following treatment of AIDS with ritonavir. AIDS 1997;11:1300–1.

57. Tavio M, Nasti G, Spina M, et al. Highly active antiretroviral therapy in HIV-related Kaposi's sarcoma. Ann Oncol 1998;9:923.

58. Lebbe C, Blum L, Pellet C, et al. Clinical and biological impact of antiretroviral therapy with protease inhibitors on HIV related Kaposi's sarcoma. AIDS 1998;12:F45–9.

59. Krischer J, Rutschman O, Hirshel B, et al. Regression of Kaposi's sarcoma during therapy with HIV-1 protease inhibitors: a prospective study. J Am Acad Dermatol 1998;38:594–8.

60. Dupin N, Rubin de Cervens V, Gorin I, et al. The influence of HAART on AIDS-associated KS. Br J Dermatol 1999; 140:875–81.

61. Nasti G, Martellotta F, Berretta M, et al. Impact of highly active antiretroviral therapy on the presenting features and outcome of patients with acquired immunodeficiency syndrome-related Kaposi sarcoma. Cancer 2003;98:2440–60.

62. Leao JC, Kumar N, McLean KA, et al. Effect of human immunodeficiency virus-1 protease inhibitors on the clearance of human herpesvirus 8 from blood of human immunodeficiency virus-1-infected patients. J Med Virol 2000;62:416–20.

63. Osman M, Kubo T, Gill J, et al. Identification of human herpesvirus 8-specific cytotoxic T-cell responses. J Virol 1999;73:6136–40.

64. Wang QJ, Jenkins FJ, Jacobson LP, et al. CD8+ cytotoxic T lymphocyte responses to lytic proteins of human herpes virus 8 in human immunodeficiency virus type 1-infected and -uninfected individuals. J Infect Dis 2000;182: 928–32.

65. Strickler HD, Goedert JJ, Bethke FR, et al. Human herpesvirus 8 cellular immune responses in homosexual men. J Infect Dis 1999;180:162–5.

66. Jung C, Bogner JR, Goebel F. Resolution of severe Kaposi sarcoma after initiation of antiretroviral triple therapy. Eur J Med Res 1998;3:439–42.

67. Krown SE. Highly active antiretroviral therapy in AIDS-associated Kaposi's sarcoma: implications for the design of therapeutic trials in patients with advanced, symptomatic Kaposi's sarcoma. J Clin Oncol 2004;22:399–402.

68. Vaccher E, di Gennaro G, Nasti G, et al. HAART is effective as anti Kaposi sarcoma therapy only after remission has been induced by chemotherapy. J Acquir Immune Defic Syndr 1999;22:407–8.

69. Walmsley S, Northfelt DW, Melosky B, et al. Treatment of AIDS-related cutaneous Kaposi's sarcoma with topical alitretinoin (9-cis-retinoic acid) gel. Panretin Gel North American Study Group. J Acquir Immune Defic Syndr 1999;22:235–46.

70. Pluda J, Broder S, Yarchoan R. Therapy of AIDS and AIDS-associated neoplasms. Cancer Chemother Biol Response Modif 1992;13:395–439.

71. Buchbinder A, Friedman-Kien A. Clinical aspect of Kaposi's sarcoma. Curr Opin Oncol 1992;4:867–74.

72. Cooper JS, Steinfeld A, Lerch I. Intentions and outcomes in the radiotherapeutic management of epidemic Kaposi's sarcoma. Int J Radiat Oncol Biol Phys 1990;20:419–22.

73. de Wit R, Smit W, Veenhof K, et al. Palliative radiation therapy for AIDS-associated Kaposi's sarcoma by using a single fraction of 800 cGy. Radiother Oncol 1990;19:131–6.

74. Nasti G, Errante D, Santarossa S, et al. A risk and benefit assessment of treatment for AIDS-related Kaposi's sarcoma. Drug Saf 1999;20:403–25.

75. Swift PS. The role of radiation therapy in the management of HIV-related Kaposi's sarcoma. Hematol Oncol Clin North Am 1996;10:1069–80.

76. Stelzer KJ, Griffin TW. A randomized prospective trial of radiation therapy for AIDS-associated Kaposi's sarcoma. Int J Radiat Oncol Biol Phys 1993;27:1057–61.

77. Poignonec S, Lachiver LD, Lamas G, et al. Intralesional bleomycin for acquired immunodeficiency syndrome-associated cutaneous KS. Arch Dermatol 1995;131:228.

78. Schwartz RA. Kaposi's sarcoma: advances and perspectives. J Am Acad Dermatol 1996;34:804–14.

79. Lilenbaum RC, Ratner S. Systemic treatment of Kaposi's sarcoma: current status and future directions. AIDS 1994; 8:141–51.

80. Boudreaux AA, Smith LL, Cosby CD, et al. Intralesional vinblastine for cutaneous Kaposi's sarcoma associated with acquired immunodeficiency syndrome. A clinical trial to evaluate efficacy and discomfort associated with infection. J Am Acad Dermatol 1993;28:61–5.

81. Gill PS, Lunardi-Iskandar Y, Louie S, et al. The effects of preparations of human chorionic gonadotropin in AIDS-related Kaposi's sarcoma. N Engl J Med 1996;335:1261–9.

82. Sheperd FA, Beaulieu R, Gelmon K, et al. Prospective randomized trial of two dose levels of interferon-α with zidovudine for the treatment of Kaposi's sarcoma associated with human immunodeficiency virus infection: a Canadian HIV Clinical Trials Network study. J Clin Oncol 1998;16:1736–42.

83. Monini P, Carlini F, Sturzl M, et al. Alpha interferon inhibits human herpesvirus 8 (HHV-8) reactivation in primary effusion lymphoma cells and reduces HHV-8 load in cultured peripheral blood mononuclear cells. J Virol 1999;73:4029–41.

84. Koster R, Blatt LM, Streubert M, et al. Consensus-interferon and platelet-derived growth factor adversely regulate proliferation and migration of Kaposi's sarcoma cells by control of c-myc expression. Am J Pathol 1996;149:1871–85.

85. Real FX, Krown SE, Oettgen HF. Kaposi's sarcoma and the acquired immunodeficiency syndrome: treatment with high and low doses of recombinant leukocyte A interferon. J Clin Oncol 1986;4:544–51.

86. Groopman JE, Gottlieb MS, Goodman J, et al. Recombinant alpha-2-interferon therapy for Kaposi's sarcoma associated with the acquired immunodeficiency syndrome. Ann Intern Med 1984;100:671–6.

87. Evans LM, Itri LM, Campion M, et al. Interferon alfa-2a in the treatment of acquired immunodeficiency syndrome-related Kaposi's sarcoma. J Immunother 1991;10:39–50.

88. Gelmann EP, Preble OT, Steis R, et al. Human lymphoblastoid

interferon treatment of Kaposi's sarcoma in the acquired immunodeficiency syndrome. Am J Med 1985;78:737–41.

89. Krown SE, Real FX, Cunningham-Rundles S, et al. Preliminary observations on the effect of recombinant leukocyte A interferon in homosexual men with Kaposi's sarcoma. N Engl J Med 1983;308:1071–6.

90. Volberding PA, Mitsuyatsu RT, Golando JP, et al. Treatment of Kaposi's sarcoma with interferon alfa-2b (Intron A). Cancer 1987;59:620–5.

91. Rios A, Mansell PWA, Newell GR, et al. Treatment of acquired immunodeficiency syndrome-related Kaposi's sarcoma with lymphoblastoid interferon. J Clin Oncol 1985;3:506–12.

92. Fischi MA, Gorowski E, Koch G, et al. Interferon alfa-n1 Wellferon™ in Kaposi's sarcoma: single agent or combination with vinblastine. In: The biology of the interferon system. 1986. Boston: Martinus Nijhoff; 1987. p. 355–62.

93. Lane HC, Kovacs JA, Feinberg J, et al. Anti-retroviral effects of interferon-alpha in AIDS-associated Kaposi's sarcoma. Lancet 1988;2:1218–22.

94. de Wit R, Schattenkerk JK, Boucher CA, et al. Clinical and virological effects of high-dose recombinant interferon-alpha in disseminated AIDS-related Kaposi's sarcoma. Lancet 1988;2:1214–7.

95. Lee FC, Mitsuyasu RT. Chemotherapy of AIDS-related Kaposi's sarcoma. Hematol Oncol Clin North Am 1996; 10:1051–68.

96. Gill PS, Wernz J, Scadden DT, et al. Randomized phase III trial of liposomal daunorubicin (DaunoXome) versus doxorubicin, bleomycin, vincristine (ABV) in AIDS-related Kaposi's sarcoma. J Clin Oncol 1996;14:2353–4.

97. Scarpe M, Easthope SE, Keating GM, Lamb HM. Polyethylene glycol-liposomal doxorubicin. Drugs 2002;62:2089–126.

98. Jie C, Tulpule A, Zheng T, et al. Treatment of epidemic (AIDS-related) Kaposi's sarcoma. Curr Opin Oncol 1997; 9:433–9.

99. Northfelt DW, Dezube BJ, Thommes JA, et al. Pegylated-liposomal doxorubicin versus doxorubicin, bleomycin and vincristine in the treatment of AIDS-related Kaposi's sarcoma: results of a randomized phase III clinical trial. J Clin Oncol 1998;16:2445–51.

100. Stewart S, Jablonowski H, Goebel FD, et al. Randomized comparative trial of pegylated liposomal doxorubicin versus bleomycin and vincristine in the treatment of AIDS-related Kaposi's sarcoma. International Pegylated Liposomal Doxorubicin Study Group. J Clin Oncol 1998;16:683–91.

101. Berry G, Billingham M, Alderman E, et al. The use of cardiac biopsy to demonstrate reduced cardiotoxicity in AIDS Kaposi's sarcoma patients treated with pegylated liposomal doxorubicin. Ann Oncol 1998;9:711–6.

102. Osoba D, Northfelt DW, Budd DW, et al. Effect of treatment on health-related quality of life in acquired immunodeficiency syndrome (AIDS)-related Kaposi's sarcoma: a randomized trial of pegylated-liposomal doxorubicin versus doxorubicin, bleomycin and vincristine. Cancer Invest 2001;19:573–80.

103. Esdaile B, Davis M, Portsmouth S, et al. The immunological effects of concomitant highly active antiretroviral therapy and liposomal anthracycline treatment of HIV-1-associated Kaposi's sarcoma. AIDS 2002;16:2344–7.

104. Holmes FA, Walters RS, Theriault RL, et al. Phase II trial of Taxol, an active drug in metastatic breast cancer. J Natl Cancer Inst 1991;83:1979–805.

105. Horwitz SB, Cohen D, Rao S, et al. Taxol: mechanisms of action and resistance. J Natl Cancer Inst Monogr 1993;15:55–62.

106. Klauber N, Parangi S, Flynn E, et al. Inhibition of angiogenesis and breast cancer in mice by the microtubule inhibitors 2-methoxyestradiol and Taxol. Cancer Res 1997;57: 81–6.

107. Rose WC. Taxol-based combination chemotherapy and other in vivo preclinical antitumor studies. J Natl Cancer Inst Monogr 1993;15:47–53.

108. Welles L, Saville MW, Lietzau J, et al. Phase II trial with dose titration of paclitaxel for the therapy of human immunodeficiency virus-associated Kaposi's sarcoma. J Clin Oncol 1998;16:1112–21.

109. Gill PS, Tulpule A, Espina BM, et al. Paclitaxel is safe and effective in the treatment of advanced AIDS-related Kaposi's sarcoma. J Clin Oncol 1999;17:1876–83.

110. Tulpule A, Groopman J, Faville MW, et al. Multicenter trial of low-dose paclitaxel in patients with advanced AIDS-related Kaposi sarcoma. Cancer 2002;95:147–54.

111. Stebbing J, Wildfire A, Portsmouth S, et al. Paclitaxel for anthracycline-resistant AIDS-related Kaposi's sarcoma: clinical and angiogenic correlations. Ann Oncol 2003;14:1660–6.

112. Evans SR, Krown SE, Testa MA, et al. Phase II evaluation of low-dose oral etoposide for the treatment of relapsed or progressive AIDS-related Kaposi's sarcoma: an AIDS Clinical Trials Group clinical study. J Clin Oncol 2002; 20:3236–41.

113. Kruse FE, Joussen AM, Rohrschneider K, et al. Thalidomide inhibits corneal angiogenesis induced by vascular endothelial growth factor. Graefes Arch Clin Exp Ophthalmol 1998;236:461–6.

114. Bauer KS, Dixon SC, Figg WD. Inhibition of angiogenesis by thalidomide requires metabolic activation, which is species-dependent. Biochem Pharmacol 1998;55:1827–34.

115. Moreira AL, Friedlander DR, Shif B, et al. Thalidomide and a thalidomide analogue inhibit endothelial cell proliferation in vitro. J Neurooncol 1999;43:109–14.

116. Keifer JA, Guttridge DC, Ashburner BP, Baldwin AS Jr. Inhibition of NFκB activity by thalidomide through suppression of IκB kinase activity. J Biol Chem 2001;276:22382–7.

117. Soler RA, Howard M, Brink NS, et al. Regression of AIDS-related Kaposi's sarcoma during therapy with thalidomide. Clin Infect Dis 1996;23:501–3.

118. Fife K, Howard MR, Gracie F, et al. Activity of thalidomide In AIDS-related Kaposi's sarcoma and correlation with HHV8 titre. Int J STD AIDS 1998;9:751–5.

119. Little RF, Wyvill KM, Pluda JM, et al. Activity of thalidomide in AIDS-related Kaposi's sarcoma. J Clin Oncol 2000;18:2593–602.

120. Miles SA, Dezube BJ, Lee JY, et al. Antitumor activity of oral 9-*cis*-retinoic acid in HIV-associated Kaposi's sarcoma. AIDS 2002;16:421–9.

121. Bernstein ZP, Chanan-Khan A, Miller KC, et al. A multicenter phase II study of the intravenous administration of liposomal tretinoin in patients with acquired immunode-

ficiency syndrome-associated Kaposi's sarcoma. Cancer 2002;95:2555–61.

122. Bikle D, Pillai S. Vitamin D, calcium and epidermal differentiation. Endocr Rev 1993;14:3–19.

123. Bar-Shavit Z, Teitelbaum SL, Reitsma P, et al. Induction of monocytic differentiation and bone resorption by 1,25-dihydroxyvitamin D$_3$. Proc Natl Acad Sci U S A 1983;80:5907–11.

124. Fukuoka M, Ogino Y, Ohta T, et al. RANTES expression in psoriatic skin and regulation of RANTES and IL-8 production in cultured epidermal keratinocytes by active vitamin D$_3$ (tacalcitol). Br J Dermatol 1998;138:63–70.

125. Koizumi H, Kaplan A, Shimizu T, Ohkawara A. 1,25-Dihydroxyvitamin D$_3$ and a new analog, 22-oxacalcitriol, modulate proliferation and interleukin-8 secretion of normal human keratinocytes. J Dermatol Sci 1997;15:207–13.

126. Larsen CG, Kristensen M, Paludan K, et al. 1,25(OH)$_2$-D$_3$ is a potent regulator of interleukin-1 induced interleukin-8 expression and production. Biochem Biophys Res Commun 1991;176:1020–6.

127. Masood R, Cai J, Tulpule A, et al. Interleukin 8 is an autocrine growth factor and a surrogate marker for Kaposi's sarcoma. Clin Cancer Res 2001;7:2693–702.

128. Masood R, Nagpal S, Zheng T, et al. Kaposi sarcoma is a therapeutic target for vitamin D$_3$ receptor agonist. Blood 2000;96:3188–94.

129. Dezube BJ, Von Roenn JH, Holden-Wiltse J, et al. Fumagillin analog in the treatment of Kaposi's sarcoma: a phase I AIDS Clinical Trial Group study. AIDS Clinical Trial Group No. 215 Team. J Clin Oncol 1998;16:1444–9.

130. IM862. Investigator brochure, 6th ed. 1998 Aug 1. Kirland (WA): Cytran Inc.; 1998.

131. Tulpule A, Scadden DT, Espina BM, et al. Results of a randomized study of IM862 nasal solution in the treatment of AIDS-related Kaposi's sarcoma. J Clin Oncol 2000;18:716–23.

132. Matrisian LM. The matrix-degrading metalloproteinases. Bioessays 1992;14:455–63.

133. Bernhard E, Gruber S, Muschel R. Direct evidence linking expression of matrix metalloproteinase 9 (92-kDa gelatinase/collagenase) to the metastatic phenotype in transformed rat embryo cells. Proc Natl Acad Sci U S A 1994;91:4293–7.

134. Ray J, Stetler-Stevenson W. Gelatinase A activity directly modulates melanoma cell adhesion and spreading. EMBO J 1995;14:908–17.

135. Kawamata H, Kameyama S, Kawai K, et al. Marked acceleration of the metastatic phenotype of a rat bladder carcinoma cell line by the expression of human gelatinase A. Int J Cancer 1995;63:568–75.

136. Mede-Tollin LC, Way D, Witte MH, et al. Expression of multiple matrix metalloproteinases and urokinase-type plasminogen activator in cultured Kaposi's sarcoma cells. Acta Histochem 1999;101:305–16.

137. Johnson MD, Kim HR, Chesler L, et al. Inhibition of angiogenesis by tissue inhibitor of metalloproteinase. J Cell Physiol 1994;160:194–02.

138. Hidalgo M, Eckhard SG. Development of matrix metalloproteinase inhibitors in cancer therapy. J Natl Cancer Inst 2001;93:178–93.

139. Cianfrocca M, Cooley TP, Lee JY, et al. Matrix metalloproteinase inhibitor COL-3 in the treatment of AIDS-related Kaposi's sarcoma: a phase I AIDS Malignancy Consortium study. J Clin Oncol 2002;20:153–9.

140. Lunardi-Iskandar Y, Bryant JT, Zeman RA, et al. Tumorigenesis and metastasis of neoplastic Kaposi's sarcoma cell line in immunodeficient mice blocked by a human pregnancy hormone. Nature 1995;375:64–9.

141. Harris PJ. Treatment of Kaposi's sarcoma and other manifestations of AIDS with human chorionic gonadotropin. Lancet 1995;346:118–9.

142. Tirelli U, Tavio M, Giacca M, et al. Human chorionic gonadotropin in the treatment of HIV-related Kaposi's sarcoma. AIDS 1997;11:387–8.

143. Kedes DH, Ganem D. Sensitivity of Kaposi's sarcoma-associated herpesvirus replication to antiviral drugs. J Clin Invest 1997;99:2082–6.

144. Medveczky M, Horvath E, Lund P, et al. In vitro antiviral drug sensitivity of the Kaposi's sarcoma-associated herpesvirus. AIDS 1997;11:1327–32.

145. Robles R, Lugo D, Gee L, Jacobson MA. Effect of antiviral drugs used to treat *Cytomegalovirus* end-organ disease on subsequent course of previously diagnosed Kaposi's sarcoma in patients with AIDS. J Acquir Immune Defic Syndr Hum Retrovirol 1999;20:34–8.

146. Martin DF, Kuppermann BD, Wolitz RA, et al. Oral ganciclovir for patients with *Cytomegalovirus* retinitis treated with a ganciclovir implant. N Engl J Med 1999;340:1063–70.

6

Castleman's Disease

GIANNA BALLON
ETHEL CESARMAN

Castleman's disease (CD) was originally described by Benjamin Castleman in 1956[1] as a solitary mediastinal lymph node hyperplasia characterized by abnormal follicles with small germinal centers (resembling Hassall's corpuscles of the thymus) and evident capillary proliferation. Our current knowledge indicates that CD actually represents several different clinicopathologic entities; thus, the literature on the topic is confusing and difficult to interpret.

Until the last decade, two histopathologic types of CD had been described: (1) the hyaline vascular (HV) variant (first described by Benjamin Castleman),[1] which is the most common form, affecting 90% of patients and usually involving a single lymph node in the mediastinum, and (2) the plasma-cell (PC) variant (described by Flendrig in 1969[2,3] and Keller and colleagues in 1972[4]), which is characterized by hyperplastic germinal centers, abundant plasma cells in the interfollicular areas, persistence of sinuses, and associated clinical and laboratory abnormalities.

Two clinical entities also have been described: (1) the localized form, which usually presents as lymph node hyperplasia in a single lymph node–bearing region (in most cases, the mediastinum) and which resolves with resection, and (2) multicentric Castleman's disease (MCD) (described by Leibetseder and Thurner in 1973[5] and by Gaba and colleagues in 1978[6]), which manifests as generalized lymphadenopathy with systemic symptoms and is characterized by a more aggressive clinical course and the potential for malignant transformation.[7,8] The histopathologic HV type tends to be localized to a single lymph node and follows a benign clinical course. The PC variant usually involves clusters of lymph nodes in a single region

and is currently thought to represent a form of localized CD. MCD resembles the PC variant histopathologically, and it is frequently described as such in the literature. However, the histologic appearance of MCD is somewhat different, and MCD should be classified separately. Besides autonomous disease (primary MCD), cases associated with other diseases (secondary MCD) are common, and MCD represents one of the most ubiquitous associations in the literature[7] (Table 6–1). Secondary MCD is a large and heterogeneous group of clinical entities and is often referred to as interleukin (IL)-6 syndrome because of evidence that an overproduction of IL-6, probably in association with other cytokines, occurs in MCD-associated diseases as well as in MCD itself, suggesting a common underlying pathogenetic mechanism.

Understanding of the pathogenesis of MCD has greatly increased since the discovery of MCD's association with Kaposi's sarcoma herpesvirus (KSHV),[9] a gammaherpesvirus first identified in a Kaposi's sarcoma (KS) lesion from a human immunodeficiency virus (HIV)–positive patient and now known to be the etiologic agent of KS.[10] KSHV, also called human herpesvirus 8, has been found in approximately half of the cases of MCD occurring in immunocompetent patients and in almost all those infected with HIV, suggesting a pathogenic role in this disease.[9] Other benign lymphoid proliferations not associated with HIV infection lack KSHV, so the association is specific to MCD.[11] Moreover, exacerbation of symptoms correlates with an increased KSHV viral load in the peripheral blood, making viral load testing a potentially useful way of monitoring therapy.[12]

Table 6–1. CLASSIFICATION OF MULTICENTRIC CASTLEMAN'S DISEASE

Primary
  Non-KSHV related
  KSHV related
Secondary
  Autoimmune diseases (rheumatoid arthritis, Sjögren's syndrome, systemic lupus erythematosus, mixed connective-tissue disease)
  HIV infection
  KSHV infection
  Kaposi's sarcoma
  Plasma-cell dyscrasias (eg, POEMS syndrome)
  Neoplasias (Hodgkin's and non-Hodgkin's lymphoma)
  Others (primary immunodeficiencies, glomerulopathy, skin diseases)

HIV = human immunodeficiency virus; KSHV = Kaposi's sarcoma herpesvirus; POEMS = polyneuropathy, organomegaly, endocrinopathy, M protein, and skin lesions.

The clinical, histopathologic, immunophenotypic, and genotypic features of Castleman's disease, as well as the current understanding of its pathogenesis, will be reviewed and discussed in this chapter (Figure 6–1).

HISTOPATHOLOGIC FEATURES

Hyaline Vascular Type

The HV type of CD is characterized by the proliferation of small hyalinized follicular centers with radially arranged capillaries penetrating the germinal center and by striking capillary proliferation in the interfollicular stroma (Figure 6–2).[13]

A large histologic review of 102 cases of CD of the HV type confirmed the main common features, which include (1) abnormal follicles with increased vascularity, poorly formed germinal centers, and predominance of the mantle zone and (2) lack of sinuses and hypervascular interfollicular tissue containing large numbers of plasmacytoid monocytes.[14] It has been suggested that the HV type of CD is a disease of stromal cells, and soft tissue sarcomas have been reported in association with this disease, as have follicular dendritic-cell tumors.[15]

Plasma-Cell Type

The PC type of CD is also characterized by lymphoid follicular proliferation; however, the follicles tend to be larger, and mature plasma cells predominate in the interfollicular stroma, which is less vascular than that in the HV variant.[13] (Figure 6–3). The nodal architecture is relatively preserved, except for the dilatation of the sinuses, which are filled with hyperchromatic lymph.[16–18] Germinal centers are numerous, and most of them are markedly abnormal, having poorly defined borders, increased vascularity, a decreased number of follicular-center cells, and a prominence of follicular dendritic cells and histiocytes.[14,19] The characteristic follicle-like structures are surrounded by concentric rings of B lymphocytes with a mantle phenotype.[20] The interfollicular tissue shows a predominant infiltration of plasma cells. Through examination of multiple sequential biopsy specimens from the same patient, an interesting dynamic phenomenon was noticed. This phenomenon consisted in a shifting from a proliferative phase characterized by an abundance of high endothelial venules with immature plasma cells, immunoblasts, and many mitoses ("starry-sky" pattern, with small plasma cells within macrophages) toward an accumulative phase with little or no evidence of increased vascularity, plasma-cell immaturity, immunoblasts, or mitoses.[21] Since this "burn-out phase" can mimic the HV variant, it has been suggested to reconsider most or all cases of MCD of the HV or "mixed" type as cases of MCD of the PC form caught in the burn-out phase.[22]

Multicentric Castleman's Disease Associated with KSHV

A plasmablastic variant of MCD characterized by the presence of medium-sized to large plasmablastic cells scattered in the mantle zones of the follicles has been described, most frequently in HIV-infected individuals (Figure 6–4). Whereas immunoglobulin (Ig) M–positive immunoblasts have been usually described in the interfollicular region in MCD,[21,23] a unique population of cells with a similar morphology was found in the mantle zone of a subset of cases of MCD in association with KSHV infection (Figure 6–5).[24] The cells harboring KSHV in MCD have been called plasmablasts, but they have been described as having classic immunoblastic features,

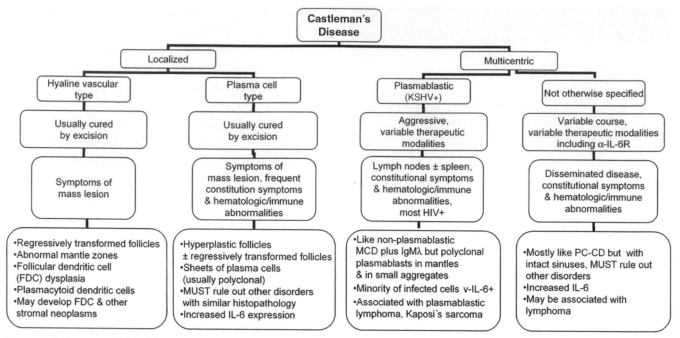

Figure 6–1. Summary of the clinicopathologic and biologic features of the major types of Castleman's disease. KSHV = Kaposi's sarcoma herpesvirus; HIV = human immunodeficiency virus; IgMlλ - immunoglobulin M heavy chain and λ light chain; IL-6 = interleukin-6; MCD = multicentric Castleman's disease; PC-CD = plasma-cell variant of Castleman's disease; v-IL-6 = viral interleukin-6. Reproduced with permission from Swerdlow SH. Castleman disease: one disease or several. In: Hematology. American Society of Hematology Program Book; 2004. p. 291–5. Copyright American Society of Hematology.

including a moderate amount of amphophilic cytoplasm and a large vesicular nucleus containing one or two prominent nucleoli.[24–26] In contrast to mature (IgG- or IgA-positive) plasma cells found in the interfollicular zone in KSHV-negative MCD cases, these KSHV-positive immunoblasts are immature cells that express cytoplasmic IgMλ, have a blastic morphology, and are predominantly seen in the mantle zones. The consistent restricted expression of λ light chain in the KSHV-positive plasmablasts (Figure 6–6) is intriguing and could be involved in the mechanism of KSHV entry in the cells or selection for those cells. These cells may be scattered or found in small confluent clusters, sometimes coalescing to form foci of "microlymphomas" or in large sheets of cells thought to represent frank plasmablastic lymphomas (discussed later in this chapter).[24,27] Analysis of clonality has revealed that despite monotypic expression of IgMlλ, the scattered plasmablasts in MCD are polyclonal; six of the eight cases with small clusters called "microlymphomas" were also polyclonal whereas the cases of MCD-associated plasmablastic lymphomas that were examined were monoclonal.[28]

IMMUNOPHENOTYPIC, GENOTYPIC, AND CYTOGENETIC FEATURES

Localized Castleman's Disease

Immunophenotypic similarities have been found in the HV and PC variants of CD, suggesting the possibility of overlapping pathogeneses.[29] The characteristic follicle-like structures are composed of B lymphocytes with a mantle zone phenotype, surrounding an inner core of follicular dendritic reticulum cells with sparse T cells.[20,30] The dendritic-cell network is abnormal; tighter and looser areas coexist, and there is no clear distribution of dark and light zones.[21] Characteristic findings are decreased germinal center proliferation and (surrounding the abnormal follicles) the presence of small B cells with a mantle zone phenotype.[20] In contrast to normal mantle cells, these cells are immunophenotypically aberrant, CD5 positive, and CD45RA negative and preferentially express the λ light chain.[31] The interfollicular tissue contains T-cell subsets in normal proportions[20,32] and a predominant population of plasma cells, which is polyclonal in most cases as

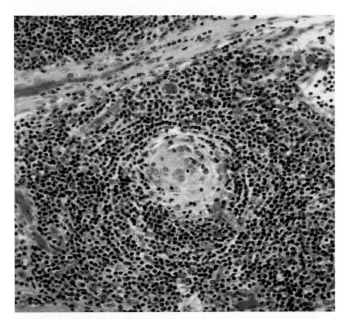

Figure 6–2. Castleman's disease: hyaline vascular type. Section of a lymph node from showing a single small hyalinized follicle. The interfollicular area contains a network of small vessels (hematoxylin-eosin; original magnification × 100). Courtesy of Amy Chadburn, MD, Weill Medical College of Cornell University/The New York Presbyterian Hospital.

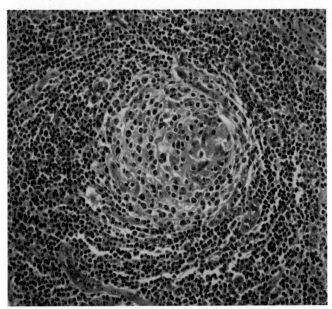

Figure 6–3. Castleman's disease: plasma cell type. Section of a lymph node from an HIV-negative but KSHV-positive patient showing an abnormal follicle and extensive plasma cell infiltration in the interfollicular stroma (hematoxylin-eosin; original magnification × 100). Courtesy of Amy Chadburn, MD, Weill Medical College of Cornell University/The New York Presbyterian Hospital.

confirmed by molecular genetic analysis of the antigen receptor genes.[16,20,31,33–36]

Multicentric Castleman's Disease

The plasmablastic variant is associated with KSHV infection, but other cases of MCD are not well understood and their diagnosis is frequently one of exclusion. In the plasmablastic variant, the cells harboring KSHV do not stain for T-cell (ie, CD3, CD45RO) or dendritic-cell (CD2, CD23) markers but stain for the B-cell marker CD20 and the memory B-cell marker CD27.[37] They lack expression of B-cell activation markers such as CD23, CD38, and

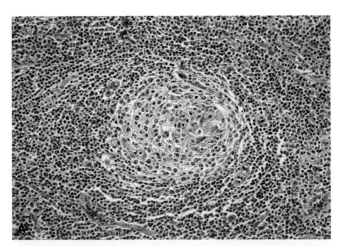

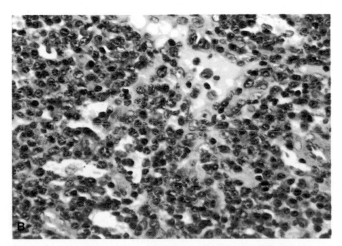

Figure 6–4. Multicentric Castleman's disease associated with HIV infection. *A,* Section of a lymph node from a patient with HIV–associated Castleman's disease, showing a single follicle with a large concentrically arranged mantle zone surrounding a germinal center. The interfollicular area contains a network of small vessels (hematoxylin-eosin; original magnification × 100). *B,* Interfollicular area showing the presence of numerous plasma cells and vascular proliferation (Hematoxylin-eosin; original magnification × 400). Courtesy of Amy Chadburn, MD, Weill Medical College of Cornell University/The New York Presbyterian Hospital.

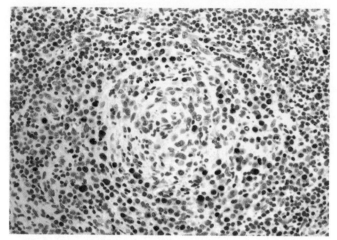

Figure 6–5. Presence of Kaposi's sarcoma herpesvirus in multicentric Castleman's disease. Immunohistochemical staining of a lymph node using mouse monoclonal antibody to KSHV latency-associated nuclear antigen (LANA) shows brown nuclear positivity in numerous cells in the mantle zone (DAB/brown; original magnification × 100). Courtesy of Elizabeth Hyjek, MD, PhD, Weill Medical College of Cornell University/The New York Presbyterian Hospital.

CD30.[37] In MCD, a monotypic plasma-cell component may be identified that is usually of IgGλ or IgAλ type, and it is associated with a serum paraprotein and with the syndrome of polyneuropathy, organomegaly, endocrinopathy, M protein, and skin lesions (POEMS syndrome).[16,38] Few cytogenetic abnormalities have been described, such as a centromeric insertion in chromosome 1[36] and t(7;14)(p22;q22).[39] The involvement of cytogenetic abnormalities at 7q21-22, where the IL-6 gene is located, is particularly interesting because it could account for the high IL-6 serum levels found in some patients and may provide a pathogenetic explanation of the disease mechanism in selected cases.[40]

PATHOGENESIS

Role of Human Interleukin-6

Several lines of evidence suggest a role for IL-6 in the pathogenesis of the PC form of localized CD and in MCD: (1) increased levels of IL-6 have been found, both in cases with localized disease and in cases of multicentric disease,[40–47] in association with increased expression of IL-6 receptor and hyper-responsiveness to IL-6[48]; (2) treatment with an anti-IL-6 antibody in some patients with localized CD[49] or with MCD[50,51] has led to normalization of IL-6 serum levels and the disappearance of clinical and laboratory abnormalities; and (3) mice overexpressing IL-6 owing to inactivation of C/EBPβ, a negative transcriptional regulator of IL-6, develop pathologic traits similar to those of MCD, with hypergammaglobulinemia, splenomegaly, and lymphadenopathy. Moreover, the simultaneous inactivation of IL-6 and C/EBPβ by generation of IL-6-/-, C/EBPβ-/- double null mice, prevents the development of such manifestations.[52,53]

IL-6 is a pleiotropic lymphokine produced by different cell types, including B and T lymphocytes,

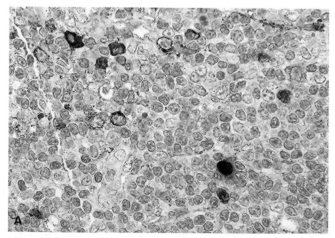

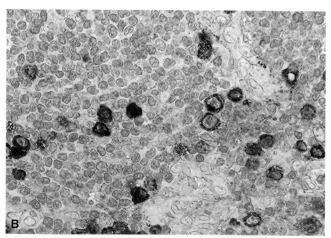

Figure 6–6. Kaposi's sarcoma herpesvirus (KSHV) is present in λ immunoglobulin light chain-positive B cells. *A,* Double immunohistochemistry for KSHV LANA and immunoglobulin κ light chain shows nuclear positivity (red staining) in cells that are negative for cytoplasmic κ (brown staining). *B,* Double immunohistochemistry for KSHV LANA and immunoglobulin λ light chain shows cells that are positive for nuclear LANA (red staining) as well as cytoplasmic λ (brown staining) (original magnification × 400). Courtesy of Elizabeth Hyjek, MD, PhD, Weill Medical College of Cornell University/The New York Presbyterian Hospital.

monocytes, macrophages, fibroblasts, endothelial cells, epidermal keratinocytes, mesangial cells, and syncytiotrophoblasts.[54,55] Human IL-6–positive cells have been found in the germinal centers[42,49] or follicular dendritic cells[56] (as well as sparsely in the marginal zone and in the interfollicular areas) and have been interpreted as immunoblasts[49] or other cells (interdigitating, lymphoid, or endothelial).[57,58]

IL-6, alone or in association with other cytokines that are also deregulated in these patients (ie, tumor necrosis factor [TNF]-α, TNF-β, interferon-γ [INF-γ], IL-1, and vascular endothelial growth factor [VEGF]),[41,59,60] may explain many clinical manifestations of MCD, including expansion of the B-cell compartment and plasmacytosis in lymphoid tissues, immune autoreactivity, the presence of B symptoms, gammaglobulinemia, hypoalbuminemia, elevated erythrocyte sedimentation rate, acute-phase reactants, and angiogenesis observed in lymph nodes and kidneys.

IL-6 is a key factor in the pathogenesis of a wide spectrum of disease, including autoimmune diseases,[61] HIV infection,[62] plasma-cell dyscrasias (ie, POEMS syndrome),[63] Kaposi's sarcoma,[64] B-cell lymphoma,[65] and Hodgkin's lymphoma.[66] Secondary MCD is frequently associated with a combination of these diseases, all of which share a common pathogenetic mechanism; therefore, the term "IL-6 syndrome" has been suggested to define this combination of diseases.

To explain the autoimmunity effect of IL-6, it has been proposed that an increased production of IL-6 in the germinal centers impairs the normal elimination of B cells with inappropriate Ig gene mutations, favoring plasma-cell differentiation and the emergence of autoreactive clones.[65] Other investigators have proposed that the CD5-positive lymphocytes localized in the mantle zone of the abnormal follicles and preferentially expressing Igλ and lacking CD45RA may correspond to long-lived memory B cells producing autoantibodies.[67]

Role of Kaposi's Sarcoma–Associated Herpesvirus

KSHV is a gammaherpesvirus etiologically linked to KS,[10] primary effusion lymphoma (also called body-cavity–based lymphoma),[68] in addition to MCD.[9]

The following pieces of evidence support the involvement of KSHV in the pathogenesis of MCD: (1) KSHV is present in approximately half of the cases of MCD occurring in immunocompetent patients and almost all of those infected with HIV, (2) KSHV sequences have also been found in the peripheral blood of patients with MCD, and (3) exacerbation of symptoms correlates with an increased KSHV viral load in the peripheral blood, making KSHV viral load assessment a potentially useful way of monitoring therapy.[9,11,12]

KSHV conforms to the replication paradigm shared by the entire lymphotropic herpesvirus family, displaying both lytic and latent replication. During latency, viral gene expression is restricted to only a few genes.[69] These latent genes are thought to maintain the viral episome in dividing cells,[70] escape host immune surveillance,[71] and provide a growth advantage to infected cells.[37,72,73] When latently KSHV-infected cells are exposed to inflammatory cytokines, especially INF-γ, the viral lytic cycle is induced, and the full repertoire of viral gene expression occurs. In contrast to latent proteins, the lytic gene products seem to be important for the inflammatory and angiogenic component of KSHV-associated lesions.

While primary effusion lymphoma (PEL) is predominantly or exclusively characterized by expression of latent KSHV genes, MCD is most likely the result of active viral infection with lytic viral gene expression in the context of a host with poor immune control (Figure 6–7).[74,75,76] Molecular analysis of KSHV-infected lymphocytes from patients with MCD shows a high degree of KSHV lytic gene activity.[74] KSHV carries at least 14 open reading frames that encode viral proteins involved in signal transduction, cell cycle regulation, and/or inhibition of apoptosis.[77] One of these is a viral homologue of human IL-6, called viral IL-6. Cells that produce viral IL-6 have been detected in the mantle zone, most likely corresponding to immunoglobulin λ-bearing plasmablasts[78,79,80] characteristically present in the plasmablastic variant of MCD.[24] In vitro, viral IL-6 mimics the effects of human IL-6[50] and may serve as an autocrine growth factor in MCD (as also described in PEL),[81,82] either by itself or via induction of other cellular cytokines (eg, human IL-6 and human IL-10). While human IL-6 requires both

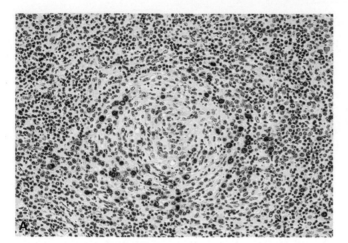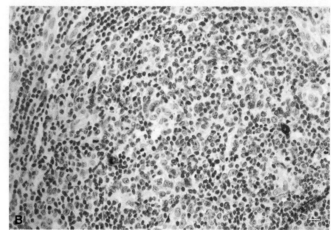

Figure 6–7. Multicentric Castleman's disease: immunohistochemistry for Kaposi's sarcoma herpesvirus (KSHV) viral antigens. *A,* Polyclonal antisera to viral interleukin-6 (vIL-6) also shows cytoplasmic positivity (diaminobenzidine/brown) in the mantle zone surrounding an atrophic germinal center. *B,* Immunohistochemistry with a monoclonal antibody to K8.1, a lytic viral antigen, shows cytoplasmic positivity (diaminobenzidine/brown) in two cells that are undergoing lytic viral replication (original magnification × 100). Courtesy of Elizabeth Hyjek, MD, PhD, Weill Medical College of Cornell University/The New York Presbyterian Hospital.

gp130 and the IL-6 receptor alpha subunits to function, viral IL-6 can bind the gp130 receptor subunit in the absence of the IL-6 receptor α chain to activate IL-6–responsive genes and promote B-cell survival.[83–85]

A variety of other virally encoded proteins are likely to play a role in MCD pathogenesis. Important, many latent and lytic genes have been found to be expressed in MCD samples, including viral cyclin D, v-*Bcl*-2, and viral G protein–coupled receptor (GPCR) genes.[86] Viral GPCR is homologous to the IL-8 receptor but does not require ligand engagement for its activation[87]; it can activate several transcriptional cascades and upregulate VEGF and a variety of other molecules, therefore inducing angiogenesis via paracrine mechanisms.[88] Another protein encoded by KSHV, called K1, can mimic signaling mediated by the B-cell antigen receptor and promote B-cell survival.[89] Viral IFN regulatory factor can inhibit IFN-induced transcriptional activation[90] and strongly reduce T cell antigen receptor (TCR)/CD3-mediated CD95 ligand induction, affecting apoptosis in T cells. The inhibition of CD95-dependent T-cell functions could contribute to immune escape of KSHV.[91] Fas-mediated apoptosis is also prevented by viral FLICE-inhibitory protein (vFLIP), recently demonstrated to be essential for the survival of PELs.[92] Viral Bcl-2 can block apoptosis as efficiently as

Bcl-2 and Bcl-XL, but it can not dimerize with other proteins (ie, Bax and Bak), which suggests that it may have evolved to escape any negative regulatory effects of cellular proteins.[93,94] Another homologue to cellular oncogenes involved in lymphomagenesis is viral cyclin D, which can associate with CDK6 and induce phosphorylation of retinoblastoma (Rb) protein and overcome Rb-mediated cell cycle arrest.[95,96]

In the context of MCD, KSHV is thought to infect naive B lymphocytes, leading to the differentiation of these cells into isolated IgMλ-restricted polyclonal plasmablasts, which may further develop into frank plasmablastic lymphoma.[97,98] This pathogenetic theory is also supported by evidence that complete remission of symptoms related to MCD can be achieved in some patients by the use of anti-CD20 monoclonal rituximab; this correlates with a decreased KSHV viral load, with a concomitant transitory but evident decrease of KSHV-harboring CD19-positive B cells.[99]

Host Factors

An impairment in the host immune system may also play a role in the pathogenesis of MCD, as suggested by the occurrence of the disease in older individuals, the frequent association with recurrent infections, and (in secondary MCD, regardless of the KSHV status) the association with a wide range of diseases that all share a common deregulation of IL-6 expression. This is also evidenced by the increased incidence of MCD in HIV-positive patients.

CLINICAL FINDINGS

Localized CD develops in most patients before the age of 30 years, and there have been infrequent case reports of presentation in children.[100–102] No sex or race predominance is seen for localized CD.

Primary MCD occurs predominantly in older age groups (range, 19–85 years; median, 55.5 years),[13] and there is a slight preference for male gender (1.4:1)[103]; it is very uncommon in children, in whom it is probably associated with a status of primary immunodeficiency.[44,101,104] The clinical onset is characterized by systemic symptoms (eg, fatigue, fever, weight loss) and lymphadenopathy, which almost invariably occurs at the peripheral lymph node regions. Mediastinal or deeper lymphadenopathy, which is the most frequent clinical presentation of the localized form, is very uncommon in MCD but eventually can occur with disease progression.[105] Hepatomegaly and splenomegaly are present in most cases. Skin and neurologic manifestations have also been described; these include characteristic numerous violaceous nodules (caused by dermal plasma cell infiltration)[106–108] and mainly sensorimotor peripheral neuropathy.[109] Rheumatologic symptoms (ie, arthralgia and myalgia, keratoconjunctivitis sicca, xerostomia, and Raynaud's phenomenon)[110] and autoimmune manifestations (ie, rheumatoid arthritis, Sjögren's syndrome, mixed connective-tissue disease, and myasthenia gravis)[101,111–113] are frequently associated and overlap with MCD, rendering it difficult to determine which is the primary underlying disease.[110,114–116] Renal abnormalities, including proteinuria and hematuria, may (uncommonly) occur[117–119] and are associated with a very heterogeneous group of pathologic patterns (ie, membranous, mesangioproliferative, or membranoproliferative glomerulopathy; interstitial nephritis; amyloidosis; renal thrombotic microangiopathy; and glomerular microangiopathy).[46,117,119–122] Of interest, serum levels of IL-6 and VEGF have been found to be markedly elevated in cases with glomerular microangiopathy. It has been reported that these drop to normal levels after successful therapy, suggesting a pathogenic role for these cytokines.[119] Amyloidosis is most commonly associated with localized CD[123]; however, MCD also has been associated with systemic, renal, or interstitial amyloidosis of the AA type[121,122,124] as a consequence of an excess of the acute-phase reactant serum amyloid A, thought to be caused by hyperproduction of IL-6.[123]

The most common laboratory findings in MCD are anemia,[22,125,126] thrombocytopenia[127] (probably of autoimmune origin), and plasmacytosis in the bone marrow. Other findings may include an elevated erythrocyte sedimentation rate, hypergammaglobulinemia,[34] and the presence of a variety of autoantibodies (including those against smooth muscle, stomach, and salivary glands; phospholipids; antinuclear antibodies; rheumatoid factor; inhibitor of factors VII and VIII; and cryoglobulins). Abnormalities in the immune function include a low number of T cells, inversion of the ratio of CD4 to CD8, and T-cell unresponsiveness to mitogens, decreased IL-2 production, increased levels of soluble IL-2 receptor, and elevated serum IL-6.[43,48]

MCD-ASSOCIATED NEOPLASIA

In the context of secondary MCD, associations with a variety of pathologic conditions have been described (see Table 6–1). As in primary MCD, infection by KSHV is present in a significant proportion of cases of secondary MCD, and most of these cases are also associated with HIV infection and POEMS syndrome.[128,129] In KSHV-positive cases, a common association is KS[9,24] and a specific variant of non-Hodgkin's lymphoma (NHL) referred to as plasmablastic lymphoma.[24] Plasmablastic lymphoma is specifically associated with KSHV and was proposed as a new KSHV-linked disease entity.[24] The plasmablastic lymphoma cells associated with MCD show exactly the same phenotypic features as the plasmablasts described in MCD, including IgMλ expression and lack of Epstein-Barr virus (EBV) infection,[24,130] suggesting that the plasmablastic variant of MCD could herald the development of frank KSHV-positive plasmablastic lymphoma. The other type of KSHV-associated lymphoma, PEL, is different from plasmablastic lymphoma in that the tumor cells frequently lack expression of B-cell antigens (including immunoglobulin) and are frequently coinfected with EBV. In addition, plasmablastic lymphomas lack somatic hypermutation of immunoglobulin genes and are therefore thought to derive from naive B cells[98] whereas PELs are frequently hypermutated and are thought to correspond to post-germinal-center B cells.[131,132]

Several other types of neoplasia are occasionally diagnosed in patients with MCD. These are most commonly lymphoid tumors, including Hodgkin's lymphoma[133] and non-Hodgkin's lymphomas (NHLs) such as diffuse large cell lymphoma,[134] immunoblastic lymphoma,[97] and NHLs of the peripheral T-cell type.[135] Associations with nonlymphoid tumors such as rectal carcinoma,[136] renal cell carcinoma,[137] and a thyroid and kidney double carcinoma[138] have also been described but are less common.

MANAGEMENT

The clinical outcome of a patient with localized CD is very favorable as resection of abnormal lymph nodes is curative in almost all cases.[139] Classic surgical resection of involved lymph nodes[103] (or much less invasive thoracoscopic surgery)[139] and radiotherapy[140] have been successfully used to treat localized CD.

In contrast, MCD can present a wide spectrum of clinical evolution according to its spread and the presence of concomitant associated diseases. The overall median survival in a historical series was 34 months.[22] MCD is a potentially lethal disease that is often refractory to systemic therapy, including corticosteroids and single- or multiagent chemotherapy.[97,141] Surgery is less frequently used in MCD cases because of systemic involvement (with the possible exception of splenectomy when indicated).[8,22]

Since IgMλ-restricted plasmablasts that are localized in the mantle zone and harboring KSHV in patients with virus-related MCD express variable levels of CD20 surface antigen,[24] the anti-CD20 monoclonal antibody rituximab was tested as a therapeutic approach in a small group of patients; there was a complete remission of CD-related symptoms in three HIV-positive patients who were monitored for up to 14 months.[99,142] In that study, clinical remission correlated with a dramatic decrease of KSHV viral load and C-reactive protein levels and with a transitory but sharp decrease of CD19-positive cells, where KSHV is harbored.[99]

INF-α and retinoid acid have also been effectively used to treat HIV-associated CD.[143,144] According to a recent case report, the administration of thalidomide, a powerful cytokine disrupter, led to a dramatic response in one patient.[145]

Antiviral therapies for KSHV have been used infrequently, and inconsistent results have been reported in different studies in the literature. Remission of HIV-associated MCD, coincident with a decline in plasma KSHV deoxyribonucleic acid (DNA) levels, was achieved in three patients treated with intravenous ganciclovir therapy, providing in vivo evidence for the usefulness of antiviral agents against KSHV in the management of MCD patients.[146] However, in a previous study, antiviral therapy had been ineffective in reducing KSHV levels, and clinical improvement was achieved only after the administration of corticosteroids in combination with chemotherapy.[147]

The beneficial effect of highly active antiretroviral therapy in HIV-positive patients with MCD is controversial; there have been both cases in which a reduction of KSHV DNA in the peripheral blood to undetectable levels was achieved along with remission of KSHV-associated clinical manifestations[148,149] and cases in which the therapy failed to clear the serum KSHV load despite immune reconstitution and sustained full suppression of HIV.[150,151] These studies suggest that the KSHV load in peripheral-blood mononuclear cells is the most accurate marker of disease, independently of HIV loads, and is a potentially useful way of monitoring therapy.[12]

Finally, dysregulated overproduction of IL-6 seems to play an important role as an autocrine or paracrine factor in MCD.[75] Humanized anti-IL-6 receptor antibody has been used in the treatment of MCD and resulted in promising marked clinical and histologic improvement.[51]

SUMMARY AND CONCLUSIONS

Castleman's disease is a disease entity that has been difficult to understand and categorize, but much light has been shed on its pathogenesis in recent years. In particular, the discovery of KSHV and its identification in MCD has made it clear that localized CD and MCD are different diseases. In addition, it is now evident that CD represents several diseases and that KSHV-associated MCD represents a distinct category that is etiologically different from KSHV-negative MCD. Detailed molecular characterization of KSHV has shed light on the function of several viral proteins and their possible roles in MCD. Targeted inhibition of one or several of these viral molecules is likely to be a much needed therapeutic approach in what is hoped to be a not-so-distant future.

REFERENCES

1. Castleman B, Iverson L, Menendez VP. Localized mediastinal lymph node hyperplasia resembling thymoma. Cancer 1956;9:822–30.
2. Flendrig JA, Schillings PHM. Benign giant lymphoma: the clinical signs and symptoms. Folia Med Neerl 1969;12:119–20.
3. Flendrig JA. Benign giant lymphoma: clinicopathologic correlation study. In: Clark RL, Cumley RW: The yearbook of cancer. Chicago: Yearbook Medical, 1970. p. 296–9.
4. Keller AR, Hochholzer L, Castleman B. Hyaline-vascular and plasma-cell types of giant lymph node hyperplasia of the mediastinum and other locations. Cancer 1972;29:670–83.
5. Leibetseder F, Thurner J. Angiofollicular lymph node hyperplasia (onion-skin lymphoma). Med Klin 1973;68:817–20.
6. Gaba AR, Stein RS, Sweet DL, Variakojis D. Multicentric giant lymph node hyperplasia. Am J Clin Pathol 1978;69:86–90.
7. Frizzera G, Peterson BA, Bayrd ED, Goldman A. A systemic lymphoproliferative disorder with morphologic features of Castleman's disease: clinical findings and clinicopathologic correlations in 15 patients. J Clin Oncol 1985;3:1202–16.
8. Peterson BA, Frizzera G. Multicentric Castleman's disease. Semin Oncol 1993;20:636–47.
9. Soulier J, Grollet L, Oksenhendler E, et al. Kaposi's sarcoma-associated herpesvirus-like DNA sequences in multicentric Castleman's disease. Blood 1995;86:1276–80.
10. Chang Y, Cesarman E, Pessin MS, et al. Identification of herpesvirus-like DNA sequences in AIDS-associated Kaposi's sarcoma. Science 1995;267:1078–80.
11. Chadburn A, Cesarman E, Nador RG, et al. Kaposi's sarcoma-associated herpesvirus sequences in benign lymphoid proliferations not associated with human immunodeficiency virus. Cancer 1997;80:788–97.
12. Oksenhendler E, Carcelain G, Aoki Y, et al. High levels of human herpesvirus 8 viral load, human interleukin-6, interleukin-10, and C reactive protein correlate with exacerbation of multicentric Castleman disease in HIV-infected patients. Blood 2000;96:2069–73.
13. Shahidi H, Myers JL, Kvale PA. Castleman's disease. Mayo Clin Proc 1995;70:969–77.
14. Danon AD, Krishnan J, Frizzera G. Morpho-immunophenotypic diversity of Castleman's disease, hyaline-vascular type, with emphasis on a stroma-rich variant and a new pathogenetic hypothesis. Virchows Arch A Pathol Anat Histopathol 1993;423:369–82.
15. Perez-Ordonez B, Rosai J. Follicular dendritic cell tumor: review of the entity. Semin Diagn Pathol 1998;15:144–54.
16. Kojima M, Sakuma H, Mori N. Histopathologic features of plasma cell dyscrasia with polyneuropathy and endocrine disturbances, with special reference to germinal center lesions. Jpn J Clin Oncol 1983;13:557–75.
17. Menke DM, Camoriano JK, Banks PM. Angiofollicular lymph node hyperplasia: a comparison of unicentric, multicentric, hyaline vascular, and plasma cell types of disease by morphometric and clinical analysis. Mod Pathol 1992;5:525–30.
18. Nguyen DT, Diamond LW, Hansmann ML, et al. Castleman's disease. Differences in follicular dendritic network in the hyaline vascular and plasma cell variants. Histopathology 1994;24:437–43.
19. Ruco LP, Gearing AJ, Pigott R, et al. Expression of ICAM-1, VCAM-1 and ELAM-1 in angiofollicular lymph node hyperplasia (Castleman's disease): evidence for dysplasia of follicular dendritic reticulum cells. Histopathology 1991;19:523–8.
20. Hall PA, Donaghy M, Cotter FE, et al. An immunohistological and genotypic study of the plasma cell form of Castleman's disease. Histopathology 1989;14:333–46, 429–32.
21. Frizzera G, Banks PM, Massarelli G, Rosai J. A systemic lymphoproliferative disorder with morphologic features of Castleman's disease. Pathological findings in 15 patients. Am J Surg Pathol 1983;7:211–31.
22. Frizzera G. Atypical lymphoproliferative disorders. In: Knowles DM, editor. Neoplastic hematopathology. 2nd ed. Philadelphia: Lippincott Williams & Wilkins 2001. p. 569–622.
23. Miller RT, Mukai K, Banks PM, Frizzera G. Systemic lymphoproliferative disorder with morphologic features of Castleman's disease. Immunoperoxidase study of cytoplasmic immunoglobulins. Arch Pathol Lab Med 1984;108:626–30.
24. Dupin N, Diss TL, Kellam P, et al. HHV-8 is associated with a plasmablastic variant of Castleman disease that is linked to HHV-8-positive plasmablastic lymphoma. Blood 2000;95:1406–12.
25. Judde JG, Lacoste V, Briere J, et al. Monoclonality or oligoclonality of human herpesvirus 8 terminal repeat sequences in Kaposi's sarcoma and other diseases. J Natl Cancer Inst 2000;92:729–36.
26. Parravicini C, Chandran B, Corbellino M, et al. Differential viral protein expression in Kaposi's sarcoma-associated herpesvirus-infected diseases: Kaposi's sarcoma, primary effusion lymphoma, and multicentric Castleman's disease. Am J Pathol 2000;156:743–9.
27. Amin HM, Medeiros LJ, Manning JT, Jones D. Dissolution of the lymphoid follicle is a feature of the HHV8+ variant of plasma cell Castleman's disease. Am J Surg Pathol 2003;27:91–100.
28. Du MQ, Liu H, Diss TC, et al. Kaposi sarcoma-associated herpesvirus infects monotypic (IgM lambda) but poly-

clonal naive B cells in Castleman disease and associated lymphoproliferative disorders. Blood 2001;97:2130–6.

29. Peh SC, Shaminie J, Poppema S, Kim LH. The immunophenotypic patterns of follicle centre and mantle zone in Castleman's disease. Singapore Med J 2003;44:185–91.

30. Weisenburger DD. Multicentric angiofollicular lymph node hyperplasia. Pathology of the spleen. Am J Surg Pathol 1988;12:176–81.

31. Menke DM, Tiemann M, Camoriano JK, et al. Diagnosis of Castleman's disease by identification of an immunophenotypically aberrant population of mantle zone B lymphocytes in paraffin-embedded lymph node biopsies. Am J Clin Pathol 1996;105:268–76.

32. Hanson CA, Frizzera G, Patton DF, et al. Clonal rearrangement for immunoglobulin and T-cell receptor genes in systemic Castleman's disease. Association with Epstein-Barr virus. Am J Pathol 1988;131:84–91.

33. Soulier J, Grollet L, Oksenhendler E, et al. Molecular analysis of clonality in Castleman's disease. Blood 1995;86:1131–8.

34. Hineman VL, Phyliky RL, Banks PM. Angiofollicular lymph node hyperplasia and peripheral neuropathy: association with monoclonal gammopathy. Mayo Clin Proc 1982;57:379–82.

35. Radaszkiewicz T, Hansmann ML, Lennert K. Monoclonality and polyclonality of plasma cells in Castleman's disease of the plasma cell variant. Histopathology 1989;14:11–24.

36. Ohyashiki JH, Ohyashiki K, Kawakubo K, et al. Molecular genetic, cytogenetic, and immunophenotypic analyses in Castleman's disease of the plasma cell type. Am J Clin Pathol 1994;101:290–5.

37. Dupin N, Fisher C, Kellam P, et al. Distribution of human herpesvirus-8 latently infected cells in Kaposi's sarcoma, multicentric Castleman's disease, and primary effusion lymphoma. Proc Natl Acad Sci U S A 1999;96:4546–51.

38. Costa A, Barosi G, Piccolo G, et al. POEMS syndrome with IgA lambda monoclonal gammopathy. Haematologica 1990;75:170–2.

39. Pauwels P, Dal Cin P, Vlasveld LT, et al. A chromosomal abnormality in hyaline vascular Castleman's disease: evidence for clonal proliferation of dysplastic stromal cells. Am J Surg Pathol 2000;24:882–8.

40. Yoshizaki K, Matsuda T, Nishimoto N, et al. Pathogenic significance of interleukin-6 (IL-6/BSF-2) in Castleman's disease. Blood 1989;74:1360–7.

41. Herbelin C, Roux-Lombard P, Herbelin A, et al. Inflammation: "a natural experiment" for the systemic pathogenicity of cytokines. Eur Cytokine Netw 1998;9:57–60.

42. Hsu SM, Waldron JA, Xie SS, Barlogie B. Expression of interleukin-6 in Castleman's disease. Hum Pathol 1993;24:833–9.

43. Ishiyama T, Nakamura S, Akimoto Y, et al. Immunodeficiency and IL-6 production by peripheral blood monocytes in multicentric Castleman's disease. Br J Haematol 1994;86:483–9.

44. Kinney MC, Hummell DS, Villiger PM, et al. Increased interleukin-6 (IL-6) production in a young child with clinical and pathologic features of multicentric Castleman's disease. J Clin Immunol 1994;14:382–90.

45. Lee M, Hirokawa M, Matuoka S, et al. Multicentric Castleman's disease with an increased serum level of macrophage colony-stimulating factor. Am J Hematol 1997;54:321–3.

46. Lui SL, Chan KW, Li FK, et al. Castleman's disease and mesangial proliferative glomerulonephritis: the role of interleukin-6. Nephron 1998;78:323–7.

47. Mandler RN, Kerrigan DP, Smart J, et al. Castleman's disease in POEMS syndrome with elevated interleukin-6. Cancer 1992;69:2697–703.

48. Ishiyama T, Koike M, Nakamura S, et al. Interleukin-6 receptor expression in the peripheral B cells of patients with multicentric Castleman's disease. Ann Hematol 1996;73:179–82.

49. Beck JT, Hsu SM, Wijdenes J, et al. Brief report: alleviation of systemic manifestations of Castleman's disease by monoclonal anti-interleukin-6 antibody. N Engl J Med 1994;330:602–5.

50. Foussat A, Fior R, Girard T, et al. Involvement of human interleukin-6 in systemic manifestations of human herpesvirus type 8-associated multicentric Castleman's disease. AIDS 1999;13:150–2.

51. Nishimoto N, Sasai M, Shima Y, et al. Improvement in Castleman's disease by humanized anti-interleukin-6 receptor antibody therapy. Blood 2000;95:56–61.

52. Screpanti I, Romani L, Musiani P, et al. Lymphoproliferative disorder and imbalanced T-helper response in C/EBP beta-deficient mice. EMBO J 1995;14:1932–41.

53. Screpanti I, Musiani P, Bellavia D, et al. Inactivation of the IL-6 gene prevents development of multicentric Castleman's disease in C/EBP beta-deficient mice. J Exp Med 1996;184:1561–6.

54. Akira S, Taga T, Kishimoto T. Interleukin-6 in biology and medicine. Adv Immunol 1993;54:1–78.

55. Yoshizaki K, Kuritani T, Kishimoto T. Interleukin-6 in autoimmune disorders. Semin Immunol 1992;4:155–66.

56. Parravicini C, Corbellino M, Paulli M, et al. Expression of a virus-derived cytokine, KSHV vIL-6, in HIV-seronegative Castleman's disease. Am J Pathol 1997;151:1517–22.

57. Leger-Ravet MB, Peuchmaur M, Devergne O, et al. Interleukin-6 gene expression in Castleman's disease. Blood 1991;78:2923–30.

58. Brousset P, Cesarman E, Meggetto F, et al. Colocalization of the viral interleukin-6 with latent nuclear antigen-1 of human herpesvirus-8 in endothelial spindle cells of Kaposi's sarcoma and lymphoid cells of multicentric Castleman's disease. Hum Pathol 2001;32:95–100.

59. Winter SS, Howard TA, Ritchey AK, et al. Elevated levels of tumor necrosis factor-beta, gamma-interferon, and IL-6 mRNA in Castleman's disease. Med Pediatr Oncol 1996;26:48–53.

60. Nishi J, Arimura K, Utsunomiya A, et al. Expression of vascular endothelial growth factor in sera and lymph nodes of the plasma cell type of Castleman's disease. Br J Haematol 1999;104:482–5.

61. Emilie D, Zou W, Fior R, et al. Production and roles of IL-6, IL-10, and IL-13 in B-lymphocyte malignancies and in B-lymphocyte hyperactivity of HIV infection and autoimmunity. Methods 1997;11:133–42.

62. Marfaing-Koka A, Aubin JT, Grangeot-Keros L, et al. In vivo role of IL-6 on the viral load and on immunological abnormalities of HIV-infected patients. J Acquir Immune Defic Syndr Hum Retrovirol 1996;11:59–68.

63. Gherardi RK, Belec L, Soubrier M, et al. Overproduction of proinflammatory cytokines imbalanced by their antagonists in POEMS syndrome. Blood 1996;87:1458–65.

64. Miles SA, Rezai AR, Salazar-Gonzalez JF, et al. AIDS Kaposi sarcoma-derived cells produce and respond to interleukin 6. Proc Natl Acad Sci U S A 1990;87:4068–72.

65. Emilie D, Coumbaras J, Raphael M, et al. Interleukin-6 production in high-grade B lymphomas: correlation with the presence of malignant immunoblasts in acquired immunodeficiency syndrome and in human immunodeficiency virus-seronegative patients. Blood 1992;80:498–504.

66. Tesch H, Jucker M, Klein S, et al. Hodgkin and Reed-Sternberg cells express interleukin 6 and interleukin 6 receptors. Leuk Lymphoma 1992;7:297–303.

67. Kasaian MT, Casali P. Autoimmunity-prone B-1 (CD5 B) cells, natural antibodies and self recognition. Autoimmunity 1993;15:315–29.

68. Cesarman E, Nador RG, Aozasa K, et al. Kaposi's sarcoma-associated herpesvirus in non-AIDS related lymphomas occurring in body cavities. Am J Pathol 1996;149:53–7.

69. Jenner RG, Alba MM, Boshoff C, Kellam P. Kaposi's sarcoma-associated herpesvirus latent and lytic gene expression as revealed by DNA arrays. J Virol 2001;75:891–902.

70. Ballestas ME, Chatis PA, Kaye KM. Efficient persistence of extrachromosomal KSHV DNA mediated by latency-associated nuclear antigen. Science 1999;284:641–4.

71. Djerbi M, Screpanti V, Catrina AI, et al. The inhibitor of death receptor signaling, FLICE-inhibitory protein defines a new class of tumor progression factors. J Exp Med 1999;190:1025–32.

72. Friborg J Jr, Kong W, Hottiger MO, Nabel GJ. *p53* inhibition by the LANA protein of KSHV protects against cell death. Nature 1999;402:889–94.

73. Radkov SA, Kellam P, Boshoff C. The latent nuclear antigen of Kaposi sarcoma-associated herpesvirus targets the retinoblastoma-E2F pathway and with the oncogene Hras transforms primary rat cells. Nat Med 2000;6:1121–7.

74. Katano H, Sato Y, Itoh H, Sata T. Expression of human herpesvirus 8 (HHV-8)-encoded immediate early protein, open reading frame 50, in HHV-8-associated diseases. J Hum Virol 2001;4:96–102.

75. Cesarman E. Kaposi's sarcoma-associated herpesvirus—the high cost of viral survival. N Engl J Med 2003;349:1107–9.

76. Damania B, Jung JU. Comparative analysis of the transforming mechanisms of Epstein-Barr virus, Kaposi's sarcoma-associated herpesvirus, and Herpesvirus saimiri. Adv Cancer Res 2001;80:51–82.

77. Russo JJ, Bohenzky RA, Chien MC, et al. Nucleotide sequence of the Kaposi sarcoma-associated herpesvirus (HHV8). Proc Natl Acad Sci U S A 1996;93:14862–7.

78. Staskus KA, Sun R, Miller G, et al. Cellular tropism and viral interleukin-6 expression distinguish human herpesvirus 8 involvement in Kaposi's sarcoma, primary effusion lymphoma, and multicentric Castleman's disease. J Virol 1999;73:4181–7.

79. Teruya-Feldstein J, Zauber P, Setsuda JE, et al. Expression of human herpesvirus-8 oncogene and cytokine homologues in an HIV-seronegative patient with multicentric Castleman's disease and primary effusion lymphoma. Lab Invest 1998;78:1637–42.

80. Cannon JS, Nicholas J, Orenstein JM, et al. Heterogeneity of viral IL-6 expression in HHV-8-associated diseases. J Infect Dis 1999;180:824–8.

81. Drexler HG, Meyer C, Gaidano G, Carbone A. Constitutive cytokine production by primary effusion (body cavity-based) lymphoma-derived cell lines. Leukemia 1999;13:634–40.

82. Jones KD, Aoki Y, Chang Y, et al. Involvement of interleukin-10 (IL-10) and viral IL-6 in the spontaneous growth of Kaposi's sarcoma herpesvirus-associated infected primary effusion lymphoma cells. Blood 1999;94:2871–9.

83. Moore PS, Boshoff C, Weiss RA, Chang Y. Molecular mimicry of human cytokine and cytokine response pathway genes by KSHV. Science 1996;274:1739–44.

84. Molden J, Chang Y, You Y, et al. A Kaposi's sarcoma-associated herpesvirus-encoded cytokine homolog (vIL-6) activates signaling through the shared gp130 receptor subunit. J Biol Chem 1997;272:19625–31.

85. Nicholas J, Ruvolo VR, Burns WH, et al. Kaposi's sarcoma-associated human herpesvirus-8 encodes homologues of macrophage inflammatory protein-1 and interleukin-6. Nat Med 1997;3:287–92.

86. Luppi M, Barozzi P, Maiorana A, et al. Expression of cell-homologous genes of human herpesvirus-8 in human immunodeficiency virus-negative lymphoproliferative diseases. Blood 1999;94:2931–3.

87. Arvanitakis L, Geras-Raaka E, Varma A, et al. Human herpesvirus KSHV encodes a constitutively active G-protein-coupled receptor linked to cell proliferation. Nature 1997;385:347–50.

88. Bais C, Santomasso B, Coso O, et al. G-protein-coupled receptor of Kaposi's sarcoma-associated herpesvirus is a viral oncogene and angiogenesis activator. Nature 1998;391:86–9.

89. Lee H, Guo J, Li M, et al. Identification of an immunoreceptor tyrosine-based activation motif of K1 transforming protein of Kaposi's sarcoma-associated herpesvirus. Mol Cell Biol 1998;18:5219–28.

90. Zimring JC, Goodbourn S, Offermann MK. Human herpesvirus 8 encodes an interferon regulatory factor (IRF) homolog that represses IRF-1-mediated transcription. J Virol 1998;72:701–7.

91. Kirchhoff S, Sebens T, Baumann S, et al. Viral IFN-regulatory factors inhibit activation-induced cell death via two positive regulatory IFN-regulatory factor 1-dependent domains in the CD95 ligand promoter. J Immunol 2002;168:1226–34.

92. Guasparri I, Keller SA, Cesarman E. KSHV vFLIP is essential for the survival of infected lymphoma cells. J Exp Med 2004;199:993–1003.

93. Cheng EH, Nicholas J, Bellows DS, et al. A Bcl-2 homolog encoded by Kaposi sarcoma-associated virus, human herpesvirus 8, inhibits apoptosis but does not heterodimerize with Bax or Bak. Proc Natl Acad Sci U S A 1997;94:690–4.

94. Sarid R, Sato T, Bohenzky RA, et al. Kaposi's sarcoma-associated herpesvirus encodes a functional bcl-2 homologue. Nat Med 1997;3:293–8.

95. Godden-Kent D, Talbot SJ, Boshoff C, et al. The cyclin encoded by Kaposi's sarcoma-associated herpesvirus stimulates cdk6 to phosphorylate the retinoblastoma protein and histone H1. J Virol 1997;71:4193–8.

96. Li M, Lee H, Yoon DW, et al. Kaposi's sarcoma-associated herpesvirus encodes a functional cyclin. J Virol 1997;71:1984–91.

97. Oksenhendler E, Duarte M, Soulier J, et al. Multicentric Castleman's disease in HIV infection: a clinical and pathological study of 20 patients. AIDS 1996;10:61–7.

98. Du MQ, Liu H, Diss TC, et al. Kaposi sarcoma-associated herpesvirus infects monotypic (IgM lambda) but polyclonal naive B cells in Castleman disease and associated lymphoproliferative disorders. Blood 2001;97:2130–6.

99. Marcelin AG, Aaron L, Mateus C, et al. Rituximab therapy for HIV-associated Castleman disease. Blood 2003;102:2786–8.

100. Zhong LP, Chen GF, Zhao SF. Cervical Castleman disease in children. Br J Oral Maxillofac Surg 2004;42:69–71.

101. Osone S, Morimoto A, Tsutsui J, et al. Systemic juvenile idiopathic arthritis mimics multicentric Castleman's disease. Clin Rheumatol 2003;22:484–6.

102. Samadi DS, Hockstein NG, Tom LW. Pediatric intraparotid Castleman's disease. Ann Otol Rhinol Laryngol 2003; 112(9 Pt 1):813–6.

103. Bowne WB, Lewis JJ, Filippa DA, et al. The management of unicentric and multicentric Castleman's disease: a report of 16 cases and a review of the literature. Cancer 1999; 85:706–17.

104. O'Reilly PE Jr, Joshi VV, Holbrook CT, Weisenburger DD. Multicentric Castleman's disease in a child with prominent thymic involvement: a case report and brief review of the literature. Mod Pathol 1993;6:776–80.

105. Frizzera G. Castleman's disease: more questions than answers. Hum Pathol 1985;16:202–5.

106. Watanabe S, Ohara K, Kukita A, Mori S. Systemic plasmacytosis. A syndrome of peculiar multiple skin eruptions, generalized lymphadenopathy, and polyclonal hypergammaglobulinemia. Arch Dermatol 1986;122:1314–20.

107. Kitamura K, Tamura N, Hatano H, et al. A case of plasmacytosis with multiple peculiar eruptions. J Dermatol 1980;7:341–9.

108. Kubota Y, Noto S, Takakuwa T, et al. Skin involvement in giant lymph node hyperplasia (Castleman's disease). J Am Acad Dermatol 1993;29(5 Pt 1):778–80.

109. Scherokman B, Vukelja SJ, May E. Angiofollicular lymph node hyperplasia and peripheral neuropathy. Case report and literature review. Arch Intern Med 1991;151:789–90.

110. Kingsmore SF, Kingsmore DB, Hall BD, et al. Cooccurrence of collagenous colitis with seronegative spondyloarthropathy: report of a case and literature review. J Rheumatol 1993;20:2153–7.

111. Ben-Chetrit E, Flusser D, Okon E, et al. Multicentric Castleman's disease associated with rheumatoid arthritis: a possible role of hepatitis B antigen. Ann Rheum Dis 1989; 48:326–30.

112. Tavoni A, Vitali C, Baglioni P, et al. Multicentric Castleman's disease in a patient with primary Sjögren's syndrome. Rheumatol Int 1993;12:251–3.

113. Nanki T, Tomiyama J, Arai S. Mixed connective tissue disease associated with multicentric Castleman's disease. Scand J Rheumatol 1994;23:215–7.

114. Gohlke F, Marker-Hermann E, Kanzler S, et al. Autoimmune findings resembling connective tissue disease in a patient with Castleman's disease. Clin Rheumatol 1997;16:87–92.

115. Suwannaroj S, Elkins SL, McMurray RW. Systemic lupus erythematosus and Castleman's disease. J Rheumatol 1999;26:1400–3.

116. Kojima M, Nakamura S, Itoh H, et al. Systemic lupus erythematosus (SLE) lymphadenopathy presenting with histopathologic features of Castleman' disease: a clinicopathologic study of five cases. Pathol Res Pract 1997; 193:565–71.

117. Chim CS, Lam KY, Chan KW. Castleman's disease with Kaposi's sarcoma and glomerulonephritis. Am J Med 1999;107:186–8.

118. Saura IM, Carreton A, Lopez Guillen E, et al. [A 21-year-old male patient with nephrotic syndrome and "idiopathic" AA amyloidosis.] Nefrologia 2004;24 Suppl 3:109–12.

119. Seida A, Wada J, Morita Y, et al. Multicentric Castleman's disease associated with glomerular microangiopathy and MPGN-like lesion: does vascular endothelial cell-derived growth factor play causative or protective roles in renal injury? Am J Kidney Dis 2004;43:E3–9.

120. Lajoie G, Kumar S, Min KW, Silva FG. Renal thrombotic microangiopathy associated with multicentric Castleman's disease. Report of two cases. Am J Surg Pathol 1995;19:1021–8.

121. Moon WK, Kim SH, Im JG, et al. Castleman disease with renal amyloidosis: imaging findings and clinical significance. Abdom Imaging 1995;20:376–8.

122. Hattori K, Irie S, Isobe Y, et al. Multicentric Castleman's disease associated with renal amyloidosis and pure red cell aplasia. Ann Hematol 1998;77:179–81.

123. Perfetti V, Bellotti V, Maggi A, et al. Reversal of nephrotic syndrome due to reactive amyloidosis (AA-type) after excision of localized Castleman's disease. Am J Hematol 1994;46:189–93.

124. Miura A, Sato I, Suzuki C. Fatal diarrhea in a patient with Castleman's disease associated with intestinal amyloidosis. Intern Med 1995;34:1106–9.

125. Liberato NL, Bollati P, Chiofalo F, et al. Autoimmune hemolytic anemia in multicentric Castleman's disease. Haematologica 1996;81:40–3.

126. Lerza R, Castello G, Truini M, et al. Splenectomy induced complete remission in a patient with multicentric Castleman's disease and autoimmune hemolytic anemia. Ann Hematol 1999;78:193–6.

127. Carrington PA, Anderson H, Harris M, et al. Autoimmune cytopenias in Castleman's disease. Am J Clin Pathol 1990;94:101–4.

128. Papo T, Soubrier M, Marcelin AG, et al. Human herpesvirus 8 infection, Castleman's disease and POEMS syndrome. Br J Haematol 1999;104:932–3.

129. Belec L, Mohamed AS, Authier FJ, et al. Human herpesvirus 8 infection in patients with POEMS syndrome-associated multicentric Castleman's disease. Blood 1999;93:3643–53.

130. Gould SJ, Diss T, Isaacson PG. Multicentric Castleman's disease in association with a solitary plasmacytoma: a case report. Histopathology 1990;17:135–40.

131. Matolcsy A, Nador RG, Cesarman E, Knowles DM. Immunoglobulin VH gene mutational analysis suggests

that primary effusion lymphomas derive from different stages of B cell maturation. Am J Pathol 1998;153: 1609–14.

132. Fais F, Gaidano G, Capello D, et al. Immunoglobulin V region gene use and structure suggest antigen selection in AIDS-related primary effusion lymphomas. Leukemia 1999;13:1093–9.

133. Brice P, Marolleau JP, D'Agay MF, et al. Autoimmune hemolytic anemia disclosing Hodgkin's disease associated with Castleman's disease. Nouv Rev Fr Hematol 1991;33:273–4.

134. Weisenburger DD, Nathwani BN, Winberg CD, Rappaport H. Multicentric angiofollicular lymph node hyperplasia: a clinicopathologic study of 16 cases. Hum Pathol 1985;16: 162–72.

135. Hanchard B, Williams N, Green M. Concurrent multicentric angiofollicular lymph node hyperplasia and peripheral T-cell lymphoma. West Indian Med J 1987;36:104–7.

136. Wengrower D, Libson E, Okon E, Goldin E. Gastrointestinal manifestations in Castleman's disease. Am J Gastroenterol 1990;85:1179–81.

137. Stelfox HT, Stewart AK, Bailey D, Harrison D. Castleman's disease in a 44-year-old male with neurofibromatosis and pheochromocytoma. Leuk Lymphoma 1997;27:551–6.

138. Mizutani N, Okada S, Tanaka J, et al. Multicentric giant lymph node hyperplasia with ascites and double cancers, an autopsy case. Tohoku J Exp Med 1989;158:1–7.

139. Seirafi PA, Ferguson E, Edwards FH. Thoracoscopic resection of Castleman disease: case report and review. Chest 2003;123:280–2.

140. Chronowski GM, Ha CS, Wilder RB, et al. Treatment of unicentric and multicentric Castleman disease and the role of radiotherapy. Cancer 2001;92:670–6.

141. Scott D, Cabral L, Harrington WJ Jr. Treatment of HIV-associated multicentric Castleman's disease with oral etoposide. Am J Hematol 2001;66:148–50.

142. Corbellino M, Bestetti G, Scalamogna C, et al. Long-term remission of Kaposi sarcoma-associated herpesvirus-related multicentric Castleman disease with anti-CD20 monoclonal antibody therapy. Blood 2001;98:3473–5.

143. Kumari P, Schechter GP, Saini N, Benator DA. Successful treatment of human immunodeficiency virus-related Castleman's disease with interferon-alpha. Clin Infect Dis 2000;31:602–4.

144. Rieu P, Droz D, Gessain A, et al. Retinoic acid for treatment of multicentric Castleman's disease. Lancet 1999;354:1262–3.

145. Lee FC, Merchant SH. Alleviation of systemic manifestations of multicentric Castleman's disease by thalidomide. Am J Hematol 2003;73:48–53.

146. Casper C, Nichols WG, Huang ML, et al. Remission of HHV-8 and HIV-associated multicentric Castleman disease with ganciclovir treatment. Blood 2004;103:1632–4.

147. Senanayake S, Kelly J, Lloyd A, et al. Multicentric Castleman's disease treated with antivirals and immunosuppressants. J Med Virol 2003;71:399–403.

148. Boivin G, Gaudreau A, Routy JP. Evaluation of the human herpesvirus 8 DNA load in blood and Kaposi's sarcoma skin lesions from AIDS patients on highly active antiretroviral therapy. AIDS 2000;14:1907–10.

149. Lebbe C, Blum L, Pellet C, et al. Clinical and biological impact of antiretroviral therapy with protease inhibitors on HIV-related Kaposi's sarcoma. AIDS 1998;12:F45–9.

150. De Jong RB, Kluin PM, Rosati S, et al. Sustained high levels of serum HHV-8 DNA years before multicentric Castleman's disease despite full suppression of HIV with highly active antiretroviral therapy. AIDS 2003;17:1407–8.

151. Loi S, Goldstein D, Clezy K, et al. Castleman's disease and HIV infection in Australia. HIV Med 2004;5:157–62.

7

Primary Effusion Lymphomas: Biology and Management

SAMIR PAREKH
JOSEPH A. SPARANO

A lymphoma syndrome characterized by pleural effusions or ascites without nodal disease was originally described by Knowles and colleagues in 1989[1] and was first called "body-cavity–based lymphoma" by Cesarman and colleagues in 1995.[2] It was subsequently called "primary effusion lymphoma" (PEL),[3] a term that has been more widely used in the literature and that is used in this chapter. The clinical, morphologic, immunophenotypic, genetic, and virologic features of PEL are summarized in Table 7–1 and are discussed in further detail in this chapter.

CLINICAL PRESENTATION AND HISTORICAL BACKGROUND

The initial report of PEL discussed three individuals with acquired immune deficiency syndrome (AIDS), two of whom had pleural effusions associated with a pleomorphic malignant neoplasm in which a precise histopathologic diagnosis could not be rendered according to established criteria.[1] The tumor cells expressed leukocyte common antigen and a variable constellation of antigens associated with B- and T-cell activation (HLA-DR, T9, T10, BL2, BL3, Ki-24, and BLAST-2) but lacked all B-cell, T-cell, myeloid, and monocyte lineage-restricted antigens. Antigen receptor gene re-arrangement analysis demonstrated that each of these three neoplasms exhibited clonal immunoglobulin heavy-chain and κ light-chain gene re-arrangements and lacked T-cell receptor β chain gene re-arrangements, suggesting

that they were B cell–derived non-Hodgkin's lymphomas (NHLs) derived from a mature stage of B-cell differentiation (see Chapter 11, Diagnosis and Management of Non-Hodgkin's Lymphoma and Hodgkin's Lymphoma in the section of this book that discusses NHL). In addition, there was consistent presence of Epstein-Barr virus (EBV) proteins and/or deoxyribonucleic acid (DNA) sequences, suggesting that EBV played a pathogenetic role. Green and colleagues reported 18 human immunodeficiency virus (HIV)-positive patients with NHL associated with pleural effusions and/or ascites.[4] In 13 of 15 patients with data available, a body cavity was the site of the initial presentation of lymphoma, and 83% exhibited a null immunophenotype.

An association between PEL and human herpesvirus 8 (HHV-8) was initially reported in 1995. Prior to this description, HHV-8 had been implicated as a cause of Kaposi's sarcoma. HHV-8-positive solid lymphomas can occur in the absence of an effusion, and these resemble PEL morphologically and molecularly.[5–7] Recently, Chadburn and colleagues described extracavitary PEL by analyzing the morphologic, immunophenotypic, and molecular features of Kaposi's sarcoma–assiciated herpesvirus (KSHV)–positive solid lymphomas occurring in eight patients with human immunodeficiency virus (HIV) infection or AIDS and comparing these features with those of 29 similarly analyzed PELs. The eight KSHV-positive solid lymphomas were virtually indistinguishable from the 29 PELs, based on mor-

Table 7–1. TYPICAL FEATURES OF PRIMARY EFFUSION LYMPHOMA	
Clinical presentation	Pleural effusion, pericardial effusion, and/or ascites without nodal mass, usually in an HIV-seropositive individual or an elderly individual with chronic heart or liver disease
Diagnostic procedure	Thoracentesis or paracentesis with cytologic examination
Morphology	Numerous atypical lymphoid cells with an immunoblastic to anaplastic appearance, most with one to three prominent nucleoli and moderate amounts of deeply basophilic cytoplasm
Immunophenotyping	No expression: B-cell markers (CD10, CD19, CD20, and CD79a), T-cell markers (CD3, CD5, and CD45RO), or myelomonocytic markers (CD11b, CD13, CD14, and CD33) Expression: CD30, EMA-1, CD138
Viral expression	KSHV always positive; EBV expression usually positive but not always
Oncogene alternations	c-*myc* re-arrangement absent; may distinguish from Burkitt's lymphoma presenting as effusion
Immunoglobulin gene re-arrangements	Heavy- or light-chain re-arrangements present
Putative cell of origin	Preplasma cell
Treatment options	No established effective treatment Because spontaneous regressions have occurred after ART, all patients should receive a course of ART. Standard cytotoxic therapy occasionally induces complete response in about 20 percent.

ART = anti-retroviral therapy; EBV = Epstein-Barr virus; HIV = human immunodeficiency virus; KSHV = Kaposi's sarcoma–associated herpesvirus.

phology (immunoblastic/anaplastic), immunophenotype (CD45 positive; T-cell antigen negative; CD30, EMA, and CD138 positive; CD10, CD15, and BCL6 negative) and genotype (100% immunoglobulin genes re-arranged; no identifiable abnormalities in c-*myc*, *bcl6*, *bcl1*, and *bcl2*; and uniformly EBV positive). The only identifiable phenotypic difference was that the KSHV-positive solid lymphomas appeared to express B-cell–associated antigens (25%) and immunoglobulin (25%) slightly more often than did the PELs (< 5% and 15%, respectively; $p = .11$ and .08, respectively). The clinical presentation and course of the patients who developed KSHV-positive solid lymphomas were also similar, except for the lack of an effusion and somewhat better survival (median of 11 months versus 3 months). However, the three KSHV-positive solid lymphoma patients alive without disease 11, 25, and 44 months after initial presentation were recently diagnosed patients and, unlike the other patients with KSHV-positive solid lymphomas, received anti-retroviral therapy.[7]

VIRAL ETIOLOGY

Human Herpesvirus 8

Because of strong epidemiologic data suggesting that Kaposi's sarcoma (KS) has an infectious etiol-

ogy of viral origin, Chang and colleagues evaluated KS lesions by representational difference analysis to isolate unique sequences.[8] They identified DNA sequences in more than 90% of KS tissues obtained from patients with AIDS and in 15% of non-KS-tissue DNA samples from AIDS patients but not in tissue DNA from patients without AIDS. The sequences are homologous to, but distinct from, capsid and tegument protein genes of Gammaherpesvirinae, herpesvirus saimiri, and EBV. Subsequently, the same group and many others analyzed DNA in tissue samples from patients with AIDS-associated KS, classic KS, and HIV-seronegative homosexual men with KS, as well as in samples of uninvolved tissue from these patients and in control tissue from healthy subjects.[9] All samples were tested blindly by polymerase chain reaction (PCR), with specific primers to amplify KS330(233), a herpesvirus-like DNA sequence. The KS330(233) PCR product was found in 20 of 21 tissue samples (95%) from the patients with KS, including 10 of the 11 samples from the patients with AIDS-associated KS, all 6 samples from the patients with classic KS, and all 4 samples from the HIV-negative homosexual men with KS. Only 1 of the 21 control samples (5%) was positive (odds ratio, 400; 95% confidence interval, 19 to 17,300). Of the 14 samples of uninvolved skin from the patients with KS, 3 were positive for KS330(233). Representative PCR product sequences were more than 98% identical for the three types of KS, suggesting that all three are caused by the same agent. The term "Kaposi's sarcoma–associated herpesvirus" (KSHV) was coined to describe these unique viral DNA sequences. These seminal studies strongly implicated the role of KSHV in the pathogenesis of all forms of KS. Because of its homology to the herpesvirus family, KSHV was subsequently known as human herpesvirus 8.[10]

HHV-8 infection is associated with PEL[2] and with other lymphoproliferative disorders, such as multicentric Castleman's disease (MCD),[2,11,12] MCD-associated plasmablastic lymphoma, and germinotrophic lymphoma.[12,13] Cesarman and colleagues first reported an association between HHV-8 and PEL after examining the DNA of 193 cases of lymphoma by Southern blot hybridization, PCR, or both methods, including 42 cases of HIV-associated lymphoma. The PCR products in the positive samples were sequenced and compared with the KSHV sequences in KS tissues from the patients with AIDS. KSHV sequences were identified in eight lymphomas, all of which came from HIV-positive patients. All eight patients (and only these eight) had a distinct clinical presentation described as a "body-cavity–based lymphoma" (BCBL) characterized by pleural, pericardial, or peritoneal lymphomatous effusions. Consistent with the original report described by Knowles, all eight cases also contained the EBV viral genome. Quantitatively, these lymphomas contained 60 to 80 copies of HHV-8 per cell, compared with one copy per cell in KS lesions. When the PCR products of KS330 were sequenced, the HHV-8 sequences in both PEL and KS were found to be highly conserved. Since this original report, a number of additional reports have described the clinical, morphologic, etiologic, and molecular characteristics of this unusual lymphoma subtype and have substantiated the association between HHV-8 and PEL. Providing further evidence for the link between HHV-8 and PEL are several reports describing PEL associated with KS occurring in both HIV-positive and HIV-negative individuals,[14,15] including after cardiac transplantation.[15]

Epstein-Barr Virus

EBV, a member of the herpesvirus family, encodes a multitude of genes that drive proliferation or confer resistance to cell death by producing proteins, such as EBV nuclear antigens (EBNAs) and latent membrane proteins (LMPs), that mimic the effects of the activated cellular signaling proteins. As with HHV-8, EBV expression occurs in virtually all cases of PEL. EBV exhibits tropism for both lymphocytes and epithelial cells and can induce both replicative (productive/lytic) and latent (persistent) infections that result in a variety of human diseases in addition to PEL. The pattern of viral gene expression varies among tumor types, different viral genes playing key roles in different tumors and conferring sensitivity to immune surveillance.[16] The latency patterns, described here in order of lesser to greater expression of latency proteins, include the following: (1) latency I (ie, EBNA1 with or without LMP2A expression), found in Burkitt's lymphoma and in the circulating mononuclear cells of healthy EBV-infected individuals; (2) latency II (ie, EBNA1 plus other LMP expression), found in undifferentiated nasopharyngeal carcinoma and Hodgkin's disease; and (3) latency III (ie, EBNA1-6, LMP1, LMP2A, and LMP2B expression), the most complete pattern of expression of latent genes, found in lymphoblastoid cell lines (LCLs), immunoblastic lymphomas, and lymphoproliferative disorders occurring in immunosuppressed populations.

Horenstein and colleagues analyzed the pattern of EBV latent gene expression in five patients with PEL confirmed to be coinfected with EBV and KSHV by reverse transcription PCR, in situ hybridization, and immunohistochemical analysis.[17] EBV-encoded ribonucleic acid 1 (EBER1) messenger ribonucleic acid (mRNA), a consistent marker of viral latency, was present in all cases although at lower levels than in the non-PEL controls. Qp-initiated mRNA, encoding only EBNA1 and characteristic of latencies I and II, was positive in all PEL cases. Wp- and Cp-initiated mRNAs, encoding all EBNAs and characteristic of latency III, were negative in all cases. LMP1 mRNA, expressed in latencies II and III, was present in three cases although at very low levels that were not detectable at the protein level by immunohistochemical analysis. Low levels of LMP2A mRNA were detected in all cases. BZLF1, an early intermediate lytic phase marker, was weakly positive in four cases, suggesting a productive viral infection in a very small proportion of cells, which was confirmed by ZEBRA antigen expression. These findings demonstrated, therefore, that PEL exhibits a restricted latency pattern. Trivedi and colleagues confirmed these findings in HHV-8-positive PEL cell lines that lacked EBV (BC-3, CRO-AP/6, and CRO-AP/3) when superinfected with the recombinant Akata EBV strain. All EBV-infected clones expressed EBER1, EBNA1, and LMP2A whereas LMP1 and LMP2B were variable, and no cell lines expressed EBNA2-6. EBV transfection was associated with down-regulation of surface markers CD30, CD74, and syndecan-1. In contrast to EBV-negative parenteral cell lines, EBV-infected BC-3 and CRO-AP/6 cells were highly tumorigenic in mice with severe combined immunodeficiency, but none expressed TCL1. The findings suggest a critical role for EBV in the pathogenesis of PEL.

CYTOMORPHOLOGY

The cytomorphology of PEL has been described by Nador and colleagues, who reported a series of 15 cases.[3] Cytologic studies of the fluid reveals numerous atypical lymphoid cells with a plasmacytoid appearance, most of which have one to three prominent nucleoli and moderate amounts of deeply basophilic cytoplasm, exhibiting features that appear to bridge those of immunoblastic and anaplastic large cell lymphoma (Figure 7–1).[3] HHV-8 protein expression is also always present and may be detected by immunohistochemical staining. Although there have been some reports indicating isolated cases of PEL not associated with HHV-8,[18] others have shown that HHV-8-negative cases usually exhibit small noncleaved histology and c-*myc* gene re-arrangements, the latter of which have not been associated with PEL.[2] Other HHV-8-negative effusion lymphomas can also occur (mostly in HIV-positive patients) and are usually EBV positive, CD20 positive, and immunoglobulin (Ig) positive. This indicates that small noncleaved and large cell lymphoma can occasionally present with a clinical syndrome that may resemble PEL.

IMMUNOPHENOTYPING

Immunohistochemical analysis, flow cytometry , or both reveal that these cells bind antibodies against the activation markers CD30, epithelial membranc antigen (EMA1), and CD138 but fail to react with antibodies against B-cell markers (CD10, CD19, CD20, and CD79a), T-cell markers (CD3, CD5, and CD45RO), myelomonocytic markers (CD11b, CD13, CD14, and CD33), or cytokeratin.[3,19] Southern blot analysis performed with DNA prepared from the cells reveals nongermline immunoglobulin gene re-arrangements (heavy chain, light chain) that are due to dominant B-lymphoid clones. Of 17 lymphomas studied, 16 exhibited clonal IgH gene re-arrangements; of 16 cases studied, 14 exhibited clonal κ light-chain gene re-arrangements; and of 11 cases studied, 4 exhibited clonal λ light-chain gene re-arrangements. One of 16 cases exhibited clonal To gene re-arrangements in addition to clonal IgH and κ light-chain gene re-arrangements, indicating bigenotypism.

CLONALITY AND CELLULAR ORIGIN

Judde and colleagues investigated the use of terminal repeat (TR) sequences flanking the long unique region as a marker of clonality in HHV-8-associated tumors, including MCD and PEL.[20] Pulsed-field gel electrophoresis and multiple-probe Southern blot analysis of the HHV-8 TR region were performed on high–molecular weight DNA obtained from tumoral KS, PEL, and MCD lesions. These analyses showed that the fused TR region contained a large but variable number of TR units (from 16 to 75) and that the viral genome was present as extrachromosomal circular DNA in these tumors in vivo. There were also occasional ladders of heterogeneous linear termini reflecting lytic replication. All PEL tumors and PEL-derived cell lines as well as some KS tumors contained monoclonal or oligoclonal fused TR fragments, in contrast with MCD tumors, which were polyclonal. These studies indicate that some HHV-8-associated lymphoproliferative disorders have a monoclonal origin (such as PEL) whereas others have a polyclonal origin (such as MCD).

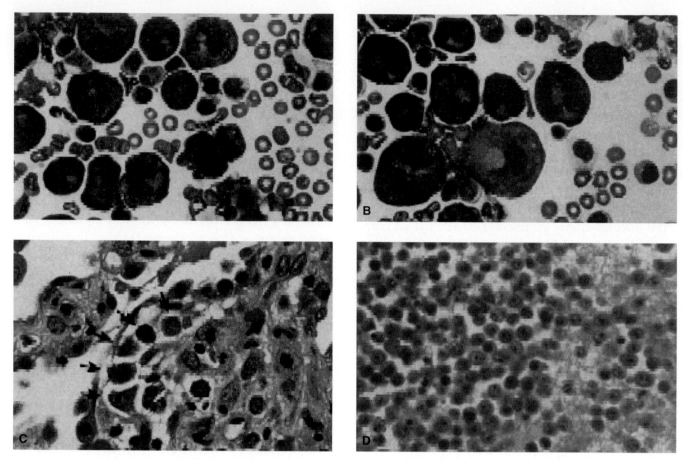

Figure 7–1.   *A* and *B*, Wright-Giemsa–stained air-dried cytocentrifuge preparation of a KSHV-positive primary effusion lymphoma. The cells are considerably larger than normal benign lymphocytes and red blood cells and exhibit cytomorphologic features that appear to bridge large cell immunoblastic lymphoma and anaplastic large cell lymphoma. The cells display variable polymorphism and generally possess moderately abundant amphophilic to deeply basophilic cytoplasm. A prominent clear perinuclear Golgi zone is frequently present. Small cytoplasmic vacuoles are occasionally present. The nuclei vary from large and round to highly irregular, multilobated and pleomorphic and often contain large prominent nucleoli (original magnification x 630). *C,* Hematoxylin and eosin-stained section of a primary effusion lymphoma involving the pulmonary lymphatics (original magnification x 630). *D,* Hematoxylin and eosin–stained pleural fluid cell block section of a KSHV-positive primary effusion lymphoma (original magnification x 400). The neoplastic cells are large but appear more uniform in size and shape and less polymorphic in these histologic sections than in the cytospin preparations. They contain moderately abundant, slightly eosinophilic cytoplasm, sometimes with a perinuclear hof, and generally large round to ovoid nuclei containing prominent nucleoli. Reproduced with permission from Nador RG et al.[3]

Klein and colleagues evaluated the cell of origin of PEL by performing gene expression analysis of PEL, various types of lymphoma, and peripheral blood lymphocytes from normal hosts.[21] The tumors evaluated in this study included samples from 9 patients with PEL, 16 patients with HIV-associated lymphomas (7 with Burkitt's lymphoma, 5 with centroblastic lymphoma, and 4 with immunoblastic lymphoma), and 37 cases of lymphoma not associated with HIV infection (6 cases of Burkitt's lymphoma, 23 cases of centroblastic lymphoma, and 8 cases of immunoblastic lymphoma). Gene expression profiles were analyzed by unsupervised cluster-ing and by supervised pattern discovery analysis. Under analysis by unsupervised clustering, PEL displayed a profile that was clearly distinguishable from those of Burkitt's lymphoma and diffuse large B-cell lymphoma. Gene expression profiling of PEL by supervised analysis confirmed that PEL was not significantly related to centroblasts or to memory B cells and that they were more related to LCLs. PEL displayed a gene expression profile that shared features of both large cell lymphoma and multiple myeloma yet was clearly distinct from both. PEL retained expression of some (*CD39, CD30, MUM-1/IRF-4*) but not all (*CD23*) of immunoblastic genes whereas PELs exhibited most myeloma markers (BLIMP1, CD138) indicative of terminal B-cell differentiation. Immunohistologic analysis showed that PEL did not express the memory B-cell marker CD27 and the B cell–specific transcription factor *PAX5*, whose expression is downregulated by BLIMP1 upon commitment to plasmacytoid differentiation. Overall, these data, together with those of the global gene expression analysis, indicate that PEL exhibits a phenotype that is intermediate between immunoblasts and plasma cells. Two upregulated genes with potential roles in receiving and transducing signals in BCLB cells were the interleukin-2 receptor and the Ras guanosine triphosphatase–activating protein–related *IQGAP2*, whose precise function is presently unknown. The most prominent among the genes specifically downregulated or absent in PEL were genes that are typically expressed in mature B cells, including the B cell specific *CD19*, *CD20*, and *CD79a/b* antigens as well as *CD22*, *CD52*, *CD72*, *BLNK*, *SHP1/PTP1C*, *SPIB*, and *BLR1/CXCR5*. A parallel study using a similar approach resulted in a similar conclusion.[22] This expression pattern further supported the notion that PEL displays a phenotype distinct from that of normal and transformed mature B cells.

TREATMENT

To more accurately describe the clinical presentation and treatment outcomes of PEL, Simonelli and colleagues retrospectively reviewed 277 patients with HIV infection and systemic lymphoma who were diagnosed at the authors' institution over a 15-year period; 11 of these cases met the criteria for PEL.[23] The clinical features and outcomes of patients with PEL were compared with those of 162 patients whose clinical information was available and who had plasmablastic lymphoma of the oral cavity (*n* = 11), immunoblastic lymphoma (*n* = 76), or centroblastic B-cell lymphoma (*n* = 75). There were no significant differences in the demographic data, CD4 count, plasma HIV viremia, or clinical characteristics of patients with PEL. Eight of the 11 PEL patients received standard combination chemotherapy regimens of cyclophosphamide, doxorubicin, and other agents (ie, regimens similar to the cyclophos-

phamide/doxorubicin/vincristine/prednisone [CHOP] regimen). Two of 11 patients who were treated with CHOP-like regimens had a complete response (CR), but one of three patients who received no cytotoxic therapy also had a CR, which may have occurred as a result of anti-retroviral therapy. Only two patients survived beyond 1 year; both had a CR after CHOP therapy or occurring spontaneously in association with anti-retroviral therapy. Spontaneous regression of PEL has been reported by others to occur after the initiation of anti-retroviral therapy.[24]

Although the great majority of cases of PEL have occurred in association with HIV infection, there have been several reports describing cases of PEL in HIV-negative individuals, including cases under unusual circumstances such as following cardiac transplantation. Ascoli and colleagues reviewed 20 cases of HIV-negative PEL reported in the literature; they called these cases "classic PEL," akin to "classic KS" reported in HIV-negative elderly Mediterranean men.[25] Typically, patients with "classic PEL" were male (all but three patients), presented at an older age (a mean age of 80 years), exhibited EBV infection less frequently (25%), and usually exhibited a less aggressive clinical course, although only six patients (30%) survived for at least 1 year. Some cases were associated with congestive heart failure (pleural presentation) and cirrhosis (ascitic presentation). The authors speculated that PEL progenitors circulating in the peripheral blood mononuclear cell fraction (like KS progenitors) may undergo viral replication when exposed to inflammatory sites or cytokine-rich environments such as the pleura or peritoneum, particularly in elderly patients who have mild age-associated immunosuppression, reside in areas endemic for HHV-8, and have chronic heart or liver disease that predisposes to pleural effusions or ascites.

Carbone and colleagues evaluated the clinical, pathologic, and molecular features of PEL occurring in four patients with HIV infection and in two patients who were not infected with HIV, as well as in an additional 10 patients who had lymphomatous effusions other than PELs.[26] KSHV was detected only in cases of PEL. The PEL cases shared common morphologic and immunophenotypic characteristics described by others and had a poorer prognosis when compared with non-PEL cases.

There are insufficient data to provide treatment recommendations for patients with PEL. Given the occasional responses reported after anti-retroviral therapy, a course of anti-retroviral therapy with the deferment of cytotoxic therapy should be considered for all patients. Responses to the anti-CD20 monoclonal antibody rituximab have been observed after treatment of MCD, a disease also associated with HHV-8 infection.[25,27,28] However, response to rituximab would not be expected in PEL, which typically lacks CD20 expression.

CONCLUSIONS

Primary effusion lymphoma is a distinct clinicopathologic entity that typically presents with a pleural effusion or ascites containing malignant lymphoma cells that have cytomorphologic, immunophenotypic, and genetic features of a lymphoma of plasmablastic origin. It usually presents in HIV-positive individuals but may occur in elderly individuals with chronic heart and liver disease. HHV-8 is always present, and EBV viral antigens are also usually expressed in a restricted latency pattern. It is believed to be a monoclonal lymphoid proliferation of aberrant plasmablasts. Treatment is unsatisfactory, but the disease may respond to the cytotoxic therapy typically administered for aggressive lymphoma although spontaneous regression may also occur, especially in patients with HIV infection treated with highly active anti-retroviral therapy.

ACKNOWLEDGMENT

The authors thank Dr. Ethel Cesarman, who reviewed this chapter and provided helpful comments.

REFERENCES

1. Knowles DM, Inghirami G, Urbiaco A, Della-Favera R. Molecular genetic analysis of three AIDS-associated neoplasms of uncertain lineage demonstrates their B-cell derivation and the possible pathogenetic role of the Epstein-Barr virus. Blood 1989;73:792–9.
2. Cesarman E, Chang Y, Moore P, et al. Kaposi's sarcoma-associated herpesvirus-like DNA sequences in AIDS-related body-cavity-based lymphomas. N Engl J Med 1995;332:1186–91.
3. Nador RG, Cesarman E, Chadbrun A, et al. Primary effusion lymphoma: a distinct clinicopathologic entity associated with the Kaposi's sarcoma-associated herpes virus. Blood 1996;88:645–56.
4. Green I, Espiritu E, Ladanyi M, et al, Primary lymphomatous effusions in AIDS: a morphological, immunophenotypic, and molecular study. Mod Pathol 1995;8:39–45.
5. Engels EA, Rosenberg PS, Frisch M, Goedert JJ. Cancers associated with Kaposi's sarcoma (KS) in AIDS: a link between KS herpesvirus and immunoblastic lymphoma. Br J Cancer 2001;85:1298–303.
6. Engels EA, Pittaluga S, Whitby D, et al. Immunoblastic lymphoma in persons with AIDS-associated Kaposi's sarcoma: a role for Kaposi's sarcoma-associated herpesvirus. Mod Pathol 2003;16:424–9.
7. Chadburn A, Hyjek E, Mathew S, et al. KSHV-positive solid lymphomas represent an extra-cavitary variant of primary effusion lymphoma. Am J Surg Pathol 2004;28:1401–16.
8. Chang Y, Cesarman E, Pessin MS, et al. Identification of herpesvirus-like DNA sequences in AIDS-associated Kaposi's sarcoma. Science 1994;266:1865–9.
9. Moore PS, Chang Y. Detection of herpesvirus-like DNA sequences in Kaposi's sarcoma in patients with and without HIV infection. N Engl J Med 1995;332:1181–5.
10. Memar OM, Rady PL, Tyring SK. Human herpesvirus-8: detection of novel herpesvirus-like DNA sequences in Kaposi's sarcoma and other lesions. J Mol Med 1995;73:603–9.
11. Palestro G, Turrini F, Pagano M, Chiusa L. Castleman's disease. Adv Clin Path 1999;3:11–22.
12. Dupin N, Diss TL, Kellam P, et al. HHV-8 is associated with a plasmablastic variant of Castleman disease that is linked to HHV-8-positive plasmablastic lymphoma. Blood 2000;95:1406–12.
13. Du MQ, Diss TC, Liu H, et al. KSHV- and EBV-associated germinotropic lymphoproliferative disorder. Blood 2002;100:3415–8.
14. Strauchen JA, Hauser AD, Burstein D, et al. Body cavity-based malignant lymphoma containing Kaposi sarcoma-associated herpesvirus in an HIV-negative man with previous Kaposi sarcoma. Ann Intern Med 1996;125:822–5.
15. Jones D, Ballestas ME, Kaye KM, et al. Primary-effusion lymphoma and Kaposi's sarcoma in a cardiac-transplant recipient. N Engl J Med 1998;339:444–9.
16. Aoki Y, Yarchoan R, Wyvill K, et al. Detection of viral interleukin-6 in Kaposi sarcoma-associated herpesvirus-linked disorders. Blood 2001;97:2173–6.
17. Horenstein MG, Nador RG, Chadburn A, et al. Epstein-Barr virus latent gene expression in primary effusion lymphomas containing Kaposi's sarcoma-associated herpesvirus/human herpesvirus-8. Blood 1997;90:1186–91.
18. Hermine O, Michel M, Buzyn-Veil A, Gessain A. Body-cavity-based lymphoma in an HIV-seronegative patient without Kaposi's sarcoma-associated herpesvirus-like DNA sequences. N Engl J Med 1996;334:272–3.
19. Gaidano G, Gloghini A, Gattei V, et al. Association of Kaposi's sarcoma-associated herpesvirus-positive primary effusion lymphoma with expression of the CD138/syndecan-1 antigen. Blood 1997;90:4894–900.
20. Judde JG, Lacoste V, Briere J, et al. Monoclonality or oligo-

clonality of human herpesvirus 8 terminal repeat sequences in Kaposi's sarcoma and other diseases. J Natl Cancer Inst 2000;92:729–36.

21. Klein U, Gloghini A, Gaidano G, et al. Gene expression profile analysis of AIDS-related primary effusion lymphoma (PEL) suggests a plasmablastic derivation and identifies PEL-specific transcripts. Blood 2003;101:4115–21.

22. Jenner RG, Maillard K, Cattini N, et al. Kaposi's sarcoma-associated herpesvirus-infected primary effusion lymphoma has a plasma cell gene expression profile. Proc Natl Acad Sci U S A 2003;100:10399–404.

23. Simonelli C, Spina M, Cinelli R, et al. Clinical features and outcome of primary effusion lymphoma in HIV-infected patients: a single-institution study. J Clin Oncol 2003; 21:3948 54.

24. Oksenhendler E, Clauvel JP,. Jouveshomme S, et al. Complete remission of primary effusion lymphoma with anti-retroviral therapy [letter]. Am J Hematol 1998;57:266.

25. Ascoli V, Lo Coco F, Torelli G, et al., Human herpesvirus 8-associated primary effusion lymphoma in HIV patients: a clinicopidemiologic variant resembling classic Kaposi's sarcoma. Haematologica 2002;87:339–43.

26. Carbone A, Gloghini A, Vaccher E, et al. Kaposi's sarcoma-associated herpesvirus DNA sequences in AIDS-related and AIDS-unrelated lymphomatous effusions. Br J Haematol 1996;94:533–43.

27. Corbellino M, Bestetti G, Scalamonga C, et al. Long-term remission of Kaposi sarcoma-associated herpesvirus-related multicentric Castleman disease with anti-CD20 monoclonal antibody therapy. Blood 2001;98:3473–5.

28. Marcelin AG, Aaron L, Mateus C, et al. Rituximab therapy for HIV-associated Castleman disease. Blood 2003;102: 2786–8.

8

Epstein-Barr Virus Infection and the Pathogenesis of Cancer: Lymphomas and Nasopharyngeal Carcinoma

PAUL G. MURRAY
LAWRENCE S. YOUNG

Epstein-Barr virus (EBV) was first identified in 1964 by electron microscopy of a cell line established from a biopsy specimen of Burkitt's lymphoma (BL); an aggressive B-cell tumor identified some 6 years earlier by Denis Burkitt. Serologic analysis then showed that BL patients had higher antibody titers to EBV antigens than healthy controls had. Subsequently, similar assays identified EBV as the etiologic agent of infectious mononucleosis (IM) and undifferentiated nasopharyngeal carcinoma (UNPC). The efficient transformation capacity of EBV was confirmed by studies that showed that the virus could convert resting B lymphocytes in vitro into permanently growing cell lines as well as induce tumors in nonhuman primates. Later studies have shown that EBV is associated with a variety of other human tumors, including B-cell malignancies such as Hodgkin's lymphoma and lymphoproliferative disease arising in immunosuppressed patients, some T-cell lymphomas, and other epithelial tumors such as gastric cancer.

EBV is a gammaherpesvirus of the *Lymphocryptovirus* (*LCV*) genus and is closely related to other *LCV* species present in Old World nonhuman primates, including EBV-like viruses of chimpanzees and rhesus monkeys. A transforming, EBV-related virus has also been isolated from spontaneous B-cell lymphomas of common marmosets and is the first EBV-like virus to be identified in a New World monkey species.[1,2] Sequencing of the genome of the marmoset *LCV* has revealed considerable divergence from the genomes of EBV and Old World primate EBV-related viruses.

EBV is a ubiquitous virus that is carried by the majority of the world's adult population as a lifelong asymptomatic infection.[3] Early in the course of primary infection, EBV infects B lymphocytes although it is not known where B lymphocytes are infected and whether this involves epithelial cells of the upper respiratory tract. To achieve long-term persistence in vivo, EBV colonizes the memory B-cell pool where it establishes latent infection, which is characterized by the expression of a limited subset of virus genes, known as "latent" genes.[4] There are several well-described forms of EBV latency, each of which is used by the virus at different stages of the normal virus life cycle and which are also reflected in the patterns of latency observed in the various EBV-associated malignancies.[3,5] Furthermore, during its life cycle, EBV must periodically enter the replicative cycle to generate infectious virus for transmission to other susceptible hosts although it is not clear where this occurs. Replicative infection is not generally a feature of EBV-associated tumors because it often results in cell death.

EBV LATENCY

The Lymphoblastoid Cell Line: A Model of EBV Latency

A minority of peripheral-blood B cells from healthy virus carriers are infected with EBV. These can give rise to the spontaneous outgrowth of EBV-transformed immortalized cell lines known as lymphoblastoid cell lines (LCLs), provided that immune T lymphocytes are either removed or inhibited by the addition of cyclosporin A to the culture.[6] LCLs can also be generated by direct infection of resting B lymphocytes with EBV derived from B-cell lines that can produce infectious virus.

Every cell in an LCL carries multiple copies of circular extrachromosomal viral DNA (known as episomes) and expresses a set of latent genes comprising genes encoding for six nuclear proteins (Epstein-Barr nuclear antigens 1, 2, 3A, 3B, 3C, and LP) and three latent membrane proteins (LMPs), namely, LMP1, LMP2A, and LMP2B (Figure 8–1). An alternative nomenclature for the EBV genes is based on the location of each gene within fragments produced by digestion with the restriction enzyme

*Bam*HI-A. Thus, an alternative designation for the *LMP1* gene is *BNLF1*, meaning that after *Bam*HI digestion, the fragment designated "N" (fragments produced after digestion are labeled "A" to "Z" in descending order of fragment size) contains the *LMP1* gene, which is the first (*1*) leftward (*L*) open reading frame (*F*). In addition to the known latent proteins, transcripts, referred to as *Bam*HI-A rightward transcripts (BARTs) are also expressed in latent infection; however, proteins from these transcripts are yet to be convincingly demonstrated.[3] LCLs also show abundant expression of the small noncoding ribonucleic acids (RNAs) known as EBV-encoded RNA (EBER) 1 and 2. The function of these transcripts is not clear, but they are believed to be expressed in all forms of latent EBV infection and have served as excellent targets for detecting EBV in tumors.

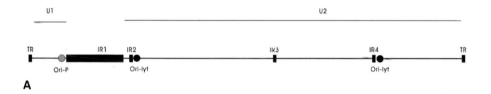

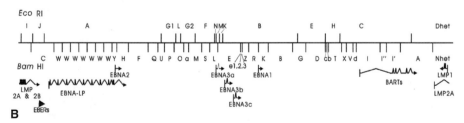

Figure 8–1. The Epstein-Barr virus (EBV) genome. *A*, General organization of linear EBV virion DNA. U1 and U2 are the short and long unique regions of the genome, respectively. These are interspersed with the four internal repeat regions IR1-4. TR represents the terminal repeats. The origin of replication (Ori-P) of the intracellular circular episomal form of the genome is indicated by the grey circle whereas the lytic origins of replication (Ori-lyt) are shown as black circles. *B*, *Eco*RI and *Bam*HI restriction endonuclease maps of EBV DNA and the positions of the genes expressed in latency. The *Bam*HI fragments are named according to the well-established B95-8 designations, with the exception of I (which is larger than its B95-8 counterpart), I', and I" (which are absent in the B95-8 strain). The splicing patterns of the latent ribonucleic acids (RNAs) through the coding regions are indicated. EBNA-LP is transcribed from variable numbers of repetitive exons. The full transcriptional patterns of the remaining *EBNA* genes are more complex than shown here (see text), and the *Bam*HI-A rightward transcripts (BARTs) consist of a number of differently spliced RNA species emanating from the same promoter.[144,145] Note that the LMP2 proteins are produced from messenger RNAs (mRNAs) that splice across the terminal repeats in the intracellular circularized EBV genome. This region has often been referred to as "Nhet" to denote the heterogeneity in this region according to the number of terminal repeats within different virus isolates.

The different Epstein-Barr nuclear antigens (EBNAs) are encoded by individual messenger ribonucleic acids (mRNAs) generated by differential splicing of the same long primary transcript expressed from one of two promoters (Cp or Wp) located close together in the *Bam*HI C and W regions of the genome.[7] The LMP transcripts are expressed from separate promoters in the *Bam*HI N region of the EBV genome, with the leftward LMP1 and rightward LMP2B mRNAs apparently controlled by the same bidirectional promoter sequence (ie, ED-L1). The LMP2A promoter is also regulated by EBNA2. Both LMP2A and LMP2B transcripts cross the terminal repeats (TRs) located at the end of each linear EBV genome. Thus, for LMP2 to be expressed, the genome must be circularized. Circularization occurs by homologous recombination of the TRs, resulting in fused termini of unique length, and this has been used as a marker of EBV clonality on the assumption that fused TRs with an identical number of repeats denote expansions of a single infected progenitor cell.[8] This contention has recently been challenged by the observation that EBV clonality post infection may be a consequence of the selective growth advantage achieved by optimal LMP2A expression over a minimal number of TRs.[9] The pattern of latent EBV gene expression observed in LCLs is referred to as latency (Lat) III and is seen in the majority of EBV-positive post-transplantation lymphomas (Figure 8–2).

The Lat III pattern of EBV gene expression has dramatic consequences for the phenotype of B cells, resulting in the high-level expression of the activation markers CD23, CD30, CD39, and CD70 and of the cellular adhesion molecules, leukocyte function associated molecule 1 (LFA-1; CD11a/18), LFA-3 (CD58), and intercellular adhesion molecule 1 (ICAM1, CD54).[10] These markers are usually absent or are expressed at low levels on resting B cells but are transiently induced when these cells are activated into short-term growth by antigenic or mitogenic stimulation; therefore, EBV-induced immortalization is elicited through the constitutive activation of the same cellular pathways that drive physiologic B-cell proliferation. The ability of EBNA2, EBNA3C, and LMP1 to induce LCL-like

phenotypic changes when expressed individually in human B-cell lines identifies these viral proteins as key effectors of the immortalization process.[11]

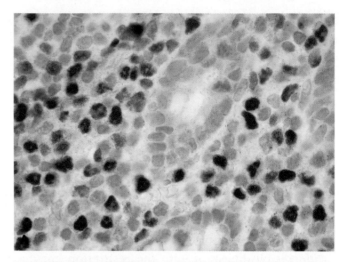

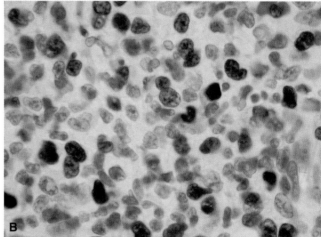

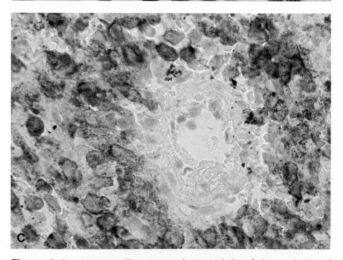

Figure 8–2. Latency III pattern characteristic of the majority of cases of post-transplantation lymphoproliferative disease. All known Epstein-Barr virus latent genes are expressed in this form of latency. *A,* EBERs. *B,* EBNA2. *C,* LMP1.

Other Forms of EBV Latency

Although the LCL model has proven valuable in identifying the role of individual EBV genes in the immortalization of B cells, it is not representative of the majority of EBV-associated tumors, which (with the exception of post-transplant lymphomas) have more restricted virus gene expression profiles. In EBV-associated primary BL, for example, EBNA1 is the only EBV protein consistently observed although there are rare reports of the expression of LMP1 and EBNA2 in some cases.[12,13] In BL, *EBNA1* is transcribed from the Qp promoter rather than from Wp or Cp.[14] In addition, the EBER and the *Bam*HI-A transcripts are also present; this form of latency is referred to as latency I (Figure 8–3).[15]

BL cells express CD10 and CD77, a phenotype most closely resembling that of centroblasts in germinal centers. When cells from EBV-positive BL tumors are cultured, the other EBNAs and LMPs may be expressed after some time, and the EBNA2- and LMP1-induced cell surface antigens, such as CD23, CD30, CD39, LFA1, LFA3, and ICAM1, may be upregulated.[12] EBNA2 and LMP1 are the major mediators of EBV-induced B-lymphocyte growth in vitro, and the lack of expression of these proteins in tumor cells suggests that they are not required for growth of BL.

Another form of EBV latency, Lat II, was originally identified in biopsy specimens of UNPC and subsequently in EBV-associated Hodgkin's lymphoma (HL).[16–19] Here, expression of the EBERs, Qp-driven EBNA1, and *Bam*HI-A transcripts is accompanied by expression of LMP1 and LMP2A/B (Figure 8–4). Transcription of LMP1 is controlled by an EBNA2-independent promoter located within the viral terminal repeats (L1-TR) and is regulated by the Janus kinase (JAK)/Signal transducer and activator of transcription (STAT) signaling pathways.[20,21] While this Lat II pattern of EBV latent gene expression is a consistent feature of virus-associated HL, LMP1 expression in nasopharyngeal carcinoma (NPC) is variable, and only about 20% of biopsy specimens are unequivocally positive for LMP1 at the protein level.[22]

The observation that the majority of UNPC tumors do not express the LMP1 and that EBNA2 can occasionally be detected in BL tumor cells emphasizes the limitations of the operational categorization of virus latency into three distinct forms.

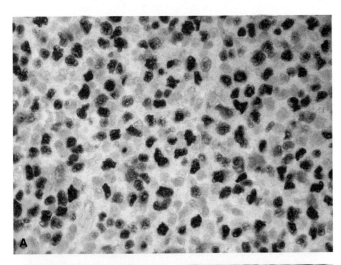

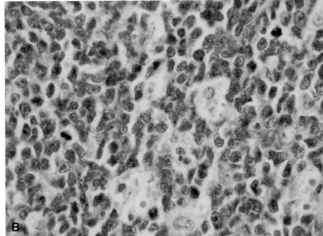

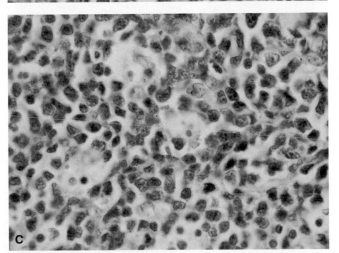

Figure 8–3. Latency I pattern in the tumor cells of Burkitt's lymphoma. Here, the only Epstein-Barr virus protein detectable is EBNA1. Shown is expression of EBERs (A) and absence of EBNA2 (B) and LMP1.

It is clear that in vivo there is often a spectrum of EBV latent gene expression within the same infected tissue. The need for caution in the rigid

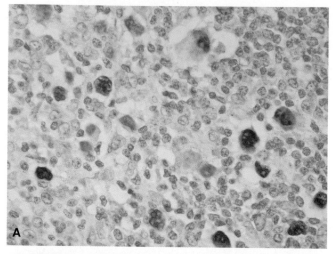

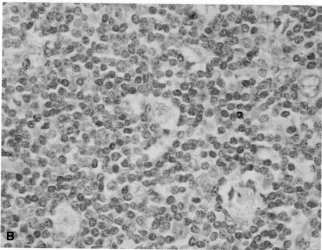

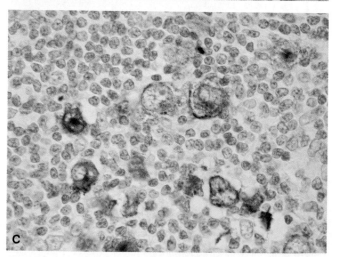

Figure 8–4. Epstein-Barr virus latency II in the Hodgkin/Reed-Sternberg cells of Hodgkin's lymphoma. *A,* Expression of EBERs. *B,* Absence of EBNA2 expression. *C,* High-level expression of LMP1.

application of these forms of EBV latency was highlighted by a recent study in which expression of the EBNA3 family has been identified in a subset of BL biopsy specimens.[23] It appears that in these tumors, the selective pressure to downregulate EBNA2 expression has occurred via deletion of the *EBNA2* gene rather than through the switch to Qp usage observed in the conventional BL scenario. Other forms of EBV latency in which the EBERs are not expressed have been reported in breast carcinoma and hepatocellular carcinoma, but here the association with EBV remains controversial.[24–26]

EBV Persistence In Vivo

B lymphocytes appear to be major site of EBV persistence in vivo. EBV-positive B lymphocytes in the peripheral blood are immunoglobulin D (IgD)–negative memory cells, gene expression in these cells being restricted to LMP2A and possibly EBNA1.[27] Healthy tonsils contain EBV-positive naive (IgD-positive) B cells, which express the Lat III program and show an activated phenotype, suggesting they have been directly infected.[28] These cells are presumably either eliminated by virus-specific cytotoxic T lymphocytes (CTLs) or differentiate to IgD-negative memory B cells that could either replenish the peripheral pool of infected memory cells or differentiate into plasma cells and enter the lytic cycle. The Lat II pattern, where both LMP1 and LMP2A are expressed, has also been detected in tonsillar memory B cells and in germinal-center B cells.[29] LMP1 acts as a surrogate for T-cell help by mimicking an activated CD40 receptor, and LMP2A substitutes for B-cell receptor engagement. Thus, the current model is one in which EBV-infected B cells enter a germinal-center reaction, re-express LMP1 and LMP2A and, in so doing, enable the antigen-independent expansion of EBV-infected B cells.[29]

Cells other than B lymphocytes can be infected by EBV in vivo. Thus, squamous epithelial cells are EBV positive in oral hairy leukoplakia (Figure 8–5), a benign lesion of the oral epithelia observed in immunosuppressed patients and characterized by intense replication of EBV in these tissues.[30,31] However, EBV is not usually detectable in normal epithelial tissues, including desquamated oropha-

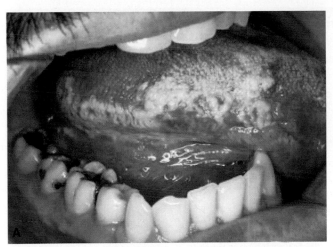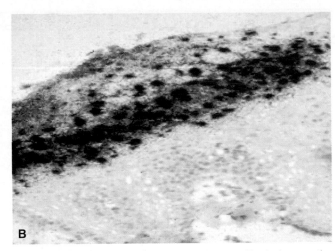

Figure 8–5. *A,* Oral hairy leukoplakia (OHL), a benign condition of the oral tissues that is characterized by white plaquelike lesions on the lateral tongue. *B,* In situ hybridization demonstrates the presence of abundant Epstein-Barr virus DNA in the upper layers of the squamous epithelium of an OHL lesion where virus replication is occurring.

ryngeal cells and tonsillar epithelium from IM patients[32–34] and normal epithelium adjacent to EBV-positive UNPCs[35] and EBV-positive gastric carcinomas.[36] It may be that epithelial infection acts to amplify EBV through viral replication during primary infection or occasionally during asymptomatic persistence and that this effect is exaggerated in hairy leukoplakia, as a consequence of immunosuppression. The establishment of latency in epithelial cells might not be a normal outcome; it may occur only if cellular genetic changes alter the cell environment. This is consistent with NPC genetics studies that demonstrate loss of heterozygosity at certain key loci occurring prior to EBV infection.[37]

Function of EBV Latent Genes

An understanding of EBV latent gene function is relevant both to the factors contributing to the establishment of persistent infection in the memory B-cell pool and to the role of the virus in the oncogenic process. The advent of recombinant EBV technology has confirmed the absolute requirement for *EBNA2* and *LMP1* in the in vitro transformation of B cells and has highlighted a role for *EBNA-LP,* *EBNA3A, EBNA3C,* and *LMP2A* in this process. These studies confirm that EBV-induced B-cell transformation requires the coordinated action of several latent genes but do not address the consequences of the more restricted patterns of EBV

latent gene expression observed in persistent infection and in certain EBV-associated tumors. More recent studies using recombinant EBV to infect either virus-negative BL cell lines or epithelial cell lines are beginning to define the contribution of more limited EBV latent gene expression to the cell phenotype and determine the mechanisms responsible for regulating virus gene expression in different cellular environments. Table 8–1 and the following text provide a brief description of EBV latent protein functions as a prelude to the consideration of the possible roles of these genes in the pathogenesis of the various EBV-associated tumors.

EBNA1

EBNA1 is a sequence-specific deoxyribonucleic acid (DNA)–binding protein that is required for the replication and maintenance of the episomal EBV genome. EBNA1 also acts as a transcriptional transactivator and upregulates the Cp and the LMP1 promoter. Furthermore, directing EBNA1 expression to B cells in transgenic mice results in B-cell lymphomas, suggesting that EBNA1 might also have a direct role in oncogenesis.[38] The EBNA1 protein contains a glycine-glycine-alanine (gly-gly-ala) repeat sequence, which varies in size in different EBV isolates and is an inhibitor of antigen processing via the ubiquitin-proteosome pathway.[39] Failure to present EBNA1-derived peptides results in inef-

Table 8-1. SUMMARY OF THE FUNCTIONS OF KNOWN EPSTEIN-BARR VIRUS LATENT PROTEINS

Protein	Function
EBNA1	DNA-binding protein required for replication and maintenance of the episomal EBV genome
EBNA2	Essential for B-cell transformation Transcriptional activator of cellular and viral genes; upregulates CD21, CD23, LMP1, LMP2, and c-*myc* oncogene Involved in the Notch pathway; interacts with DNA-binding protein RBP-Jκ
EBNA3 family	Group of three related proteins EBNA3A and EBNA3C (but not EBNA3B) essential for B-cell transformation
EBNA-LP	Not absolutely required for B-cell transformation in vitro, but necessary for efficient long-term growth of transformed B-cell lines
LMP1	Essential for B-cell transformation Activates the transcription factor NF-κB and other signaling pathways, including JNK and p38/MAPK pathways
LMP2	Gene encoding LMP2 yields two proteins (LMP2A and LMP2B). LMP2A blocks B-cell receptor–stimulated calcium mobilization, tyrosine phosphorylation, and activation of EBV lytic cycle in B cells, thus maintaining viral latency.

DNA = deoxyribonucleic acid; EBV = Epstein-Barr virus.

fective $CD8^+$ T-cell responses to EBNA1 when expressed in target cells. EBNA1 is toxic in certain epithelial cell environments, and this is associated with the processing and presentation of EBNA1 to specific CTLs.[40] These data suggest that the establishment of EBV latency is dependent on the cell background and that CTL responses to EBNA1 may contribute to the control of latent infection.

EBNA2

The inability of an EBV strain, P3HR-1 (which carries a deletion of the gene encoding EBNA2 and the last two exons of EBNA-LP), to transform B cells in vitro was the first indication of the crucial role of the EBNA2 protein in the transformation process. Restoration of the *EBNA2* gene into P3HR-1 has unequivocally confirmed the importance of EBNA2 in B-cell transformation and has allowed the functionally relevant domains of the EBNA2 protein to be identified.[41,42] EBNA2 is a transcriptional activator of both cellular and viral genes and upregulates the expression of B-cell antigens, including CD21 and CD23 as well as LMP1 and LMP2.[43] EBNA2 interacts with a ubiquitous DNA-binding protein, RBP-Jκ, and this is partly responsible for targeting EBNA2 to promoters that contain the RBP-Jκ sequence.[44] The RBP-Jκ homologue in *Drosophila* is involved in signal transduction from the Notch receptor, a pathway that is important in determining cell fate in *Drosophila* and that has also been implicated in the development of T-cell tumors in humans.[45] EBNA2 can functionally replace the intracellular region of Notch.[46] The c-*myc* oncogene is also a transcriptional target of EBNA2, a phenomenon that is likely to be important for EBV-induced B-cell proliferation.[47]

EBNA3 Family

EBNA3A and EBNA3C are essential for B-cell transformation in vitro whereas EBNA3B is dispensable. EBNA3C can induce the up-regulation of both cellular (CD21) and viral (LMP1) gene expression,[48] can repress the Cp promoter,[49] and might interact with the retinoblastoma protein pRb to promote transformation.[50] All three EBNA3 proteins can repress EBNA2-mediated transactivation by disrupting its interaction with RBP-Jκ.[51] Thus, EBNA2 and the EBNA3 proteins work together to precisely control RBP-Jκ activity, thereby regulating the expression of important cellular and viral promoters.

EBNA-LP

While not absolutely required for B-cell transformation in vitro, EBNA-LP supports the efficient outgrowth of LCLs.[52] Transient transfection of EBNA-LP and EBNA2 into primary B cells induces transition from G_0 to G_1 as measured by the up-regulation of cyclin D2 expression.[53] EBNA-LP can also cooperate with EBNA2 in upregulating transcriptional targets of EBNA2, including LMP1.[54] EBNA-LP has been shown to colocalize with pRb in LCLs, and in vitro biochemical studies have demonstrated an interaction of EBNA-LP with both pRb and *p53*.[55,56] However, this interaction has not been verified in LCLs, and unlike the situation with the human papillomavirus–encoded E6/E7 and adenovirus E1 proteins, EBNA-LP expression appears to have no effect on the regulation of the pRb and T*p53* pathways.

LMP1

LMP1 is the major transforming protein of EBV, behaving as a classic oncogene in rodent fibroblast transformation assays and being essential for EBV-induced B-cell transformation in vitro. LMP1 has pleiotropic effects when expressed in cells, resulting in the induction of cell surface adhesion molecules and activation antigens, up-regulation of anti-apoptotic proteins (Bcl-2, A20), and stimulation of cytokine production (interleukin [IL]-6, IL-8).[57] LMP1 functionally resembles a constitutively activated CD40, as evidenced by its ability to partially substitute for CD40 in vivo, providing both growth and differentiation responses in B cells.[58] LMP1 has three important domains: (1) an N-terminal cytoplasmic tail (amino acids 1 to 23), which tethers and orientates the LMP1 protein to the plasma membrane; (2) six hydrophobic transmembrane loops that are involved in self-aggregation and oligomerization (amino acids 24 to 186); and (3) a long C-terminal cytoplasmic region (amino acids 187 to 386), which possesses most of the molecule's signaling activity. Two distinct functional domains within the cytoplasmic tail (referred to as C-terminal activation regions 1 and 2 [CTAR1 and CTAR2]) have been shown to independently activate the NF-κB transcription factor pathway.[59] This effect contributes to the many phenotypic consequences of LMP1 expression described above. More recent work demonstrates that LMP1 can also regulate the processing of p100 NF-κB2 to p52 and that this is independent of the pathways responsible for controlling the canonical NF-κB pathway.[60] LMP1 is also able to engage the mitogen activated protein (MAP) kinase cascade (resulting in activation of ERK, JNK, and p38) and to stimulate the JAK/STAT pathway.[57] LMP1 can also activate the phosphatidylinositol 3 kinase (PI3-K) pathway, resulting in a variety of effects, including cell survival mediated through the Akt (PKB) kinase, actin polymerization, and cell motility.[61]

LMP2

The gene encoding LMP2 yields two distinct proteins: LMP2A and LMP2B. The structures of LMP2A and LMP2B are similar; both have 12 transmembrane domains and a 27-amino-acid cytoplasmic C-terminal. However, LMP2A has a 119-amino-acid cytoplasmic amino-terminal domain, which is absent from LMP2B. LMP2A aggregates in patches within the plasma membrane of latently infected B cells.[62] Neither LMP2A nor LMP2B are essential for B-cell transformation.[63] The LMP2A amino-terminal domain contains eight tyrosine residues, two of which (Y74 and Y85) form an immunoreceptor tyrosine-based activation motif (ITAM).[64] When phosphorylated, the ITAM in the B-cell receptor (BCR) plays a central role in mediating lymphocyte proliferation and differentiation by the recruitment and activation of the *src* family of protein tyrosine kinases (PTKs) and the *syk* PTK. LMP2A also interacts with these PTKs through its phosphorylated ITAM, and this association appears to negatively regulate PTK activity.[65] The LMP2A ITAM has been shown to block BCR-stimulated calcium mobilization, tyrosine phosphorylation, and activation of the EBV lytic cycle in B cells.[65]

Expression of LMP2A in the B cells of transgenic mice abrogates normal B-cell development, allowing immunoglobulin-negative cells to colonize peripheral lymphoid organs.[66] This suggests that LMP2A can drive the proliferation and survival of B cells in the absence of signaling through the BCR. LMP2A can also transform epithelial cells, an effect that appears to be mediated by activation of the PI3-K/Akt pathway.[67] This suggests that LMP2A-induced activation of the Akt pathway might also be relevant to the long-term survival of persistently infected memory B cells.

EBER

In addition to the latent proteins, two small non-polyadenylated (noncoding) RNAs, EBER1 and EBER2, are expressed in all known forms of latency. However, the EBERs are not essential for EBV-induced transformation of primary B lymphocytes. The EBERs assemble into stable ribonucleoprotein particles with the autoantigen La, with ribosomal protein L22 and bind the interferon-inducible double-stranded RNA-activated protein kinase PKR.[68] PKR has a role in mediating the antiviral effects of the interferons, and it has been suggested that EBER-mediated inhibition of PKR function could be important for viral persistence, perhaps by protecting cells from interferon-induced apoptosis.[68]

Reintroduction of the EBERs into EBV-negative Akata BL cells restores their capacity for growth in soft agar, tumorigenicity in severe combined immunodeficiency (SCID) mice, and resistance to apoptotic inducers, features identical to those observed in the parental EBV-positive Akata cells.[68,69] The detection of IL-10 expression in EBV-positive (but not in EBV-negative) BL tumors and the observation that the EBERs can induce IL-10 expression in BL cell lines suggest that IL-10 may be an important component in the pathogenesis of EBV-positive BL.[70] Stable expression of Bcl-2 or the EBERs in EBV-negative Akata cells significantly enhanced the tumorigenic potential of these cells, but neither Bcl-2 nor the EBERs restored tumorigenicity to the same extent as EBV.[71] Overall, these studies suggest that EBV genes previously shown to be dispensable for transformation in B-cell systems (eg, EBERs) might make more important contributions to the pathogenesis of some EBV-associated malignancies and to EBV persistence than was previously appreciated.

BARTs

BARTs were first identified in NPC tissue and subsequently in other EBV-associated malignancies such as BL, HL, and nasal T-cell lymphoma, as well as in the peripheral blood of healthy individuals.[72,73] The BARTs encode a number of potential open reading frames (ORFs), including *BARF0*, *RK-BARF0*, *A73*, and *RPMS1*. The protein products of these ORFs have not been identified, and their existence remains controversial.[73,74] However, in vitro studies have suggested potential functions, including the negative regulation of EBNA2 and Notch activity (RPMS1) and the modulation of kinase signaling (A73).[73,75,76]

EBV-ASSOCIATED TUMORS

Although subject to various interpretations, the designation of a tumor as being EBV associated usually requires unequivocal demonstration of the EBV genome or virus gene products within the tumor cell population. However, EBV might also contribute to tumorigenesis through a "hit-and-run" mechanism whereby EBV infects the tumor progenitors but is subsequently lost. A further possibility is that EBV is not involved in the early stages of tumor formation but contributes later in tumor progression; in which case its detection in tumor cells would vary according to tumor stage. Therefore, there is no single encompassing definition of EBV association. The tumors described below are those for which the virus association has usually been established by detection of virus or virus gene products in the majority of tumor cells.

EBV-Associated Lymphomas

Lymphoproliferative Disease and Post-transplantation Lymphomas

The lymphoproliferations and lymphomas that arise following iatrogenic immunosuppression for transplantation surgery are collectively known as post-transplantation lymphoproliferative disorders (PTLDs) and are related to similar lesions that can arise in inherited immunodeficiency syndromes and after infection with human immune deficiency virus (HIV). They are most often of B-cell origin and represent a family of lesions ranging from atypical polyclonal B-cell proliferations, which often regress following the withdrawal or reduction of immunosuppression), to aggressive monomorphic non-Hodgkin's lymphomas (NHLs), which generally do not resolve after immune reconstitution.

The incidence and clinical presentation of PTLDs vary with the organ transplanted, the duration of immunosuppression, and the dosage and number of agents used although there are a number of common clinical features, which include the frequent occurrence of PTLDs in numerous extranodal locations such as the gastrointestinal tract or even in the allograft organ itself. The high incidence of PTLDs in the transplanted organ suggests that chronic antigen stimulation in the graft might be important in the pathogenesis of these lesions.

The majority of PTLD cases are EBV positive, and many show a Lat III pattern of gene expression (see Figure 8-2). Thus, in many cases, PTLDs appear to represent the in vivo counterpart of in vitro immortalized LCLs and, by implication, are likely to be primarily driven by EBV. However, other forms of latency (ie, Lat I and Lat II) are occasionally observed, and EBV-negative forms of PTLD have been described, including some T-cell tumors. These EBV-negative tumors tend to be monomorphic, and they present later and are more aggressive than EBV-positive tumors.[77,78] Of interest, a proportion of these tumors respond to a decrease in immunosuppression, which might suggest the involvement of other viral agents.

Burkitt's Lymphoma

The recognition that BL in Africa was apparently restricted to areas where infection with *Plasmodium falciparum* malaria was holoendemic led to the suggestion that an infectious agent might be involved and eventually to the discovery of EBV. The so-called endemic or high-incidence form of BL has annual incidence of approximately 5 to 10 cases per 100,000 children in equatorial Africa and in parts of Papua New Guinea. By contrast, sporadic cases of BL occur worldwide but at a much lower frequency (at least 50-fold less than in the high-incidence areas).

Whereas virtually every BL tumor found in high-incidence regions is EBV positive, only about 15% of sporadic BL tumors carry the virus. In addition, certain "intermediate-incidence" areas (such as Algeria and Egypt) outside the regions of holoendemic malaria have greater numbers of cases that correlate with an increased proportion of EBV-positive tumors. BL is also observed as a consequence of HIV infection, frequently occurring

before the development of acquired immune deficiency syndrome (AIDS). Only 30 to 40% of cases of AIDS BL are associated with EBV infection. A consistent feature of all BL tumors, irrespective of geographic location or AIDS association, are chromosomal translocations involving the long arm of chromosome 8 (8q24) in the region of the c-*myc* proto-oncogene and either chromosome 14 in the region of the immunoglobulin heavy-chain gene or (less frequently) chromosome 2 or chromosome 22 in the region of the immunoglobulin light-chain genes. This translocation results in deregulated expression of the c-*myc* oncogene.

The precise role of EBV in the pathogenesis of BL remains to be established although the detection of monoclonal EBV episomes in virus-positive BL biopsy specimens suggests that EBV infection precedes proliferation of the precursor B cells.[79] The apparent origin of BL in the germinal center is based on phenotypic studies and is supported by the ability of BL risk factors such as holoendemic malaria and chronic HIV infection to stimulate the proliferation of germinal-center B cells.[3] These cells are also programmed to undergo somatic mutation of immunoglobulin genes, and this event, in conjunction with the stimulation of germinal-center proliferation and EBV infection, might be responsible for the generation and selection of B cells carrying the c-*myc* translocation.

EBNA2 and LMP1 are the major mediators of EBV-induced B-lymphocyte growth in vitro, and the lack of expression of these proteins in BL tumor cells suggests that they are not required for the maintenance of BL tumors. Altered *MYC* expression may replace EBV-driven cell proliferation and allow cells to survive and proliferate with down-regulation of the EBNAs and LMPs, which may in turn enable the infected cells to evade CTL immune surveillance. This may explain why the drift to an LCL phenotype seen in some BL lines in vitro occurs only at a low level in vivo, since "drifted" cells would be selectively removed by the CTL response. EBV-positive BL lines that have retained the tumor cell phenotype in vitro are not sensitive to lysis by EBV-specific CTLs. In addition to the down-regulation of the highly immunogenic EBNAs and LMPs, several phenotypic features contribute to decrease the immunogenicity of BL tumor cells. These include reduced expression of cell adhesion molecules, a general and allele-selective down-regulation of major histocompatibility complex (MHC) class I expression, and defects in antigen processing and peptide transport.[3]

Evidence that EBV and altered *MYC* expression can cooperate to alter B-lymphocyte growth comes from studies in which EBV was used to transform human B lymphocytes in vitro, after which a re-arranged *MYC* gene (cloned from a BL cell line) was introduced into these cells.[80] The EBV-transformed cells initially had very low cloning efficiencies in soft agar and did not form tumors in nude mice. After gene transfer of a re-arranged *MYC*, however, they grew more efficiently in soft agar and were tumorigenic. Activated *MYC* gene introduced into an EBV-transformed cell line in which EBNA2 was rendered estrogen dependent was shown to be capable of inducing continuous proliferation of these cells in the absence of functional LMP1 and EBNA2, suggesting that Myc might substitute for LMP1 and EBNA2 in BL progenitor cells.[81]

Some studies also suggest greater involvement of EBV in sporadic BL than previously documented. Thus, re-arranged defective EBV genomes have been detected in some sporadic BL tumors from the United States.[82] Such viral re-arrangements can lead to constitutive expression of the immediate early gene *BZLF1*, which by transient transfection has been shown to result in the partial elimination of EBV episomes from infected cells. The presence of these defective genomes may go undetected by conventional EBV testing (eg, EBER in situ hybridization) and suggests a process of viral DNA rearrangement and loss during malignant progression consistent with a "hit-and-run" role for EBV in the pathogenesis of at least a proportion of sporadic BL cases.

Hodgkin's Lymphoma

Although epidemiologic evidence had suggested the involvement of EBV with Hodgkin's lymphoma (HL), it was not until 1989 that EBV was first identified in the malignant Hodgkin/Reed-Sternberg (HRS) cells.[83,84] Subsequently, the demonstration of EBER expression in HRS cells provided a more sensitive method for detecting EBV-associated cases.[85]

In EBV-associated HL, the viral genomes are found in monoclonal form, indicating that infection of the tumor cells occurred prior to their clonal expansion.[83] In the majority of cases, EBV appears to persist throughout the course of HL and is also found in numerous sites of HL.[86]

The presence of EBV in HL depends on a number of factors, including the patient's country of residence, histologic subtype, sex, ethnicity, and age.[87] For example, EBV-positive HL is less common than is EBV-negative disease in developed populations; this might be due to the existence of an underlying immunosuppression in poorly developed communities, similar to that observed for African BL in a malaria-infected population. This is supported by higher EBV-positive rates in HL among HIV-infected patients.[88] Alternatively, the timing of EBV infection (which is likely to occur earlier in developing populations) might also be important.

EBV is more commonly associated with the mixed-cellularity (MC) subtype of HL and less frequently with the other forms of this disease.[87] Furthermore, it is now generally accepted that the lymphocyte-predominant form of HL, as defined by the Revised European-American Lymphoma (REAL) classification, is an EBV-negative disease.[89] HL is more likely to be EBV associated in the older age groups and in children (especially in boys under 10 years of age) than in young adults.[90] This has led to the suggestion that HL consists of three disease entities: HL of childhood (EBV positive, MC type), HL of young adults (EBV negative, nodular sclerosis type), and HL of older adults (EBV positive, MC type).[90] The infrequent association of EBV with HL in young adulthood prompted the suggestion that a second virus might be involved although there is little direct evidence to support this at present.[91] Rates of EBV positivity are generally higher in males than in females.[87] EBV-positive HL also affects more Asians and Hispanics than Whites or Blacks[87]; in the United Kingdom, it is more common among South Asian children than among non-South Asian children.[92]

It has been suggested that EBV might contribute to the pathogenesis of HL early in the transformation of the progenitor cells but might be subsequently lost in a manner analogous to that already suggested for BL; this might explain the absence of

EBV from some HL tumors. Although some investigators have detected integrated defective genomes in EBER-negative HL,[93] others have failed to find any evidence of these viral forms.[94] Furthermore, detailed analysis using quantitative polymerase chain reaction (PCR) assays that spanned the whole genome found no evidence of the deletion of EBV genomes in EBV-positive HL or the retention of EBV genomes in EBV-negative HL tissues.[95] Therefore, it seems less probable that EBV also contributes to the development of EBV-negative HL.

EBV-positive HRS cells exhibit a type II form of latency. The particularly high levels of LMP1 expression in HRS cells suggest that LMP1 plays an important role in the pathogenesis of EBV-associated cases. Activation of several signaling pathways also regulated by LMP1 is observed in HRS cells. For example, constitutive activation of NF-κB is a regular feature of HRS cells, and inhibition of this pathway in HL cell lines leads to their increased sensitivity to apoptosis after growth factor withdrawal and to impaired tumorigenicity in SCID mice.[96,97] Although NF-κB activation is a common finding in HRS cells, the molecular routes to this activation may be different between EBV-positive HL and EBV-negative HL. IκBα mutations have been reported in EBV-negative HL cells[98,99] and in 2 of 3 cases of EBV-negative primary HL but not in the two EBV-positive cases examined.[100] More recently, IκBα mutations have been found in 15 of 26 primary HL tumors, 11 of which were EBV negative.[101] In addition, comparative genomic hybridization and fluorescent in situ hybridization analysis has demonstrated frequent amplification of the NF-κB/RelA locus at 2p13-16 in HRS cells of classic HL.[102,103] This is an alternative mechanism that could lead to constitutive NF-κB activation although it is yet to be shown whether this is mutually exclusive with an EBV-positive status. Kube and colleagues demonstrated the constitutive activation of STAT3 in HRS cells.[104] STAT6 and STAT5A constitutive activation has also been reported.[105,106] Amplification of the *JAK*2 locus is observed in HRS cells, providing an explanation for the STAT activation.[107] Furthermore, it has been recently shown that HRS cells have constitutively activated AP-1 with c-Jun and JunB overexpression.[108]

The other EBV-encoded latent membrane protein, LMP2A, is also highly expressed in EBV-positive HRS cells. It has recently been shown that LMP2A expression in B cells results in the down-regulation of many of the B-cell factors previously shown to be absent or expressed at low levels in HRS cells (eg, early B-cell factor, PU.1, CD19, CD20).[109] In addition, LMP2A expression induces the up-regulation of genes involved in proliferation (eg, *Ki-67*, *PCNA*), protection from apoptosis (Bcl-xL, survivin), and suppression of cell-mediated immunity (eg, IL-13R, EBI3).[109] Many of the transcriptional changes seen in response to LMP2A are observed in EBV-negative HRS cells, which suggests that alternative mechanisms may contribute similar effects when EBV is absent.

Data from studies of the patterns of EBV gene expression during B-cell differentiation in vivo are consistent with a role for LMP1 and LMP2A in the early stages of the pathogenesis of HL. Thus, as described earlier, LMP1 and LMP2 expression in B cells might provide T-cell help and BCR signaling, respectively, enabling antigen-independent proliferation of these cells in the germinal center. The acquisition of cellular alterations that are as yet undefined could lead to the neoplastic outgrowth of EBV-infected germinal-center B cells and ultimately to the development of HL.

LMP2A (and LMP1 to a lesser extent) are targets for cytotoxic T lymphocytes in association with different MHC class I restriction elements in vitro.[110,111] The survival of EBV-infected HRS cells that express high levels of LMP1 and LMP2A in vivo suggests that mechanisms to avoid or prevent immune recognition are manifest in HL patients. These include specific immunologic defects in HL that permit the growth of the neoplastic cells as well as the development of specific immune evasion strategies by EBV-infected HRS cells. Support for the latter is provided by the finding that IL-10 is more frequently expressed in EBV-infected HRS cells when compared with their EBV-negative counterparts, and this has been suggested to account for the failure of these cells to be recognized by EBV-specific CTLs.[112] Furthermore, HRS cells express the thymus and activation-regulated chemokine (TARC), which together with other cytokines such as IL-10,

IL-13, and transforming growth factor beta (TGF-β), attract Th2 cells and contribute to a shift in the local environment away from a Th1- toward a Th2-predominate response.[113–115] The contribution of the microenvironment is underlined by the observation that tumor-derived T lymphocytes from EBV-negative HL lesions show EBV-specific cytotoxicity whereas corresponding lymphocytes from EBV-positive HL lesions do not.[116] Surprisingly, EBV-positive cases of HL have been shown to contain more activated CTLs and express relatively higher levels of MHC class I protein than do EBV-negative cases.[117–120]

T-Cell Lymphomas

EBV is also associated with a subset of T-cell NHLs; among these a very high incidence of EBV genomes has been reported in sino-nasal T-cell NHLs occurring in Japanese, Chinese, Peruvian, European, and US patients.[121] Sino-nasal T-cell NHLs display peculiar phenotypic and genotypic features, including the frequent absence of T-cell antigens, expression of natural killer (NK) cell markers, and the absence of T-cell receptor gene rearrangements.

An intriguing aspect of EBV-positive T-cell lymphomas is the frequent detection of the virus in only a fraction (5 to 50%) of the tumor cells, implying that EBV infection might have occurred subsequent to tumor development.[121] The documented increase in the proportion of EBV-positive tumor cells with T-cell lymphoma progression or recurrence suggests that the virus might provide an additional growth or survival advantage to the transformed T cells.

Most EBV-associated T-cell NHLs are extranodal and have a cytotoxic phenotype, as demonstrated by immunohistochemical staining for T-cell intracytoplasmic antigen-1 and granzyme B,[122] suggesting that these tumors might arise following an EBV infection of CTLs during the killing of EBV-infected cells by virus-specific CTLs. Of interest, EBV-positive B cells are frequently detectable in some EBV-negative T-cell lymphomas, and in contrast to the EBV-positive small lymphocytes detectable in UNPC or HL, these cells display a Lat III phenotype, suggesting that the presence of the neoplastic T cells might be a stimulus for EBV-induced B-cell transformation.[123] A further possibility is that the EBV-infected B cells present in T-cell lymphomas might contribute to the growth of the neoplastic T cells, possibly by the secretion of cytokines or perhaps more directly by interaction of their co-stimulatory molecules with partner molecules on T cells.

Nasopharyngeal Carcinoma

Although EBV is associated with other epithelial malignancies (notably gastric cancer), the most consistent association is with undifferentiated nasopharyngeal carcinoma (UNPC) (World Health Organization type III). UNPC is characterized by the presence of undifferentiated carcinoma cells together with a prominent lymphocytic infiltrate; the latter is probably important for the growth of the tumor cells.

UNPC is an uncommon disease in the West; its incidence is less than 1 per 100,000 among Caucasians from North America and other Western countries. In contrast, there is a much higher incidence in China, Southeast Asia, and some other Asian countries. The highest incidence is in southern China, particularly among Cantonese males, although a decrease in the incidence of NPC in some high-risk areas has been noted over the past 20 years, which might reflect changes in carcinogen exposure.[124] An unusually early age of onset in the high-risk populations implies that early events in life might be important. Incidence is also high among Chinese immigrants, irrespective of where they live.

Extensive serologic screening has identified elevated EBV-specific antibody titers in high-incidence areas, particularly immunoglobulin A (IgA) antibodies to EBV capsid antigen and early antigens, and these have proven useful in diagnosis and in monitoring the effectiveness of therapy.[125] EBNA1, BARTs, and the EBERs are expressed in all EBV-positive cases. LMP1 is expressed in only a minority although the detection of LMP1 in a given tumor is partly dependent on the sensitivity of the method used; reverse transcriptase PCR identifies more positive cases than does immunohistochemistry. Expression of the EBV *BARF1* gene has been observed in 85% of UNPCs and 100% of EBV-positive gastric carcinomas.[126,127] The *BARF1* ORF encodes a product of about 33 kDa that is secreted into the medium of cultured cells.[128] Although *BARF1* appears temporally as an early lytic gene in the viral life cycle, it can act as an oncogene when stably expressed in cultured murine, human, or simian cells.[129–131] In addition, Akata BL cells that have lost their tumorigenic phenotype through loss of the EBV genome regained the ability to form tumors in SCID mice following transfection with *BARF1*.[132] It has been suggested that *BARF1* may act as the viral oncogene in NPC when LMP1 is absent.

The predisposition to NPC in the southern Chinese population strongly suggests the involvement of both genetic susceptibility and environmental factors. Study of human leukocyte antigen (HLA) susceptibility among Chinese persons has found that those with HLA-A*0207 have an increased NPC risk.[133] Recent linkage analysis of Chinese NPC pedigrees has also identified susceptibility loci on chromosomes 4p15.1-q12 and 3p21.[134,135] The most relevant environmental exposure among Chinese populations is to salted fish and other preserved foods containing volatile nitrosamines. Childhood consumption of salted fish has been related to an increased risk of NPC in southern Chinese.[136] This is supported by the observation that albino rats fed a diet of salted fish develop carcinoma of the nasal cavity.[137]

Numerous genetic alterations are present in UNPC cells, including genetic losses on chromosomes 3p, 9, 11q, 13q, 14q, and 16q, whereas recurrent chromosomal gains on chromosome 12 have been observed.[37,138] These disrupt various cellular processes, including the cell cycle through interference with Rb and *p53*[138]; the *P16* gene, an important cell cycle regulator for G_1 restriction checkpoint, is inactivated in approximately two-thirds of cases and results in constitutive Rb phosphorylation and uncontrolled proliferation of NPC cells.[37,139] Although *p53* mutations are uncommon in NPC cases, the inactivation of P14 and the overexpression of a delta-N isoform of P63 are frequent, and both can abrogate *p53* function.[140,141]

High frequencies of deletions on chromosomes 3p and 9p are found in histologically normal nasopharyngeal epithelia from southern Chinese, as well as in low- and high-grade dysplastic lesions.[142,143] However, EBV infection is not present in normal nasopharyngeal epithelium nor in low-grade dysplasia. There-fore, the disruption of tumor suppressor genes such as p16 and p14 on 9p21 and RASSF1A on 3p21.3 precede EBV infection and indeed may contribute to the establishment of EBV latency in epithelial cells.

SUMMARY

Epstein-Barr virus (EBV) is a ubiquitous virus yet is involved in the development of tumors of both lymphoid and epithelial origin. In normal carriers, EBV resides in B cells, using the B-cell development program to establish long-term latency and persistence. In rare circumstances, EBV-infected B cells can become neoplastic; the cellular changes that cooperate with EBV to induce malignant transformation of B cells are not known. In contrast, epithelial cells cannot generally support latent infection unless there are preexisting cellular genetic alterations. In nasopharyngeal carcinoma, such cellular alterations probably initiate the disease, and EBV has a later tumor-promoting function. Current work is focusing on the contributions of viral infection and the individual EBV latent genes to malignancy within differing cellular contexts.

ACKNOWLEDGMENTS

We would like to thank Cancer Research UK and the Leukaemia Research Fund for supporting our research.

REFERENCES

1. Cho Y, Ramer J, Rivailler P, et al. An Epstein-Barr-related herpesvirus from marmoset lymphomas. Proc Natl Acad Sci U S A 2001;98:1224–19.

2. Rivailler P, Cho Y, Wang F. Complete genomic sequence of an Epstein-Barr virus-related herpesvirus naturally infecting a new world primate: a defining point in the evolution of oncogenic lymphocryptoviruses. J Virol 2002;76:12055–68.

3. Rickinson AB, Kieff E. Epstein-Barr virus. In: Knipe DM, Howley PM, editors. Fields virology. Philadelphia: Lippincott, Williams and Wilkins; 2001. p. 2575–627.

4. Thorley-Lawson DA. Epstein-Barr virus: exploiting the immune system. Nat Rev Immunol 2001;1:75–82.

5. Young LS, Murray PG. Epstein-Barr virus and oncogenesis: from latent genes to tumours. Oncogene 2003;22:5108–21.

6. Rickinson AB, Rowe M, Hart IJ, et al. T-cell-mediated regression of "spontaneous" and of Epstein-Barr virus-induced B-cell transformation in vitro: studies with cyclosporin A. Cell Immunol 1984;87:646–58.

7. Speck SH, Strominger JL. Transcription of Epstein-Barr virus in latently infected, growth-transformed lymphocytes. Adv Viral Oncol 1989;8:133–50.

8. Raab-Traub N, Flynn K. The structure of the termini of the Epstein-Barr virus as a marker of clonal cellular proliferation. Cell 1986;47:883–9.

9. Moody CA, Scott RS, Tao S, Sixbey JW. Length of Epstein-Barr virus termini as a determinant of epithelial cell clonal emergence. J Virol 2003;77:8555–61.

10. Rowe M, Rowe DT, Gregory CD, et al. Differences in B cell growth phenotype reflect novel patterns of Epstein-Barr virus latent gene expression in Burkitt's lymphoma cells. EMBO J 1987;6:2743–51.

11. Wang F, Gregory C, Sample C, et al. Epstein-Barr virus latent membrane protein (LMP1) and nuclear proteins 2 and 3C are effectors of phenotypic changes in B lymphocytes: EBNA-2 and LMP1 cooperatively induce CD23. J Virol 1990;64:2309–18.

12. Niedobitek G, Agathanggelou A, Rowe M, et al. Heterogeneous expression of Epstein-Barr virus latent proteins in endemic Burkitt's lymphoma. Blood 1995;86:659–65.

13. Carbone A, Gloghini A, Zagonel V, Tirelli U. Expression of Epstein-Barr virus-encoded latent membrane protein 1 in nonendemic Burkitt's lymphomas. Blood 1996;87:1202–4.

14. Nonkwelo C, Skinner J, Bell A, et al. Transcription start sites downstream of the Epstein-Barr virus (EBV) Fp promoter in early-passage Burkitt lymphoma cells define a fourth promoter for expression of the EBV EBNA-1 protein. J Virol 1996;70:623–7.

15. Gregory CD, Rowe M, Rickinson AB. Different Epstein-Barr virus-B cell interactions in phenotypically distinct clones of a Burkitt's lymphoma cell line. J Gen Virol 1990;71:1481–95.

16. Brooks L, Yao QY, Rickinson AB, Young LS. Epstein-Barr virus latent gene transcription in nasopharyngeal carcinoma cells: coexpression of EBNA1, LMP1, and LMP2 transcripts. J Virol 1992;66:2689–97.

17. Deacon EM, Pallesen G, Niedobitek G, et al. Epstein-Barr virus and Hodgkin's disease: transcriptional analysis of virus latency in the malignant cells. J Exp Med 1993;177:339–49.

18. Pallesen G, Hamilton-Dutoit SJ, Rowe M, Young LS. Expression of Epstein-Barr virus latent gene products in tumour cells of Hodgkin's disease. Lancet 1991;337:320–2.

19. Young LS, Dawson CW, Clark D, et al. Epstein-Barr virus gene expression in nasopharyngeal carcinoma. J Gen Virol 1988;69:1051–65.

20. Chen H, Lee JM, Zong YS, et al. Linkage between STAT regulation and Epstein-Barr virus gene expression in tumours. J Virol 2001;75:2929–37.

21. Chen H, Hutt-Fletcher LM, Cao L, Hayward SD. A positive autoregulatory loop of LMP1 expression and STAT activation in epithelial cells latently infected with Epstein-Barr virus. J Virol 2003;77:4139–48.

22. Niedobitek G, Young LS, Sam CK, et al. Expression of Epstein-Barr virus genes and of lymphocyte activation molecules in undifferentiated nasopharyngeal carcinomas. Am J Pathol 1992;140:879–87.

23. Kelly G, Bell A, Rickinson AB. Epstein-Barr virus-associated Burkitt lymphomagenesis selects for downregulation of the nuclear antigen EBNA1. Nat Med 2002;8:1098–104.

24. Bonnet M, Guinebretiere JM, Kremmer E, et al. Detection of Epstein-Barr virus in invasive breast cancers. J Natl Cancer Inst 1999;91:1376–81.

25. Murray PG, Lissauer D, Junying J, et al. Reactivity with a monoclonal antibody to Epstein-Barr virus (EBV) nuclear antigen 1 defines a subset of aggressive breast cancers in the absence of the EBV genome. Cancer Res 2003;63:2338–43.

26. Sugawara Y, Mizugaki Y, Uchida T, et al. Detection of Epstein-Barr virus (EBV) in hepatocellular carcinoma tissue: a novel EBV latency characterised by the absence of EBV-encoded small RNA expression. Virology 1999;256:196–202.

27. Babcock GJ, Decker LL, Volk M, Thorley-Lawson DA. EBV persistence in memory B cells in vivo. Immunity 1998;9:395–404.

28. Joseph AM., Babcock GJ, Thorley-Lawson DA. Cells expressing the Epstein-Barr virus growth program are present in and restricted to the naive B-cell subset of healthy tonsils. J Virol 2000;74:9964–71.

29. Babcock GJ, Thorley-Lawson DA. Tonsillar memory B cells, latently infected with Epstein-Barr virus, express the restricted pattern of latent genes previously found only in Epstein-Barr virus-associated tumors. Proc Natl Acad Sci U S A 2000;97:12250–5.

30. Walling DM, Ling PD, Gordadze AV, et al. Expression of Epstein-Barr virus latent genes in oral epithelium: determinants of the pathogenesis of oral hairy leukoplakia. J Infect Dis 2004;190:396–9.

31. De Souza YG, Greenspan D, Felton JR, et al. Localization of Epstein-Barr virus DNA in the epithelial cells of oral hairy leukoplakia by in situ hybridization of tissue sections. N Engl J Med 1989;320:1559–60.

32. Karajannis MA, Hummel M, Anagnostopoulos I, Stein H. Strict lymphotropism of Epstein-Barr virus during acute infectious mononucleosis in non-immunocompromised individuals. Blood 1997;89:2856–62.

33. Niedobitek G, Hamilton-Dutoit SJ, Herbst H, et al. Identification of Epstein-Barr virus-infected cells in tonsils of acute infectious mononucleosis by in situ hybridisation. Hum Pathol 1989;20:796–9.

34. Herrmann K, Frangou P, Middeldorp J, Niedobitek G. Epstein-Barr virus replication in tongue epithelial cells. J Gen Virol 2002;83:2995–8.

35. Sam CK, Brooks LA, Niedobitek G, et al. Analysis of Epstein-Barr virus infection in nasopharyngeal biopsies from a group at high risk of nasopharyngeal carcinoma. Int J Cancer 1993;53:957–62.

36. Gulley ML, Pulitzer DR, Eagan PA, Schneider BG. Epstein-Barr virus infection is an early event in gastric carcinogenesis and is independent of bcl-2 expression and p53 accumulation. Hum Pathol 1996;27:20–7.

37. Lo K-W, Huang DP. Genetic and epigenetic changes in nasopharyngeal carcinoma. Semin Cancer Biol 2002;12:451–62.

38. Wilson JB, Bell JL, Levine AJ. Expression of Epstein-Barr virus nuclear antigen-1 induces B cell neoplasia in transgenic mice. EMBO J 1996;15:3117–26.

39. Levitskaya J, Coram M, Levitsky V, et al. Inhibition of antigen processing by the internal repeat region of the Epstein-Barr virus nuclear antigen-1. Nature 1995;375:685–8.

40. Jones RJ, Smith LJ, Dawson CW, et al. Epstein-Barr virus nuclear antigen 1 (EBNA1) induced cytotoxicity in epithelial cells is associated with EBNA1 degradation and processing. Virology 2003;313:663–76.

41. Hammerschmidt W, Sugden B. Genetic analysis of immortalising functions of Epstein-Barr virus in human B lymphocytes. Nature, 1989;340:393–7.

42. Rabson M, Gradoville L, Heston L, Miller G. Non-immortalizing P3J-HR-1 Epstein-Barr virus: a deletion mutant of its transforming parent, Jijoye. J Virol 1982;44:834–44.

43. Sjoblom A, Nerstedt A, Jansson A, Rymo L. Domains of the Epstein-Barr virus nuclear antigen 2 (EBNA2) involved in the transactivation of the latent membrane protein 1 and the EBNA Cp promoters. J Gen Virol 1995;76:2669–78.

44. Grossman SR, Johannsen E, Tong R, et al. The Epstein-Barr virus nuclear antigen 2 transactivator is directed to response elements by the Jk recombination signal binding protein. Proc Natl Acad Sci U S A 1994;91:7568–72.

45. Artavanis-Tsakonas S, Matsuno K, Fortini ME. Notch signaling. Science 1995;268:225–32.

46. Zimber-Strobl U, Strobl LJ. BNA2 and Notch signalling in Epstein-Barr virus mediated immortalization of B lymphocytes. Semin Cancer Biol 2001;11:423–34.

47. Jayachandra S, Low KG, Thicke AE, et al. Three unrelated viral transforming proteins (vIRF, EBNA2, and E1A) induce the MYC oncogene through the interferon-responsive PRF element by using different transcription coadaptors. Proc Natl Acad Sci U S A 1999;96:11566–71.

48. Allday MJ, Farrell PJ. Epstein-Barr virus nuclear antigen EBNA3C/6 expression maintains the level of latent membrane protein 1 in G1-arrested cells. J Virol 1994;68:3491–8.

49. Radkov SA, Bain M, Farrell PJ, et al. Epstein-Barr virus EBNA3C represses Cp, the major promoter for EBNA expression, but has no effect on the promoter of the cell gene CD21. J Virol 1997;71:8552–62.

50. Parker GA, Crook T, Bain M, et al. Epstein-Barr virus nuclear antigen (EBNA)3C is an immortalizing oncoprotein with similar properties to adenovirus E1A and papillomavirus E7. Oncogene 1996;13:2541–9.

51. Le Roux A, Kerdiles B, Walls D, et al. The Epstein-Barr virus determined nuclear antigens EBNA-3A, -3B, and -3C repress EBNA-2-mediated transactivation of the viral terminal protein 1 gene promoter. Virology 1994;205:596–602.

52. Allan GJ, Inman GJ, Parker BD, et al. Cell growth effects of Epstein-Barr virus leader protein. J Gen Virol 1992;73:1547–51.

53. Sinclair AJ, Palmero I, Peters G, Farrell PJ. EBNA-2 and EBNA-LP cooperate to cause G0 and G1 transition during immortalisation of resting human B lymphocytes by Epstein-Barr virus. EMBO J 1994;13:3321–8.

54. Nitsche F, Bell A, Rickinson AB. Epstein-Barr virus leader protein enhances EBNA-2-mediated transactivation of latent membrane protein 1 expression: a role for the W_1W_2 repeat domain. J Virol 1997;71:6619–28.

55. Jiang WQ, Szekely L, Wendel-Hansen V, et al. Co-localisa-

tion of the retinoblastoma protein and the Epstein-Barr virus-encoded nuclear antigen EBNA-5. Exp Cell Res 1991;197:314–8.

56. Szekely L, Selivanova G, Magnusson KP, et al. EBNA-5, an Epstein-Barr virus-encoded nuclear antigen, binds to the retinoblastoma and *p53* proteins. Proc Natl Acad Sci U S A 1993;90:5455–9.

57. Eliopoulos AG, Young LS. LMP1 structure and signal transduction. Semin Cancer Biol 2001;11:435–44.

58. Uchida J, Yasui T, Takaoka-Shichijo Y, et al. Mimicry of CD40 signals by Epstein-Barr virus LMP1 in B lymphocyte responses. Science 1999;286:300–3.

59. Huen DS, Henderson SA., Croom-Carter D, Rowe M. The Epstein-Barr virus latent membrane protein-1 (LMP1) mediates activation of NF-kB and cell surface phenotype via two effector regions in its carboxy-terminal cytoplasmic domain. Oncogene 1995;10:549–60.

60. Eliopoulos AG, Caamano JH, Flavell JR, et al. Epstein-Barr virus-encoded latent infection membrane protein 1 regulates the processing of p100 NFkB2 to p52 via an IKKg/NEMO-independent signalling pathway. Oncogene 2003;22:7557–69.

61. Dawson CW, Tramountanis G, Eliopoulos AG, Young LS. Epstein-Barr virus latent membrane protein 1 (LMP1) activates the PI3-K/Akt pathway to promote cell survival and induce actin filament remodelling. J Biol Chem 2003;278:3694–704.

62. Longnecker R, Kieff E. A second Epstein-Barr virus membrane protein (LMP2) is expressed in latent infection and co-localises with LMP1. J Virol 1990;64:2319–26.

63. Longnecker R. Epstein-Barr virus latency: LMP2, a regulator or means for Epstein-Barr virus persistence? Adv Cancer Res 2000;79:175–200.

64. Fruehling S, Longnecker R. The immunoreceptor tyrosine-based activation motif of Epstein-Barr virus LMPA2 is essential for blocking BCR-mediated signal transduction. J Virol 1997;235:241–51.

65. Miller CL, Burkhardt AL, Lee JH, et al. Integral membrane protein 2 of Epstein-Barr virus regulates reactivation from latency through dominant negative effects on protein-tyrosine kinases. Immunity 1995;2:155–66.

66. Caldwell RG, Wilson JB, Anderson SJ, Longnecker R. Epstein-Barr virus LMP2A drives B cell development and survival in the absence of normal B cell receptor signals. Immunity 1998;9:405–11.

67. Scholle F, Bendt KM, Raab-Traub N. Epstein-Barr virus LMP2A transforms epithelial cells, inhibits cell differentiation, and activates Akt. J Virol 2000;74:10681–9.

68. Nanbo A, Takada K. The role of Epstein-Barr virus-encoded small RNAs (EBERs) in oncogenesis. Rev Med Virol 2002;12:321–6.

69. Komano J, Maruo S, Kurozumi K, et al. Oncogenic role of Epstein-Barr virus-encoded RNAs in Burkitt's lymphoma cell line Akata. J Virol 1999;73:9827–31.

70. Kitagawa N, Goto M, Kurozumi K, et al. Epstein-Barr virus-encoded poly(A)(-) RNA supports Burkitt's lymphoma growth through interleukin-10 induction. EMBO J 2000;19:6742–50.

71. Ruf IK, Rhyne PW, Yang C, et al. Epstein-Barr virus small RNAs potentiate tumourigenicity of Burkitt lymphoma

cells independently of an effect on apoptosis. J Virol 2000;74:10223–8.

72. Chen H, Smith P, Ambinder RF, Hayward SD. Expression of Epstein-Barr virus BamHI-A rightward transcripts in latently infected B cells from peripheral blood. Blood 1999;93:3026–32.

73. Smith P. Epstein-Barr virus complementary strand transcripts (CSTs/BARTs) and cancer. Semin Cancer Biol 2001; 11:469–76.

74. van Beek J, Brink AA, Vervoort MB, et al. In vivo transcription of the Epstein-Barr virus (EBV) BamHI-A region without associated in vivo BARF0 protein expression in multiple EBV-associated disorders. J Gen Virol 2003; 84:2647–59.

75. Zhang J, Chen H, Weinmaster G, Hayward SD. Epstein-Barr virus BamHi-a rightward transcript-encoded RPMS protein interacts with the CBF1-associated corepressor CIR to negatively regulate the activity of EBNA2 and NotchIC. J Virol 2001;75:2946–56.

76. Smith PR, de Jesus O, Turner D, et al. Structure and coding content of CST (BART) family RNAs of Epstein-Barr virus. J Virol 2000;74:3082–92.

77. Dotti G, Fiocchi R, Motta T, et al. Epstein-Barr virus-negative lymphoproliferative disorders in long-term survivors after heart, kidney, and liver transplant. Transplantation 2000;69:827–33.

78. Nelson BP, Nalesnik MA, Bahler DW, et al. Epstein-Barr virus-negative post-transplant lymphoproliferative disorders: a distinct entity? Am J Surg Pathol 2000;24:375–85.

79. Neri A, Barriga F, Inghirami G, et al. Epstein-Barr virus infection precedes clonal expansion in Burkitt's and acquired immunodeficiency syndrome-associated lymphoma. Blood 1991;77:1092–5.

80. Lombardi L, Newcomb EW, Dalla-Favera R. Pathogenesis of Burkitt lymphoma: expression of an activated c-myc oncogene causes the tumorigenic conversion of EBV-infected human B lymphoblasts. Cell 1987;49:161–70.

81. Polack A, Hortnagel K, Pajic A., et al. C-myc activation renders proliferation of Epstein-Barr virus (EBV)-transformed cells independent of EBV nuclear antigen 2 and latent membrane protein 1. Proc Natl Acad Sci U S A 1996;93:10411–6.

82. Razzouk BI, Srinivas S, Sample CE, et al. Epstein-Barr virus DNA recombination and loss in sporadic Burkitt's lymphoma. J Infect Dis 1996;173:529–35.

83. Anagnostopoulos I, Herbst H, Niedobitek G, Stein H. Demonstration of monoclonal EBV genomes in Hodgkin's disease and Ki-1 positive anaplastic large cell lymphoma by combined Southern blot and in situ hybridization. Blood 1989;74:810–6.

84. Weiss LM, Movahed LA, Warnke RA, Sklar J. Detection of Epstein-Barr viral genomes in Reed-Sternberg cells of Hodgkin's disease. New Engl J Med 1989;320:502–6.

85. Wu TC, Mann RB, Charache P, et al. Detection of EBV gene expression in Reed-Sternberg cells of Hodgkin's disease. Int J Cancer 1990;46:801–4.

86. Coates PJ, Slavin G, D'Ardenne AJ. Persistence of Epstein-Barr virus in Reed-Sternberg cells throughout the course of Hodgkin's disease. J Pathol 1991;164:291–7.

87. Glaser SL, Lin RJ, Stewart SL, et al. Epstein-Barr virus-associated Hodgkin's disease: epidemiologic characteristics in international data. Int J Cancer 1997;70:375–82.

88. Uccini S, Monardo F, Stoppacciaro A, et al. High frequency of Epstein-Barr virus-genome detection in Hodgkin's disease of HIV-positive patients. Int J Cancer 1990;46:581–5.

89. Chan WC. Cellular origin of nodular lymphocyte-predominant Hodgkin's lymphoma: immunophenotypic and molecular studies. Semin Hematol 1999;36:242–52.

90. Armstrong AA, Alexander FE, Cartwright R, et al. Epstein-Barr virus and Hodgkin's disease: further evidence for the three disease hypothesis. Leukemia 1998;12:1272–6.

91. Armstrong AA, Shield L, Gallagher A, Jarrett RF. Lack of involvement of known oncogenic DNA viruses in Epstein-Barr virus-negative Hodgkin's disease. Brit J Cancer 1998;77:1045–7.

92. Flavell KJ, Biddulph JP, Powell JE, et al. South Asian ethnicity and material deprivation increase the risk of Epstein-Barr virus infection in childhood Hodgkin's disease. Br J Cancer 2001;85:350–6.

93. Gan YJ, Razzouk BI, Su T, Sixbey JW. A defective, rearranged Epstein-Barr virus genome in EBER-negative and EBER-positive Hodgkin's disease. Am J Pathol 2002;160:781–6.

94. Staratschek-Jox A, Kotkowski S, Belge G, et al. Detection of Epstein-Barr virus in Hodgkin-Reed-Sternberg cells: no evidence for the persistence of integrated viral fragments in latent membrane protein-1 (LMP-1)-negative classical Hodgkin's disease. Am J Pathol 2000;156:209–16.

95. Gallagher A, Perry J, Freeland J, et al. Hodgkin lymphoma and Epstein-Barr virus (EBV): no evidence to support hit-and-run mechanism in cases classified as non-EBV-associated. Int J Cancer 2003;104:624–30.

96. Bargou RC, Leng C, Krappmann D, et al. High-level nuclear NF-kappa B and Oct-2 is a common feature of cultured Hodgkin/Reed-Sternberg cells. Blood 1996;87:4340–7.

97. Bargou RC, Emmerich F, Krappmann D, et al. Constitutive nuclear factor-kappaB-RelA activation is required for proliferation and survival of Hodgkin's disease tumor cells. J Clin Invest 1997;100:2961–9.

98. Emmerich F, Meiser M, Hummel M, et al. Overexpression of I kappa B alpha without inhibition of NF-kappaB activity and mutations in the I kappa B alpha gene in Reed-Sternberg cells. Blood 1999 94:3129–34.

99. Cabannes E, Khan G, Aillet F, et al. Mutations in the IkBa gene in Hodgkin's disease suggest a tumour suppressor role for IkappaBalpha. Oncogene 1999;18:3063–70.

100. Jungnickel B, Staratschek-Jox A, Bräuninger A, et al. Clonal deleterious mutations in the IkappaBalpha gene in the malignant cells in Hodgkin's lymphoma. J Exp Med 2000;191:395–401.

101. Jarrett RF, Lake A, Andrew L, et al. Somatic IkBa mutations are a frequent occurrence in Hodgkin's lymphoma [abstract]. Blood 2002;100:4333.

102. Martin-Subero JI, Gesk S, Harder L, et al. Recurrent involvement of the REL and BCL11A loci in classical Hodgkin lymphoma. Blood 2002;99:1474–7.

103. Barth TF, Martin-Subero JI, Joos S, et al. Gains of 2p involving the REL locus correlate with nuclear c-Rel protein accumulation in neoplastic cells of classical Hodgkin lymphoma. Blood 2003;101:3681–6.

104. Kube D, Holtick U, Vockerodt M, et al. STAT3 is constitutively activated in Hodgkin cell lines. Blood 2001;98: 762–70.

105. Skinnider BF, Elia AJ, Gascoyne RD, et al. Signal transducer and activator of transcription 6 is frequently activated in Hodgkin and Reed-Sternberg cells of Hodgkin lymphoma. Blood 2002;99:618–26.

106. Hinz M, Lemke P, Anagnostopoulos I, et al. Nuclear factor kappaB-dependent gene expression profiling of Hodgkin's disease tumor cells, pathogenetic significance, and link to constitutive signal transducer and activator of transcription 5a activity. J Exp Med 2002;196:605–17.

107. Joos S, Granzow M, Holtgreve-Grez H, et al. Hodgkin's lymphoma cell lines are characterized by frequent aberrations on chromosomes 2p and 9p including REL and JAK2. Int J Cancer 2003;103:489–95.

108. Mathas S, Hinz M, Anagnostopoulos I, et al. Aberrantly expressed c-Jun and JunB are a hallmark of Hodgkin lymphoma cells, stimulate proliferation and synergize with NF-kappa B. EMBO J 2001;21:4104–13.

109. Portis T, Dyck P, Longnecker R. Epstein-Barr virus (EBV) LMP2A induces alterations in gene transcription similar to those observed in Reed-Sternberg cells of Hodgkin lymphoma. Blood 2003;102:4166–78.

110. Khanna R, Burrows SR, Nicholls J, Poulsen LM. Identification of cytotoxic T cell epitopes within Epstein-Barr virus (EBV) oncogene latent membrane protein 1 (LMP1): evidence for HLA A2 supertype-restricted immune recognition of EBV-infected cells by LMP1-specific cytotoxic T lymphocytes. Eur J Immunol 1998;28:451–8.

111. Lee SP, Tierney RJ, Thomas WA, et al. Conserved CTL epitopes within EBV latent membrane protein 2: a potential target for CTL-based tumor therapy. J Immunol 1997; 158:3325–34.

112. Herbst H, Foss HD, Samol J, et al. Frequent expression of interleukin-10 by Epstein-Barr virus-harboring tumor cells of Hodgkin's disease. Blood 1996;87:2918–29.

113. Poppema S, Potters M, Visser L, van den Berg AM. Immune escape mechanisms in Hodgkin's disease. Ann Oncol 1998;9 Suppl 5:S21–4.

114. Kapp U, Yeh W-C, Patterson B, et al. Interleukin 13 is secreted by and stimulates the growth of Hodgkin and Reed-Sternberg cells. J Exp Med 1999;189:1939–46.

115. van den Berg A, Visser L, Poppema S. High expression of the CC chemokine TARC in Reed-Sternberg cells. A possible explanation for the characteristic T-cell infiltrate in Hodgkin's lymphoma. Am J Pathol 1999;154: 1685–91.

116. Frisan T, Sjoberg J, Dolcetti R, et al. Local suppression of Epstein-Barr virus (EBV)-specific cytotoxicity in biopsies of EBV-positive Hodgkin's disease. Blood 1995;86: 1493–501.

117. Oudejans JJ, Jiwa NM, Kummer JA, et al. Analysis of major histocompatibility complex class I expression on Reed-Sternberg cells in relation to the cytotoxic T-cell response in Epstein-Barr virus-positive and -negative Hodgkin's disease. Blood 1996;87:3844–51.

118. Murray PG, Constandinou CM, Crocker J, et al. Analysis of major histocompatibility complex class I, TAP expression, and LMP2 epitope sequence in Epstein-Barr virus-positive Hodgkin's disease. Blood 1998;92:2477–83.

119. Oudejans JJ, Jiwa NM, Kummer JA, et al. Activated cytotoxic T cells as prognostic marker in Hodgkin's disease Blood 1997;89:1376–82.

120. Lee SP, Constandinou CM, Thomas WA, et al. Antigen presenting phenotype of Hodgkin Reed-Sternberg cells: analysis of the HLA class I processing pathway and the effects of interleukin-10 on Epstein-Barr virus-specific cytotoxic T-cell recognition. Blood 1998;92:1020–30.

121. Niedobitek G, Young LS. In: Magrath I, editor. The non-Hodgkin's lymphomas. 2nd ed. London: Edward Arnold; 1997. p. 309–29.

122. Brink AA, ten Berge RL, van den Brule AJ, et al. Epstein-Barr virus is present in neoplastic cytotoxic T cells in extranodal, and predominantly in B cells in nodal T non-Hodgkin lymphomas. J Pathol 2000;191:400–6.

123. Niedobitek G, Baumann I, Brabletz T, et al. Hodgkin's disease and peripheral T-cell lymphoma: composite lymphoma with evidence of Epstein-Barr virus infection. J Pathol 2000;191:394–9.

124. Lee AW, Foo W, Mang O, et al. Changing epidemiology of nasopharyngeal carcinoma in Hong Kong over a 20-year period (1980-99): an encouraging reduction in both incidence and mortality. Int J Cancer 2003;103:680–5.

125. Deng H, Zeng Y, Lei Y, et al. Serological survey of nasopharyngeal carcinoma in 21 cities of south China. Chin Med J 1995;108:300–3.

126. Decaussin G, Sbih-Lammali F, de Turenne-Tessier M, et al. Expression of BARF1 gene encoded by Epstein-Barr virus in nasopharyngeal carcinoma biopsies. Cancer Res 2000;60:5584–8.

127. zur Hausen H, Brink AA, Craanen ME, et al. Unique transcription pattern of Epstein-Barr virus (EBV) in EBV-carrying gastric adenocarcinomas: expression of the transforming BARF1 gene. Cancer Res 2000;60:2745–8.

128. Strockbine LD, Cohen JI, Farrah T, et al. The Epstein-Barr virus BARF1 gene encodes a novel, soluble colony-stimulating factor-1 receptor. J Virol 1998;72:4014–21.

129. Wei MX, de Turenne-Tessier M, Decaussin G, et al. Establishment of a monkey kidney epithelial cell line with the BARF1 open reading frame from Epstein-Barr virus. Oncogene 1997;14:3073–81.

130. Wei MX, Moulin JC, Decaussin G, et al. Expression and tumorigenicity of the Epstein-Barr virus BARF1 gene in human Louckes B-lymphocyte cell line. Cancer Res 1994;54:1843–8.

131. Wei MX, Ooka T. A transforming function of the BARF1 gene encoded by Epstein-Barr virus. EMBO J 1989;8: 2897–903.

132. Sheng W, Decaussin G, Ligout A, et al. Malignant transformation of Epstein-Barr virus-negative Akata cells by introduction of the BARF1 gene carried by Epstein-Barr virus. J Virol 2003;77:3859 65.

133. Hildesheim A, Apple RJ, Chen CJ, et al. Association of HLA class I and II alleles and extended haplotypes with nasopharyngeal carcinoma in Taiwan. J Natl Cancer Inst 2002;94:1780–9.

134. Xiong W, Zeng ZY, Xia JH, et al. A susceptibility locus at chromosome 3p21 linked to familial nasopharyngeal carcinoma. Cancer Res 2004;64:1972–4.

135. Feng BJ, Huang W, Shugart YY, et al. Genome-wide scan for familial nasopharyngeal carcinoma reveals evidence of linkage to chromosome 4. Nat Genet 2002;31:395–9.

136. Yu MC, Yuan JM. Epidemiology of nasopharyngeal carcinoma. Semin Cancer Biol 2002;12:421–9.

137. Huang DP, Ho JH, Saw D, Teoh TB. Carcinoma of the nasal and paranasal regions in rats fed Cantonese salted marine fish. IARC Sci Publ 1978;20:315–28.

138. Lo KW, To KF, Huang DP. Focus on nasopharyngeal carcinoma. Cancer Cell 2004;5:423–8.

139. Lo KW, Cheung ST, Leung SF, et al. Hypermethylation of the p16 gene in nasopharyngeal carcinoma. Cancer Res 1996;56:2721–5.

140. Crook T, Nicholls JM, Brooks L, et al. High level expression of deltaN-p63: a mechanism for the inactivation of *p53* in undifferentiated nasopharyngeal carcinoma (NPC)? Oncogene 2000 Jul 13;19:3439–44.

141. Melino G, Lu X, Gasco M, Crook T, Knight RA. Functional regulation of p73 and p63: development and cancer. Trends Biochem Sci 2003;28:663–70.

142. Chan AS, To KF, Lo KW, et al. Frequent chromosome 9p losses in histologically normal nasopharyngeal epithelia from southern Chinese. Int J Cancer 2002;102:300–3.

143. Chan AS, To KF, Lo KW, et al. High frequency of chromosome 3p deletion in histologically normal nasopharyngeal epithelia from southern Chinese. Cancer Res 2000;60: 5365–70.

144. Smith PR, de Jesus O, Turner D, et al. Structure and coding content of CST (BART) family RNAs of Epstein-Barr virus. J Virol 2000;74:3082–92.

145. de Jesus O, Smith PR, Spender LC, et al. Updated Epstein-Barr virus (EBV) DNA sequence and analysis of a promoter for the BART (CST, BARFO) RNAs of EBV. J Gen Virol 2003;84(Pt 6):1443–50.

9

Nasopharyngeal Cancer Diagnosis and Management

SING-FAI LEUNG
PHILIP J. JOHNSON
ANTHONY T. C. CHAN

Although rare in the West, nasopharyngeal carcinoma (NPC) is a major public health problem throughout southern China, where it is the fifth commonest form of malignancy in men. Several features, including a consistent association with a virus (Epstein-Barr virus), a practical serologic marker, and sensitivity to treatment such that cure is possible even in patients with advanced disease, make this a model tumor of wide interest to workers in many fields of oncology.

EPIDEMIOLOGY

NPC occurs sporadically in the West, where it is associated with the risk factors common to most other head and neck cancers, excessive alcohol consumption, and tobacco smoking. In southern China, NPC is endemic, having incidence rates of 15 to 50 per 100,000 persons. There is an intermediate incidence in populations living in the Mediterranean basin, and in Alaskan Eskimos. The rate of incidence rises after age 20 years and decreases after age 60 years, and males are more often affected (a male-female ratio of 3:1).[1] The median age at presentation is 40 to 50 years, a significantly younger age than that observed for other head and neck cancers.

ETIOLOGY

There is a stepwise progression of histologic features that reflect underlying genetic events. Dysplas-tic areas of the nasopharynx are the earliest recognizable lesions, probably caused by some environmental carcinogen. These are associated with allelic losses on the short arms of chromosomes 3 and 9 that result in the inactivation of several tumor suppressor genes, including *p14*, *p15*, and *p16*.[2–5] The relevant carcinogens have not been established, but a very strong link between the consumption of salted fish and the development of NPC has been established.[1] These dysplastic areas themselves are unlikely to lead to further progression, but at this stage, latent Epstein-Barr virus (EBV) infection becomes established and may lead to the development of severe dysplasia. Gains of genes on chromosome 12 and allelic loss on 11q, 13q, and 16q accompany the development of invasive carcinoma; metastasis is associated with mutation of *P53* and aberrant expression of cadherins.[6,7]

PATHOLOGY

Three histopathologic types are recognized in the World Health Organization (WHO) classifications[8]: type I, squamous cell carcinoma (SCC) with varying degrees of differentiation; type II, nonkeratinizing carcinoma; and type III, undifferentiated carcinoma. The latter is often referred to as a "lymphoepithelioma" although the lymphocytic infiltration is reactive and not neoplastic. There are similarities in the epidemiologic, serologic, clinical, and natural history features of WHO types II and III, and it has been suggested that NPC be divided into only two categories,[9] namely, SCC and undifferentiated carcinoma of the nasopharyngeal type. Undifferentiated and poorly differentiated nonkeratinizing carcinomas probably have a higher local control rate and a better prognosis than do keratinizing SCCs because keratinizing SCCs are more radioresistant.[10,11] Furthermore, whereas keratinizing squamous NPCs (WHO type I) fail more locally than distantly, poorly differentiated NPCs (WHO types II and III) fail more distantly than locally.

PRESENTING SYMPTOMS AND SIGNS

Overview

As noted above, NPC is much more common among persons of certain ethnic groups, such as southern Chinese, North Africans, and Eskimos.[11–14] The physician should be particularly alert to the diagnosis in patients from these ethnic backgrounds. The cancer may rarely present in children, especially in North Africa.[14] The symptoms and signs[15] can be readily explained by the anatomic location of the nasopharynx: at the posterior end of the nasal passage, containing the medial opening of the eustachian tube (Figures 9–1 and 9–2), and immediately below the skull base (Figure 9–3), with lymphatic drainage to the upper and then to the middle and lower parts of the neck (Figure 9–4). Distant metastases are rare at presentation (being found in only about 5% of cases) and are almost never the presenting symptom.[16] Paraneoplastic syndromes are uncommon, but dermatomyositis is one well-recognized example.[17–19] Table 9–1 summarizes the more common presenting symptoms.

Practice Point: Neck Lump

Nodal metastases from NPC follow an orderly pattern in a cephalad to caudal direction; thus, the initially involved node is found in the upper neck, followed by nodes of smaller size at the middle and lower levels of the neck[20] (see Figure 9–4). It is usually painless and unilateral, but bilateral involvement is not uncommon (Figure 9–5).

Ultrasonography is the preferred imaging modality for assessment because it has high accuracy in

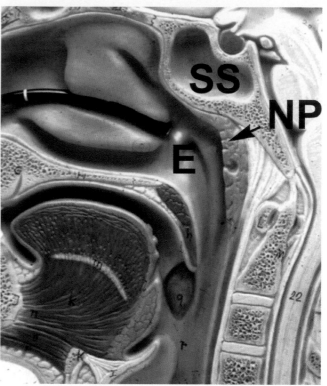

Figure 9–1. Sagittal section of the head, showing the posterior part of the nasal cavity and oral cavity. A flexible endoscope has been advanced to the nasopharynx (NP). A tumor at this location can partially block the nasal passage and cause nasal obstruction. Bleeding from the tumor can give rise to epistaxis (nose bleed) or dripping down to the oropharynx (throat) as postnasal drip. "E" denotes the opening of the eustachian tube (which connects the middle ear)on the lateral wall of the nasopharynx. When involved by tumor, middle ear symptoms (impaired hearing, tinnitus) may result. "SS" denotes the sphenoid sinus, which forms part of the "base of the skull" that, when involved, may cause headache. NP = posterior wall of nasopharynx.

distinguishing nodal masses from non-nodal masses. Under gray-scale and Doppler ultrasonography, most of the nonmalignant masses, such as branchial cysts and lipomas, have diagnostic features.[21] Benign and malignant nodes can be distinguished on the basis of characteristic ultrasonographic features.[22,23] For a malignant node, distinction between lymphoma and nasopharyngeal carcinoma is also possible.[24,25]

Fine-needle aspiration for cytology (FNAC) can be readily applied under ultrasonographic guidance, to confirm the malignant nature of the node and to distinguish it from lymphoma. Excisional biopsy of the neck node should not be undertaken lightly, as it is invasive and unnecessary in most situations. The malignant nature of the node can be readily shown by ultrasonography with or without FNAC; the potential

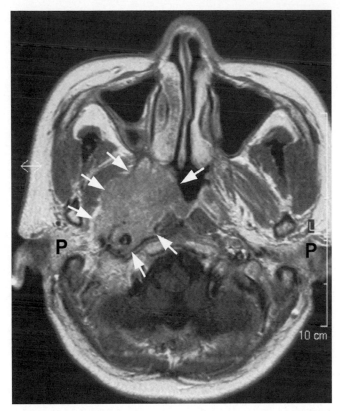

Figure 9–2. Magnetic resonance imaging scan (axial section) showing nasopharyngeal tumor (outlined by *white arrows*) with right-sided parapharyngeal extension. Nasal blockage and ear symptoms on the right side are expected. "P" denotes the parotid glands, which are subject to incidental irradiation during radiation therapy.

primary sites of cancer should be sought by endoscopy, and a definitive diagnosis can be obtained by biopsy of the primary tumor. Whether pretreatment nodal biopsy has a negative prognostic impact is controversial.[26] If the primary site of cancer is not apparent on endoscopy and imaging, and the malignant nature of the node is proven by FNAC, the cytology specimen can be stained for EBV markers such as EBV-encoded ribonucleic acid (EBER) (Figure 9–6)[27] or EBV deoxyribonucleic acid.[28] Positivity for EBER favors the diagnosis of NPC.

Practice Point:
Ear and Nasal Symptoms

Recent-onset unilateral impairment of hearing in an adult or recurrent otitis media due to conductive hearing loss from eustachian tube dysfunction raises the possibility of NPC[29,30] (Figure 9–7). This is more probable if there is parapharyngeal extension of tumor

on the involved side[31] (see Figure 9–2). Tinnitus occurs in about one-third of patients with NPC, but otalgia is rare.[15] The distinction between NPC, allergic rhinitis, and other diseases is difficult on the basis of nasal symptoms. While nasal discharge and obstruction can be caused by rhinitis and sinusitis, blood in postnasal discharge is particularly suspicious.

Practice Point:
Pattern of Cranial Nerve Involvement

Cranial nerve involvement indicates advanced local disease. Some cranial nerves pass close to the nasopharynx as they pass through the skull base, especially in the cavernous sinus region (Figure 9–8; see also Figure 9–3). Cranial nerves V and VI are most commonly involved (Figure 9–9) owing to their greater proximity to the nasopharynx as compared to other cranial nerves.[32,33] Nerves III and VII are involved very late in the natural history of disease, and their involvement is invariably associated with other cranial nerves. Thus, a patient presenting with *isolated* nerve III or VII palsy (eg, a picture similar to that of Bell's palsy) is unlikely to have NPC.

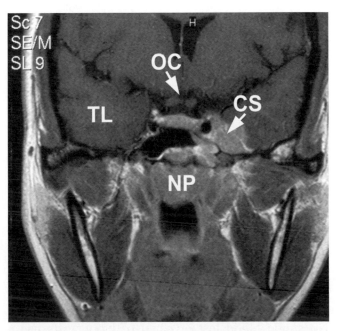

Figure 9–3. Magnetic resonance imaging scan (coronal section) showing nasopharyngeal tumor with extension to the skull base and involvement of the left cavernous sinus (Cs) (potentially involving cranial nerves VI, V, IV, and III) and, the adjacent brain. "TL" denotes the of the brain. Skull base involvement may cause headache. OC = Optic chiasm.

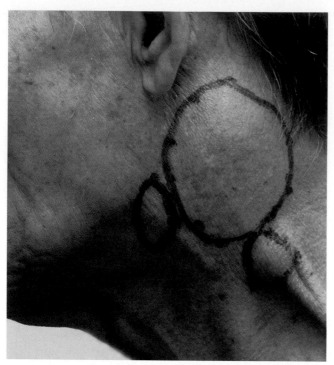

Figure 9–4. Photograph of the left side of the neck of a patient with nodal metastases from nasopharyngeal carcinoma; nodes are denoted by skin marks. The largest node was located at the upper cervical region. In this case, the node was mostly underneath the sternocleidomastoid muscle. It is also common for the node to be located more anteriorly in front of the anterior border of the muscle. Submandibular nodal metastasis is uncommon.

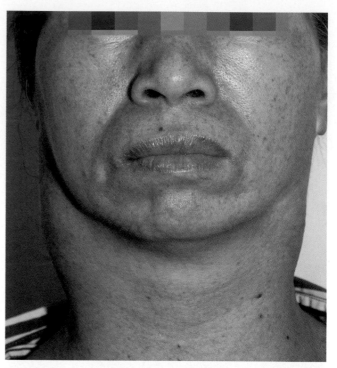

Figure 9–5. Bilateral nodal metastases are not uncommon. This female patient had very bulky bilateral upper cervical nodal metastases; the nodal mass on the right side was bulkier than that on the left side.

CONFIRMATION OF DIAGNOSIS

Definitive diagnosis relies on endoscopically guided nasopharyngeal biopsy (Figures 9–10 and 9–11). This can be done with the patient under topical anesthesia, in the sitting or supine position. A practical arrangement is for a flexible endoscope to be passed through the side of the nose opposite to the suspected tumor site, leaving the ipsilateral side clear for passage of the biopsy forceps.[34] The use of tiny forceps, such as might be used through the operating channel of a flexible endoscope, is discouraged because unrepresentative samples might be obtained.

ROLE OF BLOOD TESTING IN DIAGNOSIS

No single blood test or panel of blood tests has a diagnostic accuracy of 100% for NPC; thus, no single blood test or panel of blood tests can be relied on to exclude or confirm the diagnosis of NPC. Almost all serologic markers of NPC are based on the detec-

tion of antibodies to EBV[35] or on the detection of EBV genetic material.[36,37] These EBV markers may not be applicable to patients with well-differentiated tumors (WHO type 1 histology), irrespective of the ethnic background of the patient.[38–40] The most widely used test—and the one with the longest track record—measures the immunoglobulin A (IgA) antibody to the viral capsid antigen of the EBV.[35] It has been used in countries both endemic[35] and nonendemic[39] to the disease. It has a sensitivity ranging from 80 to 90%[35,38,39] when measured by the semi-

Table 9–1. PRESENTING SYMPTOMS OF NASOPHARYNGEAL CANCER
Common Symptoms
Lump in upper neck (lymph node) (see Figures 9–4 and 9–5) Blood-stained nasal or postnasal discharge, nasal obstruction Unilateral hearing loss, tinnitus (middle ear dysfunction) (see Figure 9–7)
Less common symptoms (related to advanced-stage disease)
Headache (skull base involvement) Diplopia, altered facial sensation (VI and V nerve palsies) (see Figure 9–3)

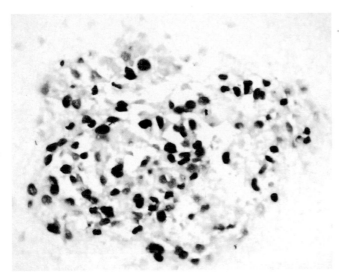

Figure 9–6. Fine-needle aspiration cytology specimen from neck nodal metastases, with immunohistochemical staining for Epstein-Barr virus.

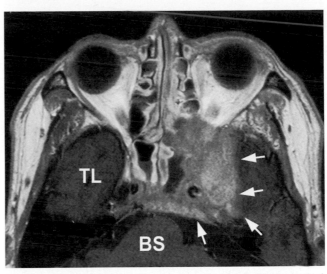

Figure 9–8. Magnetic resonance imaging scan (axial section) showing an advanced tumor (*white arrow*) infiltrating the left cavernous sinus and temporal lobe. (TL = temporal lobe of opposite side; BS = brainstem.)

quantitative indirect immunofluorescent method, with a cutoff titer of 1 in 10.

Few single-marker blood tests have been reported to have both diagnostic sensitivity and specificity of more than 90%. Exceptional examples include assay of circulating EBV deoxyribonucleic acid (DNA) by quantitative polymerase chain reaction,[41] antibodies to EBV thymidine kinase,[42] and antibody to the EBV transactivator protein (ZEBRA).[43] A rather large number of other EBV-based blood markers with lower sensitivities and specificities have been reported in case-control studies.[44–55] A combination of tests in a

panel increases diagnostic accuracy[41,44,49–51,54–57]; some of these panels have been shown to have accuracies higher than 90%.[43,53,55]

WORK-UP AND STAGING

Since NPC is regularly treated by nonsurgical modalities, clinical rather than pathologic staging is regularly used. The International Union Against Cancer and the American Joint Committee on Cancer share the same stage classification system for NPC[58,59] (Table 9–2), based on consensus and review of treatment outcomes of patients in both endemic and nonendemic disease regions. Currently, different therapeutic strategies are used for early-stage and advanced-stage NPC.[60]

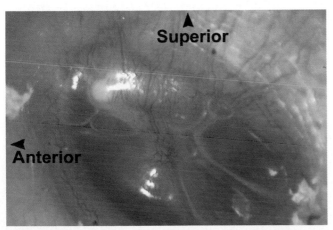

Figure 9–7. Photograph of the left eardrum of a patient with middle ear effusion (note swelling of the tympanic membrane with air bubbles) from eustachian tube dysfunction resulting from nasopharyngeal carcinoma. The eustachian tube connects the nasopharynx and middl ear

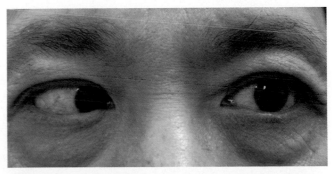

Figure 9–9. A man with left-sided VI nerve palsy due to nasopharyngeal carcinoma with skull base involvement. Photograph was taken with the patient gazing to the left side.

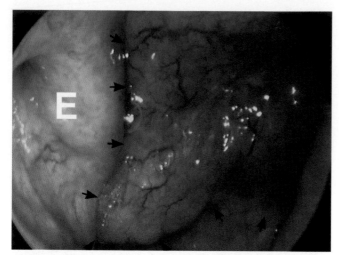

Figure 9–10. Endoscopic view of a nasopharynx with tumor. *Arrows* indicate the border of the tumor. "E" denotes the eustachian tube opening on the right lateral wall of the nasopharynx.

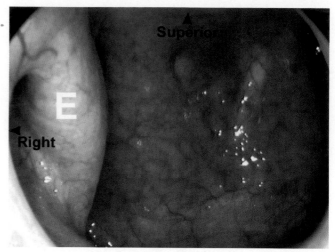

Figure 9–11. Endoscopic view of a normal nasopharynx. "E" denotes the eustachian tube opening on the right lateral wall of the nasopharynx.

Staging Tools for Primary Tumor and Nodal and Distant Metastases

Although the imaging modalities to be used in staging are not specified in the staging system, magnetic resonance imaging (MRI) is currently the main staging tool because it is superior to computed tomography (CT) in assessing the involvement of soft-tissue, skull base, and perineural spread.[61–63] It also facilitates high-precision radiation therapy planning.[64] Endoscopic assessment is complementary to imaging in mapping the extent of mucosal disease.[61]

MRI is also suitable for assessing nodal metastases[61,65] although nodal staging is commonly based

Table 9–2. STAGING SYSTEM FOR NASOPHARYNGEAL CARCINOMA			
Nasopharynx (T)			
T1	Nasopharynx		
T2	Soft tissue of oropharynx and/or nasal fossa		
T2a	Without parapharyngeal extension		
T2b	With parapharyngeal extension		
T3	Invades bony structure and/or paranasal sinuses		
T4	Intracranial extension, involvement of cranial nerves, infratemporal fossa, hypopharynx, orbit		
Regional lymph node (N)			
N1	Unilateral metastasis in lymph node(s), 6 cm or less in greatest dimension, above supraclavicular fossa		
N2	Bilateral metastasis in lymph node(s), 6 cm or less in greatest dimension, above supraclavicular fossa		
N3	Metastasis in lymph node(s), greater than 6 cm in dimension, in the supraclavicular fossa		
Distant metastasis (M)			
M0	No distant metastasis		
M1	Distant metastasis		
Stage grouping			
Stage 0	Tis	N0	M0
Stage I	T1	N0	M0
Stage IIA	T2a	N0	M0
Stage IIB	T2b	N0	M0
	T1, T2a, T2b	N1	M0
Stage III	T3	N0,N1	M0
	T1, T2, T3	N2	M0
Stage IVA	T4	N0, N1, N2	M0
Stage IVB	Any T	N3	M0
Stage IVC	Any T	Any N	M1

Adapted from Union Internationale Contre le Cancer[58]; American Joint Committee on Cancer.[59]

on hand palpation. Distant-metastasis screening can be considered for those in high-risk groups, such as patients with advanced nodal-stage disease.[66,67] The role of positron emission tomography (PET) has not been fully evaluated for staging NPC.

Implications of Specific Stages

NPC commonly extends laterally to the parapharyngeal space (denoted by T2b stage), a significant degree of posterolateral extension (see Figure 9–2) would make two-dimensional radiation therapy (2D-RT) planning problematic as the posterior limit of cancer is close to the brainstem and spinal cord, which may be exposed to incidental irradiation. Extension superior to the skull base (denoted by T3 and T4 stages) carries adverse prognostic impact in terms of local and distant failure,[68] and constitutes an indication for combined modality treatment.[60] 2D-RT planning also tends to be problematic when the tumor is close to the optic pathway and brainstem[69] (see Figures 9–3 and 9–8). Tumor extension to the anterior part of skull base, such as ethmoid sinus and orbit, may necessitate the sacrifice of vision by radiation therapy (see Figure 9–8). Increasing N stage correlates with increased risk of distant failure[68]; combined-modality treatment should be considered for N2 to N3 stage disease.[60]

TREATMENT

Radiation therapy (RT) is the mainstay of treatment and is an essential component of curative-intent treatment of nondisseminated NPC. Stages I and II disease are treated by RT alone whereas stages III and IV disease are treated by RT with concurrent chemotherapy.[60] The role of concurrent chemotherapy in stage II disease is less well defined because some patients with stage II disease had been categorized under stage III disease (in the pre-1997 stage-classification) and included in the American Intergroup study showing benefit of concurrent chemotherapy.[60] Surgery is not a primary treatment modality for the following reasons: its nonapplicability to T3,T4 tumors, its morbidity, problematic bilateral neck dissection for nodal metastases, the need for postoperative RT as a result of close surgical margins, and the relative effectiveness of RT.

Radiation Therapy

RT is based on the ability of high-energy photons from linear accelerators to kill cancer cells. The radiation is targeted to the imaging-visible tumor and metastatic neck nodes plus a surrounding margin of tissue at risk of microscopic tumor spread[70] (Figure 9–12). The tissue considered at risk commonly includes (besides the nasopharynx) the parapharyngeal region (laterally), the posterior part of the nasal passage and maxillary antrum (anteriorly), the sphenoid sinus (superiorly), and the oropharynx (inferiorly).[70] The full length of both sides of the neck is irradiated. For nodal stage 0 disease, elective neck irradiation is also commonly given. The safety of omitting elective neck irradiation in patients defined to have uninvolved cervical lymphatics by present-day imaging tools is still under investigation.[71] The final part of the treatment is sometimes targeted to a smaller volume that includes only the gross tumor and a small margin.

The total irradiation dose to the imaging-visible tumor is usually between 60 and 80 Gy and is typically in the range of 66 to 72 Gy; 2 Gy are given each day, 5 days a week (conventional fractionation) for 1.5 to

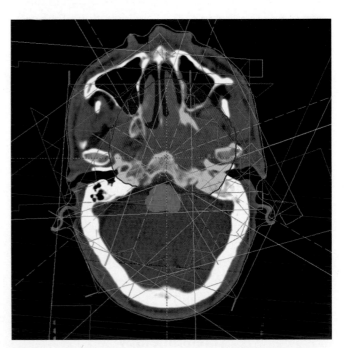

Figure 9–12. Axial computed tomography image showing that the area to be treated (in red paint and including the nasopharynx, the paranasopharyngeal region on the lateral sides, and the clivus at the back of the nasopharynx) is in close proximity to the brainstem.

2 months. The biologic effect of irradiation could be increased by increasing the total dose (dose escalation), shortening the overall treatment duration (eg, by treating for 6 days instead of 5 days a week [accelerated fractionation]), giving two treatments a day during part of the course (hyperfractionation, concomitant boost),[72] or adding chemotherapy. A limited amount of clinical data suggests a benefit of accelerated fractionation in NPC.[73] Hyperfractionated RT has been shown to be advantageous in some studies[74,75] (but not in others)[76] and may be associated with complications if the time interval between the fractions is short.[76]

In conventional RT, the nasopharynx and adjacent region is treated by radiation beams from the left and right sides and sometimes also from the front. The borders of the irradiation ports are determined with reference to landmarks on plain radiographs.[68,77,78] The neck is usually irradiated by a separate anterior radiation beam. Since the 1990s, three-dimensional conformal RT (3D-CRT) planning and delivery have been increasingly used.[79] This involves the acquisition of serial cross-sectional images of the head and neck by CT with the patient in the treatment position, followed by virtual reconstruction of three-dimensional images of the tumor and adjacent anatomic organs, and evaluation of the use of radiation beams from different directions (using the "beam's-eye view" function of the software), to determine the optimal dose distribution (Figure 9–13). Intensity-modulated RT (IMRT) represents a further step forward in improving dose distribution by introducing a matrix of partial transmission blocks in each radiation beam under computer control (intensity modulation), resulting in even higher conformity of the dose distribution to the tumor geometry[80] (Figure 9–14). Early clinical results of IMRT reveal a very high rate of local tumor control of over 90%, even for advanced T-stage disease.[70] In some centers, a booster dose of radiation is given routinely during the last part of the course of RT. This can be delivered as 2D-RT,[81] conformal RT,[82] stereotactic RT,[83,84] IMRT,[85] or brachytherapy (ie, placing radioactive sources inside the nasopharyngeal cavity).[86–88]

Chemotherapy

Patients with stage III–IV disease are usually treated with current chemotherapy.[60] Chemotherapy can

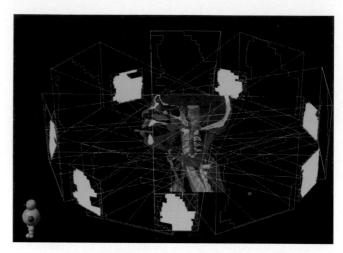

Figure 9–13. Computer graphic representation of a three-dimensional radiation therapy set-up. In this example, seven radiation beams are directed at the nasopharyngeal region; normal organs, outlined on serial computed tomography images and reconstructed for visualization (eyeballs, optic nerves, and chiasm in purple; brainstem in blue), are shielded from individual radiation beams. Intensity-modulated radiation therapy is a special form of three-dimensional conformal radiation therapy in which a matrix of partial shielding blocks are inserted in the radiation beams under computer control to modulate the intensity of the irradiation and to achieve even better conformity of the irradiation to the tumor target.

potentially be given in three modes in relation to the timing of RT: concurrently, as neoadjuvant therapy, and as adjuvant therapy.

Concurrent chemotherapy (ie, during the period of RT), or "chemoradiation," is the standard therapy for advanced-stage NPC.[60,89–91] Randomized trials have shown benefit in terms of overall survival, progression-free survival, and reduction of local and distant failures. The main cytotoxic agents used are cisplatin and 5-fluorouracil.

Chemotherapy given as adjuvant therapy (given after completion of RT, is attractive because distant metastases represent the major mode of relapse of NPC, implying the presence of subclinical residual disease at completion of initial therapy in at-risk patients. However, there is little evidence that adjuvant chemotherapy alone can improve survival or reduce distant relapse in NPC patients.[90,92–94] Although adjuvant therapy was given as part of a chemoradiation protocol in the American Intergroup Study,[60] toxicity is of concern. Patients often have considerable difficulty in tolerating chemotherapy when it is given after a full course of RT or chemoradiation.[60,92,94]

The benefit of chemotherapy given as neoadjuvant therapy (ie, given before the commencement of

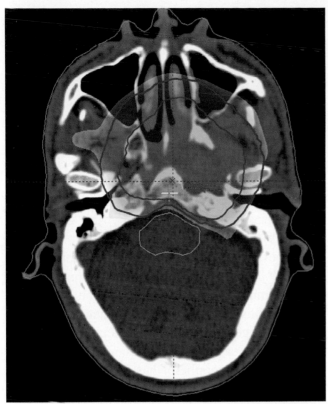

Figure 9–14. Axial computed tomography image showing radiation dose distribution from seven "intensity-modulated" radiation beams. *Inner red circle* denotes the extent of gross tumor treated to a high uniform radiation dose; *outer red circle* denotes an additional margin treated to a slightly lower dose to cover microscopic extension of tumor plus a margin for set-up error. The brainstem is spared from the high radiation dose. This is difficult to achieve if only two lateral radiation beams are used in two-dimensional conventional radiation therapy.

RT), in terms of improving progression-free survival and local control[95,96] and reducing distant failure,[96] has been shown by some (but not all)[94,97] randomized trials. No randomized trial has shown an improved overall survival. Currently, this is not regarded as standard therapy.

The Influence of Histology on Treatment Strategy

There is a question as to whether treatment strategies for patients with the well-differentiated histology should be different from those for patients with the undifferentiated or poorly differentiated histology.

It is recognized that the biologic behavior of the disease and the treatment outcomes of the two histologic types are different.[97–100] Compared to undiffer-

entiated and poorly differentiated tumors, well-differentiated tumors tend to present with less advanced disease and have a lower rate of distant metastases but a less favorable outcome after therapy. Randomized trials in nonendemic regions, such as the American Intergroup study,[60] consist of an appreciable proportion of patients with the well-differentiated histology whereas trials in Southeast Asia consist almost exclusively of patients with the undifferentiated histology.[89,90,91] Although these trials have concordant conclusions supporting the benefit of chemoradiation over RT alone, the treatment outcomes for the same treatment modality were quite different among different studies, and the relative impact on local control and distant failure also differs among studies. Some retrospective matched-cohort studies in endemic regions have failed to demonstrate improvement with chemoradiation.[101,102] Whether these discordant findings can be explained by difference in the mix of histologic types in the different studies remains unclear.

POSTTREATMENT ASSESSMENT

Nasopharyngoscopy is performed several weeks after the completion of therapy, when the inflammatory changes resulting from radiation have partly settled. During the first 10 to 12 weeks after RT, endoscopic appearance[103] and biopsy results[104] may be difficult to interpret because a residual swelling found during this period, even if biopsy-positive, might later go into complete remission; similarly, residual neck nodes may also take several weeks to regress completely. Imaging is of limited value in the early post-RT period for assessment of local and nodal disease status.[105,106] PET has been shown to be more accurate than MRI in distinguishing residual/recurrent tumor when performed 4 months after therapy.[107,108] In the early post-therapy period, serum EBV DNA has been shown to be a powerful predictor of the risks of recurrence and persistent disease.[109,110]

TREATMENT TOXICITIES

Range of Toxicities

A wide spectrum of potential treatment toxicities arises from RT and chemotherapy.[111] Radiation toxicities are categorized as acute or late. Acute toxicities occur during and immediately after RT and are characterized by temporary inflammatory changes in irradiated tissue (eg, pharyngitis, dermatitis). Late toxicities emerge months to years after RT and are characterized by irreversible atrophy, fibrosis, and dysfunction of irradiated organs. The toxicities of chemotherapy are mainly short-term effects. Chemotherapy also augments the severity of some acute and late radiation toxicities.[60,112] The spectrum and severity of toxicities are understandably related to the context in which treatment is delivered. Tissues regularly involved by the gross tumor and its potential microscopic extension (such as the mucosa of the nasopharynx and oropharynx, part of the eustachian tubes, or the soft tissue of the neck) are expected to sustain irradiation effects in all cases although the effects are largely acceptable (eg, mucosal dryness, fibrosis of the soft tissue of the neck, and middle ear effusion). The parotid glands are immediately outside the irradiation target but are unavoidably subject to incidental irradiation; this could be minimized by RT delivery systems with high conforming capacity, such as IMRT. Irradiation of advanced T-stage tumors not only involves a larger volume of tissue but also risks irradiation of the more peripheral organs (such as the optic pathway and the brainstem) and also exposure to the toxicities of concurrent chemotherapy. Re-irradiation for recurrent tumors would also give rise to exceptionally severe toxicities.[113,114] The more worrisome late toxicities are related to the irradiation of neurologic organs such as the optic nerves and optic chiasm (leading to impaired vision or blindness), temporal lobes (leading to impaired memory and intracranial edema from the necrotic foci of brain tissue), brainstem (leading to quadriparesis), and spinal cord (resulting in paraparesis). These critical organs can be readily protected when treating T1 and T2 tumors, but they may be very close to T3 and T4 tumors and are thus at some risk of injury in such circumstances.

Reduction and Management

Conceptually, toxicities of irradiation could be minimized by a physical approach (ie, by precisely conforming the irradiation dose distribution to the tumor and minimizing the irradiation of adjacent organs) or by a biologic approach (ie, by modulating the biologic effect of irradiation on tissues by using radioprotectors, for example, or by manipulating the size of each irradiation dose).

Xerostomia (dryness of the oral cavity) resulting from incidental irradiation of the salivary gland affects almost all patients to a certain extent. This could be minimized by using IMRT to physically spare part of the parotid glands from irradiation, or by using the radioprotector amifostine.[115] For established xerostomia, alleviation by the cholinergic agent pilocarpine has been reported[116,117] although the role of pilocarpine in prevention is more controversial.[118] Middle and inner ear problems are relatively common.[119–121] Because of the associated complications, prophylactic placement of ventilation tubes is generally not recommended for prevention of middle ear effusion.[122] A combination of pentoxifylline and tocopherol has been reported to be effective in reversing severe radiation-induced soft-tissue fibrosis and radiation-induced ulcers.[123] Trismus may also be helped.[124]

Brain injury is uncommon, but may be encountered when treating advanced T-stage tumors when the lower portions of the temporal lobes are subject to high-dose incidental irradiation.[125] The injury is typically represented by necrotic foci at the lowermost part of the temporal lobes; these foci induce an edematous effect in the surrounding brain tissue.[126,127] Temporal-lobe epileptic symptoms may also occur.[127] The natural history of the lesions is unpredictable, and the lesions may remain static then regress, progress then regress, or wax and wane.[128] The changes usually occur over months to years. The main risk is an increase in intracranial pressure in the progressive edema phase, and a course of high-dose steroid[127] and/or surgical intervention[129] may be required. Acute hemorrhage is an uncommon but recognized risk.[130] Tocopherol has been reported to improve cognitive function in some patients with temporal-lobe injury.[131] Patients with advanced T-stage tumors are more likely to have the hypothalamus and pituitary included within the irradiation ports, and some patients may develop hypopituitarism on follow-up. Most cases are subclinical, and the gonadal and thyroidal axes are the more commonly affected axes.[132–134] Patients with suspicious symptoms, such as unexplained fatigue, on follow-up should alert the treating physician. Hormonal replacement is indicated if deficiency is confirmed.

RECURRENCES

Local Recurrence

Small local recurrences are potentially curable, and the main issue is choice of the most appropriate therapeutic option. Options include surgery (nasopharyngectomy),[135–138] brachytherapy,[139,140] radiosurgery or stereotactic RT,[141] IMRT,[142] a combination of surgery and RT (brachytherapy or external RT), and a combination of external RT and brachytherapy. There is a lack of randomized studies comparing the treatment options, and interpretation of relative efficacy on the basis of different studies is difficult owing to variation in selection criteria. The best 5-year survival rates reported are from brachytherapy with radioactive iridium mold[139] and implantation of radioactive gold grain.[140] Treatment decisions are tailored to the specific situation of individual cases in regard to the volume, location, and extent of the recurrent tumor. For advanced-stage local recurrence, the difficult decision is whether to treat or not to treat. Therapeutic options are few because those of surgery and brachytherapy are inappropriate. Experiences with re-irradiation by 2D-RT generally have not been very rewarding, being characterized by rather low cure rates and high complication rates.[111,113,114] Selected cases may be suitable for stereotactic RT, and the role of IMRT is being explored. The volume of the recurrent tumor and the time lapse after the initial RT are important considerations.[113,143]

Regional Recurrence

Regional recurrence is managed by radical neck dissection (if resectable) with or without intraoperative placement of catheters for postoperative brachytherapy.[144] Patients are at risk of both local recurrence and distant relapse,[145] and these sites should be screened before surgery. The prognosis of synchronous local and regional recurrence is poor.[146]

Distant Metastases

The median survival time a patient with distant metastasis is about 9 months and is influenced by the disease and the patient's characteristics.[147,148] Although there is a lack of randomized studies that address the impact of therapy on survival and quality of life, palliative chemotherapy is often considered for patients whose performance status is adequate. A small percentage of patients appeared to be cured by therapy.[147–150] Platinum-containing regimens are commonly used as first-line therapy.[150–155] Nonplatinum-based regimens are also used, especially when patients have had prior exposure to cisplatin-based chemoradiation for advanced-stage disease.[156] Newer active agents include paclitaxel,[157–159] docetaxel,[160] gemcitabine,[161–163] and capecitabine[164]; these can be used as single agents[157,161,164] or in combination.[158–160,162,163] Response rates improved with more intensive chemotherapy, but the added treatment toxicities remain of concern.[165,166]

NOVEL THERAPIES

Overexpression of the epidermal growth factor receptor (EGFR) has been shown to correlate with poor survival in advanced-stage NPC patients.[167] Encouraging preliminary data on the use of C225 (cetuximab), an antibody to EGFR, in combination with cisplatin for head and neck cancers have been reported,[168] and studies on its use for NPC are under way. Cytotoxic T lymphocytes (CTLs) play a major role in controlling EBV infections, and EBV latent membrane protein (LMP)–specific CTL responses can be detected in untreated NPC patients.[169] Immunization with LMP2 peptide epitopes presented on autologous dendritic cells is a potential strategy for treating metastatic NPC. The presence of hypermethylated EBV DNA in NPC tumor cells provides an opportunity to use a DNA methylation inhibitor to effect demethylation and gene reexpression to facilitate immune-mediated destruction of tumor cells. 5-Azacytidine has been shown to bring about demethylation in tumor tissue in NPC patients.[170] Several other molecular pathology parameters have been identified as having prognostic bearing in NPC cases and might be potential targets for gene therapy.[171,172] Preclinical work has examined some of these targets, paving the way for clinical studies.[173]

ACKNOWLEDGMENTS

The authors would like to acknowledge the contribution of the following members at the Chinese University of Hong Kong, Hong Kong for their contribution of original photos, diagrams and references to the work: Anil Ahuja, MD FRCR and Ann King, FRCR of Department of Diagnostic Radiology and Organ Imaging; Ricky Chau, MSc of Department of Clinical Oncology; KF To, FRCPath of Department of Anatomical and Cellular Pathology; and John KS Woo, FRCS of Department of Surgery.

REFERENCES

1. Ho JHC. An epidemiologic and clinical study of nasopharyngeal carcinoma. Int J Radiat Oncol Biol Phys 1978;4: 183–205.
2. Lo KW, Cheung ST, Leung SF, et al. Hypermethylation of the p16 gene in nasopharyngeal carcinoma. Cancer Res 1996;56:2721–5.
3. Chan AS, To KF, Lo KW, et al. High frequency of chromosome 3p deletion in histologically normal nasopharyngeal epithelia from southern Chinese. Cancer Res 2000;60: 5365–70.
4. Lo KW, Teo PM, Hui AB, et al. High resolution allelotype of microdissected primary nasopharyngeal carcinoma. Cancer Res 2000;60:3348–53.
5. Lo KW, Kwong J, Hui AB, et al. High frequency of promoter hypermethylation of RASSF1A in nasopharyngeal carcinoma. Cancer Res 2001;61:3877–81.
6. Huang DP, Lo KW, van Hasselt CA, et al. A region of homozygous deletion on chromosome 9p21-22 in primary nasopharyngeal carcinoma. Cancer Res 1994;54:4003–6.
7. Hui AB, Lo KW, Leung SF, et al. Detection of recurrent chromosomal and losses in primary nasopharyngeal carcinoma by comparative genomic hybridization. Int J Cancer 1999;82:498–503.
8. Shanmugaratnam K, Sobin LH. The World Health Organization histological classification of tumours of the upper respiratory tract and ear. A commentary on the second edition. Cancer 1993;71:2689–97.
9. Krueger GR, Wustrow J. Current histological classification of nasopharyngeal carcinoma at Cologne University. In: Grundmann E, editor. Nasopharyngeal carcinoma, Cancer campaign: nasopharyngeal carcinoma. Vol 5. Stuttgart: G Fischer Verlag; 1981. p. 11–15.
10. Reddy SP, Raslan WF, Gooneratne S, et al. Prognostic significance of keratinization in nasopharyngeal carcinoma. Am J Otolaryngol 1995;16:103–8.
11. Marks JE, Phillips JL, Menck HR. The National Cancer Data Base report on the relationship of race and national origin to the histology of nasopharyngeal carcinoma. Cancer 1998;83:582–8.
12. Fandi A, Altun M, Azli N, et al., Nasopharynx cancer: epidemiology, staging, and treatment. Semin Oncol 1994;21: 382–97.
13. Easton JE, Levin PH, Hyarns VJ. Nasopharyngeal carcinoma in the United States: a pathological study of 177 US and 30 foreign cases. Arch Otolaryngol 1980;106:88–91.
14. Ellouz R, Cammoun M, Attia RB, Bahi J. Nasopharyngeal carcinoma in children and adolescents in Tunisia: clinical aspects and the paraneoplastic syndrome. IARC Sci Publ 1978;(20):115–29.
15. Skinner DW, Van Hasselt CA, Tsao SY. Nasopharyngeal carcinoma: modes of presentation Ann Otol Rhinol Laryngol 1991;100:544–51.
16. Teo PM, Kwan WH, Lee WY, et al. Prognosticators determining survival subsequent to distant metastasis from nasopharyngeal carcinoma. Cancer 1996;77:2423–31.
17. Teo P, Tai TH, Choy D. Nasopharyngeal carcinoma with dermatomyositis. Int J Radiat Oncol Biol Phys 1989;16:471–4.
18. Ang P, Sugeng MW, Chua SH. Classical and amyopathic dermatomyositis seen at the National Skin Centre of Singapore: a 3-year retrospective review of their clinical characteristics and association with malignancy. Ann Acad Med Singapore 2000;29:219–23.
19. Cvitkovic E, Bachouchi M, Boussen H, et al. Leukemoid reaction, bone marrow invasion, fever of unknown origin, and metastatic pattern in the natural history of advanced undifferentiated carcinoma of nasopharyngeal type: a review of 255 consecutive cases. J Clin Oncol 1993; 11:2434–42.
20. Sham JS, Choy D, Wei WI. Nasopharyngeal carcinoma: orderly neck node spread. Int J Radiat Oncol Biol Phys 1990;19:929–33.
21. Koischwitz D, Gritzmann N. Ultrasound of the neck. Radiol Clin North Am 2000;38:1029–45.
22. Ahuja A, Ying M. Sonography of neck lymph nodes. Part II: abnormal lymph nodes. Clin Radiol 2003;58:359–66.
23. Ahuja A, Ying M. Sonographic evaluation of cervical lymphadenopathy: is power Doppler sonography routinely indicated? Ultrasound Med Biol 2003;29:353–9.
24. Ahuja A, Ying M, Yang WT, et al. The use of sonography in differentiating cervical lymphomatous lymph nodes from cervical metastatic lymph nodes. Clin Radiol 1996;51: 186–90.
25. Ho SS, Ahuja AT, Kew J, Metreweli C. Differentiation of lymphadenopathy in different forms of carcinoma with Doppler sonography. Clin Radiol 2000;55:627–31.
26. Leung SF, Teo PM, Foo WW, et al. Pretreatment neck node biopsy, distant metastases, and survival in nasopharyngeal carcinoma. Head Neck 1993;15:296–9.
27. Huang DP, Ho HC, Henle W et al. Presence of EBNA in nasopharyngeal carcinoma and control patient tissues related to EBV serology. Int J Cancer. 1978;22:266–74.
28. Macdonald MR, Freeman JL, Hui MF. Role of Epstein-Barr virus in fine-needle aspirates of metastatic neck nodes in the diagnosis of nasopharyngeal carcinoma. Head Neck 1995;17:487–93.
29. Sham JS, Wei WI, Lau SK. Serous otitis media. An opportu-

nity for early recognition of nasopharyngeal carcinoma. Arch Otolaryngol Head Neck Surg 1992;118:794–7.

30. Dempster JH, Simpson DC. Nasopharyngeal neoplasms and their association with adult onset otitis media with effusion. Clin Otolaryngol 1988;13:363–5.

31. Sham JS, Wei WI, Lau SK. Serous otitis media and paranasopharyngeal extension of nasopharyngeal carcinoma. Head Neck 1992;14:19–23.

32. Leung SF, Tsao SY, Teo P, Foo W. Cranial nerve involvement by nasopharyngeal carcinoma: response to treatment and clinical significance. Clin Oncol (R Coll Radiol) 1990;2: 138–41.

33. Sham JS, Cheung YK, Choy D. Cranial nerve involvement and base of the skull erosion in nasopharyngeal carcinoma. Cancer 1991;68:422–6.

34. Waldron J, Van Hasselt CA, Wong KY. Sensitivity of biopsy using local anesthesia in detecting nasopharyngeal carcinoma. Head Neck 1992;14:24–7.

35. Henle G, Henle W. Epstein-Barr virus-specific IgA serum antibodies as an outstanding feature of nasopharyngeal carcinoma. Int J Cancer 1976;17:1–7.

36. Lo YMD, Chan LYS, Lo KW, et al. Quantitative analysis of cell-free Epstein-Barr virus DNA in plasma of patients with nasopharyngeal carcinoma. Cancer Res 1999;59:1188–91.

37. Wong TS, Kwong DL, Sham JS, et al. Quantitative plasma hypermethylated DNA markers of undifferentiated nasopharyngeal carcinoma. Clin Cancer Res 2004;10: 2401–6.

38. Neel IIB III, Pearson GR, Weiland LH, et al. Anti-EBV serologic tests for nasopharyngeal carcinoma. Laryngoscope 1980;90:1981–90.

39. Neel HB III, Pearson GR, Taylor WF. Antibodies to Epstein-Barr virus in patients with nasopharyngeal carcinoma and in comparison groups. Ann Otol Rhinol Laryngol 1984; 93:477–82.

40. Pratesi C, Bortolin MT, D'Andrea M, et al. Quantitative plasma/serum EBV DNA load by LMP2A determination in an Italian cohort of NPC patients. J Clin Virol 2003;28: 155–64.

41. Leung SF, Tam JS, Chan AT, et al. Improved accuracy of detection of nasopharyngeal carcinoma by combined application of circulating Epstein-Barr virus DNA and anti-Epstein-Barr viral capsid antigen IgA antibody. Clin Chem 2004;50:339–45.

42. Connolly Y, Littler E, Sun N, et al. Antibodies to Epstein-Barr virus thymidine kinase: a characteristic marker for the serological detection of nasopharyngeal carcinoma. Int J Cancer 2001;91:692–7.

43. Dardari R, Khyatti M, Benider A, et al. Antibodies to the Epstein-Barr virus transactivator protein (ZEBRA) as a valuable biomarker in young patients with nasopharyngeal carcinoma. Int J Cancer 2000;86:71–5.

44. Cai WM, Li YW, Wu B, et al. A double-blind study of four EB virus antibodies with evaluation by sequential discrimination. Int J Radiat Oncol Biol Phys 1983;9:1763–8.

45. Chien YC, Chen JY, Liu MY, et al. Serologic markers of Epstein-Barr virus infection and nasopharyngeal carcinoma in Taiwanese men. N Engl J Med 2001;345:1877–82.

46. Zhu XX, Zeng Y, Wolf H. Detection of IgG and IgA antibodies to Epstein-Barr virus membrane antigen in sera from

patients with nasopharyngeal carcinoma and from normal individuals. Int J Cancer 1986;37:689–91.

47. Ginsburg M. Antibodies against the large subunit of the EBV-encoded ribonucleotide reductase in patients with nasopharyngeal carcinoma. Int J Cancer 1990;45: 1048–53.

48. Baylis SA, Purifoy DJ, Littler E. High-level expression of the Epstein-Barr virus alkaline deoxyribonuclease using a recombinant baculovirus: application to the diagnosis of nasopharyngeal carcinoma. Virology 1991;181:390–4.

49. Cheng HM, Foong YT, Mathew A, et al. Screening for nasopharyngeal carcinoma with an ELISA using the Epstein-Barr virus nuclear antigen, EBNA 1: a complementary test to the IgA/VCA immunofluorescence assay. J Virol Methods 1993;42:45–51.

50. Liu MY, Chang YL, Ma J, et al. Evaluation of multiple antibodies to Epstein-Barr virus as markers for detecting patients with nasopharyngeal carcinoma. J Med Virol 1997;52:262–9.

51. Chow KC, Ma J, Lin LS, et al. Serum responses to the combination of Epstein-Barr virus antigens from both latent and acute phases in nasopharyngeal carcinoma: complementary test of EBNA-1 with EA-D. Cancer Epidemiol Biomarkers Prev 1997;6:363–8.

52. Liu MY, Shih YY, Chou SP, et al. Antibody against the Epstein-Barr virus BHRF1 protein, a homologue of Bcl-2, in patients with nasopharyngeal carcinoma. J Med Virol 1998;56:179–85.

53. Chen MR, Liu MY, Hsu SM, et al. Use of bacterially expressed EBNA-1 protein cloned from a nasopharyngeal carcinoma (NPC) biopsy as a screening test for NPC patients. J Med Virol 2001;64:51–7.

54. Hsu MM, Hsu WC, Sheen TS, Kao CL. Specific IgA antibodies to recombinant early and nuclear antigens of Epstein-Barr virus in nasopharyngeal carcinoma. Clin Otolaryngol 2001;26:334–8.

55. Cheng WM, Chan KH, Chen HL, et al. Assessing the risk of nasopharyngeal carcinoma on the basis of EBV antibody spectrum. Int J Cancer 2002;97:489–92.

56. Chan KH, Gu YL, Ng F, et al. EBV specific antibody-based and DNA-based assays in serologic diagnosis of nasopharyngeal carcinoma. Int J Cancer 2003;105:706–9.

57. Dardari R, Hinderer W, Lang D, et al. Antibody responses to recombinant Epstein-Barr virus antigens in nasopharyngeal carcinoma patients: complementary test of ZEBRA protein and early antigens p54 and p138. J Clin Microbiol 2001;39:3164–70.

58. Union Internationale Contre le Cancer. Sobin L, Wittekind C, editors. TNM classification of malignant tumours. 5th ed. New York: Wiley-Liss; 1997.

59. American Joint Committee on Cancer. Fleming I, Cooper J, Henson D, et al, editors. Manual for staging of cancer. 5th ed. Philadelphia: Lippincott-Raven; 1997.

60. Al-Sarraf M, LeBlanc M, Giri PG, et al. Chemoradiotherapy versus radiotherapy in patients with advanced nasopharyngeal cancer: phase III randomized intergroup study 0099. J Clin Oncol 1998;16:1310–7.

61. Chong VF, Mukherji SK, Ng SH, et al. Nasopharyngeal carcinoma: review of how imaging affects staging. J Comput Assist Tomogr 1999;23:984–93.

62. Ng SH, Chang TC, Ko SF, et al. Nasopharyngeal carcinoma: MRI and CT assessment. Neuroradiology 1997;39:741–6.

63. Chong VFH, Fan YF, Khoo JBK. Nasopharyngeal carcinoma with intracranial spread: CT and MRI characteristics. J Comput Assist Tomogr 1996;20:563–69.

64. Emami B, Sethi A, Petruzzelli GJ. Influence of MRI on target volume delineation and IMRT planning in nasopharyngeal carcinoma. Int J Radiat Oncol Biol Phys 2003; 57:481–8.

65. Curtin HD, Ishwaran H, Mancuso AA, et al. Comparison of CT and MR imaging in staging neck metastases. Radiology 1998;207:123–30.

66. Kumar MB, Lu JJ, Loh KS, et al. Tailoring distant metastatic imaging for patients with clinically localized undifferentiated nasopharyngeal carcinoma. Int J Radiat Oncol Biol Phys 2004;58:688–93.

67. Leung S, Cheung H, Teo P, Lam WW. Staging computed tomography of the thorax for nasopharyngeal carcinoma. Head Neck 2000;22:369–72.

68. Lee AW, Au JS, Teo PM, et al. Staging of nasopharyngeal carcinoma: suggestions for improving the current UICC/ AJCC staging system. Clin Oncol (R Coll Radiol) 2004; 16:269–76.

69. Waldron J, Tin MM, Keller A, et al. Limitation of conventional two dimensional radiation therapy planning in nasopharyngeal carcinoma. Radiother Oncol 2003;68:153–61.

70. Lee N, Xia P, Quivey JM, et al. Intensity-modulated radiotherapy in the treatment of nasopharyngeal carcinoma: an update of the UCSF experience. Int J Radiat Oncol Biol Phys 2002;53:12–22.

71. Lee AW, Sham JS, Poon YF, Ho JH. Treatment of stage I nasopharyngeal carcinoma: analysis of the patterns of relapse and the results of withholding elective neck irradiation. Int J Radiat Oncol Biol Phys 1989;17:1183–90.

72. Fu KK, Pajak TF, Trotti A, et al. A Radiation Therapy Oncology Group (RTOG) phase III randomized study to compare hyperfractionation and two variants of accelerated fractionation to standard fractionation radiotherapy for head and neck squamous cell carcinomas: first report of RTOG 9003. Int J Radiat Oncol Biol Phys 2000;48:7–16.

73. Lee AW, Sze WM, Yau TK, et al. Retrospective analysis on treating nasopharyngeal carcinoma with accelerated fractionation (6 fractions per week) in comparison with conventional fractionation (5 fractions per week): report on 3-year tumor control and normal tissue toxicity. Radiother Oncol 2001;58:121–30.

74. Wang CC. Accelerated hyperfractionation radiation therapy for carcinoma of the nasopharynx. Techniques and results. Cancer 1989;63:2461–7.

75. Jen YM, Lin YS, Su WF, et al. Dose escalation using twice-daily radiotherapy for nasopharyngeal carcinoma: does heavier dosing result in a happier ending? Int J Radiat Oncol Biol Phys 2002;54:14–22.

76. Teo PM, Leung SF, Chan AT, et al. Final report of a randomized trial on altered-fractionated radiotherapy in nasopharyngeal carcinoma prematurely terminated by significant increase in neurologic complications. Int J Radiat Oncol Biol Phys 2000;48:1311–22.

77. Sanguineti G, Geara FB, Garden AS, et al. Carcinoma of the nasopharynx treated by radiotherapy alone: determinants of local and regional control. Int J Radiat Oncol Biol Phys 1997;37:985–96.

78. Lee AW, Poon YF, Foo W, et al. Retrospective analysis of 5037 patients with nasopharyngeal carcinoma treated during 1976-1985: overall survival and patterns of failure. Int J Radiat Oncol Biol Phys 1992;23:261–70.

79. Kutcher GJ, Fuks Z, Brenner H, et al. Three-dimensional photon treatment planning for carcinoma of the nasopharynx. Int J Radiat Oncol Biol Phys 1991;21:169–82.

80. Leibel SA, Fuks Z, Zelefsky MJ et al. Intensity-modulated radiotherapy. Cancer J 2002;8:164–76.

81. Yan JH, Xu GZ, Hu YH, et al. Management of local residual primary lesion of nasopharyngeal carcinoma. II. Results of prospective randomized trial on booster dose. Int J Radiat Oncol Biol Phys 1990;18:295–8.

82. Wolden SL, Zelefsky MJ, Hunt MA, et al. Failure of a 3D conformal boost to improve radiotherapy for nasopharyngeal carcinoma. Int J Radiat Oncol Biol Phys 2001; 49:1229–34.

83. Tate DJ, Adler JR Jr, Chang SD, et al. Stereotactic radiosurgical boost following radiotherapy in primary nasopharyngeal carcinoma: impact on local control. Int J Radiat Oncol Biol Phys 1999;45:915–21.

84. Le QT, Tate D, Koong A, et al. Improved local control with stereotactic radiosurgical boost in patients with nasopharyngeal carcinoma. Int J Radiat Oncol Biol Phys 2003; 56:1046–54.

85. Butler EB, Teh BS, Grant WH III, et al. Smart (simultaneous modulated accelerated radiation therapy) boost: a new accelerated fractionation schedule for the treatment of head and neck cancer with intensity modulated radiotherapy. Int J Radiat Oncol Biol Phys 1999;45:21–32.

86. Teo PM, Leung SF, Lee WY, Zee B. Intracavitary brachytherapy significantly enhances local control of early T-stage nasopharyngeal carcinoma: the existence of a dose-tumor-control relationship above conventional tumoricidal dose. Int J Radiat Oncol Biol Phys 2000;46:445–58.

87. Levendag PC, Schmitz PI, Jansen PP, et al. Fractionated high-dose-rate brachytherapy in primary carcinoma of the nasopharynx. J Clin Oncol 1998;16:2213–20.

88. Wang CC. Improved local control of nasopharyngeal carcinoma after intracavitary brachytherapy boost. Am J Clin Oncol 1991;14:5–8.

89. Lin JC, Jan JS, Hsu CY, et al. Phase III study of concurrent chemoradiotherapy versus radiotherapy alone for advanced nasopharyngeal carcinoma: positive effect on overall and progression-free survival. J Clin Oncol 2003;21:631–7.

90. Kwong DL, Sham JS, Au GK, et al. Concurrent and adjuvant chemotherapy for nasopharyngeal carcinoma: a factorial study. J Clin Oncol 2004;22:2643–53.

91. Chan ATC, Teo PML, Ngan RK, et al: Concurrent chemotherapy-radiotherapy compared with radiotherapy alone in locoregionally advanced nasopharyngeal carcinoma: progression-free survival analysis of a phase III randomized trial. J Clin Oncol 2002;20:2038–44.

92. Rossi A, Molinari R, Boracchi P, et al. Adjuvant chemotherapy with vincristine, cyclophosphamide, and doxorubicin after radiotherapy in local-regional nasopharyngeal cancer: results of a 4-year multicenter randomized study. J Clin Oncol 1988;6:1401–10.

93. Chi KH, Chang YC, Guo WY, et al. A phase III study of adjuvant chemotherapy in advanced nasopharyngeal carcinoma patients. Int J Radiat Oncol Biol Phys 2002;52:1238–44.

94. Chan AT, Teo PM, Leung TW, et al. A prospective randomized study of chemotherapy adjunctive to definitive radiotherapy in advanced nasopharyngeal carcinoma. Int J Radiat Oncol Biol Phys 1995;33:569–77.

95. Preliminary results of a randomized trial comparing neoadjuvant chemotherapy (cisplatin, epirubicin, bleomycin) plus radiotherapy vs. radiotherapy alone in stage IV(> or = N2, M0) undifferentiated nasopharyngeal carcinoma: a positive effect on progression-free survival. International Nasopharynx Cancer Study Group. VUMCA I trial. Int J Radiat Oncol Biol Phys 1996;35:463–9.

96. Ma J, Mai HQ, Hong MH, et al. Results of a prospective randomized trial comparing neoadjuvant chemotherapy plus radiotherapy with radiotherapy alone in patients with locoregionally advanced nasopharyngeal carcinoma. J Clin Oncol 2001;19:1350–7.

97. Chua DT, Sham JS, Choy D, et al. Preliminary report of the Asian-Oceanian Clinical Oncology Association randomized trial comparing cisplatin and epirubicin followed by radiotherapy versus radiotherapy alone in the treatment of patients with locoregionally advanced nasopharyngeal carcinoma. Asian-Oceanian Clinical Oncology Association Nasopharynx Cancer Study Group. Cancer 1998;83: 2270–83.

98. Su CK, Wang CC. Prognostic value of Chinese race in nasopharyngeal cancer. Int J Radiat Oncol Biol Phys 2002;54:752–8.

99. Shi W, Pataki I, MacMillan C, et al. Molecular pathology parameters in human nasopharyngeal carcinoma. Cancer 2002;94:1997–2006.

100. Hoppe RT, Williams J, Warnke R, et al. Carcinoma of the nasopharynx— the significance of histology. Int J Radiat Oncol Biol Phys 1978;4:199–205.

101. Chow E, Payne D, O'Sullivan B, et al. Radiotherapy alone in patients with advanced nasopharyngeal cancer: comparison with an intergroup study. Is combined modality treatment really necessary? Radiother Oncol 2002;63:269–74.

102. Chua DT, Sham JS, Au GK, Choy D. Concomitant chemoirradiation for stage III-IV nasopharyngeal carcinoma in Chinese patients: results of a matched cohort analysis. Int J Radiat Oncol Biol Phys 2002;53:334–43.

103. Kwong DL, Nicholls J, Wei WI, et al. Correlation of endoscopic and histologic findings before and after treatment for nasopharyngeal carcinoma. Head Neck 2001;23:34–41.

104. Kwong DL, Nicholls J, Wei WI, et al. The time course of histologic remission after treatment of patients with nasopharyngeal carcinoma. Cancer 1999;85:1446–53.

105. Ng SH, Liu HM, Ko SF, et al. Posttreatment imaging of the nasopharynx. Eur J Radiol 2002;44:82–95.

106. Ahuja A, Ying M, Leung SF, Metreweli C. The sonographic appearance and significance of cervical metastatic nodes following radiotherapy for nasopharyngeal carcinoma. Clin Radiol 1996;51:698–701.

107. Yen RF, Hung RL, Pan MH, et al. 18-Fluoro-2-deoxyglucose positron emission tomography in detecting residual/recurrent nasopharyngeal carcinomas and comparison with magnetic resonance imaging. Cancer 2003;98:283–7.

108. Kao CH, Shian YC, Shen YY, Yen RF. Detection of recurrent or persistent nasopharyngeal carcinomas after radiotherapy with technetium-99m methoxyisobutylisonitrile single photon emission computed tomography and computed tomography: comparison with 18-fluoro-2-deoxyglucose. Cancer 2002;94:1981–6.

109. Chan AT, Lo YM, Zee B, et al. Plasma Epstein-Barr virus DNA and residual disease after radiotherapy for undifferentiated nasopharyngeal carcinoma. J Natl Cancer Inst 2002;94:1614–9.

110. Lin JC, Wang WY, Chen KY, et al. Quantification of plasma Epstein-Barr virus DNA in patients with advanced nasopharyngeal carcinoma. N Engl J Med 2004;350:2461–70.

111. Lee AW, Law SC, Ng SH, et al. Retrospective analysis of nasopharyngeal carcinoma treated during 1976-1985: late complications following megavoltage irradiation. Br J Radiol 1992;65:918–28.

112. Peters LJ, Harrison ML, Dimery IW, et al. Acute and late toxicity associated with sequential bleomycin-containing chemotherapy regimens and radiation therapy in the treatment of carcinoma of the nasopharynx. Int J Radiat Oncol Biol Phys 1988;14:623–33.

113. Lee AW, Foo W, Law SC, et al. Reirradiation for recurrent nasopharyngeal carcinoma: factors affecting the therapeutic ratio and ways for improvement. Int J Radiat Oncol Biol Phys 1997;38:43–52.

114. Teo PM, Kwan WH, Chan AT, et al. How successful is high-dose (> or = 60 Gy) reirradiation using mainly external beams in salvaging local failures of nasopharyngeal carcinoma? Int J Radiat Oncol Biol Phys 1998;40:897–913.

115. Schuchter LM, Hensley ML, Meropol NJ, Winer EP. 2002 update of recommendations for the use of chemotherapy and radiotherapy protectants: clinical practice guidelines of the American Society of Clinical Oncology. J Clin Oncol 2002;20:2895–903.

116. Johnson JT, Ferretti GA, Nethery WJ, et al. Oral pilocarpine for post-irradiation xerostomia in patients with head and neck cancer. N Engl J Med 1993;329:390–5.

117. Horiot JC, Lipinski F, Schraub S, et al. Post-radiation severe xerostomia relieved by pilocarpine: a prospective French cooperative study. Radiother Oncol 2000;55:233–9.

118. Warde P, O'Sullivan B, Aslanidis J, et al. A phase III placebo-controlled trial of oral pilocarpine in patients undergoing radiotherapy for head-and-neck cancer. Int J Radiat Oncol Biol Phys 2002;54:9–13.

119. Ho WK, Wei WI, Kwong DL, et al. Long-term sensorineural hearing deficit following radiotherapy in patients suffering from nasopharyngeal carcinoma: a prospective study. Head Neck 1999;21:547–53.

120. Wang LF, Kuo WR, Ho KY, et al. A long-term study on hearing status in patients with nasopharyngeal carcinoma after radiotherapy. Otol Neurotol 2004;25:168–73.

121. Kwong DL, Wei WI, Sham JS, et al. Sensorineural hearing loss in patients treated for nasopharyngeal carcinoma: a prospective study of the effect of radiation and cisplatin treatment. Int J Radiat Oncol Biol Phys 1996;36:281–9.

122. Ho WK, Wei WI, Kwong DL, et al. Randomized evaluation of the audiologic outcome of ventilation tube insertion for middle ear effusion in patients with nasopharyngeal carcinoma. J Otolaryngol 2002;31:287–93.

123. Delanian S, Porcher R, Balla-Mekias S, Lefaix JL. Randomized, placebo-controlled trial of combined pentoxifylline and tocopherol for regression of superficial radiation-induced fibrosis. J Clin Oncol 2003;21:2545–50.

124. Chua DT, Lo C, Yuen J, Foo YC. A pilot study of pentoxifylline in the treatment of radiation-induced trismus. Am J Clin Oncol 2001;24:366–9.

125. Lee AW, Kwong DL, Leung SF, et al. Factors affecting risk of symptomatic temporal lobe necrosis: significance of fractional dose and treatment time. Int J Radiat Oncol Biol Phys 2002;53:75–85.

126. Chan YL, Leung SF, King AD, et al. Late radiation injury to the temporal lobes: morphologic evaluation at MR imaging. Radiology 1999;213:800–7.

127. Lee AW, Ng SH, Ho JH, et al. Clinical diagnosis of late temporal lobe necrosis following radiation therapy for nasopharyngeal carcinoma. Cancer 1988;61:1535–42.

128. Hu JQ, Guan YH, Zhao LZ, et al. Delayed radiation encephalopathy after radiotherapy for nasopharyngeal cancer: a CT study of 45 cases. J Comput Assist Tomogr 1991;15:181–7.

129. Lee AW, Ng SH, Tse VK, et al. Bilateral temporal lobectomy for necrosis induced by radiotherapy for nasopharyngeal carcinoma. Acta Oncol 1993;32:343–4.

130. Cheng KM, Chan CM, Fu YT, et al. Acute hemorrhage in late radiation necrosis of the temporal lobe: report of five cases and review of the literature. J Neurooncol 2001;51:143–50.

131. Chan AS, Cheung MC, Law SC, Chan JH. Phase II study of alpha-tocopherol in improving the cognitive function of patients with temporal lobe radionecrosis. Cancer 2004; 100:398–404.

132. Lam KS, Ho JH, Lee AW, et al. Symptomatic hypothalamic-pituitary dysfunction in nasopharyngeal carcinoma patients following radiation therapy: a retrospective study. Int J Radiat Oncol Biol Phys 1987;13:1343–50.

133. Samaan NA, Vieto R, Schultz PN, et al. Hypothalamic, pituitary and thyroid dysfunction after radiotherapy to the head and neck. Int J Radiat Oncol Biol Phys 1982;8:1857–67.

134. Sham J, Choy D, Kwong PW, et al. Radiotherapy for nasopharyngeal carcinoma: shielding the pituitary may improve therapeutic ratio. Int J Radiat Oncol Biol Phys 1994;29:699–704.

135. Wei WI, Ho CM, Yuen PW, et al. Maxillary swing approach for resection of tumors in and around the nasopharynx. Arch Otolaryngol Head Neck Surg 1995;121:638–42.

136. Morton RP, Liavaag PG, McLean M, Freeman JL. Transcervico-mandibulo-palatal approach for surgical salvage of recurrent nasopharyngeal cancer. Head Neck 1996;18: 352–8.

137. To EW, Teo PM, Ku PK, Pang PC. Nasopharyngectomy for recurrent nasopharyngeal carcinoma: an innovative transnasal approach through a mid-face deglove incision with stereotactic navigation guidance. Br J Oral Maxillofac Surg 2001;39:55–62.

138. Fee WE Jr, Moir MS, Choi EC, Goffinet D. Nasopharyngectomy for recurrent nasopharyngeal cancer: a 2- to 17-year follow-up. Arch Otolaryngol Head Neck Surg 2002;128: 280–4.

139. Law SC, Lam WK, Ng MF, et al. Reirradiation of nasopharyngeal carcinoma with intracavitary mold brachytherapy: an effective means of local salvage. Int J Radiat Oncol Biol Phys 2002;54:1095–113.

140. Kwong DL, Wei WI, Cheng AC, et al. Long term results of radioactive gold grain implantation for the treatment of persistent and recurrent nasopharyngeal carcinoma. Cancer 2001;91:1105–13.

141. Chua DT, Sham JS, Kwong PW, et al. Linear accelerator-based stereotactic radiosurgery for limited, locally persistent, and recurrent nasopharyngeal carcinoma: efficacy and complications. Int J Radiat Oncol Biol Phys 2003;56:177–83.

142. Lu TX, Mai WY, Teh BS, et al. Initial experience using intensity-modulated radiotherapy for recurrent nasopharyngeal carcinoma. Int J Radiat Oncol Biol Phys 2004;58:682–7.

143. Hsu MM, Hong RL, Ting LL, et al. Factors affecting the overall survival after salvage surgery in patients with recurrent nasopharyngeal carcinoma at the primary site: experience with 60 cases. Arch Otolaryngol Head Neck Surg 2001;127:798–802.

144. Wei WI, Ho WK, Cheng AC, et al. Management of extensive cervical nodal metastasis in nasopharyngeal carcinoma after radiotherapy: a clinicopathological study. Arch Otolaryngol Head Neck Surg 2001;127:1457–62.

145. King WW, Teo PM, Li AK. Patterns of failure after radical neck dissection for recurrent nasopharyngeal carcinoma. Am J Surg 1992;164:599–602.

146. Chua DT, Wei WI, Sham JS, et al. Treatment outcome for synchronous locoregional failures of nasopharyngeal carcinoma. Head Neck 2003;25:585–94.

147. Teo PM, Kwan WH, Lee WY, et al. Prognosticators determining survival subsequent to distant metastasis from nasopharyngeal carcinoma. Cancer 1996;77:2423–31.

148. Ong YK, Heng DM, Chung B, et al. Design of a prognostic index score for metastatic nasopharyngeal carcinoma. Eur J Cancer 2003;39:1535–41.

149. Fandi A, Bachouchi M, Azli N, et al. Long-term disease-free survivors in metastatic undifferentiated carcinoma of nasopharyngeal type. J Clin Oncol 2000;18:1324–30.

150. Choo R, Tannock I. Chemotherapy for recurrent or metastatic carcinoma of the nasopharynx. A review of the Princess Margaret Hospital experience. Cancer 1991;68:2120–4.

151. Decker DA, Drelichman A, Al-Sarraf M, et al. Chemotherapy for nasopharyngeal carcinoma. A ten-year experience. Cancer 1983;52:602–5.

152. Boussen H, Cvitkovic E, Wendling JL, et al. Chemotherapy of metastatic and/or recurrent undifferentiated nasopharyngeal carcinoma with cisplatin, bleomycin, and fluorouracil. J Clin Oncol;9:1675–81.

153. Su WC, Chen TY, Kao RH, Tsao CJ. Chemotherapy with cisplatin and continuous infusion of 5-fluorouracil and bleomycin for recurrent and metastatic nasopharyngeal carcinoma in Taiwan. Oncology 1993;50:205–8.

154. Chi KH, Chan WK, Cooper DL, et al. A phase II study of outpatient chemotherapy with cisplatin, 5-fluorouracil, and leucovorin in nasopharyngeal carcinoma. Cancer 1994;73:247–52.

155. Yeo W, Leung TW, Leung SF, et al. Phase II study of the combination of carboplatin and 5-fluorouracil in metastatic nasopharyngeal carcinoma. Cancer Chemother Pharmacol 1996;38:466–70.

156. Chua DT, Kwong DL, Sham JS, et al. A phase II study of ifos-

famide, 5-fluorouracil and leucovorin in patients with recurrent nasopharyngeal carcinoma previously treated with platinum chemotherapy. Eur J Cancer 2000;36:736–41.

157. Au E, Tan EH, Ang PT. Activity of paclitaxel by three-hour infusion in Asian patients with metastatic undifferentiated nasopharyngeal cancer. Ann Oncol 1998;9:327–9.

158. Yeo W, Leung TW, Chan AT, et al. A phase II study of combination paclitaxel and carboplatin in advanced nasopharyngeal carcinoma. Eur J Cancer 1998;34:2027–31.

159. Tan EH, Khoo KS, Wee J, et al. Phase II trial of a paclitaxel and carboplatin combination in Asian patients with metastatic nasopharyngeal carcinoma. Ann Oncol 1999; 10:235–7.

160. McCarthy JS, Tannock IF, Degendorfer P, et al. A phase II trial of docetaxel and cisplatin in patients with recurrent or metastatic nasopharyngeal carcinoma. Oral Oncol 2002;38:686–90.

161. Foo KF, Tan EH, Leong SS, et al. Gemcitabine in metastatic nasopharyngeal carcinoma of the undifferentiated type. Ann Oncol 2002;13:150–6.

162. Ngan RK, Yiu HH, Lau WH, et al. Combination gemcitabine and cisplatin chemotherapy for metastatic or recurrent nasopharyngeal carcinoma: report of a phase II study. Ann Oncol 2002;13:1252–8.

163. Ma BB, Tannock IF, Pond GR, et al. Chemotherapy with gemcitabine-containing regimens for locally recurrent or metastatic nasopharyngeal carcinoma. Cancer 2002;95: 2516–23.

164. Chua DT, Sham JS, Au GK. A phase II study of capecitabine in patients with recurrent and metastatic nasopharyngeal carcinoma pretreated with platinum-based chemotherapy. Oral Oncol 2003;39:361–6.

165. Azli N, Fandi A, Bachouchi M, et al. Final report of a phase II study of chemotherapy with bleomycin, epirubicin, and cisplatin for locally advanced and metastatic/recurrent undifferentiated carcinoma of the nasopharyngeal type Cancer J Sci Am 1995;1:222–9.

166. Siu LL, Czaykowski PM, Tannock IF. Phase I/II study of the CAPABLE regimen for patients with poorly differentiated carcinoma of the nasopharynx. J Clin Oncol 1998;16: 2514–21.

167. Chua DT, Nicholls JM, Sham JS, Au GK. Prognostic value of epidermal growth factor receptor expression in patients with advanced stage nasopharyngeal carcinoma treated with induction chemotherapy and radiotherapy. Int J Radiat Oncol Biol Phys 2004;59:11–20.

168. Herbst RS, Hong WK. IMC-C225, an anti-epidermal growth factor receptor monoclonal antibody for treatment of head and neck cancer. Semin Oncol 2002;29(5 Suppl 14): 18–30.

169. Lee SP, Chan AT, Cheung ST, et al. CTL control of EBV in nasopharyngeal carcinoma (NPC): EBV-specific CTL responses in the blood and tumors of NPC patients and the antigen-processing function of the tumor cells. J Immunol 2000;165:573–82.

170. Chan AT, Tao Q, Robertson KD, et al. Azacitidine induces demethylation of the Epstein-Barr virus genome in tumors. J Clin Oncol 2004;22:1373–81.

171. Shi W, Pataki I, MacMillan C, et al. Molecular pathology parameters in human nasopharyngeal carcinoma. Cancer 2002;94:1997–2006.

172. Ma BB, Poon TC, To KF, et al. Prognostic significance of tumor angiogenesis, Ki 67, p53 oncoprotein, epidermal growth factor receptor and HER2 receptor protein expression in undifferentiated nasopharyngeal carcinoma—a prospective study. Head Neck 2003;25:864–72.

173. Liu FF. Novel gene therapy approach for nasopharyngeal carcinoma. Semin Cancer Biol 2002;12:505–15.

10

Management of Primary Central Nervous System Lymphoma and Primary Intraocular Lymphoma

JAMES L. RUBENSTEIN
MITCHEL S. BERGER

Neurologic complications of non-Hodgkin's lymphoma (NHL) are associated with an adverse prognosis.[1] Central nervous system (CNS) involvement by lymphomas occurs by two distinct pathways: dissemination of systemic lymphoma, or development within the brain as a primary tumor. When, at diagnosis, NHL is confined to the cranial-spinal axis, the condition is known as primary central nervous system lymphoma (PCNSL).

PCNSL is a relatively rare type of NHL, representing only 1 to 2% of all NHLs and < 5% of all primary brain tumors. The estimated incidence of PCNSL is approximately 1 in 100,000 persons per year in the United States of America. The incidence of this disease is increasing: almost threefold over the last three decades, in parallel with a rise in the number of cases of systemic NHL. Moreover, this rise cannot be completely explained by the human immunodeficiency virus (HIV) epidemic and does not appear to be a consequence of technologic advances that facilitate more precise diagnosis.[2,3]

PRESENTATION AND DIAGNOSTIC WORK-UP IN PCNSL

The mean age of diagnosis of PCNSL is 55 years for immunocompetent patients and 30 years for patients with acquired immune deficiency syndrome (AIDS). There is a slight male predominance in incidence.

Risk factors for the development of PCNSL are similar to those associated with other types of NHL. Profound immunodeficiency associated with AIDS, the Wiskott-Aldrich syndrome, immunoglobulin-A deficiency syndrome, and severe combined immunodeficiency or even subtle immunodeficiency states such as those associated with rheumatoid arthritis and systemic lupus erythematosus, clearly predispose individuals to the development of PCNSL. In patients with AIDS, PCNSL tends to be a manifestation of advanced disease and is associated with a CD4 count of < 50 cells/mm^3.[4,5]

The clinical presentation of PCNSL may occur by disruption of virtually any aspect of normal CNS function. At least 50% of patients present with focal neurologic deficits such as hemiparesis or aphasia, 35% exhibit alteration in cognition or personality, 11% present with seizure, and 32% present with headache, nausea, vomiting, and papilledema as a manifestation of increased intracranial pressure. Approximately 10 to 20% of patients present with ocular lymphoma manifest by the presence of floaters, or blurry or cloudy vision. Less than 10% of patients exhibit spinal dissemination marked by cauda equina syndrome, back pain, or radiculopathy.

Magnetic resonance imaging (MRI) is the standard imaging modality for initial detection and evaluation of PCNSL. Usually, PCNSL images are hypointense to isointense on T1-weighted images with intense homogeneous contrast enhancement. The majority of these lesions exhibit periventricular localization (Figure 10–1). Peritumoral edema is often less than that of contrast-enhancing high-grade gliomas or brain metastases. In AIDS-related PCNSL, lesions are often ring enhancing on T1-weighted images and may be associated with hemorrhage or necrosis. PCNSL lesions are unifocal in approximately 60% of cases and multifocal in 40% of cases, by MRI. More than 90% of AIDS patients have multifocal PCNSL on radiographic imaging.[5,6] The majority of PCNSL cases at necropsy exhibit multifocal involvement.[7] This biologic invasiveness is a significant factor in terms of therapeutic management, as this tumor usually proves to be refractory to attempts at surgical resection or focal radiotherapy.

When NHL presents with only neurologic signs and symptoms and a pathologic diagnosis of NHL is established by detection of tumor within the CNS, then there is an approximate 90% chance that the diagnosis is PCNSL. A thorough staging work-up is indicated to definitively rule out systemic disease as well as to define the extent of CNS involvement. This process requires evaluation of distinct compartments within the CNS axis. An ophthalmologic evaluation including slit-lamp examination is mandated to evaluate concomitant vitreous disease, and an MRI with contrast is needed to evaluate the brain and spine. Lumbar puncture is appropriate in all patients, unless contraindicated because of increased intracranial pressure. In addition, staging bone marrow biopsy as well as computed tomography scans of the chest, abdomen, and pelvis are indicated. Because approximately 30% of testicular lymphomas metastasize to the brain, a testicular examination is recommended to rule out subclinical testicular lymphoma as a primary tumor. In addition, an HIV antibody test is appropriate both for prognostic reasons and to help determine therapy. As with systemic NHL, a serum lactate dehydrogenase (LDH) measurement is appropriate to define prognosis. Ultimately, only 10% of patients who present with a tentative diagnosis of

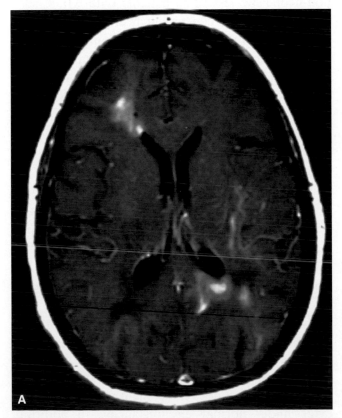 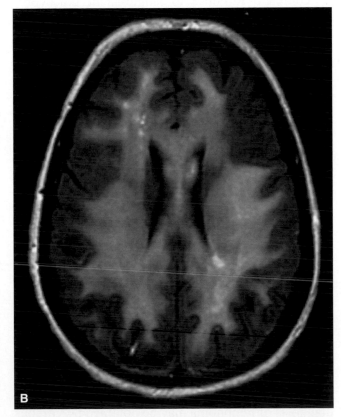

Figure 10–1. Magnetic resonance (MR) imaging of primary central nervous system lymphoma. *A,* The transverse contrast-enhanced T1-weighted MR image shows multiple foci of periventricular enhancement. *B,* The transverse T2-weighted transverse image shows extensive T2 abnormality, far greater than T1 enhancement.

PCNSL will be found to have occult systemic NHL on rigorous systemic staging evaluation.[3,8]

Establishing the diagnosis of PCNSL may be a significant challenge in the patient who presents with neurologic complaints and suspicious findings on radiographic imaging. The differential diagnosis is often relatively broad and includes glioma, metastatic malignancy, vasculitis, sarcoid, infection, or multiple sclerosis. There is often significant diagnostic latency in the presentation of PCNSL; in particular, in immunocompetent patients in whom the disease may present with a smoldering course. A critical problem in the initial diagnostic work-up of patients with PCNSL is the common practice of administering glucocorticoids as an early intervention to attenuate or reverse progressive neurologic decline in the patient at first presentation, before diagnosis. Because glucocorticoids usually induce tumor regression, probably by apoptosis in PCNSL, administration of steroids such as dexamethasone before diagnosis increases the risk for a nondiagnostic specimen at the time of initial work-up. The rate of complete response to single-agent glucocorticoids may be as high as 20%.[9] The ideal approach, therefore, is to withhold corticosteroids prior to biopsy, unless there is active clinical decompensation mandating this intervention before diagnosis.

Stereotactic biopsy is the preferred method for obtaining a tissue diagnosis in patients suspected of having PCNSL. There is an up to 4% risk of significant intracranial hemorrhage associated with stereotactic biopsy.[10] In addition, stereotactic biopsy is associated with an 8 to 9% rate of failure, defined as a biopsy in which a definitive histologic diagnosis is not achieved based on the tissue obtained.[11] Unlike malignant gliomas, aggressive surgical resection in PCNSL has no proven therapeutic value, unless immediate surgical decompression is required because of impending herniation or critical neurologic deterioration. Failed stereotactic biopsies are frequently associated with antecedent use of glucocorticoids or failure to use intraoperative pathologic examination.[12]

In subsets of patients who present with signs and symptoms of intraocular lymphoma, pathologic diagnosis of lymphoma may be obtained by vitreous biopsy after detection of a suspicious vitreous infiltrate by slit-lamp examination, fluorescein angiography, or ocular ultrasonography. Another means of establishing tissue diagnosis is by evaluation of the cerebrospinal fluid (CSF): 10 to 20% of patients with PCNSL present with overt leptomeningeal lymphoma. In these patients, diagnostic information may be achieved from lumbar puncture with cytologic analysis and/or flow cytometric analysis to identify kappa or lambda light-chain restriction in lymphoma cells. Pathologic diagnosis of an intraocular, leptomeningeal, or brain parenchymal lymphoma is essentially equivalent to establish the diagnosis of PCNSL.

Recent evidence suggests that diagnostic brain biopsy may be obviated in the setting of suspected AIDS-associated PCNSL. The association between Epstein-Barr virus (EBV) infection and AIDS-related PCNSL is well established, and the detection of EBV DNA in CSF by polymerase chain reaction has been shown to be a useful biomarker, with specificity in excess of 95%. Because single-photon emission computed tomography (SPECT) is also able to differentiate between cerebral lymphoma and non-neoplastic lesions in patients with AIDS, such as toxoplasmosis, concordant positive SPECT and EBV DNA polymerase chain reaction results obviate the need for brain biopsy and facilitate immediate clinical intervention in the treatment of AIDS-associated PCNSL.[13] Positron emission tomography has also been shown to facilitate the distinction between CNS lymphoma and cerebral toxoplasmosis in AIDS patients with contrast-enhancing lesions.[14] Unfortunately, there is at present no CSF marker to facilitate the noninvasive diagnosis of PCNSL arising in immunocompetent patients, and definitive diagnosis is usually dependent upon histopathologic analysis.

PATHOLOGY AND PROGNOSIS IN PCNSL

At least 95% of PCNSL are B-cell neoplasms that express the B-cell marker CD20 (Figure 10–2). A central puzzle in the pathogenesis of this disorder is why a lymphoma should present in the CNS, an organ system that does not contain resident lymphocytes under normal circumstances. In addition, although the lymphoma spreads aggressively within the CNS, these tumors rarely metastasize elsewhere

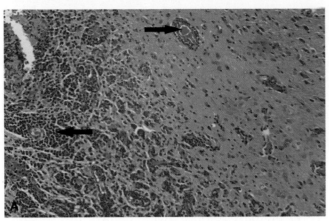
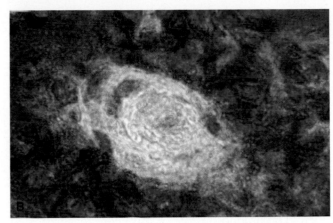

Figure 10–2. *A,* Example of angiotropic growth pattern of primary central nervous system large B-cell lymphoma (hematoxylin-eosin; original magnification ×400). *B,* At higher magnification, immunohistochemical localization of the B-cell marker CD20 (reddish brown color) to lymphoma cells but not endothelial cells (hematoxylin counterstain; original magnification ×1000).

in the body. At least two hypotheses may explain this biology: (1) the lymphoma develops as a consequence of malignant transformation of an inflammatory process that has developed in situ within the CNS; and (2) malignant B lymphocytes acquire selective adhesion receptors for ligands expressed by the brain; in particular, the cerebral vascular endothelium. In support of the latter is the observation that lymphoma cells in PCNSL exhibit angiotropism (see Figure 10–2). To date, no unique adhesion receptors have been identified that distinguish CNS lymphomas from systemic lymphoma. A recent study established the expression in PCNSL tumors of a lymphoid chemokine, CXCL13, which is involved in B-cell compartmental homing within secondary lymphoid organs, suggesting that this chemokine may influence CNS localization.[15] This chemokine was shown to be synthesized by tumor cells in PCNSLs, but not by tumor-associated blood vessels.[15]

The vast majority of PCNSLs in immunocompetent individuals are large B-cell neoplasms that express the transcription factor *BCL6* as well as the oncogene *BCL2*.[16] Molecular genetic studies have revealed that the *P14 ARF* gene and *p16INK4a* gene are frequently inactivated by either homozygous deletion or by hypermethylation in approximately 56% of cases of PCNSL.[17] In addition to *BCL6* expression, there is genetic evidence that primary CNS lymphomas originate from germinal centers, based upon shared genetic properties including a high frequency of mutations in the immunoglobulin variable gene region.[18] The notion that primary CNS

lymphomas can be categorized as germinal center large B-cell lymphomas is in a sense paradoxical, given that the prognosis associated with PCNSL is significantly worse than that for most cases of systemic stage IE NHL. This is clearly at odds with data showing that germinal center large-cell lymphomas are associated with a favorable prognosis relative to the activated B-cell type.[19] Recent gene expression profile data in large-cell PCNSL tumors obtained from immunocompetent patients provide evidence for germinal center ontogeny, but also demonstrate that PCNSL represents a distinct molecular subclass of large B-cell lymphoma that is related to germinal center lymphoma.[20] In AIDS, the majority of PCNSL are EBV-driven neoplasms of either Burkitt's or large-cell histology.

There is increasing evidence for the existence of biologically distinct risk groups within histologically similar types of NHL, including PCNSL.[16,19,20] Recently, the International Extranodal Lymphoma Study Group conducted a multicenter evaluation of prognostic indicators in PCNSL, to derive a prognostic scoring system for immunocompetent patients.[21] The potential prognostic role of patient-, lymphoma-, and treatment-related variables were studied in a series of 378 patients with PCNSL seen at 23 cancer centers from five different countries. Age of more than 60 years, Eastern Cooperative Oncology Group (ECOG) performance status > 1, elevated serum LDH level, elevated CSF protein concentration, and involvement of deep regions of the brain (periventricular regions, basal ganglia, brainstem, and/or cerebellum) were significantly and independently associated with a worse survival. Each of these five factors, when considered as discrete variables added together, constitute the prognostic score, according to this system. Each variable was assigned a value of either 0, if favorable, or 1, if unfavorable. The cumulative prognostic score was then tested in 105 assessable PCNSL patients for whom complete data for all five variables were available (Figure 10–3). The 2-year overall survival was 80%, 48%, and 15% ($p = .00001$) for patients with 0 to 1, 2 to 3, and 4 to 5 unfavorable features, respectively. The prognostic role of this score was validated by analysis of PCNSL patients who were treated with high-dose methotrexate-based chemotherapy. The histologic type of NHL, presence of leptomeningeal disease, or ocular disease, had no impact on survival in PCNSL. The only treatment-related variable that has been shown to reproducibly impact survival is the use of high-dose systemic methotrexate-containing regimens.[22] Use of intrathecal chemotherapy, high-dose cytarabine, or anthracyclines did not impact survival in the multivariate analysis.

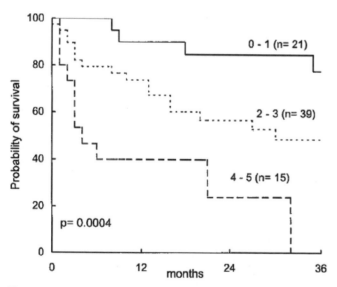

Figure 10–3. Survival according to the prognostic scoring system for primary central nervous system lymphoma, proposed by the International Extranodal Lymphoma Study Group. Age, performance status, cerebrospinal fluid protein, serum lactate dehydrogenase, and presence or absence of tumor in deep brain structures were each analyzed as discrete variables. Patients with 0 to 1 negative prognostic factor survived significantly longer than patients with 4 to 5 negative prognostic variables in a group of 75 patients in whom complete data for all five variables were available and who received high-dose methotrexate-based therapy with or without radiation. Adapted from Ferreri AJ et al.[21]

THERAPY OF PCNSL

Immunocompetent PCNSL

The optimal therapy for PCNSL has yet to be defined. A number of therapeutic principles have emerged in the time that clinical experience in this disease has begun to mature. When considering treatment options, clinicians must realize that PCNSL is an aggressive brain tumor; without treatment, most patients will die within 3 months.

In the past 5 to 10 years, clinical investigators have recognized that unlike the vast majority of malignant gliomas, long-term lymphoma-free survival is possible in PCNSL, with rates of 5-year overall survival approaching 30%.[23] On the other hand, it has also become clear that in virtually every clinical series, approximately 15 to 20% of patients exhibit refractory disease within the first 6 months of therapy and succumb to tumor progression.

Glucocorticoids

Glucocorticoids represent an important first-line intervention in the treatment of PCNSL, not only to diminish tumor-associated edema, but also because of their direct lymphocytotoxic effects. There is evidence that the oncolytic effect of glucocorticoids may be more marked in PCNSL than in systemic lymphomas, with single-agent response rates approaching 70% in PCNSL.[9] As mentioned above, a common problem is that initial complete responses yielded by glucocorticoids may increase the risk for nondiagnostic biopsies, resulting in significant delays in the diagnosis and initiation of definitive therapy.

Radiation Therapy

PCNSL is a radiation-sensitive disease: response rates to whole-brain irradiation exceed 90%, and rates of complete response are approximately 60%. Whole-brain radiation therapy has historically been a cornerstone in therapeutic management of this disease and has been associated with improved survival compared to no therapy; median survival with radiation alone is between 12 and 18 months.[24] Approaches using focal irradiation are not recommended because of the multifocal, highly infiltrative nature of this tumor. There are currently no data to support the use of a radiation boost to the tumor bed, as most patients exhibit tumor progression at sites of previous tumor involvement.[25] Total radiation dose may also be a significant factor, as indicated in a recent study by Bessell and colleagues that compared outcomes in patients who received identical chemotherapy programs followed by whole-brain irradiation at 4,500 cGy as opposed to 3,060 cGy.[26] Reduction in the radiation dose from 4,500 cGy to 3,060 cGy was associated with significantly increased risk of relapse and lower overall survival.[26] For this reason, the standard dose of whole-brain irradiation is still considered to be between 4,000 and 4,500 cGy. There is no evidence that craniospinal axis irradiation provides therapeutic advantage, unless there is evidence of spinal dissemination or meningeal drop metastases; spinal cord irradiation may even compromise later therapeutic options because of radiation-induced bone marrow suppression.[5]

Chemotherapy

Conventional therapy for systemic large B-cell lymphoma includes combination chemotherapy, usually with cyclophosphamide, doxorubicin, vincristine, and prednisone (CHOP). Multicenter studies of CHOP (or CHO plus dexamethasone) followed by cranial radiation demonstrated that these agents are ineffective for PCNSL and do not improve survival over whole-brain irradiation alone.[27,28] The biologic basis for this differential sensitivity may relate to the blood-brain barrier, because the majority of compounds in the CHOP regimen penetrate poorly into the CNS, due to tight junctions in the CNS vasculature. Molecular distinctions between PCNSL and systemic lymphomas may also contribute to the differential chemotherapeutic sensitivity.[20]

Methotrexate administered intravenously at 1 g/m^2 or more is able to penetrate an intact blood-brain barrier and achieve cytotoxic levels in the CSF.[29] Dramatic antilymphoma effects in the CNS were first demonstrated in case reports and anecdotal experience in CNS lymphomas in the 1970s.[30,31] Bokstein and colleagues found that the rate of complete response to high-dose intravenous methotrexate for metastatic NHL within the brain was twofold higher than the rate of response for systemic lymphoma in the same patients.[32] As mentioned above, the use of high-dose methotrexate has emerged in multivariate analyses as the most important treatment-related prognostic variable in PCNSL.[21]

Combined-Modality Therapy

The first successful combined-modality therapy for PCNSL was pioneered by the Memorial Sloan-Kettering group in the 1980s. The Memorial Sloan-Kettering approach was to use methotrexate, administered both by intrathecal injection through an Ommaya reservoir and intravenously at doses $\geq 1 \text{ g/m}^2$ body surface area, before the initiation of whole-brain irradiation. The pre-irradiation chemotherapy regimen also included procarbazine plus vincristine. Finally, high-dose intravenous cytarabine was administered at the completion of irradiation. The success of this combined-modality approach was realized in marked prolongation of survival, with a median overall survival of 42 months and a 5-year survival of 22.3 months, compared with the 3 to 5% rate of 5-year survival in historic controls treated with whole-brain irradiation alone.[23]

With the awareness that long-term survival can be expected in a significant fraction of PCNSL patients, there has been an accumulation of interest and data regarding the problem of late treatment-related neurotoxicity. In at least 80% of patients who are over 60 years of age at diagnosis, whole-brain irradiation has been associated with delayed neurotoxicity characterized by a syndrome of progressive dementia, gait ataxia, and urinary incontinence, presenting with an average latency of 13 months.[23] Because this syndrome of profound neurotoxicity was not detected in a subset of patients who received chemotherapy alone, there has been increased interest in developing more effective chemotherapy programs to minimize or eliminate the need for radiation treatment.

Late neurotoxicity was formally evaluated in a European Organization for Research and Treatment of Cancer (EORTC) study in PCNSL patients treated with combined-modality therapy involving high-dose methotrexate and whole-brain irradiation.[33] An extensive neuropsychologic assessment including quality-of-life measures was conducted in 19 patients; results were compared with age- and sex-matched control subjects with systemic hematologic malignancies, who received similar chemotherapy regimens and non-CNS radiotherapy. The mean age of patients in this study was 44 years. Cognitive impairment was found in 63% of patients with PCNSL compared with only 11% of control subjects. Only 42% of surviving PCNSL patients resumed work compared with 81% of control subjects. The results of this formal neurocognitive evaluation extended the conclusions of Abrey and colleagues, in that significant cognitive impairment was commonly detected in patients aged 60 years or less, who were treated with combined-modality therapy.[23,33]

The Memorial Sloan-Kettering regimen was recently studied in a multicenter evaluation involving the RTOG, in 102 immunocompetent patients with PCNSL. The rate of complete response to pre-irradiation chemotherapy (methotrexate, procarbazine, and vincristine) was 58%; the median overall survival was 36.9 months (Figure 10–4). There was a 15% rate of severe delayed neurologic toxicity that was detected in 12 patients, 8 of whom died, confirming the potential for severe neurotoxicity with combined-modality therapy.[23,34]

Intrathecal Methotrexate

The role of intrathecal methotrexate during the induction chemotherapy for PCNSL has yet to be determined. A recent study of high-dose intravenous methotrexate that evaluated matched CSF and serum pharmacokinetic data demonstrated that cytotoxic CSF and serum methotrexate concentrations were maintained much longer after intravenous administration compared with intrathecal dosing of methotrexate.[29] Outcomes in 16 patients, who received high-dose intravenous methotrexate at 8 g/m^2 over 4 hours for solid tumor neoplastic meningitis malignancies, were compared retrospectively with a reference group of patients treated only with intrathecal methotrexate. The median survival in the group treated with high-dose methotrexate was significantly longer than the group treated with intrathecal methotrexate, being 13.8 months versus 2.3 months ($p = .003$), respectively.[29] At present, there is no evidence to support the routine administration of intrathecal methotrexate in newly diagnosed PCNSL patients who receive intensive high-dose methotrexate therapy of at least 1 g/m^2 body surface area.[35]

High-Dose Methotrexate

In parallel with the development of combined-modality therapy for PCNSL, clinical investigators at Massachusetts General Hospital performed eval-

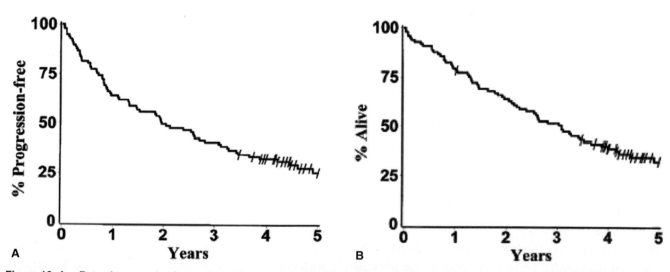

Figure 10–4.   Rate of progression-free and overall survival among 102 immunocompetent primary central nervous system lymphoma patients treated on Radiation Therapy Oncology Group protocol 93-10, the first multicenter trial for primary central nervous system lymphoma to demonstrate a marked survival benefit using combined modality therapy. Median overall survival was 36.9 months. Adapted from Khan RB et al.[35]

uations of intensive intravenous methotrexate monotherapy with deferral of radiotherapy until progression.[36] Methotrexate at 8 g/m² was given every 2 weeks until complete response, followed by four more cycles every 2 weeks, and then monthly methotrexate treatments through 1 year of therapy. The initial responses in 31 patients were extremely promising, with an overall rate of response of 100% and a complete response rate of 65%. The treatment was demonstrated to be well tolerated, with a minimal rate of myelosuppression and mucositis. Quality-of-life assessment in 11 long-term survivors was similar to normative groups and there was no evidence of methotrexate-induced encephalopathy.[36] This pilot experience led to a recent multicenter study of intensive high-dose methotrexate at 8 g/m² administered every 2 weeks, through the New Approaches to Brain Tumor Therapy (NABTT) Consortium.[37] The rate of complete response to high-dose methotrexate in the multicenter study was 52%; no delayed neurotoxicity was detected in this multicenter study. Median progression-free survival was 12.8 months (Figure 10–5).

Because there is evidence that the blood-brain barrier is a significant factor contributing to therapeutic failure in brain tumors, there has been considerable interest in developing methods to disrupt the tight junctions and specializations of CNS endothelia that restrict entry of macromolecules into the brain. One approach has been to use osmotic agents to disrupt the blood-brain barrier followed by intra-arterial or intravenous chemotherapy. In a review of 74 PCNSL patients treated with such an approach over a 15-year period, the rate of complete response was 65% and the estimated median survival was 40.7 months.[38] Although each disruption procedure requires general anesthesia and is associated with significant acute toxicities including stroke and seizure, comprehensive neuropsychologic testing performed in 36 patients who achieved a durable complete response (> 1 year) revealed no evidence of cognitive loss in those patients who did not receive whole-brain irradiation.[38]

Autologous Stem Cell Transplant

Because high-dose chemotherapy with autologous stem cell transplantation (ASCT) is an effective treatment approach for some patients with high-risk or relapsed systemic NHL, this strategy is being evaluated in PCNSL in an attempt to maximize the potential benefit of chemotherapy and to avoid the toxicity of whole-brain irradiation in patients with newly diagnosed PCNSL.[39] Abrey and colleagues were among the first to conduct a trial involving ASCT in this disease.[40] Their approach was an induction therapy with high-dose methotrexate and cytarabine followed by high-dose BEAM (carmustine, etoposide, cytarabine, and melphalan) and ASCT. Fourteen of the 28 patients enrolled exhibited sufficient response to the induction regimen to warrant ASCT. The median progression-free survival for transplanted

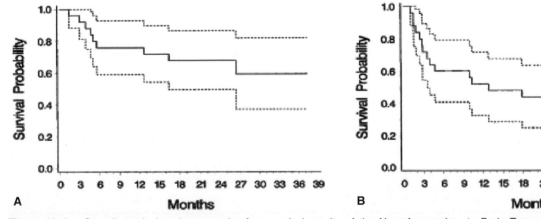

Figure 10–5. Overall survival and progression-free survival results of the New Approaches to Brain Tumor Therapy trial of high-dose methotrexate monotherapy in 25 patients with primary central nervous system lymphoma (PCNSL). This multicenter study demonstrated that high-dose methotrexate monotherapy at 8 g/m² induced durable remissions in a population of immunocompetent patients with PCNSL. Adapted from Batchelor T et al.[37]

patients was only 9.3 months; 8 of 14 patients who received ASCT developed progressive disease at a median of 2.3 months after transplantation.[40]

Although these results demonstrate that ASCT is feasible for patients with PCNSL, the unacceptable rate of early relapse in the study using the BEAM combination raises the question of what the optimal induction and transplantation regimen for this disease is. Soussain and colleagues used a conditioning regimen consisting of busulfan, thiotepa, and cyclophosphamide in 22 patients with recurrent ($n = 10$) or refractory ($n = 12$) PCNSL and/or ocular lymphoma.[41] Transplant was associated with a 53% probability of 3-year event-free survival and only a 20% rate of relapse in this heavily pretreated population. Patients over 60 years of age did poorly, with 71% resulting in a treatment-related mortality. The efficacy of the combination of high-dose cytarabine plus high-dose etoposide as salvage therapy before ASCT was an unexpected finding of this study. Combination high-dose cytarabine plus high-dose etoposide resulted in 12 responses (8 complete) among 14 treated patients.[41]

Several principles have thus emerged with respect to therapeutic options in PCNSL. One is that there is an accumulation of evidence demonstrating that long-term survival and cure is now possible in PCNSL. Although approximately 20% of patients exhibit early refractory disease in response to cytotoxic therapy, a significant fraction of patients (between 20 and 30%) may exhibit durable responses and long-term survival with simple high-dose methotrexate-based chemotherapy without whole-brain irradiation.[37] In addition, there is increasing evidence that augmentation of high-dose methotrexate with other chemotherapeutic and/or biologic agents may result in durable responses for a greater fraction of patients with acceptable toxicity (Table 10–1).[42–44]

Immunotherapy

The current goal in treating relapsed disease in many cases is not only to palliate symptoms but also perhaps to achieve remission. Management of relapsed or refractory disease is an area of active clinical study. A number of agents are under investigation, including the anti-CD20 monoclonal antibody rituximab. Rituximab is the first monoclonal antibody to receive Food and Drug Administration approval in the treatment of cancer. CD20 is a cell-surface protein that occurs almost exclusively on mature B cells and is not found in normal brain. Rituximab is a chimeric human immunoglobulin G1, in which the CD20-binding region was derived by genetic engineering from a mouse monoclonal antibody.

Although rituximab has activity as a single agent in the treatment of relapsed large-cell lymphoma,

Table 10–1.								
Lead Author	Ref. No.	N	Chemotherepeutic Regimen	% CR to Induction Chemotherapy	WB-XRT	Median PFS	Median OS	% TRM
Batchelor	38	25	HD-MTX	52	No	12.8 months	Not reacted	0
Sandor	46	14	HD-MTX, Thiotepa, Vinc	79	No	16.5 months	Not reacted	0
Abrey	44	28	Induction (HD-MTX, HD-Ara-C) + ASCT (BEAM)	29	No	5.6 months	Not reacted	3.60
McAllister	39	74	MTX-based BBBD	65	No	Not reported	40.7 months	5
DeAngelis	35	102	HD-MTX, Procarb, Vinc, HD-Ara-C + IT M	58	45 Gy	24 months	36.9 months	7.80
Pels	47	65	HD-MTX, HD-Ara-C, Dex, Vind, Vic, Ifos, Cy + IT M, IT A, IT MP	61	No	21 months	50	9

ASCT = autologous stem cell transplant; BBBD = blood brain barrier disruption; BEAM = carmustine, etoposide, cytarabine, and melphalan; Cy = cyclophosphamide; Ifos = ifosfamide; HD-Ara-C = high-dose cytarabine; HD-MTX = high-dose methotrexate; IT A = intrathecal cytarabine; IT M = intrathecal methotrexate; IT MP = intrathecal methylprednisilone; Procarb = procarbazine; TRM = treatment-related mortality; Vinc = vincristine; Vind = vindesine; WB-XRT = whole-brain irradiation.

there is an accumulation of data demonstrating synergistic interaction with chemotherapy. Randomized data generated by the Groupe d'Etude des Lymphomes de l'Adulte (GELA) comparing CHOP chemotherapy plus rituximab versus CHOP alone in 399 elderly patients with systemic non-CNS diffuse large B-cell lymphoma revealed that the rate of complete response was significantly higher in the group that received CHOP plus rituximab than in the group that received CHOP alone (76% versus 63%; p = .005). The addition of rituximab to standard CHOP chemotherapy also significantly reduced the risk of treatment failure and death.[45]

These data are likely relevant to PCNSL, as large B-cell lymphoma is the most common type of histology to involve the CNS.[45] For this reason, a number of studies are exploring the use of rituximab in this disease, both as a single agent and in combination with chemotherapeutic agents.[44,46] One of the limitations of the systemic administration of rituximab is that only 0.1% of this monoclonal antibody is able to penetrate the blood-brain barrier to enter CSF.[47] Although anecdotal responses in the CNS have been described after the systemic administration of rituximab, retrospective analysis of the GELA data demonstrated that systemic administration of rituximab did not affect the rate of CNS relapse in this population of patients.[48] For these reasons, there is current interest in studying the intrathecal administration of rituximab, both in the treatment of PCNSL and in the prophylaxis against CNS dissemination of NHL.[49,50]

Other Investigational Therapy

A number of other chemotherapeutic agents that have been shown to have activity in the treatment of PCNSL are under clinical investigation. One example is the alkylating agent temozolomide, a congener of dacarbazine (DTIC), recently approved for the treatment of malignant glioma. Temozolomide is administered orally and exhibits excellent CNS penetrance as well as a favorable adverse-effect profile. Its use is associated with benefit in health-related quality-of-life in brain tumor patients.[51] There is increasing evidence that temozolomide has activity in PCNSL, both at diagnosis and at relapse,

with response rates in the order of 26%.[52] The administration of temozolomide in combination with rituximab is also under investigation.[46] At the University of California, San Francisco, the combination of high-dose methotrexate plus temozolomide and intravenous rituximab is currently under investigation as an intensive induction regimen, followed by high-dose cytarabine plus etoposide as consolidation (Figure 10–6).

Another chemotherapeutic agent being studied in PCNSL is the topoisomerase I inhibitor topotecan, a derivative of camptothecan. Fischer and colleagues treated 16 immunocompetent patients with refractory or relapsed PCNSL: 6 patients exhibited responses, 4 of which were complete.[53]

Leptomeningeal dissemination represents a common pathway of relapse and dissemination in PCNSL. Standard treatment of lymphomatous meningitis consists of radiation to sites of radiographically visible disease, and the intrathecal administration of chemotherapy with either cytarabine or methotrexate. A recent randomized trial evaluating intrathecal administration of a long-acting form of cytarabine, DepoCyt, in the treatment of lymphomatous meningitis demonstrated that this drug had a significantly more favorable response rate (71%) compared with free cytarabine (15%).[54]

Intraventricular administration of chemotherapy drugs such as cytarabine or methotrexate using an Ommaya reservoir device is sometimes favored in neoplastic meningitis, because of evidence suggesting more reliable efficacy compared with intrathecal administration of drugs by lumbar puncture.[55] Ommaya reservoir placement requires a neurosurgical procedure and is associated with an approximate 10% risk of complications such as infection.[56] Therefore, the decision to place such a device should be balanced with respect to the probability of benefit and anticipated survival. A significant and avoidable complication may occur when there is tumor-associated obstruction in the ventricular system; delayed clearance of chemotherapy drugs from the cerebral ventricles can result in severe neurotoxicity. For this reason, a radionuclide CSF flow study may be indicated, to evaluate patency of the ventricular outflow system before administration of cytotoxic agents using an Ommaya reservoir.[57]

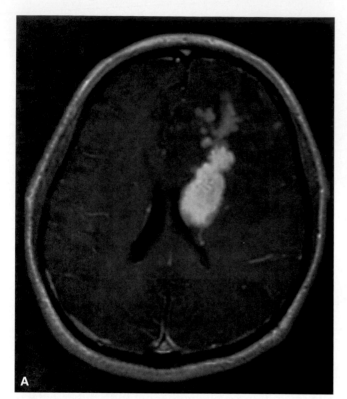 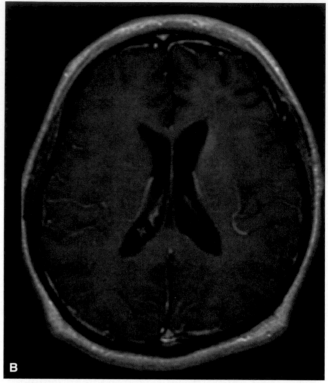

Figure 10–6. Radiographic complete response in primary central nervous system lymphoma (PCNSL). *A*, PCNSL at diagnosis. The transverse T1-weighted magnetic resonance image shows a multicentric, homogeneously contrast-enhancing tumor associated with moderate frontal midline shift and compression of adjacent lateral ventricle. *B*, The transverse T1-weighted image shows no residual enhancing mass after treatment with combination high-dose methotrexate, temozolomide, and rituximab.[24] The patient remains disease free, with a normal performance status 3.5 years later, without receipt of whole-brain irradiation.

AIDS-ASSOCIATED PCNSL

AIDS-associated PCNSL has, until recently, been associated with a dismal prognosis and a median survival of only 3 months.[5] The standard approach in treating AIDS-associated PCNSL has been to use whole-brain irradiation, largely because of concern that patients with this condition have significant comorbidities that contradict the use of chemotherapy. A recent pilot study from France evaluated the use of high-dose intravenous methotrexate at 3 g/m^2, given every 14 days, yielded encouraging results. Seven out of 15 patients exhibited radiographic complete responses and the median overall survival was 290 days. Importantly, the treatment was generally well tolerated and the median Karnofsky score improved from 50 to 80, results that have not been achieved using whole-brain irradiation monotherapy.[58] There is increasing evidence that the recent emergence of highly active antiretroviral therapy (HAART) has resulted in a decreased incidence of

AIDS-related PCNSL and that use of HAART is associated with a survival benefit in this disease.[59,60]

PRIMARY INTRAOCULAR LYMPHOMA

Primary intraocular lymphoma is characterized by the involvement of malignant lymphoid cells in the retina, vitreous, and/or optic nerve head and is closely related to PCNSL. In 80% of cases the disease is bilateral. Intraocular lymphoma complicates up to 20% of cases of primary CNS lymphoma, and 60 to 80% of patients who present with primary intraocular lymphoma will develop primary CNS lymphoma within 2 years. Intraocular lymphoma is a distinct entity from systemic lymphomas that metastasize via the circulation to the uvea and/or develop de novo in the external eye (conjunctiva, lacrimal gland, or orbit).

Treatment options for intraocular lymphoma are somewhat limited because of the blood-ocular barrier which is derived from tight junctions between vascular endothelial cells and pigmented epithelial cells of the anterior uvea and retina. The optimal therapeutic approach for intraocular lymphoma has not been defined. However, both intravenous methotrexate and intravenous cytarabine are able to penetrate the blood-ocular barrier and have activity in intraocular lymphoma.[61,62] Radiotherapy alone has long been used to treat patients with isolated ocular lymphoma.[63] Radiation-associated ocular toxicities include retinopathy, visual loss, and cataracts. Moreover, this treatment cannot be repeated, should tumor relapse in the irradiated eye. For this reason, intravitreous administration of methotrexate is being evaluated on an experimental basis for isolated and recurrent ocular disease.

One approach to treatment of PCNSL with ocular involvement is to use combined-modality therapy with systemic high-dose methotrexate-based chemotherapy and with radiation to the ocular globes.[64] Recurrence of intraocular lymphoma alone may be treated with intravitreous methotrexate as a single agent at some centers. There is evidence that intrathecal rituximab also has activity in recurrent ocular lymphoma.[50]

REFERENCES

1. van Besien K, Forman A, Champlin R. Central nervous system relapse of lymphoid malignancies in adults: the role of high-dose chemotherapy. Ann Oncol 1997;8:515–24.
2. Olson JE, Janney CA, Rao RD, et al. The continuing increase in the incidence of primary central nervous system non-Hodgkin lymphoma: a surveillance, epidemiology, and end results analysis. Cancer 2002;95:1504–10.
3. Corn BW, Marcus SM, Topham A, et al. Will primary central nervous system lymphoma be the most frequent brain tumor diagnosed in the year 2000? Cancer 1997;79:2409–13.
4. Levine A. Acquired immunodeficiency syndrome-related lymphoma. Blood 1992;80:8–20.
5. Fine HA, Mayer RJ. Primary central nervous system lymphoma. Ann Intern Med 1993;119:1093–104.
6. Cha S, Knopp EA, Johnson G, et al. Intracranial mass lesions: dynamic contrast-enhanced susceptibility-weighted echo-planar perfusion MR imaging. Radiology 2002;223:11–29.
7. Lai R, Rosenblum MK, DeAngelis L. Primary CNS lymphoma: a whole-brain disease? Neurology 2002;59:1557–62.
8. O'Neill BP, Dinapoli RP, Kurtin PJ, Habermann T. Occult systemic non-Hodgkin's lymphoma (NHL) in patients initially diagnosed as primary central nervous system lymphoma (PCNSL): how much staging is enough? J Neurooncol 1995;25:67–71.
9. Weller M. Glucocorticoid treatment of primary CNS lymphoma. J Neurooncol 1999;43:237–9.
10. Kulkarni AV, Guha A, Lozano A, Bernstein M. Incidence of silent hemorrhage and delayed deterioration after stereotactic brain biopsy. J Neurosurg 1998;89:31–5.
11. Soo TM, Bernstein M, Provias J, et al. Failed stereotactic biopsy in a series of 518 cases. Stereotact Funct Neurosurg 1995;64:183–96.
12. Bernstein M, Berger MS, editors. In: Neuro-oncology: the essentials. New York: Thieme; 2000. p. 122–34.
13. Antinori A, De Rossi G, Ammassari A, et al. Value of combined approach with thallium-201 single-photon emission computed tomography and Epstein-Barr virus DNA polymerase chain reaction in CSF for the diagnosis of AIDS-related primary CNS lymphoma. J Clin Oncol 1999;17:554–60.
14. Pierce MA, Johnson MD, Maciunas RJ, et al. Evaluating contrast-enhancing brain lesions in patients with AIDS by using positron emission tomography. Ann Intern Med 1995;123:594–8.
15. Smith JR, Braziel RM, Paoletti S, et al. Expression of B-cell-attracting chemokine 1 (CXCL13) by malignant lymphocytes and vascular endothelium in primary central nervous system lymphoma. Blood 2003;101:815–21.
16. Braaten KM, Betensky RA, de Leval L, et al. BCL-6 expression predicts improved survival in patients with primary central nervous system lymphoma. Clin Cancer Res 2003;9:1063–9.
17. Nakamura M, Sakaki T, Hashimoto H, et al. Frequent alterations of the p14(ARF) and p16(INK4a) genes in primary central nervous system lymphomas. Cancer Res 2001;61:6335–9.
18. Larocca LM, Capello D, Rinelli A, et al. The molecular and phenotypic profile of primary central nervous system lymphoma identifies distinct categories of the disease and is consistent with histogenetic derivation from germinal center-related B cells. Blood 1998;92:1011–9.
19. Alizadeh AE, Davis M, Ma R, et al. Distinct types of diffuse large B-cell lymphoma identified by gene expression profiling. Nature 2000;403:503–11.
20. Rubenstein JL, Shen A, Fridlyand J, et al. Gene expression profile analysis of primary CNS lymphoma: class distinction and outcome prediction. In: Proceedings of the 2004 Annual Meeting of the American Association for Cancer Research. Vol 45. 2004. p. 4433.
21. Ferreri AJ, Blay JY, Reni M, et al. Prognostic scoring system for primary CNS lymphomas: the International Extranodal Lymphoma Study Group experience. J Clin Oncol 2003;21:266–72.
22. Blay JY, Conroy T, Chevreau C, et al. High-dose methotrexate for the treatment of primary cerebral lymphomas: analysis of survival and late neurologic toxicity in a retrospective series. J Clin Oncol 1998;16:864–71.
23. Abrey LE, DeAngelis LM, Yahalom J. Long-term survival in primary CNS lymphoma. J Clin Oncol 1998;16:859–63.
24. Deangelis L. Current management of primary central nervous system lymphoma. Oncology 1995;9:63–71.
25. Nelson DF, Martz KL, Bonner H, et al. Non-Hodgkin's lymphoma of the brain: can high dose, large volume radiation therapy improve survival? Report on a prospective trial by the Radiation Therapy Oncology Group (RTOG): RTOG 83. Int J Radiat Oncol Biol Phys 1992;23:9–17.
26. Bessell EM, Lopez-Guillermo A, Villa S, et al. Importance of

radiotherapy in the outcome of patients with primary CNS lymphoma: an analysis of the CHOD/BVAM regimen followed by two different radiotherapy treatments. J Clin Oncol 2002;20:231–6.

27. Schultz C, Scott C, Sherman W, et al. Preirradiation chemotherapy with cyclophosphamide, doxorubicin, vincristine, and dexamethasone for primary CNS lymphomas: initial report of radiation therapy oncology group protocol 88-06. J Clin Oncol 1996;14:556–64.

28. O'Neill BP, O'Fallon JR, Earle JD, et al. Primary central nervous system non-Hodgkin's lymphoma: survival advantages with combined initial therapy? Int J Radiat Oncol Biol Phys 1995;33:663–73.

29. Glantz MJ, Cole BF, Recht L, et al. High-dose intravenous methotrexate for patients with nonleukemic leptomeningeal cancer: is intrathecal chemotherapy necessary? J Clin Oncol 1998;16:1561–7.

30. Ervin T, Canellos GP. Successful treatment of recurrent primary central nervous system lymphoma with high-dose methotrexate. Cancer 1980;45:1556–7.

31. Skarin AT, Zuckerman KS, Pitman SW, et al. High-dose methotrexate with folinic acid in the treatment of advanced non-Hodgkin lymphoma including CNS involvement. Blood 1977;50:1039–47.

32. Bokstein F, Lossos A, Lossos IS, Siegal T. Central nervous system relapse of systemic non-Hodgkin's lymphoma: results of treatment based on high-dose methotrexate combination chemotherapy. Leuk Lymphoma 2002;43:587–93.

33. Harder H, Holtel H, Bromberg JEC, et al. Cognitive status and quality of life after treatment for primary CNS lymphoma. Neurology 2004;62:544–7.

34. DeAngelis LM, Seiferheld W, Schold SC, et al. Combination chemotherapy and radiotherapy for primary central nervous system lymphoma: Radiation Therapy Oncology Group Study 93-10. J Clin Oncol 2002;20:4643–8.

35. Khan RB, Shi W, Thaler HT, et al. Is intrathecal methotrexate necessary in the treatment of primary CNS lymphoma? J Neurooncol 2002;58:175–8.

36. Guha-Thakurta N, Damek D, Pollack C, Hochberg F. Intravenous methotrexate as initial treatment for primary central nervous system lymphoma: response to therapy and quality of life of patients. J Neurooncol 1999;43:259–68.

37. Batchelor T, Carson K, O'Neill A, et al. Treatment of primary CNS lymphoma with methotrexate and deferred radiotherapy: a report of NABTT 96-07. J Clin Oncol 2003;21:1044–9.

38. McAllister LD, Doolittle ND, Guastadisegni PE, et al. Cognitive outcomes and long-term follow-up results after enhanced chemotherapy delivery for primary central nervous system lymphoma. Neurosurgery 2000;46:51–60.

39. Van Besien K, Ha CS, Murphy S, et al. Risk Factors, Treatment and Outcome of Central Nervous Recurrence in Adults with Intermediate-Grade and Immunoblastic Lymphoma. Blood 1998;91:1174–84.

40. Abrey LE, Moskowitz CH, Mason WP, et al/ Intensive methotrexate and cytarabine followed by high-dose chemotherapy with autologous stem-cell rescue in patients with newly diagnosed primary CNS lymphoma: an intent-to-treat analysis. J Clin Oncol 2003;21:4151–6.

41. Soussain C, Suzan F, Hoang-Xuan K, et al. Results of inten-sive chemotherapy followed by hematopoietic stem-cell rescue in 22 patients with refractory or recurrent primary CNS lymphoma or intraocular lymphoma. J Clin Oncol 2001;19:742–9.

42. Sandor V, Stark-Vancs V, Pearson D, et al. Phase II trial of chemotherapy alone for primary CNS and intraocular lymphoma. J Clin Oncol 1998;16:3000–6.

43. Pels H, Schmidt-Wolf IG, Glasmacher A, et al. Primary central nervous system lymphoma: results of a pilot and phase II study of systemic and intraventricular chemotherapy with deferred radiotherapy. J Clin Oncol 2003;21:4489–95.

44. Rubenstein J, L, Trager M, et al. Clinical and biological prognostic factors in primary CNS and ocular lymphoma: the UCSF experience. In preparation

45. Coiffier B, Lepage E, Briere J, et al. CHOP chemotherapy plus rituximab compared with CHOP alone in elderly patients with diffuse large-B-cell lymphoma. N Engl J Med 2002;346:235–42.

46. Wong ET, Tishler R, Barron L, Wu JK. Immunochemotherapy with rituximab and temozolomide for central nervous system lymphomas. Cancer 2004;101:139–45.

47. Rubenstein JL, Combs D, Rosenberg J, et al. Rituximab therapy for CNS lymphomas: targeting the leptomeningeal compartment. Blood 2003;101:466–8.

48. Feugier P, Virion JM, Tilly H, et al. Incidence and risk factors for central nervous system occurrence in elderly patients with diffuse large-B-cell lymphoma: influence of rituximab. Ann Oncol 2004;15:129–33.

49. Schulz H, Pels H, Schmidt-Wolf I, et al. Intraventricular treatment of relapsed central nervous system lymphoma with the anti-CD20 antibody rituximab. Haematologica 2004;89:753–4.

50. Rubenstein JL, Shen A, Abrey L, et al. Results from a phase I study of intraventricular administration of rituximab in patients with recurrent lymphomatous meningitis. In: Proceedings of the 2004 Annual Meeting of the American Society of Clinical Oncology. 2004. p. 6593.

51. Osoba D, Brada M, Yung WK, Prados M. Health-related quality of life in patients treated with temozolomide versus procarbazine for recurrent glioblastoma multiforme. 2000;18:1481–91.

52. Reni M, Mason W, Zaja F, et al. Salvage chemotherapy with temozolomide in primary CNS lymphomas: preliminary results of a phase II trial. Eur J Cancer 2004;40:1682–8.

53. Fischer L, Thiel E, Klasen HA, et al. Response of relapsed or refractory primary central nervous system lymphoma (PCNSL) to topotecan. Neurology 2004;62:1885–7.

54. Glantz MJ, LaFollette S, Jaeckle KA, et al. Randomized trial of a slow-release versus a standard formulation of cytarabine for the intrathecal treatment of lymphomatous meningitis. J Clin Oncol 1999;17:3110–6.

55. Bleyer WA, Poplack DG. Intraventricular versus intralumbar methotrexate for central-nervous-system leukemia: prolonged remission with the Ommaya reservoir. Med Pediatr Oncol 1979;6:207–13.

56. Sandberg DI, Bilsky MH, Souweidane MM, et al. Ommaya reservoirs for the treatment of leptomeningeal metastases. Neurosurgery 2000;47:49–54.

57. Mason WP, Yeh SD, DeAngelis L. 111Indium-diethylenetri-amine pentaacetic acid cerebrospinal fluid flow studies

predict distribution of intrathecally administered chemotherapy and outcome in patients with leptomeningeal metastases. Neurology 1998;50:438–44.

58. Jacomet C, Girard PM, Lebrette MG, et al. Intravenous methotrexate for primary central nervous system non-Hodgkin's lymphoma in AIDS. AIDS 1997;11:1725–30.

59. Inungu J, Melendez MF, Montgomery J. AIDS-related primary brain lymphoma in Michigan, January 1990 to December 2000. AIDS Patient Care STDS 2002;16:107–12.

60. Skiest D, Crosby C. Survival is prolonged by highly active antiretroviral therapy in AIDS patients with primary central nervous system lymphoma. AIDS 2003;17:1787–93.

61. Baumann MA, Ritch PS, Hande KR, et al. Treatment of intraocular lymphoma with high-dose Ara-C. Cancer 1986;57:1273–5.

62. Batchelor TT, Kolak G, Ciordia R, et al. High-dose methotrexate for intraocular lymphoma. Clin Cancer Res 2003;9:711–5.

63. Margolis L, Fraser R, Lichter A, Char D. The role of radiation therapy in the management of ocular reticulum cell sarcoma. Cancer 1980;45:688–92.

64. Hormigo A, DeAngelis L. Primary ocular lymphoma: clinical features, diagnosis, and treatment. Clin Lymphoma 2003; 4:22–9.

11

Diagnosis and Management of Non-Hodgkin's Lymphoma and Hodgkin's Lymphoma

AJAI CHARI
LAWRENCE KAPLAN

Lymphomas originate when a lymphocyte undergoes malignant transformation resulting in lymphadenopathy or involvement of virtually any organ system. Lymphomas are subdivided into two major categories: non-Hodgkin's lymphoma (NHL) and Hodgkin's lymphoma (HL). NHL is not a single disease, but rather, it represents a diverse group of cancers that are distinguished by the histologic characteristics of the cancerous cells. The subgroups of NHL have different natural histories and, accordingly, are treated differently. HL is a specialized form of lymphoma that is distinguished by the presence of a large abnormal cell, called the Reed-Sternberg cell.

In the United States in 2004, when patients with active lymphoma and those in remission were combined, there were 346,749 people living with NHL and 123,181 people living with HL for a total of 469,930.[1] In addition, 62,250 individuals in the United States would be newly diagnosed with lymphoma in 2004 (54,370 cases of NHL and 7,880 cases of HL). Even among children, lymphomas are common, following only leukemia and nervous system tumors in frequency.

NON-HODGKIN'S LYMPHOMA

Epidemiology

Non-Hodgkin's lymphoma is the sixth most common cancer diagnosis in the United States. From 1976 to 2001, the incidence of NHL has risen annually by 2.6%. Although the association with the human immunodeficiency virus (HIV) is a contributing factor, the reason for the increase in age-adjusted incidence by 249% from 1950 to 2001 and by 71% from 1976 to 2001 is not completely clear.

The incidence of NHL increases with age, from 2.3 per 100,000 persons in 20- to 24-year-olds, to 43.8 per 100,000 persons by age 60 years and > 100 per 100,000 persons after age 75 years (Figure 11–1). Age-adjusted incidence rates for NHL are also higher among males, with rates of 3.0 per 100,000 persons for males and 1.7 per 100,000 persons for females aged 20 to 24 years. By ages 60 to 64 years, the rates are 52.2 per 100,000 persons for males and 36.1 per 100,000 persons for females. Whites generally have higher incidence rates than Blacks (except during the second through fourth decades).

Classification

Based on the 1994 Revised European-American Lymphoma (REAL) system, the World Health Organization (WHO) published a classification of lymphoid neoplasms (Table 11–1).[2] This classification system incorporates a combination of morphology, immunophenotypes, genetic features, and clinical features. As shown in Table 11–2, nearly 90% of NHLs are of B-cell origin, with the diffuse large B cell and follicular histologies alone accounting for more than 50%.[3] The advent of gene expression profiling will undoubtedly result in further modifications to this classification schema. Although the schema represents a current worldwide pathologic and clinical consensus, organization by clinical behavior makes the nearly 40 histologically distinct variants of NHL much more manageable.

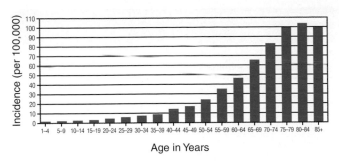

Figure 11–1. Age-specific incidence rates for non-Hodgkin's lymphoma, 1997–2001. Reproduced with permission from National Cancer Institute.[1]

the most rapidly proliferative human malignancies, with a proliferation rate of nearly 100%), and associated with short disease-free survivals if refractory to chemotherapy or if relapse occurs. However, these aggressive lymphomas are also more curable with chemotherapy. Conversely, the indolent lymphomas tend to be incurable, but associated with less rapid growth and longer overall survival. Of note, mantle cell lymphoma, although considered to be in the low-grade group of the Working Formulation, behaves more as an aggressive NHL.

Etiology and Risk Factors

Based in part on the Working Formulation that divided NHL by morphology into low-, intermediate-, and high-grade groups, NHL can be divided by clinical behavior into three categories: indolent, aggressive, and highly aggressive (Table 11–3).[4] Generally speaking, the more aggressive the NHL, the more fulminant the presentation and behavior (eg, Burkitt's lymphoma is considered to be amongst

For lymphomas originating from B cells, the transforming event is believed to occur in the germinal center, where cells undergo a number of DNA-modifying events such as class switching and somatic hypermutation. Alteration in these events can result in inappropriate translocations (eg, onco-

Table 11–1. WORLD HEALTH ORGANIZATION CLASSIFICATION OF LYMPHOID NEOPLASMS		
B-Cell Neoplasms	**T-Cell and NK-Cell Neoplasms**	**Hodgkin's Lymphoma (Hodgkin's Lymphoma)** Nodular lymphocyte-predominant Hodgkin's lymphoma
Precursor B-cell neoplasm Precursor B lymphoblastic leukemia/lymphoma	**Precursor T-cell neoplasm** Precursor T lymphoblastic lymphoma/leukemia Blastic NK-cell lymphoma	
Mature B-cell neoplasms B-cell chronic lymphocytic leukemia/ small lymphocytic lymphoma B-cell prolymphocytic leukemia Lymphoplasmacytic lymphoma Splenic marginal-zone lymphoma Hairy cell leukemia Plasma cell myeloma Solitary plasmacytoma of bone Extraosseous plasmacytoma Extranodal marginal-zone B-cell lymphoma of mucosa-associated lymphoid tissue (MALT-lymphoma) Nodal marginal-zone lymphoma Follicular lymphoma Mantle cell lymphoma Diffuse large B-cell lymphoma Mediastinal (thymic) large B-cell lymphoma Primary effusion lymphoma Burkitt's lymphoma/leukemia	**Mature T-cell neoplasms** T-cell prolymphocytic leukemia T-cell granular lymphocytic leukemia Aggressive NK-cell leukemia Adult T-cell lymphoma/leukemia Extranodal NK/T-cell lymphoma, nasal type Enteropathy-type T-cell lymphoma Hepatosplenic T-cell lymphoma Subcutaneous panniculitis-like T-cell lymphoma Mycosis fungoides Sézary syndrome Primary cutaneous anaplastic large-cell lymphoma Peripheral T-cell lymphoma, unspecified Angioimmunoblastic T-cell lymphoma Anaplastic large-cell lymphoma	*Classical Hodgkin's lymphoma* Nodular sclerosis Hodgkin's lymphoma Lymphocyte-rich classical Hodgkin's lymphoma Mixed cellularity Hodgkin's lymphoma Lymphocyte depleted Hodgkin's lymphoma
B-cell proliferations of uncertain malignant potential Lymphomatoid granulomatosis Posttransplant lymphoproliferative disorder, polymorphic	**T-cell proliferation of uncertain malignant potential** Lymphomatoid papulosis	

Adapted from Jaffe ES et al.[2]

Table 11–2. NON-HODGKIN'S LYMPHOMA FREQUENCY AND ASSOCIATED KARYOTYPES, ONCOGENES, AND INFECTIOUS AGENTS

Diagnosis	Frequency	Karyotype [% with abnormality]	Oncogene	Infectious Agent
Diffuse large B cell	30.6	t (8;14) [20–30%], ch 3 translocation	BCL2, BCL6	SV40*
Follicular	22.1	t (14;18) [90%]	BCL2	
Marginal zone B cell, MALT	7.6	t (11;18), t (1;14)	API2/MALT1, BCL10	H. pylori
Peripheral T cell	7			
Small B-lymphocytic (SLL)	6.7	13q14 deletion [50%]†		
Mantle cell	6	t (11;14)	cyclin d1	
Medium-sized, mixed, and large	3.7	t (3;14)l; t (3;v), t (14;18)	BCL6 (in large cell)	
Primary mediastinal large B cell	2.4			
Anaplastic large T/null cell	2.4	t (2;5)(p23;q35)	ALK‡	
High-grade B cell, Burkitt-like	2.1			
Marginal zone B cell, nodal	1.8			
Precursor T lymphoblastic	1.7			
Angiocentric, nasal	1.4			
Angioimmunoblastic	1.2			
Lymphoplasmacytoid	1.2			
Marginal zone B cell, splenic	< 1			Hepatitis C
Mycosis fungoides	< 1			
Burkitt's	< 1	t (8;14), t (2;8), t (8;22)	c-myc	EBV (> 95% endemic versus 20% sporadic)
Intestinal	< 1			
Lymphoepithelioid	< 1			
Hepatosplenic	< 1			
Adult T-cell leukemia/lymphoma	< 1			HTLV-1
All other types	6.1			
Primary effusion lymphoma				HHV-8
Nasal NK/T cell				EBV

ALK = anaplastic lymphoma kinase; EBV = Epstein-Barr virus; HHV-8 = human herpes virus 8; HTLV-1 = human T-cell lymphotropic virus 1; MALT = mucosa-associated lymphoid tissue; SV40 = simian virus 40.
*SV40 DLBCL, data from Nakatsuka et al[171]
†13q14 SLL, data from Kalachikov et al[172]
‡ALK, data from Morris et al[173]
Adapted from Simon R et al.[168]

gene to immunoglobulin switch region) or point mutations in oncogenes. Table 11–2 lists the translocations and oncogenes identified to date that are associated with lymphomas.

A major risk factor for the development of lymphoma is any abnormality of the immune system, either immunodeficiency (HIV infection, immunosuppressive medications to prevent graft rejection posttransplantation, or primary immunodeficiencies),

or autoimmune disorders. The relative risk of developing NHL is 14- to 652-fold increased in the presence of HIV, 6.6-fold after solid organ transplantation, and 33- to 44-fold in patients with Sjögren's syndrome.[5–8]

Lymphoproliferative disease associated with solid organ transplantation is associated with Epstein-Barr virus (EBV) in a large majority of cases, whereas EBV positivity has been associated with about 60% of HIV-associated NHL.[2,9,10] Even in patients without

Table 11–3. NON-HODGKIN'S LYMPHOMA CLASSIFICATION BY CLINICAL BEHAVIOR

Indolent	Aggressive	Highly Aggressive
Follicular lymphoma	Diffuse large B-cell lymphoma	Burkitt's lymphoma
Small lymphocytic lymphoma	Peripheral T-cell lymphoma	Precursor B-lymphoblastic lymphoma/ leukemia
Marginal zone lymphoma	Anaplastic large cell lymphoma, T/null cell	Adult T-cell lymphoma/leukemia
Lymphoplasmacytic lymphoma	Mantle cell lymphoma	Precursor T-lymphoblastic lymphoma/leukemia
Mycosis fungoides/Sézary syndrome		
Splenic marginal zone lymphoma		

Adapted from Armitage JO and Weisenburger DD.[4]

a known history of immunodeficiency, EBV is detectable in more than 95% of cases of the endemic variant of Burkitt's lymphoma (BL) found in sub-Saharan Africa, and 15 to 20% of sporadic cases in other parts of the world.[11,12] A review of five large case series involving various subtypes of NHL found that EBV could be detected at the molecular level in 25% of 284 T-cell NHL tested and 11% of 932 B-cell NHL. Higher-grade NHLs were more associated with EBV than lower grade (16% versus 8%, respectively).[13]

The human T-cell lymphocytotropic virus type I (HTLV-1) is another virus that is also associated with T-cell lymphoma, particularly in Southern Japan, the Caribbean, South America, and Africa.[14] The human herpesvirus 8 (HHV-8) is strongly associated with HIV-associated body-cavity–based lymphomas, although EBV is detected in most cases as well.[15,16] Hermine and colleagues showed that treatment of hepatitis C with interferon resulted in partial or complete responses of the splenic lymphoma with villous lymphocytes in 9 of 9 patients.[17] The simian virus 40 has also been implicated in NHL.[18,19] Other infectious agents associated with NHL include *Helicobacter pylori* and *Borrelia* species.[20–22]

The increasing incidence of lymphoma even before the entry and spread of HIV in the human population has led to a search for other factors. A meta-analysis found that the relative risk of NHL was 1.34 in farmers.[23] A strong dose response was found for the polychlorinated biphenyls, an organochlorine used as a pesticide, with the highest quartile having a relative risk of 4.5 of developing NHL.[24]

Diagnosis

The "B" symptoms of NHL include unexplained fever greater than 38°C, drenching night sweats, and unexplained weight loss of more than 10% of baseline during the preceding 6 months.[25] Approximately 40% of patients with NHL present with a B symptom.[26] Other manifestations include pruritus, lymphadenopathy, hepatosplenomegaly, and symptoms due to either bulky disease or involvement of other organ systems such as the brain, bone, gastrointestinal tract, testes, or skin. Potential infectious etiologies for these symptoms must be excluded.

Complete blood counts may reveal cytopenias from bone marrow involvement, hypersplenism,

immune-mediated thrombocytopenia (ITP), or anemia of chronic disease. Hypercalcemia is seen, particularly in patients with adult T-cell lymphoma, and the highly aggressive NHL subtypes sometimes present with evidence of spontaneous tumor lysis. In the absence of lymphadenopathy detected on physical examination, computed tomography (CT) scans of the neck (if clinically indicated), chest, abdomen, and pelvis can help identify a lesion amenable to biopsy.

Ideally, a lymph node chosen for tissue diagnosis should be easily accessible and persistently enlarged/enlarging. Supraclavicular nodes typically have the highest yield of a diagnosis, whereas inguinal nodes have the lowest.[27] A fine-needle aspiration (FNA) is often performed initially, to determine if there is any evidence of lymphoma. With the additional information gained from immunophenotyping (Table 11–4), sometimes an FNA can yield a pathologic diagnosis. However, an excisional biopsy, unlike an FNA, allows the pathologist to discern not only the histologic grade but also the pattern of lymph node involvement (nodular versus diffuse), and thus provides the greatest amount of information. If an excisional biopsy is not feasible, then a core needle biopsy may also provide sufficient tissue. Molecular genetics and cytogenetics can further help identify the specific type of NHL (see Table 11–2).

Staging

After a diagnosis of NHL has been made, the extent of the disease must be determined. Staging evaluation includes CT scans of the chest and abdomen and any other area of concern due to symptoms or signs (eg, skeletal imaging may be indicated for bone pain). Endoscopic evaluation may be complementary to CT scans in patients suspected to have gastrointestinal tract involvement.

Table 11–4. IMMUNOPHENOTYPING OF CD20⁺ SMALL B-CELL NON-HODGKIN'S LYMPHOMA				
	Follicular	**Mantle Cell**	**Marginal Zone**	**Small Lymphocytic**
CD5	−	+	−	+
CD10	+	−	−	−
CD23	±	−	−	+

Adapted from Young NA and Al-Saleem T.[169]

Radionuclide imaging can also be useful in the staging of NHL, particularly when CT scans are equivocal or suboptimal (eg, due to the inability to use intravenous contrast). Gallium-67 citrate binds to transferrin receptors in some lymphomas, and when combined with single-photon emission computed tomography (SPECT), it then detects intermediate and high-grade NHLs with 70 to 85% sensitivity.[28] The sensitivity of gallium scans tends to be lower for low-grade lymphomas, being approximately 70%, and lower still for marginal-zone lymphomas.[29]

Fluorodeoxyglucose-positron emission tomography (FDG-PET) has a similar disparity, being able to detect disease in only 67% of marginal-zone lymphomas and 40% of peripheral T-cell lymphomas, but nearly 100% of patients with large B-cell lymphoma, mantle cell lymphoma, and even follicular lymphoma.[30] Studies directly comparing gallium and PET scans have consistently found PET to be more sensitive, typically detecting disease in 15 to 30% more anatomic sites and patients than with gallium (Figures 11–2 and 11–3).[31–33] PET scans also tend to be particularly better at detecting splenic involvement of NHL. PET and gallium scans in staging are particularly helpful in ensuring that patients who receive only local treatment for presumed limited-stage disease are not being inadvertently undertreated.

Radionuclide imaging is also useful in monitoring response to therapy, as conventional CT scans do not reliably differentiate residual lymphoma from

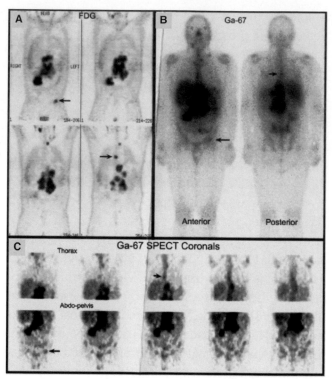

Figure 11–3. In a patient with diffuse large cell non-Hodgkin's lymphoma, the arrows in panel *A* indicate disease in the posterior mediastinum and L inguinal area discernible by PET scan. These areas are not clearly distinguishable from background marrow activity on gallium imaging (*B* and *C*). Reproduced with permission from Wirth A et al.[33]

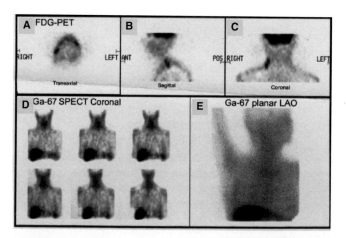

Figure 11–2. In a patient with diffuse large cell non-Hodgkin's lymphoma, the PET scan clearly demonstrates disease in the right neck (*A, B, C*) that is not discernible on gallium scanning (*D, E*). FDG-PET = fluorodeoxyglucose positron emission tomography; Ga-67 SPECT = Gallium 67 single photon emission computed tomography; LAO = left anterior oblique view. Reproduced with permission from Wirth A et al.[33]

the fibrosis or necrosis that can be seen after lymphoma therapy. Indeed, persistent gallium positivity during or after chemotherapy is associated with a significantly increased risk of early relapse and/or decreased survival.[28,34–36] The same is true for persistently positive PET scans during and after treatment.[37–40] For example, in one study, 11 of 67 patients with a negative PET scan after chemotherapy relapsed, with a median progression-free survival (PFS) of 404 days. In contrast, all 26 patients with persistently abnormal PET scans relapsed, with median PFS of 73 days.[40] Persistent radionuclide abnormalities therefore identify high-risk patients who may need additional or alternative treatments.

A bone marrow biopsy is a routine part of the staging process, since marrow involvement of NHL signifies the most advanced stage (IV) of NHL. Typically, the marrow involvement is focal and more often detected on a core biopsy than on aspiration. Approximately 40% of indolent NHL have marrow involvement versus 20% involvement for higher grade lymphomas.[41] Historically, bilateral posterior iliac crest biopsies were performed; however, the detection rate of bone marrow involvement in one study increased with increasing trephine length/examination of multiple levels, but was not dependent on the number of sites sampled.[42] Thus, a unilateral 20 mm biopsy is likely sufficient.

For certain patients, staging also includes a lumbar puncture with cytologic examination of the cerebrospinal fluid. Such patients include those with HIV and patients with aggressive NHL involving the bone marrow, testes, periorbital/paranasal sinuses, or parameningeal/ paravertebral areas, as all of these sites are thought to be associated with an increased risk of central nervous system (CNS) relapse. However, in a study of 605 patients, multivariate analysis identified only increased lactate dehydrogenase (LDH) and the involvement of more than one extranodal site as predictors of CNS relapse, with associated relative risks of 7.0 and 5.5, respectively.[43]

The following baseline blood tests are often useful for prognosis, disease monitoring, or guiding therapy: LDH, β_2-microglobulin, erythrocyte sedimentation rate (ESR), complete blood count (CBC) with differential, liver function tests, blood urea nitrogen, creatinine, calcium, phosphorus, uric acid, and HIV testing.

Once the extent of disease has been fully characterized, the patient can be assigned a stage (I through IV) according to the modified Ann Arbor staging system (Table 11–5).[44]

Prognosis

The Ann Arbor staging system is one component of the international prognostic index (IPI; Table 11–6A), a very well-validated prognostic tool. This system is based upon the identification of five independent prognostic features in patients with aggressive histology lymphomas. Poor prognostic factors include age > 60 years, abnormal LDH, ≥ 2 extranodal sites of disease, an Eastern Cooperative Oncology Group (ECOG) performance score of ≥ 2, and stage III or IV disease. An IPI score of 0 is associated with 73% 5-year survival, whereas a score of 4 or 5 is associated with only a 26% survival (Table 11–6B). An age-adjusted IPI is used for patients under the age of 60 years (Tables 11–6 C and D). The IPI was created for the initial diagnosis of aggressive NHL. Since then, it has been validated for patients with HIV and also for patient who relapse after initial therapy.[45–47]

Application of the IPI to indolent NHL produces mixed results, in part because only 10 to 15% of patients fall into the high-risk category. Recently, a new prognostic index, follicular lymphoma international prognostic index (FLIPI), was developed using data from 1,795 patients with follicular lymphoma and validated with 919 other patients (Table 11–7). Patients with a FLIPI score of 0 to 1 have a 71% 10-year survival, whereas a score of 3 or more is associated with only 36% survival to 10 years. The FLIPI was found to be simple, reproducible, and better at predicting the risk of death than the IPI score.[48]

More recently, there has been interest in the use of gene expression profiling to predict outcomes. Rosenwald and colleagues found that the survival of patients with diffuse large B-cell lymphoma after chemotherapy was associated with the subgroup that their gene expression profile belonged to: germinal center B cell-like, activated B cell-like or type 3 (Figure 11–4).[49] Those with the germinal center B-cell–like pattern had the highest 5-year survival.[49]

Table 11–5. MODIFIED ANN ARBOR STAGING SYSTEM	
Stage	**Area of Involvement**
I	Single lymph node group
II	Multiple lymph node groups on same side of diaphragm
III	Multiple lymph node groups on both sides of diaphragm
IV	Multiple extranodal sites or lymph nodes and extranodal disease
Modifiers	
X	Bulk > 10 cm
E	Extranodal extension or single isolated site of extranodal diseasethat can be encompassed in a single radiation port
A/B	B symptoms: weight loss > 10%, fever, drenching night sweats

Adapted from Lister TA et al.[44]

Table 11–6A. INTERNATIONAL PROGNOSTIC INDEX (IPI) RISK FACTORS AND ECOG PERFORMANCE STATUS

IPI Risk Factors	ECOG Performance Status
Age > 60 years	0: Asymptomatic
LDH > normal	1: Symptomatic; fully ambulatory
ECOG performance status 2–4	2: Symptomatic; ambulatory > 50% of day
Ann Arbor stage III or IV	3: Symptomatic; ambulatory < 50% of day
Two or more extranodal sites of disease	4: Bedridden

ECOG = Eastern Cooperative Oncology Group; LDH = lactate dehydrogenase.
Adapted from The International Non-Hodgkin's Lymphoma Prognostic Factors Project.[170]

Table 11–6B. IPI INDEX

Risk Group	Risk Factors (Sum)	CR (%)	5-Year OS (%)
Low	0–1	87	73
Low-intermediate	2	67	51
High-intermediate	3	55	43
High	4–5	44	26

CR = complete remission; OS = overall survival.
Adapted from The International Non-Hodgkin's Lymphoma Prognostic Factors Project.[170]

Table 11–6C. AGE-ADJUSTED IPI RISK FACTORS

Age-Adjusted IPI for Age < 60 Years
Lactate dehydrogenase > normal
ECOG performance status 2–4
Ann Arbor stage III or IV

ECOG = Eastern Cooperative Oncology Group.
Adapted from The International Non-Hodgkin's Lymphoma Prognostic Factors Project.[170]

Table 11–6D. AGE-ADJUSTED IPI INDEX

Risk Group	Risk Factors (Sum)	CR (%)	5-Year OS (%)
Low	0	92	83
Low-intermediate	1	78	69
High-intermediate	2	57	46
High	3	46	32

CR = complete remission; OS = overall survival.
Adapted from The International Non-Hodgkin's Lymphoma Prognostic Factors Project.[170]

Because it is difficult to standardize such tests on a large scale, Lossos and colleagues limited the measurements to the expression of six genes by polymerase chain reaction, including the genes *BCL2* and *BCL6* (Figure 11–5). Their multivariate model could predict overall survival in patients with DLBCL, independent of the IPI. For example, even for patients with a low-risk IPI score, the six-gene model could identify patients with a 5-year survival rate of only 57%.[50]

Treatment

The choice of treatment is based on the NHL subtype, cell of origin (B versus T/NK), and prognostic score.

Indolent Lymphomas

Grades 1 to 2 follicular lymphoma (FL), small lymphocytic lymphoma, and marginal-zone lymphoma are generally treated in a similar fashion. Only approximately 15% of individuals with indolent lym-

Table 11–7. FOLLICULAR LYMPHOMA INTERNATIONAL PROGNOSTIC INDEX (FLIPI)

Parameter	Adverse Factor
Age	≥ 60 years
Ann Arbor stage	III-IV
Hemoglobin level	< 120 g/L
Serum LDH level	> ULN
Number of nodal sites	> 4

Risk Group	No. of Factors	Distribution of Patients (%)	5-Year OS (%)	10-Year OS (%)
Low	0–1	36	90.6	70.7
Intermediate	2	37	77.6	50.9
High	≥ 3	27	52.5	35.5

LDH = lactate dehydrogenase; OS = overall survival; ULN = upper limit normal.
Adapted from Solal-Celigny P et al.[48]

phoma will present with early-stage disease. For these patients, long-term disease-free survival has been observed. Therefore, it is generally recommended that individuals with stages I to II indolent NHL without bulky disease receive 30 to 36 Gy involved field radiation therapy with a curative intent. The Stanford experience demonstrates that at 10 years, treatment with radiation alone is associated with a 44% relapse-free survival, 64% overall survival, and a median survival of 13.7 years.[51] Few relapses occurred after 10 years, suggesting a significant number of cures. The addition of chemotherapy and extended field radiation does not improve overall survival, but can improve event-free survival (EFS).

Gastric mucosa-associated lymphoid tissue lymphomas and splenic marginal-zone lymphomas represent special cases. Durable remissions are possible in some patients with marginal-zone lymphoma limited to the stomach, treated with therapy to eradicate *H. pylori.* Similarly, splenectomy for patients with marginal-zone lymphoma limited to the spleen can be highly successful therapy.

Currently, stages II–X (ie, bulky stage II), III, or IV follicular NHL cannot be cured. Therefore, the indications for therapy include symptoms or patient preference, massive bulk, NHL-related cytopenias (autoimmune or due to marrow involvement), or threatened organ function.

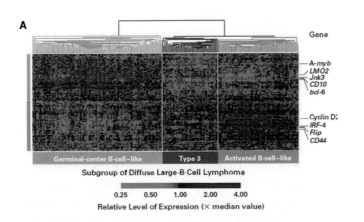

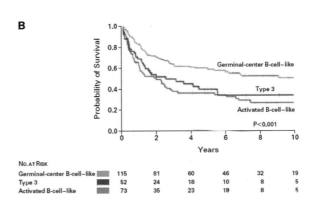

Figure 11–4. Gene expression profiles were performed on biopsies of 240 patients with newly diagnosed diffuse large B-cell lymphoma and 34 patients who had been previously treated or had a preexisting history of low grade lymphoma. Shown in panel *A* is hierarchical clustering of 100 genes, with each row representing a single gene and each column representing a patient specimen. Red indicates overexpression and green decreased expression. Genes characteristically expressed by germinal-center B cells and activated B cell are indicated, whereas the type 3 group did not highly express either set of genes.
Shown in panel *B* are the Kaplan-Meyer overall survival estimates for the 240 newly diagnosed patients who all received anthracycline based chemotherapy (predominantly CHOP). Reproduced with permission from Rosenwald A et al.[49]

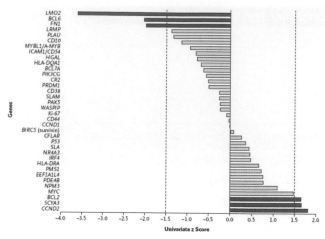

Figure 11–5. Quantitative polymerase chain reaction analyses of 36 genes was performed in 66 patients with newly diagnosed diffuse large B-cell lymphoma. Using a *z* score from univariate analysis with overall survival (OS) as a dependent variable, the genes are ranked here on the basis of their predictive power. A negative score is associated with longer OS whereas a positive score is associated with shorter OS. The six genes that were the strongest predictors (*LMO2, BCL6, FN1, CCND2, SCYA3,* and *BCL2*) were then used to create a multivariate prediction model. Reproduced with permission from Lossos IS et al.[50]

If the decision is made to treat, then single-agent front-line possibilities include rituximab, chlorambucil, cyclophosphamide, or fludarabine. Single-agent rituximab has been associated with a 70 to 80% response rate (RR) and approximately 20% complete remission rate (CR).[52] Options for multiagent therapy include the addition of rituximab to the other single agents mentioned or to combination regimens such as CVP (cyclophosphamide, vincristine, prednisone), CHOP (cyclophosphamide, doxorubicin, vincristine, and prednisone), and FND (fludarabine, mitoxantrone, dexamethasone). It is worth noting that there has been no proven survival benefit from early anthracycline exposure in follicular NHL.[53]

In a recently published trial, patients with stage III or IV follicular lymphoma were randomly assigned to receive either 8 cycles of CVP plus rituximab (R-CVP) or CVP alone. Without any increase in toxicity, all outcomes were superior with R-CVP, including overall response rate (81% versus 57%), CR (41% versus 10%), and time to progression (median 32 months versus 15 months).[54] Studies conducted combining rituximab with either CHOP or fludarabine showed better outcomes than with R-CVP; however, these were both phase II studies.[55,56] In a recent randomized study, fludara-

bine and mitoxantrone followed by rituximab therapy was associated with a 71% molecular CR versus 51% for CHOP followed by rituximab.[57] Despite these impressive CR rates, no regimen has been found to improve overall survival in FL, which admittedly will be difficult to demonstrate in an indolent disorder unless better risk stratification (eg, the FLIPI score) is employed in future clinical trials.

In addition to upfront therapy, there are data supporting maintenance therapy with rituximab. In one study, 151 patients with responding or stable FL at week 12 after rituximab monotherapy were randomized to either no further treatment or 4 additional doses of rituximab at 8-week intervals.[58] The median EFS was 36 and 19 months, respectively.[58] Similar benefits were noted in a phase III Swiss Intergroup study.[59] However, it is unclear how this compares to retreatment with rituximab at the time of progression, which is associated with a 40% response rate.

In a prospective, multicenter trial, patients with relapsed disease after chemotherapy, but with responding/stable disease with rituximab monotherapy, were subsequently randomized to either retreatment at the time of lymphoma progression or maintenance rituximab weekly × 4, repeated at 6-month intervals for a total of four courses.[60] Declining accrual led to trial termination, but of the 90 patients randomized, all outcomes favored maintenance, with overall response rate of 52% versus 35%, CR of 27% versus 4%, and median PFS of 31 versus 8 months. However, the median duration of rituximab benefit was similar for both groups (31 versus 27 months).[60] Many questions therefore remain regarding the dose, schedule, cost-effectiveness, and possible drug resistance of maintenance rituximab therapy.

Radioimmunotherapy has also become part of the armamentarium in the treatment of indolent NHL (Figure 11–6). Treatment of patients with relapsed or refractory follicular NHL with the yttrium 90 conjugated murine anti-CD20 monoclonal antibody (Zevalin) resulted in 80% RR, including 30% CR in a phase III study.[61] Studies with the murine anti-CD20 monoclonal antibody conjugated to [131]I (Bexxar) have found similar RR (55 to 71%) and CR (20 to 35%).[62,63] Importantly, radioimmunotherapy does not preclude stem cell

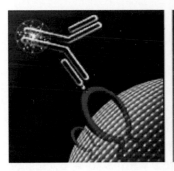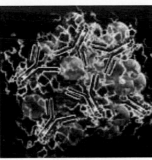

Figure 11–6. Antibodies directed against the CD20 antigen can be tagged with radioactive isotopes such as yttrium 90 (ibritumomab tiuxetan–Zevalin™) or iodine 131 (tositumomab–Bexxar™) resulting in damage to the targeted cell and other nearby cells.

collection for transplantation and is also being incorporated into some preparative transplant regimens.

Few randomized studies are published on the use of stem cell transplantation (SCT) in indolent NHL. In the European CUP trial, 89 patients with relapsed FL responding to salvage chemotherapy and with limited bone marrow involvement were randomized to further chemotherapy or SCT. The outcomes favored SCT, with 2-year PFS (26% versus 58%) and 4-year OS (46% versus 71%).[64] In a recent larger German Low Grade Lymphoma Study Group (GLSG) study, a similar benefit in 5-year PFS (33% versus 64.7% for interferon maintenance versus SCT) was noted, without sufficient events or follow-up to compare OS. However, both the GLSG study and the Groupe Ouest-Est des Leucemies et des Autres Maladies du Sang (GOELAMS) study evaluating SCT as front-line therapy have found an increased incidence of secondary hematologic malignancies that may obscure any benefit in overall survival from disease control.[65,66]

A comparison of autologous and myeloablative allogenic transplants performed in patients with FL found the decrease in relapse to be offset by the increase in transplant-related mortality (TRM).[67] There are numerous trials investigating reduced intensity conditioning regimens. The largest published so far found that 52 patients with relapsed indolent lymphoma, who received nonmyeloablative allogenic transplants, had a 100-day TRM of 11% and 2-year OS of 65%.[68]

At this time, autologous SCT is recommended for patients who have a good performance status and chemotherapy-sensitive disease in second relapse, or patients in first relapse whose first remission duration is < 1 year. Nonmyeloablative allogenic transplants are being performed primarily in the context of clinical trials.

Another novel approach to therapy capitalizes on the fact that vaccination with the unique tumor-specific immunoglobulin idiotype (Id) protein, which is expressed in a clonal fashion by each patient with B-cell lymphoma, induces humoral and/or cellular anti-Id immune responses. Of the 136 patients with FL who had received Id vaccination, those who mounted humoral immune responses (35%) had a longer PFS than those who did not (8.21 versus 3.38 years). Also predictive of improved outcome was the genotype of the immunoglobulin Fc gamma receptor.[69] Sponsored by the National Cancer Institute, a multicenter randomized phase III anti-Id vaccine trial is ongoing.

Mantle Cell Lymphomas

The management of mantle cell lymphoma (MCL) is challenging in that the disease shares morphologic features with indolent lymphomas and is incurable; however, it also exhibits the clinical behavior of aggressive lymphomas. As shown in Tables 11–2 and 11–4, it is typically characterized by coexpression of CD20 and CD5 but not CD23 or CD10. Many cases are associated with t(11;14)(q13;q32) translocation and cyclin D1 overexpression. In one study of 151 cases of lymphoma with morphology consistent with MCL, 85% demonstrated positive nuclear staining for cyclin D1 by immunohistochemistry. Relative to the cyclin D1-negative group, the cyclin D1-positive group was associated with a higher IPI score and worse 5-year survival (86% versus 30%).[70] Gene expression profiling has also identified a cohort lacking molecular expression of cyclin D1.[71]

Most patients will have advanced-stage disease, with 70% presenting with stage IV disease, and will require systemic therapy.[4] Due to the absence of a standard of care, patients with MCL should be preferentially treated on clinical trials. Treatment with single-agent alkylators such as chlorambucil results in approximately 40% RR, with 10 to 15% CR but a median duration of response of only 8 to 12 months.[72] Results with single-agents fludarabine and rituximab are comparable.[73–75] The combination of rituximab with CHOP resulted in better overall response rates of 96%, including a 48% CR. However, the median time to progression was only 16.6 months and even in patients demonstrating a molecular CR was not significantly prolonged.[76]

The underwhelming results from conventional therapy led to interest in high-dose chemotherapy with autologous stem cell rescue. Data from two studies have found the 5-year OS to be 50 to 77% and DFS at 33 to 43%.[77,78] Therefore, patients with MCL in first remission should undergo high-dose chemotherapy with SCT for the possibility of a more durable remission. Nonmyeloablative allogenic transplants appear promising as well.[79] One of the most promising therapies for relapsed disease has been the proteasome inhibitor bortezomib, for which a 50% RR was observed in heavily pretreated populations.[80,81] Other options for relapsed disease include radioimmunotherapy (with or without chemotherapy), anti-idiotype vaccines, flavoperidol to target the cyclin D1 activity, antisense *BCL2*, and thalidomide.

Aggressive Lymphomas

DLBCL, grade 3 follicular lymphoma, and anaplastic large cell lymphoma (ALCL) are all treated in the same fashion; the only exception is that ALCL is not treated with the anti-CD20 antibody rituximab that is specific for B-cell lymphomas. Nearly 50% of patients with DLBCL can be cured with anthracycline-based induction therapy, with CHOP proven to be as efficacious and safer than other combination chemotherapy regimens.[82]

Prior to treatment with CHOP, it is recommended that patients (particularly the elderly) have a baseline evaluation of the cardiac ejection fraction. Every attempt should be made to administer the standard dosages on time (every 21 days). Attention should also be given to minimizing sequelae of tumor lysis with initial therapy by aggressive hydration, use of allopurinol, and if necessary, the use of rasburicase, a recombinant urate-oxidase enzyme.

Treatment guidelines for patients with nonbulky stages I to II DLBCL are guided by the results of the Miller study, where approximately 400 patients were randomized to receive either eight cycles of CHOP alone or three cycles of CHOP followed by involved-field radiotherapy (40 to 55 Gy).[83] The 5-year PFS was 64% versus 77%, respectively, and OS was 72% versus 82%. In addition, fewer life-threatening toxic effects and decreases in left ventricular ejection fraction were seen with combined-modality therapy.[83] Therefore, patients with stage I to II nonbulky DLBCL, who also lack adverse IPI risk factors, can be treated with 3 to 4 cycles of CHOP, followed by involved-field radiation (30 to 40 Gy). The benefit of adding rituximab (R) is unclear, but most would do so. If any of the adverse IPI risk factors are present or there is bulky disease, then patients should receive a full course (6 to 8 cycles) of R-CHOP with or without adjuvant radiation therapy.

For patients with higher stages DLBCL, the Groupe d'Etude des Lymphomes de l'Adulte (GELA) study showed that relative to CHOP, the addition of rituximab (R-CHOP) improved CR (63% versus 76%), 2-year EFS (39% versus 57%), and OS (57% versus 70%).[84] Outcome improvement in all age groups was noted in a retrospective British Columbia study as well as the randomized MabThera International Trial (MInT) trial involving patients younger than 60.[85] The latter was terminated early with CR rates of 66% versus 84.7% for CHOP versus R-CHOP, respectively, and 15-month EFS of 62.5% versus 84%.[86] Thus, for patients with stages III to IV DLBCL falling into the low or low-intermediate IPI risk group, a full course of R-CHOP is indicated for patients of all ages.

When CHOP became the standard of care for DLBCL (prior to the advent of rituximab), the Germans started several prospective randomized trials to determine whether CHOP could be improved. One approach was to add etoposide to CHOP (CHOEP) at 100 mg/m^2 on days 1 through 3. In young low-risk patients, when compared to CHOP, CHOEP was associated with higher CR (87.6% versus 79.4%) and 5-year EFS (69.2% versus 57.6%), but not OS. In addition, CHOEP was also associated with increased cytopenias, transfusion requirements, intravenous antibiotic use, and cost (due to granulocyte colony stimulating factor or GCSF).[87] In patients 61 to 75 years of age, CHOEP was associated with increased toxicity.[88]

Another variable examined by the German group was decreasing the time between cycles of CHOP, from the standard 21 days to 14 days (CHOP-14) with mandatory administration of GCSF starting day 4 of each 14-day cycle. CHOP-14 was associated with better OS (85.0% versus 79.2%), but no difference in EFS was noted.[87] For CHOP-14 and CHOP-21 in elderly patients, improvement was noted in all outcomes, including CR (76.1% versus 60.1%), 5-year EFS (43.8% versus 32.5%), and OS (53.3% versus 43.8%, respectively). Although encouraging, before making CHOEP-21 in young patients or CHOP-14 in the elderly the standard of care, direct comparisons with rituximab and CHOP (both 21 and 14) are required, which are ongoing.[88]

The role of high-dose chemotherapy with ASCT as part of initial therapy for high-risk individuals remains controversial, but recent studies suggest there may be clinical benefit to this approach. One trial in Milan randomized patients with high-risk IPI scores to combination chemotherapy versus high-dose chemotherapy with bone marrow transplantation, and found superior CR and EFS with transplantation but no statistically significant difference in OS.[89] The recent study by Milpied and colleagues found at 5 years not only improved estimated EFS (55% versus 37%), but also improved OS (74 versus 44%) for those patients with a high-intermediate-risk age-adjusted IPI score.[90] However, the increased morbidity, mortality, and cost of high-dose chemotherapy with ASCT was not justified for nearly two-thirds of patients, thereby highlighting the role of better risk stratification, perhaps with gene expression profiling. Moreover, no randomized studies have yet compared upfront high-dose chemotherapy with ASCT to the current standard of care, rituximab with CHOP. The indication and timing of ASCT is an area of active clinical research, and patients with high-intermediate- or high-risk IPI scores should be treated in the context of a clinical trial.

Patients receiving induction chemotherapy should have radiologic evaluation repeated after 3 to 4 cycles. After the disease becomes undetectable by radiologic studies, two additional cycles of R-CHOP should be administered to ensure elimination of any microscopic disease. The functional imaging modalities (ie, gallium and PET scans) are very useful in following patients' responses to treatment, particularly in distinguishing whether an abnormality on CT scan represents residual disease as opposed to fibrotic or necrotic tissue.

Patients with either disease relapse or refractory to primary therapy should be treated with a salvage noncross-resistant regimen. Second-line regimens include ICE (ifosfamide, carboplatin, etoposide), DHAP (dexamethasone, high-dose cytarabine, cisplatin), or EPOCH (96-hour continuous intravenous etoposide, vincristine, doxorubicin with bolus cytoxan and daily prednisone). Rituximab can also be added for patients with CD20-positive diseases. Those patients with a response to a salvage regimen should then receive high-dose therapy with stem cell rescue. This was confirmed in the PARMA trial, where the 5-year OS was 46% for patients with relapsed disease randomized to receive high-dose chemotherapy with ASCT versus 12% in the group treated with chemotherapy alone.[91] However, chemosensitivity to second-line therapy correlates with outcomes, with 3-year OS of 19% versus 48% for patients with resistant versus sensitive disease in another trial.[92] Patients with high IPI scores at initiation of salvage therapy, or chemoresistance to salvage regimens, should therefore be considered for investigational treatment.[47]

Highly Aggressive Lymphomas

Lymphoblastic lymphomas and BL have a high risk of tumor lysis, so the appropriate prophylactic measures described above for aggressive lymphomas should be employed and the first cycle of chemotherapy should be administered in a monitored, inpatient setting. Lymphoblastic lymphomas are treated in the same way as acute lymphoblastic leukemias, the details of which are beyond the scope of this chapter.

Patients with limited-stage BL have an excellent prognosis, even with limited chemotherapy and without radiation. However, adults with advanced-stage disease, when treated with large-cell lymphoma regimens such as CHOP, have had poor outcomes, with OS < 15% at 3 years.[93,94] This has led to the investigation of more intensive treatments, initially taken from pediatric regimens.

Phase II trials have suggested that significantly better outcomes can be achieved with regimens containing multiple alternating cycles of noncross-resistant agents including augmented doses of alkylating agents and high-dose methotrexate. One such regimen is CODOX-M (cyclophosphamide, vincristine, doxorubicin, high-dose methotrexate) alternating with IVAC (ifosfamide, etoposide, high-dose cytarabine), which even in high-risk patients was associated with a 2-year EFS of 60% and OS of 70%.[95,96] At 3 years, the OS for patients treated with the French Lymphomes Malins B (LMB) regimens was approximately 75%.[97] An alternative dose-intensive regimen is hyperCVAD (hyperfractionated cyclophosphamide, vincristine, doxorubicin, dexamethasone with alternating high-dose methotrexate and cytarabine), used also in patients with HIV and with or without rituximab.[98,99] Efforts are also underway to shorten the duration of intensive chemotherapy, such as the Cancer and Leukemia Group B (CALGB) 9251 regimen, which includes triple intrathecal therapy with or without cranial irradiation.[100] Patients with relapsed or refractory BL should be treated on clinical trials.

AIDS-Related Lymphomas

The majority of NHLs that develop in patients with HIV are systemic lymphomas, either DLBCL or BL, but approximately 15% are primary CNS lymphoma (PCNSL), and approximately 4% are primary effusion lymphomas (PEL).[101] Whereas BL is generally found in patients with higher CD4 counts, patients with CD4 < 100 cells/µL are at increased risk of PEL, and those with CD4 < 50 are at increased risk for PCNSL.[102] Highly active anti-retroviral therapy (HAART) should be started on all patients with AIDS-related lymphoma (ARL), as immune reconstitution is a key component of treatment.

Generally, the treatment of systemic lymphomas is similar to that for patients without HIV, with a few exceptions. Intrathecal chemotherapy prophylaxis is crucial, as patients with HIV are at higher risk for CNS involvement. The use of rituximab in the treatment of ARL is controversial. Preliminary information from two studies suggests that rituximab may increase the risk of neutropenia and infection.[103,104]

The added benefit of rituximab in HIV-associated lymphoma is also not clear, as the benefit of rituximab in HIV-negative patients is seen particularly in patients with BCL2 overexpression. Little and colleagues found less BCL2 expression in patients with HIV than in those without (16% versus 41%).[105]

In the same study, the dose-adjusted continuous infusion regimen EPOCH (etoposide, prednisone, vincristine, cyclophosphamide, and doxorubicin) resulted in 74% CR, and at 53 months, DFS and OS of 92% and 60%, respectively. These outcomes seem significantly better than standard CHOP, which has been associated with 40% OS at 36 months.[106] Trials are ongoing to compare the importance of both rituximab and infusional therapy.

PEL can present with symptoms due to malignant effusions in the pericardium, pleura, peritoneum, joints, or meninges. Masses and nodal involvement are typically absent. In one case series, complete remission was obtained in 3 out of 7 patients treated with combination chemotherapy including high-dose methotrexate.[107] In another study, 42% of the 8 patients treated with a CHOP-like regimen had a complete remission.[101] Unfortunately, the median survival was 6 months, thus illustrating the need for clinical trials.[101]

Complications

Patients with NHL can experience complications due to disease involvement of various organ systems, including lymphomatous meningitis and/or CNS mass lesions; spinal cord compression; obstruction of airway, vena cava, intestines, or ureters (hydronephrosis); sequelae of serosal involvement, such as pericardial tamponade; gastrointestinal perforation or fistulas; splenic rupture; hepatic, adrenal, or renal insufficiency due to organ replacement; leukocytosis or hyperviscosity syndrome; paraneoplastic conditions including hypercalcemia; tumor lysis syndrome; autoimmune hemolytic anemia or thrombocytopenia.

Additional complications can occur from therapy, such as radiation-induced damage to normal tissue near the field of radiation; bone marrow aplasia or anemia or thrombocytopenia; myelodysplasia or second malignancies; infertility; intolerance of steroids; motor or sensory or autonomic neuropathy from vinca alkaloids; and cardiotoxicity from anthracyclines.

HODGKIN'S LYMPHOMA

Epidemiology

Thomas Hodgkin has been credited with first identifying this disease, which has subsequently been identified as a lymphoma. The incidence of HL is consistently lower than that of NHL and has decreased over the past 30 years. As shown in Figure 11–7, the age-specific incidence of HL has a bimodal distribution in the United States, with one peak at age 25 years and another at age 80 years. After the age of 25 years, males tend to have higher incidence rates than females.

Classification

As shown in Table 11–1, the WHO classifies HL into two distinct entities: nodular lymphocyte-predominant HL (NLPHL) and classical HL. The unifying feature is the presence of a large single and multinucleated neoplastic cell, called the Reed-Sternberg cell (Figure 11–8), which is outnumbered by surrounding non-neoplastic inflammatory and accessory cells. Based on immunoglobulin rearrangement studies, Reed-Sternberg cells represent clonal tumor-cell populations derived from germinal center B cells in 95% of cases.[108,109] In rare cases, they represent transformed T lymphocytes.

NLPHL comprises approximately 5% of all HLs.[2] As implied by the name, nodularity and the presence of many small lymphocytes and occasional Reed-Sternberg cells are characteristic (Figure

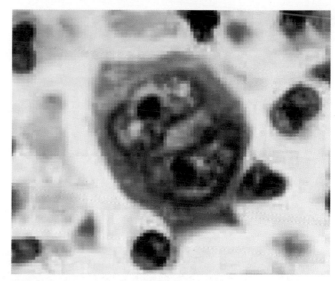

Figure 11–8. A typical Reed-Sternberg cell with a clear area surrounding the nucleoli.

11–9A). Furthermore, many popcorn or L and H (lymphocytic and/or histocytic) Reed-Sternberg variants are seen that have small peripheral nucleoli resulting in the appearance of a popped kernel of corn. Approximately 75% of patients are male, and most present with low-stage disease and generally have a good prognosis.[110]

Nodular sclerosis (NS) is the most common subtype and derives its name from the fact that fibrosis in the tumor divides it into nodules (Figure 11–9B). Typically seen in young females, the prognosis is generally favorable. Tissue eosinophilia appears to signify poor prognosis in this variant.[111] It is also the most frequent subtype found in children, accounting for 98% of pediatric HL cases.

Mixed cellularity has an infiltrate that includes plasma cells, eosinophils, lymphocytes, histiocytes, and Reed-Sternberg cells. Relative to NS, there is an increased incidence of B symptoms, extranodal disease, and subdiaphragmatic disease, all of which may account for a worse prognosis. It is the second most common variant in the Western world and is common in the elderly.

The lymphocyte-depleted variant has an increased reticular network and thus fewer cells (Figure 11–9C). Associated with advanced age and B symptoms, it has the worst prognosis. The number of cases identified as this subtype has decreased in recent years, partly due to immunophenotyping clas-

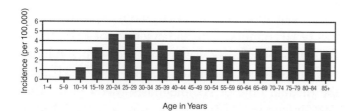

Figure 11–7. Age-specific incidence rates for Hodgkin's lymphoma, 1997–2001. Reproduced with permission from National Cancer Institute.[1]

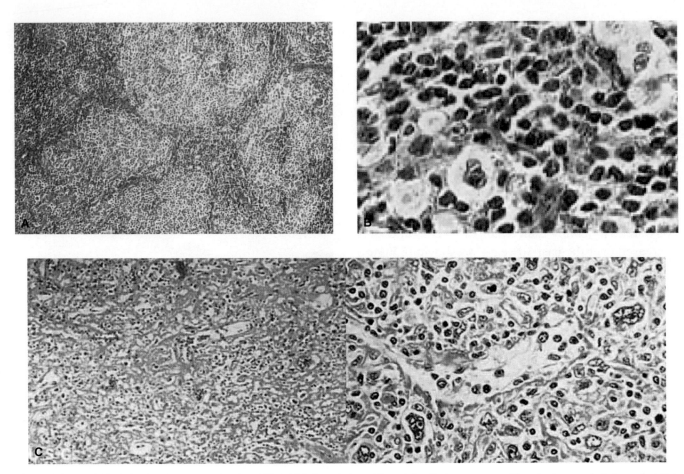

Figure 11–9. *A,* Nodular lymphocyte predominant Hodgkin's lymphoma with nodules that are apparent in a background of dense lymphocytic infiltrate. *B,* Nodular sclerosis. Reed-Sternberg cells with cytoplasmic retraction during fixation giving the appearance of a clear space or lacuna around the RS cell. *C,* Lymphocyte depleted, with few inflammatory cells present, findings are essentially cells and fibrosis.

sifying as T-cell lymphomas what might otherwise have been called lymphocyte-depleted HL.

Reed-Sternberg cells in NLPHL are unique in that they express mature B-cell antigens. In the other subtypes, most of the typical B-cell gene expression is lost and neither B- nor T-cell markers are expressed.[109] Reed-Sternberg cells in classical HL are characterized, however, by surface expression of CD30, a lymphoid antigen, in nearly all cases, and by expression of CD15, the myeloid antigen part of the tumor necrosis factor receptor superfamily, in 75 to 85% of cases.[2,112]

Etiology and Risk Factors

Several studies have found that in the young, a higher socioeconomic status (SES) is associated with an increased risk of HL, particularly the NS subtype.[113,114] Some have suggested that this risk

suggests a delayed exposure to an infectious agent. Other subtypes, however, such as mixed cellularity, are inversely correlated with SES.[115] In older adults, there appears to be no association with SES.[116]

The EBV, associated with approximately one-third of HL cases, is a postulated infectious agent.[117] EBV genomes and gene products detected in the Reed-Sternberg cells are frequently monoclonal, suggesting a causative role.[118] Recently, cases of HL that developed in nearly 40,000 patients with serologic evidence of an acute EBV infection had serologic evaluation of EBV in HL biopsy specimens. Of the 29 HL tumors, 55% had evidence of EBV. Infectious mononucleosis was associated with a relative risk of 4.0 for the diagnosis of EBV-positive HL, and the median time of HL diagnosis was 4 years after EBV infection.[119] EBV association varies by HL subtype, with 75 to 95% of mixed cellularity cases, 30% of NS cases, and only 10% of NLPHL cases having evidence of EBV.[118,120] The complex epidemiologic data regarding age, SES, EBV, and HL subtype lend credence to the idea that HL may actually be comprised of several different disease entities.[116,121]

Genetic factors have also been implicated. A recent large population study found that the relative risk of HL in relatives of patients with HL was 3.11 and was especially increased in families of affected individuals age < 40 years, in males, and in siblings.[122] Adding to a genetic contribution is the twin study that found the risk of HL to be nearly 100 times increased in monozygotic twins over dizygotic twins.[123]

Another major risk factor for HL is immunosuppression. Found in HIV-positive patients, both early with high CD4 counts and in advanced AIDS, the relative risk of developing HL in patients with HIV is 7.6 over the general population.[124] The majority of cases are mixed cellularity subtype and patients often present with B symptoms. From 75 to 90% of patients have widely disseminated extranodal disease, and 40 to 50% present with bone marrow involvement.[125,126]

Although much more rare than NHL, HL has occurred in patients receiving immunosuppressive therapy after organ transplantation, typically of the mixed cellularity subtype. Also, unlike posttransplant lymphoproliferative disorders (PTLD) and NHL, which are seen most often in the first year posttransplant, HD is seen 2 to 4 years later.[127,128] Like PTLD, however, EBV is detected in virtually all cases of HL found in transplant patients but also in patients with HIV.[126,127,129,130]

Diagnosis and Staging

The most common presentation of HL is a painless mass. Sixty to 70% of patients have cervical adenopathy, 50 to 60% have mediastinal adenopathy, and 25 to 35% have axillary node involvement.[131] In addition to pruritus and pain after alcohol ingestion, at sites of HL nodal involvement the typical constitutional B symptoms of weight loss, night sweats, and fevers may also be present. Cyclical fevers occurring at intervals of days to weeks, known as Pel-Ebstein fevers, are uncommon but nearly pathognomonic for HL.[132] In addition to the list of complications described above for NHL, HL has

been associated with rare but specific paraneoplastic conditions, including cerebellar degeneration and nephrotic syndrome.[133,134]

The discussion of tests for diagnosis and staging in NHL applies in its entirety to HL as well. In addition to the tests already mentioned, the serum albumin concentration should measured for patients with HL, as it has prognostic value. With respect to staging, HL typically progresses in an anatomically contiguous fashion, making the appearance of distant discrete sites of disease much rarer than for NHL. Table 11–5 shows the modifications made to the Ann Arbor staging system at the Cotswolds meeting.[44]

Historically, patients diagnosed with HL had staging laparotomies, which included splenectomy, liver biopsies, and excisional biopsies of retroperitoneal nodes. Particularly for those patients found to have limited disease by clinical staging, and therefore would be treated with radiation alone, a staging laparotomy was important in detecting occult disease, which would change the treatment plan.

Several studies have shown that with modern imaging techniques and the increased use of chemotherapy with earlier stage disease, laparotomy does not improve overall or relapse-free survival.[135,136] In fact, the morbidity and mortality of a staging laparotomy is sometimes associated with inferior outcomes.[137] Since the laparotomy is typically no longer performed, patients with early-stage HL should have in addition to CT scans either a PET or gallium scan to ensure that there is no subdiaphragmatic disease. PET scans appear to be more sensitive than gallium scans, particularly for splenic involvement.[31,138,139]

Since many patients are diagnosed with HL while in their reproductive years, fertility issues should be discussed early with patients. In particular, patients requiring either chemotherapy or pelvic radiation should be offered semen cryopreservation or oophoropexy. If splenic radiation is being contemplated, vaccination for pneumococcous, H. flu, and mengiococcus is recommended.

Prognosis

As with most malignancies, age is a prognostic factor. Age > 50 years at time of HL diagnosis is associated with decreased survival. This has been attributed to both increased comorbidities or sequelae of HL treatment and decreased efficacy of salvage treatment at relapse.[140,141]

For localized (stages I to II) HL, the unfavorable prognostic factors are indicated in Table 11–8. These include bulky diseases, which for a mediastinal mass is defined as having a diameter greater than one-third of the maximum intrathoracic diameter at the level of T5/T6 interspace. For any other mass, it is a diameter > 10 cm.[142] B symptoms and an ESR > 30 mm/h, or an ESR > 50 mm/h without B symptoms, is another poor prognostic factor.[143] Finally, having > 3 sites of involvement is associated with inferior outcomes.[144] Although approximately 60% of patients fall into the favorable-risk group, the use of chemotherapy in addition to radiation therapy in all patients with limited-stage disease makes the significance of these prognostic factors less clear.

In the International Prognostic Factors Project (IPFP) on advanced Hodgkin's disease, the outcomes of 5,141 patients with advanced HL (defined by the participating institutions' local guidelines) were evaluated. Patients were treated with at least four planned cycles of combination chemotherapy (preferably containing doxorubicin) with or without radiotherapy. As shown in Table 11–9, multivariate analysis identified seven risk factors that had hazard ratios ranging from 0.23 to 0.40. This model risk-stratified patients into six groups, with 5-year relapse free rates ranging from 82 to 42%.[145]

The prognostic value of the B-cell marker CD20, which is expressed in 10 to 30% of HL, is unclear. For HL patients treated with ABVD (doxorubicin, bleomycin, vinblastine, and dacarbazine), one study found both time to treatment failure and OS to be significantly decreased in those patients who had CD20 expression compared to those who did not.[146] However, two other studies found no difference in outcomes.[147,148] A prospective trial with a large number of patients is necessary to settle this issue.

Treatment of Limited-Stage Classical Hodgkin's Lymphomas

For patients with stages I to II HL, a meta-analysis of 13 trials comparing combined-modality therapy

Table 11–8. UNFAVORABLE FACTORS FOR LIMITED STAGE HODGKIN'S LYMPHOMA[142–144]

Bulky Disease
  Mediastinal mass maximum width > ⅓ of maximum
    intrathoracic diameter
  Any other mass > 10 cm
Erythrocyte sedimentation rate (ESR)
  > 30 if B symptoms present
  > 50i f no B symptoms
> 3 sites of disease

(CMT) to radiation therapy (RT) alone found no survival differences. However, CMT, which typically involved a MOPP-like regimen (mechlorethamine, vincristine, procarbazine, prednisone; Table 11–10) was associated with a lower risk of relapse at 10 years than RT alone (15.8% versus 32.7% respectively).[149]

Since patients with HL have amongst the best outcomes of any malignancy, recent efforts have been directed toward decreasing toxicity. Three randomized trials have been performed using ABVD-based regimens (see Table 11–10) instead of MOPP, because the alkylator exposure in the latter regimen is associated with increased myelosuppression, gonadal toxicity, and delayed secondary hematologic malignan-

Table 11–9A. RISK FACTORS IDENTIFIED FOR ADVANCED HODGKIN'S LYMPHOMA

Risk Factors Identified
Age > 45 years
Male sex
Stage IV disease
White blood cell (WBC) > 15k
Absolute Lymphocyte Count (ALC)
< 600 or < 8% WBC or both
Hg <10.5 g/dL
Albumin < 4 g/dL

Adapted from Hasenclever D and Diehl V.[145]

Table 11–9B. RISK FACTORS IDENTIFIED FOR ADVANCED HODGKIN'S LYMPHOMA

No. of Risk Factors	% Freedom from Disease Progression
0	84
1	77
2	67
3	60
4	51
≥ 5	42

Adapted from Hasenclever D and Diehl V.[145]

Table 11–10. TREATMENT MODALITIES IN HODGKIN'S LYMPHOMA

Chemotherapy Guidelines
ABVD[174]
    Doxorubicin 25 mg/m² IV d1, 15
    Bleomycin 10 mg/m² IV d1, 15
    Vinblastine 6 mg/m² IV d1, 15
    Dacarbazine 375 mg/m² IV d1, 15

MOPP[175]
    Mechlorethamine 6.0 mg/m² IV d1, 8
    Vincristine 1.4 mg/m² IV d1, 8 (uncapped)
    Procarbazine 100 mg/m² PO d1-14
    Prednisone 40 mg/m² PO d1-14 (only cycle 1,4)

Stanford V[176]
    Doxorubicin 25 mg/m² IV d1, 15
    Vinblastine 6 mg/m²* IV d1, 15
    Mechlorethamine 6 mg/m² IV d1
    Vincristine 1.4 mg/m²* IV (max 2 mg) d8, 22
    Bleomycin 5 units/m² IV d8, 22
    Etoposide 60 mg/m² IV d15, 16
    Prednisone 40 mg/m²* PO qid, every other day for 10 weeks then taper weeks 11 to 12

q28d × 3 cycles, then XRT to sites > 5 cm or macroscopic splenic disease
Vinblastine dose to 4 mg/m² for cycle 3 if patient > 50 years old
Vincristine dose to 1 mg/m² for cycle 3 if patient > 50 years old
Prednisone tapered by 10 mg qid, starting week 10

	Standard Dose (mg/m²)	Increased Dose (mg/m²)	Day Given
BEACOPP[177]			
Bleomycin	10	10	8
Etoposide	100	200	1–3
Doxorubicin	25	35	1
Cyclophosphamide	650	1,200	1
Vincristine	1.4	1.4	8
Procarbazine	100	100	1–7
Prednisone	40	40	1–4

ABVD = doxorubicin, bleomycin, vinblastine, and dacarbazine; BEACOPP = bleomycin, etoposide, doxorubicin, cyclophosphamide, vincristine, procarbazine, and prednisone; IV = intravenously; MOPP = mechlorethamine, vincristine, procarbazine, prednisone; PO = per os; XRT = irradiation.

cies.[150] In these studies, CMT consisted of either 2 cycles of ABVD plus extended-field RT, 3 cycles of ABV plus extended-field RT, or 3 cycles of MOPP-ABV plus involved-field RT.[136,151,152] All three studies compared outcomes with patients randomized to extended-field RT alone. At time points ranging from 2 to 4 years in the different studies, EFS rates for CMT ranged from 94 to 99% versus 77 to 84% for RT. In each study, DFS was significantly better for the CMT arm than the RT arm, and in the European Organisation for Research and Treatment of Cancer (EORTC)-GELA study, OS at 4 years improved from 95% with RT alone to 99% with CMT.[152] Although the longer term follow-up from these studies has yet to be published, CMT with ABVD plus involved-field RT, has become the standard treatment approach for patients with limited-stage HL.

Extended-field RT is associated with an increased risk of secondary solid tumors. In an effort to reduce radiotherapy doses and fields, a nonrandomized prospective study found that even for tumors > 6 cm, in-field recurrence was equivalent whether patients received more or less than 35 Gy.[153] The German Hodgkin's Lymphoma Study Group's (GHSG) randomized multicenter HD8 study compared extended-field with involved-field radiation after chemotherapy in patients with unfavorable stages I to II HL. There was no difference in CR rates, 5-year OS or EFS, or secondary neoplasia in the two arms; however, marrow suppression and gastrointestinal toxicity were more frequent in the extended-field arm.[154]

Whereas four cycles of ABVD followed by IFRT have become the standard of care for most individuals with stages I to II HL, those with bulky mediastinal disease usually receive a full six cycles of ABVD followed by involved-field RT. The ongoing HD10 trial of the GHSG is investigating not only whether involved-field doses can be further reduced, but also whether fewer cycles of chemotherapy can be used. In this study, patients with favorable stages I to II HL were randomized in a two-by-two design to receive either 2 or 4 cycles of ABVD followed by either 20 or 30 Gy of involved-field RT. With a median follow up of 2 years, the OS and DFS rates were 98.5% and 96.6%, respectively, and there have been no difference in outcomes in the four arms of the study.[155] Thus, while CMT has been established as the standard of care for limited stage HL, the emerging trend appears to be toward using lower doses and smaller fields of radiation, with possibly fewer cycles of chemotherapy as well.

Treatment of Advanced-Stage Classical Hodgkin's Lymphomas

For patients with advanced (stages III to IV) HL, the mainstay of treatment is chemotherapy, with or without RT. A randomized trial comparing ABVD and MOPP in advanced disease found MOPP to be associated with inferior response rates relative to ABVD (67% versus 82%) and DFS at 5 years (50% versus 61%). There was no significant difference in OS, estimated at 70% at 5 years.[156] When combined with the increased toxicities seen with MOPP, as described above, ABVD is the standard regimen for the treatment of advanced HL.

One of the concerns of using ABVD, however, is the cardiotoxicity of doxorubicin and the pulmonary toxicity of bleomycin being potentially followed by radiation damage to the same organs. The Stanford V regimen (see Table 11–10) is a briefer, but more intense, chemotherapy regimen, and is followed by radiation to sites of disease > 5 cm. For 142 patients with advanced HL treated with this regimen, failure-free progression was 89% at 5 years and OS was 96%.[157,158] Similar results were obtained by an Italian group, with 48 patients.[158] The advantage of this regimen is lower cumulative exposure to doxorubicin and bleomycin, suggesting a reduced risk of infertility and secondary neoplasms. A randomized,

multicenter phase III trial comparing Stanford V to ABVD is now underway.

In another randomized trial, patients with advanced HL were assigned to receive either eight cycles of cyclophosphamide, vincristine, procarbazine, and prednisone alternating with doxorubicin, bleomycin, vinblastine, and dacarbazine (COPP-ABVD); bleomycin, etoposide, doxorubicin, cyclophosphamide, vincristine, procarbazine, and prednisone (BEACOPP; see Table 11–10); or increased-dose BEACOPP; each followed by local RT when indicated. With nearly 2,000 patients enrolled, the 5-year freedom from treatment failure was 69% in the COPP-ABVD group, 76% in the BEACOPP group, and 87% in the increased-dose BEACOPP group. The five-year rates of OS were 83%, 88%, and 91%, respectively. Therefore, dose-escalated BEACOPP improved both tumor control and OS when compared with COPP-ABVD.[159] However, it is important to recognize that significant benefit was only observed in those with ≥ 4 IPFP risk factors (see Table 11–9), and these are the only individuals in whom this regimen should be considered. This regimen may be associated with a greater risk of secondary myelodysplasia or acute myeloid leukemia relative to the other treatments used in this trial.

A critical aspect of the treatment of HL is restaging at all sites of initial disease to determine the response to the first four cycles of ABVD or MOPP therapy. Gallium or PET scans are particularly helpful in distinguishing residual disease from fibrotic or necrotic remnants of initially bulky disease. In one study, a negative PET scan was 95% accurate in predicting remission at 1 year, whereas a positive PET scan was 60% accurate at predicting relapse.[160]

The general principle here is that evidence of a complete or near-complete response upon restaging after four cycles means that consolidation can be initiated. For stages I to II disease, this would be radiation therapy, and for stages III to IV, this would mean an additional two cycles of chemotherapy. With advanced-stage disease, two cycles of chemotherapy are always given after radiologic resolution of disease (to a maximum of eight cycles). RT at 20 to 36 Gy may then be administered to sites of bulky disease at diagnosis. For the Stanford V regimen, as mentioned above, 36 Gy should be delivered to sites > 5 cm at diagnosis.

In the event of < 50% decrease in initial disease or persistently positive PET or gallium scans, a repeat biopsy may be indicated to confirm the diagnosis of presumed persistent HL. The treatment options for persistent HL would then include secondary chemotherapy, RT, or high-dose therapy with ASCT.

Treatment of Nodular Lymphocyte-Predominant Hodgkin's Lymphoma

For patients with stage I NLPHL whose site of disease is unilateral and above the hyoid bone, involved-field or regional RT is recommended. Patients with stage Ia disease in other sites or IIa disease can either be treated in the same fashion, or alternatively, with chemotherapy combined with involved-field RT. Patients with stage IIb disease have the same options or treatment with locoregional RT or chemotherapy alone. Relapse-free survival at 8 years for early-stage disease is 71 to 85% and OS approximately 95%.[110]

In one study, stage IV NLPHL disease was associated with an OS of only 40%, although this was derived from a retrospective study with a variety of therapeutic regimens.[110] However, compared with Classical Hodgkin's Lymphoma, patients with NLPHL appear to have more relapses (27% had more than one relapse) but seem to have better salvage rates at time of relapse. In addition, treatment for NLPHL was associated with more deaths from secondary malignancies than from recurrent HL (32% versus 26%).

Since some patients with NLPHL have an indolent, multiply relapsing course, and the late toxicities of treatment appear to be substantial, some authors have suggested that (analogous to indolent NHL) patients with asymptomatic stage III or IVa disease should either be observed or treated with chemotherapy alone. Once symptomatic, chemotherapy with or without RT is recommended. In an effort to develop systemic therapies with less long-term toxicity, rituximab has been studied for NLPHL, which is characterized by CD20-positive tumor cells. In both the de novo and relapsed setting, significant responses have been seen in phase II trials, albeit sometimes of short duration when used as a single agent.[161-163]

Follow-Up

Five-year relative survival is 96% for HL in those under 20 years of age. For adults, the 5-year relative survival rate for patients with HL has doubled from 40% in whites in 1960, to more than 85% today. With longer follow-up, however, the most frequent cause of death is not recurrent HL. An international collaboration evaluated the outcomes of 9,041 patients with limited-stage HL, beginning in the early 1960s and approximately 20 years of follow-up. The cause of death of the 22% of patients who died was predominantly HL during the first 10 years of follow-up, but by 13 years, other causes of death had surpassed HL.[164] Subsequently, randomized trials have confirmed that nearly 60% of deaths in patients with HL were from causes other than HL, even at median follow-up periods of 2 to 4 years.[151,165]

Cardiovascular events and second cancers are the most common causes of death other than HL. A recent review of studies evaluating the occurrence of secondary malignancies found that solid tumors accounted for 59 to 89% of cases, and were more strongly associated with radiation or CMT. Leukemia and NHL accounted for much fewer numbers. While younger patients had a higher relative risk of developing secondary cancers, older patients had a higher absolute risk. With respect to cardiovascular events, the risk of death from coronary artery disease in patients with HL increases from 2 to 6% at 10 years to 10 to 12% at 15 to 25 years. The risks of carotid or subclavian vascular events and valvular heart disease are also increased.[166]

As described above, studies are ongoing to determine whether less intensive therapy can decrease toxicity without sacrificing efficacy. While awaiting these results, patients with HL require careful long-term follow-up to detect late treatment effects. For the year or two after treatment completion, history, physical examination, CBC, ESR, and chemistry profile should be done every 3 months. The interval should be increased to every 6 months for 5 years and then annually. Chest radiography or CT should be done every 3 to 6 months during the first 2 to 3 years and annually thereafter, whereas abdominal or pelvic CT should be checked every 6 to 12 months for the first 2 to 3 years and annually for the subsequent 2 years.

Thyroid-stimulating hormone should be checked annually for patients receiving RT to the neck. Chest radiation or bleomycin treatment warrants an annual influenza vaccination. For women receiving RT above the diaphragm, a mammography should be initiated at age 40 years or 8 years after therapy completion, whichever occurs sooner. Finally, for patients treated with splenic radiation, vaccinations for encapsulated organisms should be repeated every 6 years.[167]

REFERENCES

1. Surveillance, Epidemiology and End Results (SEER) Program, 1975–2001. National Cancer Institute; 2004.
2. Jaffe ES, Harris NL, Stein H, Vardiman JW, editors. Pathology and genetics of tumours of haematopoietic and lymphoid tissues. IARC Press; 2001.
3. A clinical evaluation of the International Lymphoma Study Group classification of non-Hodgkin's lymphoma. The Non-Hodgkin's Lymphoma Classification Project. Blood 1997;89:3909–18.
4. Armitage JO, Weisenburger DD. New approach to classifying non-Hodgkin's lymphomas: clinical features of the major histologic subtypes. Non-Hodgkin's Lymphoma Classification Project. J Clin Oncol 1998;16:2780–95.
5. Cote TR, Biggar RJ, Rosenberg PS, et al. Non-Hodgkin's lymphoma among people with AIDS: incidence, presentation and public health burden. AIDS/Cancer Study Group. Int J Cancer 1997;73:645–50.
6. Adami J, Gabel H, Lindelof B, et al. Cancer risk following organ transplantation: a nationwide cohort study in Sweden. Br J Cancer 2003;89:1221–7.
7. Kassan SS, Thomas TL, Moutsopoulos HM, et al. Increased risk of lymphoma in sicca syndrome. Ann Intern Med 1978;89:888–92.
8. Valesini G, Priori R, Bavoillot D, et al. Differential risk of non-Hodgkin's lymphoma in Italian patients with primary Sjögren's syndrome. J Rheumatol 1997;24:2376–80.
9. Nelson BP, Nalesnik MA, Bahler DW, et al. Epstein-Barr virus-negative post-transplant lymphoproliferative disorders: a distinct entity? Am J Surg Pathol 2000;24:375–85.
10. Shibata D, Weiss LM, Hernandez AM, et al. Epstein-Barr virus-associated non-Hodgkin's lymphoma in patients infected with the human immunodeficiency virus. Blood 1993;81:2102–9.
11. Miller G. Epstein-Barr virus: biology, pathogenesis, and medical aspects. New York: Raven Press; 1990.
12. Ziegler JL. Burkitt's lymphoma. N Engl J Med 1981;305:735–45.
13. Birmann B, Chang E, Mueller N. Epidemiology of lymphoma. Hamilton (ON): BC Decker Inc; 2002.
14. Hinuma Y, Komoda H, Chosa T, et al. Antibodies to adult T-cell leukemia-virus-associated antigen (ATLA) in sera from patients with ATL and controls in Japan: a nationwide sero-epidemiologic study. Int J Cancer 1982;29:631–5.
15. Cesarman E, Chang Y, Moore PS, et al. Kaposi's sarcoma-associated herpesvirus-like DNA sequences in AIDS-related body-cavity-based lymphomas. N Engl J Med 1995;332:1186–91.
16. Horenstein MG, Nador RG, Chadburn A, et al. Epstein-Barr virus latent gene expression in primary effusion lymphomas containing Kaposi's sarcoma-associated herpesvirus/human herpesvirus-8. Blood 1997;90:1186–91.
17. Hermine O, Lefrere F, Bronowicki JP, et al. Regression of splenic lymphoma with villous lymphocytes after treatment of hepatitis C virus infection. N Engl J Med 2002;347:89–94.
18. Shivapurkar N, Harada K, Reddy J, et al. Presence of simian virus 40 DNA sequences in human lymphomas. Lancet 2002;359:851–2.
19. Vilchez RA, Madden CR, Kozinetz CA, et al. Association between simian virus 40 and non-Hodgkin lymphoma. Lancet 2002;359:817–23.
20. Steinbach G, Ford R, Glober G, et al. Antibiotic treatment of gastric lymphoma of mucosa-associated lymphoid tissue. An uncontrolled trial. Ann Intern Med 1999;131:88–95.
21. Jelic S, Filipovic-Ljeskovic I. Positive serology for Lyme disease borrelias in primary cutaneous B-cell lymphoma: a study in 22 patients; is it a fortuitous finding? Hematol Oncol 1999;17:107–16.
22. Cerroni L, Zochling N, Putz B, Kerl H. Infection by Borrelia burgdorferi and cutaneous B-cell lymphoma. J Cutan Pathol 1997;24:457–61.
23. Keller-Byrne JE, Khuder SA, Schaub EA, McAfee O. A meta-analysis of non-Hodgkin's lymphoma among farmers in the central United States. Am J Ind Med 1997;31:442–4.
24. Rothman N, Cantor KP, Blair A, et al. A nested case-control study of non-Hodgkin lymphoma and serum organochlorine residues. Lancet 1997;350:240–4.
25. Shipp MA. Prognostic factors in aggressive non-Hodgkin's lymphoma: who has "high-risk" disease? Blood 1994;83:1165–73.
26. Anderson T, Chabner BA, Young RC, et al. Malignant lymphoma. 1. The histology and staging of 473 patients at the National Cancer Institute. Cancer 1982;50:2699–707.
27. Doberneck RC. The diagnostic yield of lymph node biopsy. Arch Surg 1983;118:1203–5.
28. Front D, Israel O, Epelbaum R, et al. Ga-67 SPECT before and after treatment of lymphoma. Radiology 1990;175:515–9.
29. Ben-Haim S, Bar-Shalom R, Israel O, et al. Utility of gallium-67 scintigraphy in low-grade non-Hodgkin's lymphoma. J Clin Oncol 1996;14:1936–42.
30. Elstrom R, Guan L, Baker G, et al. Utility of FDG-PET scanning in lymphoma by WHO classification. Blood 2003;101:3875–6.
31. Kostakoglu L, Leonard JP, Kuji I, et al. Comparison of fluorine-18 fluorodeoxyglucose positron emission tomography and Ga-67 scintigraphy in evaluation of lymphoma. Cancer 2002;94:879–88.
32. Shen YY, Kao A, Yen RF. Comparison of 18F-fluoro-2-deoxyglucose positron emission tomography and gallium-

67 citrate scintigraphy for detecting malignant lymphoma. Oncol Rep 2002;9:321–5.

33. Wirth A, Seymour JF, Hicks RJ, et al. Fluorine-18 fluorodeoxyglucose positron emission tomography, gallium-67 scintigraphy, and conventional staging for Hodgkin's disease and non-Hodgkin's lymphoma. Am J Med 2002; 112:262–8.

34. Kaplan WD, Jochelson MS, Herman TS, et al. Gallium-67 imaging: a predictor of residual tumor viability and clinical outcome in patients with diffuse large-cell lymphoma. J Clin Oncol 1990;8:1966–70.

35. Israel O, Mor M, Epelbaum R, et al. Clinical pretreatment risk factors and Ga-67 scintigraphy early during treatment for prediction of outcome of patients with aggressive non-Hodgkin lymphoma. Cancer 2002;94:873–8.

36. Zinzani PL, Magagnoli M, Franchi R, et al. Diagnostic role of gallium scanning in the management of lymphoma with mediastinal involvement. Haematologica 1999;84:604–7.

37. Torizuka T, Nakamura F, Kanno T, et al. Early therapy monitoring with FDG-PET in aggressive non-Hodgkin's lymphoma and Hodgkin's lymphoma. Eur J Nucl Med Mol Imaging 2004;31:22–8.

38. Spaepen K, Stroobants S, Dupont P, et al. Early restaging positron emission tomography with (18)F-fluorodeoxyglucose predicts outcome in patients with aggressive non-Hodgkin's lymphoma. Ann Oncol 2002;13:1356–63.

39. Jerusalem G, Beguin Y, Fassotte MF, et al. Whole-body positron emission tomography using 18F-fluorodeoxyglucose for posttreatment evaluation in Hodgkin's disease and non-Hodgkin's lymphoma has higher diagnostic and prognostic value than classical computed tomography scan imaging. Blood 1999;94:429–33.

40. Spaepen K, Stroobants S, Dupont P, et al. Prognostic value of positron emission tomography (PET) with fluorine-18 fluorodeoxyglucose ([18F]FDG) after first-line chemotherapy in non-Hodgkin's lymphoma: is [18F]FDG-PET a valid alternative to conventional diagnostic methods? J Clin Oncol 2001;19:414–9.

41. Conlan MG, Bast M, Armitage JO, Weisenburger DD. Bone marrow involvement by non-Hodgkin's lymphoma: the clinical significance of morphologic discordance between the lymph node and bone marrow. Nebraska Lymphoma Study Group. J Clin Oncol 1990;8:1163–72.

42. Campbell JK, Matthews JP, Seymour JF, et al. Optimum trephine length in the assessment of bone marrow involvement in patients with diffuse large cell lymphoma. Ann Oncol 2003;14:273–6.

43. van Besien K, Ha CS, Murphy S, et al. Risk factors, treatment, and outcome of central nervous system recurrence in adults with intermediate-grade and immunoblastic lymphoma. Blood 1998;91:1178–84.

44. Lister TA, Crowther D, Sutcliffe SB, et al. Report of a committee convened to discuss the evaluation and staging of patients with Hodgkin's disease: Cotswolds meeting. J Clin Oncol 1989;7:1630–6.

45. Rossi G, Donisi A, Casari S, et al. The International Prognostic Index can be used as a guide to treatment decisions regarding patients with human immunodeficiency virus-related systemic non-Hodgkin lymphoma. Cancer 1999;86:2391–7.

46. Moskowitz CH, Nimer SD, Glassman JR, et al. The international prognostic index predicts for outcome following autologous stem cell transplantation in patients with relapsed and primary refractory intermediate-grade lymphoma. Bone Marrow Transplant 1999;23:561–7.

47. Hamlin PA, Zelenetz AD, Kewalramani T, et al. Age-adjusted international prognostic index predicts autologous stem cell transplantation outcome for patients with relapsed or primary refractory diffuse large B-cell lymphoma. Blood 2003;102:1989–96.

48. Solal-Celigny P, Roy P, Colombat P, et al. Follicular lymphoma international prognostic index. Blood 2004;104: 1258–65.

49. Rosenwald A, Wright G, Chan WC, et al. The use of molecular profiling to predict survival after chemotherapy for diffuse large-B-cell lymphoma. N Engl J Med 2002; 346:1937–47.

50. Lossos IS, Czerwinski DK, Alizadeh AA, et al. Prediction of survival in diffuse large-B-cell lymphoma based on the expression of six genes. N Engl J Med 2004;350: 1828–37.

51. Mac Manus MP, Hoppe RT. Is radiotherapy curative for stage I and II low-grade follicular lymphoma? Results of a long-term follow-up study of patients treated at Stanford University. J Clin Oncol 1996;14:1282–90.

52. Colombat P, Salles G, Brousse N, et al. Rituximab (anti-CD20 monoclonal antibody) as single first-line therapy for patients with follicular lymphoma with a low tumor burden: clinical and molecular evaluation. Blood 2001; 97:101–6.

53. Dana BW, Dahlberg S, Nathwani BN, et al. Long-term follow-up of patients with low-grade malignant lymphomas treated with doxorubicin-based chemotherapy or chemoimmunotherapy. J Clin Oncol 1993;11:644–51.

54. Marcus R, Imrie K, Belch A, et al. CVP chemotherapy plus Rituximab compared with CVP as first-line treatment for advanced follicular lymphoma. Blood 2005;105:1417-23.

55. Czuczman MS, Fallon A, Mohr A, et al. Rituximab in combination with CHOP or fludarabine in low-grade lymphoma. Semin Oncol 2002;29:36–40.

56. Czuczman MS, Fallon A, Mohr A. Phase II study of rituximab plus fludarabine in patients (pts) with low-grade lymphoma (LGL) [abstract]. Blood 2001;98:601a

57. Zinzani PL, Pulsoni A, Perrotti A, et al. Fludarabine plus mitoxantrone with and without rituximab versus CHOP with and without rituximab as front-line treatment for patients with follicular lymphoma. J Clin Oncol 2004; 22:2654–61.

58. Ghielmini M, Schmitz SF, Cogliatti SB, et al. Prolonged treatment with rituximab in patients with follicular lymphoma significantly increases event-free survival and response duration compared with the standard weekly × 4 schedule. Blood 2004;103:4416–23.

59. Van Oers MH, Hagenbeek A, Van Glabbeke M, Teodorovic I. Chimeric anti-CD20 monoclonal antibody (Mabthera) in remission induction and maintenance treatment of relapsed follicular non-Hodgkin's lymphoma: a phase III randomized clinical trial—Intergroup Collaborative Study. Ann Hematol 2002;81:553–7.

60. Hainsworth J, Litchy SF, Greco A. Scheduled rituximab

maintenance therapy versus rituximab retreatment at progression in patients with indolent non-Hodgkin's lymphoma (NHL) responding to single-agent rituximab: a randomized trial of the Minnie Pearl Cancer Research Network. Blood 2003;102: Abstract no. 321.

61. Witzig TE, Gordon LI, Cabanillas F, et al. Randomized controlled trial of yttrium-90-labeled ibritumomab tiuxetan radioimmunotherapy versus rituximab immunotherapy for patients with relapsed or refractory low-grade, follicular, or transformed B-cell non-Hodgkin's lymphoma. J Clin Oncol 2002;20:2453–63.

62. Kaminski MS, Estes J, Zasadny KR, et al. Radioimmunotherapy with iodine (131)I tositumomab for relapsed or refractory B-cell non-Hodgkin lymphoma: updated results and long-term follow-up of the University of Michigan experience. Blood 2000;96:1259–66.

63. Kaminski MS, Zelenetz AD, Press OW, et al. Pivotal study of iodine I 131 tositumomab for chemotherapy-refractory low-grade or transformed low-grade B-cell non-Hodgkin's lymphomas. J Clin Oncol 2001;19:3918–28.

64. Schouten HC, Qian W, Kvaloy S, et al. High-dose therapy improves progression-free survival and survival in relapsed follicular non-Hodgkin's lymphoma: results from the randomized European CUP trial. J Clin Oncol 2003;21:3918–27.

65. Lenz D, Unterhalt M, Haferlach T, et al. Significant increase of secondary myelodysplasia and acute myeloid leukemia after myeloablative radiochemotherapy followed by autologous stem cell transplantation in indolent lymphoma patients: results of a prospective randomized study for the GLSG. Blood 2003;102: Abstract #3671.

66. Deconinck E, Foussard C, Bertrand PP, et al. Value of autologous stem cell transplantation in first line therapy of follicular lymphoma with high tumor burden: final results of the randomized GOELAMS 064 Trial. Blood 2003;102: Abstract no. 865.

67. van Besien K, Loberiza FR Jr, Bajorunaite R, et al. Comparison of autologous and allogeneic hematopoietic stem cell transplantation for follicular lymphoma. Blood 2003; 102:3521–9.

68. Robinson SP, Goldstone AH, Mackinnon S, et al. Chemoresistant or aggressive lymphoma predicts for a poor outcome following reduced-intensity allogeneic progenitor cell transplantation: an analysis from the Lymphoma Working Party of the European Group for Blood and Bone Marrow Transplantation. Blood 2002;100:4310–6.

69. Weng WK, Czerwinski D, Timmerman J, et al. Clinical outcome of lymphoma patients after idiotype vaccination is correlated with humoral immune response and immunoglobulin G Fc receptor genotype. J Clin Oncol 2004;22:4717–24.

70. Yatabe Y, Suzuki R, Tobinai K, et al. Significance of cyclin D1 overexpression for the diagnosis of mantle cell lymphoma: a clinicopathologic comparison of cyclin D1-positive MCL and cyclin D1-negative MCL-like B-cell lymphoma. Blood 2000;95:2253–61.

71. Rosenwald A, Wright G, Wiestner A, et al. The proliferation gene expression signature is a quantitative integrator of oncogenic events that predicts survival in mantle cell lymphoma. Cancer Cell 2003;3:185–97.

72. Evans LS, Hancock BW. Non-Hodgkin lymphoma. Lancet 2003;362:139–46.

73. Foran JM, Rohatiner AZ, Coiffier B, et al. Multicenter phase II study of fludarabine phosphate for patients with newly diagnosed lymphoplasmacytoid lymphoma, Waldenstrom's macroglobulinemia, and mantle-cell lymphoma. J Clin Oncol 1999;17:546–53.

74. Ghielmini M, Schmitz SF, Burki K, et al. The effect of rituximab on patients with follicular and mantle-cell lymphoma. Swiss Group for Clinical Cancer Research (SAKK). Ann Oncol 2000;11 Suppl 1:123–6.

75. Foran JM, Rohatiner AZ, Cunningham D, et al. European phase II study of rituximab (chimeric anti-CD20 monoclonal antibody) for patients with newly diagnosed mantle-cell lymphoma and previously treated mantle-cell lymphoma, immunocytoma, and small B-cell lymphocytic lymphoma. J Clin Oncol 2000;18:317–24.

76. Howard OM, Gribben JG, Neuberg DS, et al. Rituximab and CHOP induction therapy for newly diagnosed mantle-cell lymphoma: molecular complete responses are not predictive of progression-free survival. J Clin Oncol 2002; 20:1288–94.

77. Khouri IF, Saliba RM, Okoroji GJ, et al. Long-term follow-up of autologous stem cell transplantation in patients with diffuse mantle cell lymphoma in first disease remission: the prognostic value of beta2-microglobulin and the tumor score. Cancer 2003;98:2630–5.

78. Vandenberghe E, Ruiz de Elvira C, Loberiza FR, et al. Outcome of autologous transplantation for mantle cell lymphoma: a study by the European Blood and Bone Marrow Transplant and Autologous Blood and Marrow Transplant Registries. Br J Haematol 2003;120:793–800.

79. Maris MB, Sandmaier BM, Storer BE, et al. Allogeneic hematopoietic cell transplantation after fludarabine and 2 Gy total body irradiation for relapsed and refractory mantle cell lymphoma. Blood 2004;104:3535–42.

80. Goy A, Younes A, McLaughlin P, et al. Update on a phase (ph) 2 study of bortezomib in patients (pts) with relapsed or refractory indolent or aggressive non-Hodgkin's lymphomas (NHL). J Clin Oncol 2004;22:6581.

81. O'Connor OA. Marked clinical activity of the novel proteasome inhibitor bortezomib in patients with relapsed follicular (RL) and mantle cell lymphoma (MCL). J Clin Oncol 2004;22:6582.

82. Fisher RI, Gaynor ER, Dahlberg S, et al. Comparison of a standard regimen (CHOP) with three intensive chemotherapy regimens for advanced non-Hodgkin's lymphoma. N Engl J Med 1993;328:1002–6.

83. Miller TP, Dahlberg S, Cassady JR, et al. Chemotherapy alone compared with chemotherapy plus radiotherapy for localized intermediate- and high-grade non-Hodgkin's lymphoma. N Engl J Med 1998;339:21–6.

84. Coiffier B, Lepage E, Briere J, et al. CHOP chemotherapy plus rituximab compared with CHOP alone in elderly patients with diffuse large-B-cell lymphoma. N Engl J Med 2002;346:235–42.

85. Sehn LH, Donaldson J, Chhanabhai M, et al. Introduction of combined CHOP-rituximab therapy dramatically improved outcome of diffuse large B-cell lymphoma (DLBC) in British Columbia (BC) [abstract]. Blood 2003;102:29a.

86. Pfreundschuh MG, Trümper L, Ma D. Randomized intergroup trial of first line treatment for patients 60 years with diffuse large B-cell non-Hodgkin's lymphoma (DLBCL) with a CHOP-like regimen with or without the anti-CD20 antibody rituximab: early stopping after the first interim analysis. J Clin Onc 2004;22:6500.

87. Pfreundschuh M, Trumper L, Kloess M, et al. Two-weekly or 3-weekly CHOP chemotherapy with or without etoposide for the treatment of young patients with good-prognosis (normal LDH) aggressive lymphomas: results of the NHL-B1 trial of the DSHNHL. Blood 2004;104:626–33.

88. Pfreundschuh M, Trumper L, Kloess M, et al. Two-weekly or 3-weekly CHOP chemotherapy with or without etoposide for the treatment of elderly patients with aggressive lymphomas: results of the NHL-B2 trial of the DSHNHL. Blood 2004;104:634–41.

89. Gianni AM, Bregni M, Siena S, et al. High-dose chemotherapy and autologous bone marrow transplantation compared with MACOP-B in aggressive B-cell lymphoma. N Engl J Med 1997;336:1290–7.

90. Milpied N, Deconinck E, Gaillard F, et al. Initial treatment of aggressive lymphoma with high-dose chemotherapy and autologous stem-cell support. N Engl J Med 2004; 350:1287–95.

91. Philip T, Guglielmi C, Hagenbeek A, et al. Autologous bone marrow transplantation as compared with salvage chemotherapy in relapses of chemotherapy-sensitive non-Hodgkin's lymphoma. N Engl J Med 1995;333: 1540–5.

92. Stiff PJ, Dahlberg S, Forman SJ, et al. Autologous bone marrow transplantation for patients with relapsed or refractory diffuse aggressive non-Hodgkin's lymphoma: value of augmented preparative regimens—a Southwest Oncology Group trial. J Clin Oncol 1998;16:48–55.

93. Bernstein JI, Coleman CN, Strickler JG, et al. Combined modality therapy for adults with small noncleaved cell lymphoma (Burkitt's and non-Burkitt's types). J Clin Oncol 1986;4:847–58.

94. Magrath IT, Janus C, Edwards BK, et al. An effective therapy for both undifferentiated (including Burkitt's) lymphomas and lymphoblastic lymphomas in children and young adults. Blood 1984;63:1102–11.

95. Magrath I, Adde M, Shad A, et al. Adults and children with small non-cleaved-cell lymphoma have a similar excellent outcome when treated with the same chemotherapy regimen. J Clin Oncol 1996;14:925–34.

96. Mead GM, Sydes MR, Walewski J, et al. An international evaluation of CODOX-M and CODOX-M alternating with IVAC in adult Burkitt's lymphoma: results of United Kingdom Lymphoma Group LY06 study. Ann Oncol 2002;13:1264–74.

97. Soussain C, Patte C, Ostronoff M, et al. Small noncleaved cell lymphoma and leukemia in adults. A retrospective study of 65 adults treated with the LMB pediatric protocols. Blood 1995;85:664–74.

98. Kantarjian HM, O'Brien S, Smith TL, et al. Results of treatment with hyper-CVAD, a dose-intensive regimen, in adult acute lymphocytic leukemia. J Clin Oncol 2000; 18:547–61.

99. Cortes J, Thomas D, Rios A, et al. Hyperfractionated cyclophosphamide, vincristine, doxorubicin, and dexamethasone and highly active antiretroviral therapy for patients with acquired immunodeficiency syndrome-related Burkitt lymphoma/leukemia. Cancer 2002;94:1492–9.

100. Rizzieri DA, Johnson JL, Niedzwiecki D, et al. Intensive chemotherapy with and without cranial radiation for Burkitt leukemia and lymphoma: final results of Cancer and Leukemia Group B Study 9251. Cancer 2004;100: 1438–8.

101. Simonelli C, Spina M, Cinelli R, et al. Clinical features and outcome of primary effusion lymphoma in HIV-infected patients: a single-institution study. J Clin Oncol 2003;21: 3948–54.

102. Pluda JM, Venzon DJ, Tosato G, et al. Parameters affecting the development of non-Hodgkin's lymphoma in patients with severe human immunodeficiency virus infection receiving antiretroviral therapy. J Clin Oncol 1993;11: 1099–107.

103. Kaplan LD, Lee J, Scadden DT, et al. No benefit form rituximab in a randomized phase III trial of CHOP with or wihtout rituximab for patients with HIV-associated non-Hodgkins lymphoma: updated data from AIDS Malignancies Consortium Study 010 [abstract]. Blood 2003:409a.

104. Little R, Dunleavy K, Grant N, et al. Phase II study of abbreviated treatment (short-course) with EPOCH and rituximab (EPOCH-R) in AIDS-related lymphoma (ARL): preliminary results on the role of rituximab in treatment [abstract]. Blood 2003;102:411a.

105. Little RF, Pittaluga S, Grant N, et al. Highly effective treatment of acquired immunodeficiency syndrome-related lymphoma with dose-adjusted EPOCH: impact of antiretroviral therapy suspension and tumor biology. Blood 2003;101:4653–9.

106. Besson C, Goubar A, Gabarre J, et al. Changes in AIDS-related lymphoma since the era of highly active antiretroviral therapy. Blood 2001;98:2339–44.

107. Boulanger E, Daniel MT, Agbalika F, Oksenhendler E. Combined chemotherapy including high-dose methotrexate in KSHV/HHV8-associated primary effusion lymphoma. Am J Hematol 2003;73:143–8.

108. Kuppers R. Molecular biology of Hodgkin's lymphoma. Adv Cancer Res 2002;84:277–312.

109. Kuppers R, Schwering I, Brauninger A, et al. Biology of Hodgkin's lymphoma. Ann Oncol 2002;13 Suppl 1:11–8.

110. Diehl V, Sextro M, Franklin J, et al. Clinical presentation, course, and prognostic factors in lymphocyte-predominant Hodgkin's disease and lymphocyte-rich classical Hodgkin's disease: report from the European Task Force on Lymphoma Project on Lymphocyte-Predominant Hodgkin's Disease. J Clin Oncol 1999;17:776–83.

111. von Wasielewski R, Seth S, Franklin J, et al. Tissue eosinophilia correlates strongly with poor prognosis in nodular sclerosing Hodgkin's disease, allowing for known prognostic factors. Blood 2000;95:1207–13.

112. Haluska FG, Brufsky AM, Canellos GP. The cellular biology of the Reed-Sternberg cell. Blood 1994;84:1005–19.

113. Gutensohn N, Cole P. Epidemiology of Hodgkin's disease in the young. Int J Cancer 1977;19:595–604.

114. Glaser SL. Regional variation in Hodgkin's disease incidence by histologic subtype in the US. Cancer 1987;60:2841–7.

115. Cozen W, Katz J, Mack TM. Risk patterns of Hodgkin's disease in Los Angeles vary by cell type. Cancer Epidemiol Biomarkers Prev 1992;1:261–8.

116. Gutensohn NM. Social class and age at diagnosis of Hodgkin's disease: new epidemiologic evidence for the "two-disease hypothesis." Cancer Treat Rep 1982;66:689–95.

117. Jarrett RF. Risk factors for Hodgkin's lymphoma by EBV status and significance of detection of EBV genomes in serum of patients with EBV-associated Hodgkin's lymphoma. Leuk Lymphoma 2003;44 Suppl 3:S27–32.

118. Gulley ML, Eagan PA, Quintanilla-Martinez L, et al. Epstein-Barr virus DNA is abundant and monoclonal in the Reed-Sternberg cells of Hodgkin's disease: association with mixed cellularity subtype and Hispanic American ethnicity. Blood 1994;83:1595–602.

119. Hjalgrim H, Askling J, Rostgaard K, et al. Characteristics of Hodgkin's lymphoma after infectious mononucleosis. N Engl J Med 2003;349:1324–32.

120. Pallesen G, Hamilton-Dutoit SJ, Rowe M, Young LS. Expression of Epstein-Barr virus latent gene products in tumour cells of Hodgkin's disease. Lancet 1991;337:320–2.

121. Armstrong AA, Alexander FE, Cartwright R, et al. Epstein-Barr virus and Hodgkin's disease: further evidence for the three disease hypothesis. Leukemia 1998;12:1272–6.

122. Goldin LR, Pfeiffer RM, Gridley G, et al. Familial aggregation of Hodgkin lymphoma and related tumors. Cancer 2004;100:1902–8.

123. Mack TM, Cozen W, Shibata DK, et al. Concordance for Hodgkin's disease in identical twins suggesting genetic susceptibility to the young-adult form of the disease. N Engl J Med 1995;332:413–8.

124. Goedert JJ, Cote TR, Virgo P, et al. Spectrum of AIDS-associated malignant disorders. Lancet 1998;351:1833–9.

125. Levine AM. HIV-associated Hodgkin's disease. Biologic and clinical aspects. Hematol Oncol Clin North Am 1996;10:1135–48.

126. Herndier BG, Sanchez HC, Chang KL, et al. High prevalence of Epstein-Barr virus in the Reed-Sternberg cells of HIV-associated Hodgkin's disease. Am J Pathol 1993;142:1073–9.

127. Garnier JL, Lebranchu Y, Dantal J, et al. Hodgkin's disease after transplantation. Transplantation 1996;61:71–6.

128. Bierman PJ, Vose JM, Langnas AN, et al. Hodgkin's disease following solid organ transplantation. Ann Oncol 1996;7:265–70.

129. Audouin J, Diebold J, Pallesen G. Frequent expression of Epstein-Barr virus latent membrane protein-1 in tumour cells of Hodgkin's disease in HIV-positive patients. J Pathol 1992;167:381–4.

130. Timms JM, Bell A, Flavell JR, et al. Target cells of Epstein-Barr-virus (EBV)-positive post-transplant lymphoproliferative disease: similarities to EBV-positive Hodgkin's lymphoma. Lancet 2003;361:217–23.

131. Friedberg JW, Dipiro PJ. Staging and pretreatment evaluation of Hodgkin's disease. Hamilton (ON): American Cancer Society; 2002.

132. Good GR, DiNubile MJ. Images in clinical medicine. Cyclic fever in Hodgkin's disease (Pel-Ebstein fever). N Engl J Med 1995;332:436.

133. Hammack J, Kotanides H, Rosenblum MK, Posner JB. Paraneoplastic cerebellar degeneration. II. Clinical and immunologic findings in 21 patients with Hodgkin's disease. Neurology 1992;42:1938–43.

134. Dabbs DJ, Striker LM, Mignon F, Striker G. Glomerular lesions in lymphomas and leukemias. Am J Med 1986;80:63–70.

135. Gomez GA, Reese PA, Nava H, et al. Staging laparotomy and splenectomy in early Hodgkin's disease. No therapeutic benefit. Am J Med 1984;77:205–10.

136. Press OW, LeBlanc M, Lichter AS, et al. Phase III randomized intergroup trial of subtotal lymphoid irradiation versus doxorubicin, vinblastine, and subtotal lymphoid irradiation for stage IA to IIA Hodgkin's disease. J Clin Oncol 2001;19:4238–44.

137. Carde P, Hagenbeek A, Hayat M, et al. Clinical staging versus laparotomy and combined modality with MOPP versus ABVD in early-stage Hodgkin's disease: the H6 twin randomized trials from the European Organization for Research and Treatment of Cancer Lymphoma Cooperative Group. J Clin Oncol 1993;11:2258–72.

138. Friedberg JW, Fischman A, Neuberg D, et al. FDG-PET is superior to gallium scintigraphy in staging and more sensitive in the follow-up of patients with de novo Hodgkin lymphoma: a blinded comparison. Leuk Lymphoma 2004;45:85–92.

139. Rini JN, Manalili EY, Hoffman MA, et al. F-18 FDG versus Ga-67 for detecting splenic involvement in Hodgkin's disease. Clin Nucl Med 2002;27:572–7.

140. Specht L, Nordentoft AM, Cold S, et al. Tumor burden as the most important prognostic factor in early stage Hodgkin's disease. Relations to other prognostic factors and implications for choice of treatment. Cancer 1988;61:1719–27.

141. Mauch PM, Kalish LA, Marcus KC, et al. Long-term survival in Hodgkin's disease. Cancer J Sci Am 1995;1:33–42.

142. Mauch P, Goodman R, Hellman S. The significance of mediastinal involvement in early stage Hodgkin's disease. Cancer 1978;42:1039–45.

143. Henry-Amar M, Friedman S, Hayat M, et al. Erythrocyte sedimentation rate predicts early relapse and survival in early-stage Hodgkin disease. The EORTC Lymphoma Cooperative Group. Ann Intern Med 1991;114:361–5.

144. Tubiana M, Henry-Amar M, Hayat M, et al. Prognostic significance of the number of involved areas in the early stages of Hodgkin's disease. Cancer 1984;54:885–94.

145. Hasenclever D, Diehl V. A prognostic score for advanced Hodgkin's disease. International Prognostic Factors Project on Advanced Hodgkin's Disease. N Engl J Med 1998;339:1506–14.

146. Portlock CS, Donnelly GB, Qin J, et al. Adverse prognostic significance of CD20 positive Reed-Sternberg cells in classical Hodgkin's disease. Br J Haematol 2004;125:701–8.

147. Tzankov A, Krugmann J, Fend F, et al. Prognostic significance of CD20 expression in classical Hodgkin lymphoma: a clinicopathological study of 119 cases. Clin Cancer Res 2003;9:1381–6.

148. Rassidakis GZ, Medeiros LJ, Viviani S, et al. CD20 expression in Hodgkin and Reed-Sternberg cells of classical Hodgkin's disease: associations with presenting features and clinical outcome. J Clin Oncol 2002;20:1278–87.

149. Specht L, Gray RG, Clarke MJ, Peto R. Influence of more

extensive radiotherapy and adjuvant chemotherapy on long-term outcome of early-stage Hodgkin's disease: a meta-analysis of 23 randomized trials involving 3,888 patients. International Hodgkin's Disease Collaborative Group. J Clin Oncol 1998;16:830–43.

150. Viviani S, Santoro A, Ragni G, et al. Gonadal toxicity after combination chemotherapy for Hodgkin's disease. Comparative results of MOPP vs ABVD. Eur J Cancer Clin Oncol 1985;21:601–5.

151. Sieber M, Franklin J, Tesch H, et al. Two cycles ABVD plus extended field radiotherapy is superior to radiotherapy alone in early stage Hodgkin's disease: results of the German Hodgkin's Lymphoma Study Group (GHSG) Trial HD7 [abstract]. Blood 2002;100:93a.

152. Hagenbeek A, Eghbali H, Ferme C, al. E. Three cycles of MOPP/ABV hybrid and involved-field irradiation is more effective than subtotal nodal irradiation in favorable supradiaphragmatic clinical stages I-II Hodgkin's disease: preliminary results of the EORTC-GELA H8-F randomized trials in 543 patients [abstract]. Blood 2000;96:575a.

153. Mendenhall NP, Rodrigue LL, Moore-Higgs GJ, et al. The optimal dose of radiation in Hodgkin's disease: an analysis of clinical and treatment factors affecting in-field disease control. Int J Radiat Oncol Biol Phys 1999;44:551–61.

154. Engert A, Schiller P, Josting A, et al. Involved-field radiotherapy is equally effective and less toxic compared with extended-field radiotherapy after four cycles of chemotherapy in patients with early-stage unfavorable Hodgkin's lymphoma: results of the HD8 trial of the German Hodgkin's Lymphoma Study Group. J Clin Oncol 2003;21:3601–8.

155. Diehl V, Brillant C, Engert A, et al. Reduction of combined modality treatment intensity in early stage Hodgkin's lymphoma: interim analysis of the HD 10 trial of the GHSG [abstract]. Blood 2004;104:1307a.

156. Canellos GP, Anderson JR, Propert KJ, et al. Chemotherapy of advanced Hodgkin's disease with MOPP, ABVD, or MOPP alternating with ABVD. N Engl J Med 1992; 327:1478–84.

157. Horning SJ, Hoppe RT, Breslin S, et al. Stanford V and radiotherapy for locally extensive and advanced Hodgkin's disease: mature results of a prospective clinical trial. J Clin Oncol 2002;20:630–7.

158. Aversa SM, Salvagno L, Soraru M, et al. Stanford V regimen plus consolidative radiotherapy is an effective therapeutic program for bulky or advanced-stage Hodgkin's disease. Acta Haematol 2004;112:141–7.

159. Diehl V, Franklin J, Pfreundschuh M, et al. Standard and increased-dose BEACOPP chemotherapy compared with COPP-ABVD for advanced Hodgkin's disease. N Engl J Med 2003;348:2386–95.

160. Weihrauch MR, Re D, Scheidhauer K, et al. Thoracic positron emission tomography using 18F-fluorodeoxyglucose for the evaluation of residual mediastinal Hodgkin disease. Blood 2001;98:2930–4.

161. Ekstrand BC, Lucas JB, Horwitz SM, et al. Rituximab in lymphocyte-predominant Hodgkin disease: results of a phase 2 trial. Blood 2003;101:4285–9.

162. Ibom VK, Prosnitz RG, Gong JZ, et al. Rituximab in lymphocyte predominance Hodgkin's disease: a case series. Clin Lymphoma 2003;4:115–8.

163. Rehwald U, Schulz H, Reiser M, et al. Treatment of relapsed CD20+ Hodgkin lymphoma with the monoclonal antibody rituximab is effective and well tolerated: results of a phase 2 trial of the German Hodgkin Lymphoma Study Group. Blood 2003;101:420–4.

164. Henry-Amar M, Aeppli D, Anderson J, et al. Long term survival and study of causes of death. In: Somers R, Henry-Amar M, Meerwaldt J, Carde P, editors. Treatment strategy in Hodgkin's disease. London: John Libbey and Co; 1990. p. 381–418.

165. Meyer RM, Gospodarowicz M, Connors J, et al. A randomized phase II comparison of single-modlaity ABVD with a strategy that includes radiation therapy in patients with early-stage Hodgkin's disease: the HD-6 trial of the National Cancer Institute of Canada Clinical Trials Group (Eastern Cooperative Oncology Group Trial JHD06) [abstract]. Blood 2003;102:26a.

166. Meyer RM, Ambinder RF, Stroobants S. Hodgkin's lymphoma: evolving concepts with implications for practice. Hematology (Am Soc Hematol Educ Program) 2004:184–202.

167. Hoppe RT, Abrams RA, Alam RA, et al. NCCN clinical practice guidelines in oncology: Hodgkin's disease. Vol version 1.2004. National Comprehensive Cancer Network; 2004.

168. Simon R, Durrleman S, Hoppe RT, et al. The Non-Hodgkin Lymphoma Pathologic Classification Project. Long-term follow-up of 1153 patients with non-Hodgkin lymphomas. Ann Intern Med 1988;109:939–45.

169. Young NA, Al-Saleem T. Diagnosis of lymphoma by fine-needle aspiration cytology using the revised European-American classification of lymphoid neoplasms. Cancer 1999;87:325–45.

170. A predictive model for aggressive non-Hodgkin's lymphoma. The International Non-Hodgkin's Lymphoma Prognostic Factors Project. N Engl J Med 1993;329:987–94.

171. Nakatsuka S, Liu A, Dong Z et al. Simian virus 40 sequences in malignant lymphomas in Japan. Cancer Res 2003;63: 7606–8.

172. Kalachikov S, Migliazza A, Cayanis E, ret al. Cloning and gene mapping of the chromosome 13q14 region deleted in chronic lymphocytic leukemia. Genomics 1997;42:369–77.

173. Morris SW, Xue L, Ma Z, Kinney MC. Alk+ CD30+ lymphomas: a distinct molecular genetic subtype of non-Hodgkin's lymphoma. Br J Haematol 2001;113:275–95.

174. Santoro A, Bonfante V, Bonadonna G. Salvate chemotherapy with ABVD in MOPP-resistant Hodgkin's disease. Ann Intern Med 1982;96:139–43.

175. Devita VT Jr., Serpick AA, Carbone PP. Combination chemotherapy in the treatment of advanced Hodgkin's disease. Ann Intern Med 1970;73:881–95.

176. Bartlett NL, Rosenberg SA, Hoppe RT, et al. Brief chemotherapy, Stanford V, and adjuvant radiotherapy for bulky or advanced-stage Hodgkin's disease: a preliminary report. J Clin Oncol 1995;May:1080–88.

177. Diehl V, Franklin J, Pfreundschuh M, et al. Standard and increased-dose BEACOPP chemotherapy compared with COPP-ABVD for advanced Hodkin's disease. N Engl J Med 2003;348:2386–95.

Pathogenesis of Human Papillomavirus–Related Malignancies

KAREN SMITH-McCUNE

Human papillomavirus (HPV) is a double-stranded deoxyribonucleic acid (DNA) virus in the papovavirus family. The virion is a nonenveloped protein-coated icosahedron. The HPV genome is approximately 8,000 base pairs in size, with an open reading frame on one strand. Over 100 HPV types have been identified to date, and new types are constantly being identified on the basis of sequence comparisons to types that are already classified. HPV infects stratified squamous epithelium (ie, skin and mucosal surfaces). Each HPV type has restricted tropism as to the type of epithelium it can infect. For example, HPV-1 and HPV-2 infect skin cells, causing common warts and plantar warts. Approximately 30 of the known HPV types infect genital epithelium, including that of the cervix, the vulva, the vagina, the perianal region, and the anal canal. New HPV types continue to be discovered. A new HPV type is designated when its sequence is 50% different from any existing HPV sequence. Genital HPV types are classified according to their association with cervical cancer. There are 18 types that have been found worldwide to be associated with invasive cervical cancer; these are types 16, 18, 26, 31, 33, 35, 39, 45, 51, 52, 53, 56, 58, 59, 66, 68, 73, and 82.[1,2] The most common HPV type in cancer is HPV-16, but HPV-16 also accounts for the majority of HPV infections in asymptomatic individuals; hence, HPV infection clearly is necessary but not sufficient for the development of cancer. Among the HPV types found in cervical cancer, some types (HPV-31, -33, -35, -51, -52, and -58) are considered

to be intermediate risk because they are more commonly associated with precancerous changes than with actual invasive cancer.[2] The remaining genital HPV types are considered to be low risk because they are not associated with cervical cancer although they can cause other clinical manifestations (discussed below). The most common HPV type in almost every epidemiologic study is HPV-16, which accounts for 50 to 70% of incident infections regardless of age group.

LIFE CYCLE OF HUMAN PAPILLOMAVIRUSES

As with other viruses of the papovavirus family, the viral life cycle of HPV consists of an orderly process of infection of susceptible host cells (in this case, epithelial cells), followed by replication of viral genomes within the host cells and the assembly and release of new infectious particles. Several components of the HPV life cycle are unknown because there is no in vitro system for studying viral replication. Hence, key issues such as the identification of the viral receptor on the epithelial cell surface, the determinants of tropism, and the mechanisms governing viral latency are unknown. Nevertheless, the fundamentals of the HPV life cycle are understood.[3] The HPV genome encodes an early region and a late region, with distinct functions in the viral life cycle. A third region, the long control region, regulates viral gene expression. The early region is important for viral replication within the host cell. HPV replicates within intermediate cells in the middle layers of the stratified squamous epithelium; these cells normally undergo terminal differentiation and, as such, are nonreplicating. Therefore, the early region encodes genes required for the initiation of DNA synthesis, an essential step in the viral life cycle. The names and functions of early-region viral genes are summarized in Table 12–1 and are discussed in more detail below. The late region encodes the viral capsid proteins L1 and L2, whose assembly into the icosahedral virion is the last step in viral assembly prior to host-cell shedding and the release of new infectious viral particles. The virus replicates in the intermediate cell layers of stratified squamous epithelium, and infected cells traverse toward the top of the epithelium during the viral replicative life cycle, resulting in the release of infectious virions at the surface of the epithelium. Hence, the life cycle is designed to optimize the infectious capacity of the virus.

CLINICAL MANIFESTATIONS OF HUMAN PAPILLOMAVIRUS INFECTION

The biologic effects of HPV infection on epithelia are broad (Figure 12–1). The most common sequela is a subclinical infection with no detectable manifestations. Genital warts are the most common clinical manifestation of HPV infection. Genital warts usually resolve spontaneously although the warts occasionally cause symptoms or concerns that bring the patient to clinical attention and treatment. HPV infection can also cause dysplasia or cervical intraepithelial neoplasia (CIN), a form of abnormal growth characterized by cellular proliferation, genetic instability, and induction of new blood vessels. CIN 3 has been established as a definitive pre-

cancerous lesion; 12% or more of CIN3 cases progress to invasive disease.[4] The development of cervical cancer from CIN3 is thought to take many years, presumably reflecting an accumulation of genetic events leading to a fully invasive tumor phenotype. In rare instances, infection with HPV can result in frank invasive cancer: the abnormally dividing squamous cells acquire the ability to invade through the basement membrane into the underlying stroma and spread laterally and into lymph nodes and vessels. Intraepithelial lesions caused by HPV at other genital sites (such as vaginal, vulvar, anal, perianal, and penile intraepithelial neoplasias) are also thought to be cancer precursors. These lesions underscore the multifocal nature of HPV infection although the frequencies of cancers at these sites are orders of magnitude lower than that of cancer at the cervix. The mechanisms by which HPV infection can result in cancer (and speculation as to why the cervix is the most susceptible site) are discussed in this chapter.

EPIDEMIOLOGIC DATA LINKING HUMAN PAPILLOMAVIRUS INFECTION TO CERVICAL CANCER

Cervical cancer is a leading cause of cancer morbidity in women worldwide, and more than 500,000 cases are diagnosed annually.[5,6] The potential role of an infectious agent in its etiology was suspected from epidemiologic data indicating that the risk factors for cervical cancer includes numbers of sexual partners, age at first intercourse, and herpesvirus infection. The pivotal role of HPV in cervical carcinogenesis has emerged through a confluence of extensive epidemiologic and molecular investiga-

Table 12–1. HUMAN PAPILLOMAVIRUS GENES AND FUNCTIONS	
HPV Gene	**Function**
E1	Replication of DNA; binds to replication origin, helicase
E2	Facilitates E1 binding to replication origin; regulates *E6* and *E7* gene expression
E4	Disruption of cytokeratin network
E5	Transformation; acidification of endosomes
E6	Transformation; binds to p53
E7	Transformation; binds to pRB
L1	Major capsid protein
L2	Minor capsid protein

DNA - deoxyribonucleic acid; HPV = human papillomavirus.

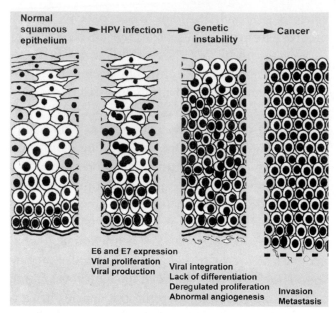

Figure 12–1. Progressive changes in human papillomavirus (HPV)–infected squamous epithelium, leading to invasive cancer.

tions that were launched by observations in the 1980s that cervical cancers contain integrated HPV genomes.[7–9] By far the highest risk factor for cervical cancer is the presence of HPV (with an odds ratio [OR] of 24, the highest OR reported for any linkages by cancer research, even surpassing ORs for smoking and lung cancer). That HPV genomes can be detected in more than 95% of cervical cancers worldwide argues compellingly that HPV has an important role in cervical cancer.[10] Other risk factors include smoking (OR, 1.5), early age at first intercourse (OR, 4.3 [for age < 16 years versus ≥ 24 years]), early age at first birth (OR, 5.0 [for age < 16 years versus ≥ 24 years]), low educational level (OR, 2.5), high parity (OR, 3.8 [for ≥ 7 births versus 0 births), long-term use of oral contraceptives (OR, 4.0 [for ≥ 10 years of use]; OR, 6.5 [for ever using versus never using]), and immunocompromised status (acquired immunodeficiency syndrome patients, organ transplant recipients, etc).[11–13] Infection with other sexually transmitted infectious organisms, such as *Chlamydia* or herpesviruses, also confers some risk.[14–16] Of interestingly, circumcision of the male partner is protective against cervical cancer (OR, 0.4); this is attributed to lower rates of HPV detection in circumcised men.[17] In addition, cesarean section (OR, 0.4) and prior screening by Pap smear (OR, 0.1–0.7) reduce the risk of cervical cancer.[11]

PATHOGENESIS OF CERVICAL CANCER

Human Papillomavirus Oncogenes

HPV normally replicates in the middle layer of the stratified squamous epithelium, which is composed of terminally differentiated growth-arrested keratinocytes. Hence, the virus has evolved mechanisms to jump-start DNA replication in the process of initiating viral genome replication. It accomplishes this through the action of the proteins encoded by genes in the early region; these proteins bind to tumor suppressor genes and inhibit the activity of critical cell cycle checkpoints. Normally, differentiated cells exhibit cell cycle checkpoints that restrict unscheduled DNA proliferation and maintain the cell in a resting or differentiated state (G_0/G_1). The virus contains genes in the early region, specifically *E6* and *E7*, that are pivotal for the induction of DNA synthesis as required for its life cycle. Together these genes are able to transform cells in culture and to immortalize primary keratinocytes.[18,19] In addition, overexpression of these genes results in skin and cervical cancer in transgenic models in which their expression is targeted to the basal cells of the epidermis and epithelium.[20–23] *E7* appears to be the primary oncogene as demonstrated in an animal model of estrogen-stimulated HPV-induced cervical cancer. In that model, expression of E6 alone resulted in low-grade dysplasias but no progression to cancer over a 6-month period; expression of E7 alone resulted in precancers and cancer, and expression of E6 and E7 together resulted in larger cancers.[24]

An important component of the viral life cycle in precancerous lesions is that the virus can integrate into the human genome. Integration appears to preferentially interrupt the viral E2 open reading frame, indicating a selective advantage of cells in which E2 expression is checked. One of the key mechanisms by which E2 loss promotes carcinogenesis is the function of E2 as a transcriptional repressor of the early-region promoter. Hence, cells containing integrated HPV express higher levels of the HPV oncogenes E6 and E7. Indeed, re-introduction of E2 into the HPV-18–positive cervical cancer cell line HeLa results in the down-regulation of E6 and E7 and subsequent cellular senescence,[25] indicating that sustained expression of HPV oncogenes is required for maintenance of the malignant phenotype. The integration of HPV into the genome has been studied in an in vitro model system, and it has been demonstrated that expression of numerous genes that were not previously implicated in carcinogenesis is altered upon viral integration and may contribute to carcinogenesis.[26] Sites of HPV integration are random throughout the genome,[27] dispelling a model in which HPV carcinogenesis is promoted by insertional mutagenesis of a host gene. Integration of the viral genome and enhanced host chromosomal instability are linked events, and in a model system, integration appears to precede chromosomal instability.[28] However, data from human lesions suggest that aneuploidy precedes integration.[29] Given that viral integration appears to be an important event in the progression of premalignant lesions to cancer, markers of viral integration are being studied as potential biomarkers for cervical cancer screening.[30]

Cervical cancer is associated with a constellation of chromosomal aberrations. During cell immortalization, deletions of 3p, 6, and 10p are common whereas gain of chromosome 3q and loss of chromosome 11 are later events associated with invasive tumors.[31] E6 and E7 play important and different roles in generating chromosomal instability (elaborated below).[32] The viral oncogenes E6 and E7 target cell cycle checkpoints and contribute to genomic instability by different mechanisms; in concert, these functions contribute to the generation of potentially carcinogenic cell clones and explain the role of HPV in the multistep pathway to cervical cancer.

Functional Properties of E7

E7 is a small protein (97–110 amino acids) with several functional domains determined by mutational analysis to be important to its function in cellular transformation. E7 contains a zinc-binding domain consisting of two copies of a CysXXCys motif.[33] This domain is required for extending the life span of primary keratinocytes and is also required for the activation of genes in the late region during virion replication.[34] E7 is a phosphoprotein and contains a phosphorylation site required for transformation.[35] E7 is phosphorylated by

casein kinase early in the cell cycle and by an unidentified kinase in the S phase.[36] E7 is a nuclear protein that lacks a classic nuclear localization signal and appears to enter through nuclear pores by using an unconventional pathway requiring the guanosine triphosphate–binding protein Ran.[37]

However, the most intensively studied and most crucial function of E7 derives from its ability to bind to pRB and its family members (p107 and p130)[38,39] through an LXCXE motif. In quiescent cells, the pRB proteins interact with the E2F family of transcription factors; phosphorylation of pRB by cyclin D cyclin-dependent kinase (CDK) complexes results in the release of E2F and the transcription of rate-limiting genes for progression into the S phase, such as cyclin E, CDK2, and enzymes involved in DNA synthesis.[40] E7 binding to pRB similarly results in release of E2F[41] and regulation of E2F transcriptional targets, allowing progression through the cell cycle independently of cyclin-D CDK phosphorylation of pRB. As a result of E7 binding to pRB, E2F alters gene transcription of a host of genes involved in DNA replication and cell cycle progression through G_1 into S phase and also for mitosis.[42–44] E7 binding also results in reduced levels of pRB through enhanced degradation of pRB, a function that requires a conserved N-terminal domain of E7.[45] Therefore, E7 targets the pRB checkpoint by two mechanisms. E7 binding and destabilization of pRB and its family members promote cell cycle reentry (important for viral propagation) and also contribute to the malignant potential of the virus. Indeed, E7 from low-risk HPV types has a lower binding affinity to pRB than E7 from high-risk HPV types has,[46] indicating a direct correlation between pRB binding and carcinogenic potential. However, the situation is more complex, as evident from studies demonstrating that E7 from noncarcinogenic HPV-1 can bind to pRB with high affinity and transforms rodent cell lines[47] (but not primary cells).[48] These data indicate that pRB binding alone is not sufficient for transformation.

Cellular senescence occurs when primary cells are placed in culture; presumably, it mimics a physiologic state in which normal cells lose their ability to divide after a finite number of cell divisions. A recently discovered function of E7 with relevance to cancer is the ability of E7 to overcome cellular senescence. This function also appears to be mediated through the pRB-binding function of E7. When HeLa cells (cells of the HPV-18–positive cervical cancer cell line) are forced to express high levels of HPV-18 E2, they demonstrate an increased activity of pRB and undergo senescence. This effect of E2 can be negated by overexpression of wild-type E7 but not by E7 containing mutations in the pRB-binding domain, suggesting that the ability of HeLa cells to overcome senescence requires E7 inactivation of pRB.[49] In a different system, which used the promyelocytic leukemia gene (*PML*) to induce senescence in primary human fibroblasts, E7 was able to overcome senescence via both pRB-dependent and pRB-independent mechanisms[50]; however, the relevance of this system to cervical cancer is as yet unknown.

E7 is able to overcome cell cycle checkpoints with another mechanism complementary to the ability to bind to the pRB family of proteins. E7 from high-risk viral types also has the ability to bind to and inactivate cell cycle inhibitors. The proteins P21 and P27 bind to and inactivate the kinase activities of cyclin-E CDK2 and cyclin-A CDK2, respectively. E7 from high-risk HPV types overcomes the inhibitory effects for P21 and P27,[51–53] allowing G_1- to S-phase transitions as well as progress through mitosis.

E7 also has the ability to interfere with P53-induced cell cycle arrest.[54] While E6 has direct effects on P53 (discussed below), the ability of E7 alone to alter P53 function was unexpected. E7 can interfere with the transcriptional activity of P53; this has been attributed to the ability of E7 to bind to the TATA binding protein.[55,56] E7 binds to a numerous other cellular proteins, which results in additional functional properties of E7,[44,57] among which is a role in cellular metabolism. M2 pyruvate kinase is a pivotal enzyme in cell glucose use and determines the equilibrium between glycolysis versus glycogen synthesis; cancer cells display a unique propensity to the less active dimeric form of the enzyme.[58] E7 binds to M2 pyruvate kinase, resulting in the persistence of the dimeric form under conditions in which the more active tetrameric form would normally be favored.[59] This function is more pronounced in E7 from transforming HPV types than in nontransforming HPV types, which suggests that the ability to

bind to M2 pyruvate kinase is important in transformation.[59] In addition, E7 induces the expression of catalase, resulting in resistance to oxidative stress, possibly leading to protection from apoptosis in the local tumor environment.[60]

Another recently recognized property of E7 is its pleiotropic effects on mitosis. Expression of E7 in primary human fibroblasts results in the development of polyploid cells.[61,62] This effect of E7 on the mitotic spindle checkpoint was surprising, given that the genomic instability associated with HPV had previously been attributed to E6, as discussed below. Further investigation revealed that E7 causes abnormal centrosome synthesis, resulting in multipolar mitotic plates.[63] Chromosomal tetrasomy induced by E7 in keratinocytes in culture is not dependent on pRb binding[64,65] but rather may depend on the ability of E7 to bind to cyclin A and to activate CDK2.[66] CDK2 activity is a major determinant for the initiation of centrosome duplication. Thus, centrosome instability caused by E7 may be due to the effect of E7 on dysregulation of CDK2 activity.[32] In addition, E7 can induce anaphase bridges.[65] Thus, E7 has more than one mechanism by which it contributes to genetic instability.

In summary, E7 has numerous effects on the host cell that result in DNA synthesis, progression through the cell cycle, polyploidy, and alterations in cellular metabolism, all of which are important in the viral life cycle but which also contribute to a carcinogenic potential and partly explain the association between HPV infection and human cancers.[67–69]

Functional Properties of Human Papillomavirus E6

The early gene *E6* encodes a small hydrophobic protein (149–158 amino acids) with numerous functions that are important in the viral life cycle but that also confer risk of malignancy. A crucial function of E6 appears to inactivate the tumor suppressor gene *P53* by increasing P53 turnover through protein degradation.[70,71] A principal function of P53 is to cause cell cycle arrest or cell death in the presence of DNA damage, through the induction of cell cycle control genes such as *P21* or through the induction of proapoptotic genes such as bax 1 and the fas receptor.

Loss of P53 function therefore results in DNA replication in the face of damaged DNA, resulting in genomic instability and the accumulation of mutations, thereby driving cells toward a malignant phenotype. During replication, DNA tumor viruses generate nonphysiologic levels of DNA ends and episomal DNA, which are interpreted by the cell as damaged and extrachromosomal DNA; hence, DNA viruses have evolved mechanisms to evade the P53 DNA damage checkpoint. In the case of HPV, E6 binds to P53 and to an E6-associated protein (E6-AP),[72] forming a trimolecular complex. E6-AP was subsequently identified as an E3 ubiquitin ligase that transfers ubiquitin to the target protein (in this case, P53), resulting in its degradation in the 26S proteasome.[73,74] This function of E6 is thought to explain the ability of E6 to bypass the G_1 checkpoint[75] and mitotic checkpoints[76] in the presence of DNA damage; indeed, in a mutational analysis of E6, the functional domains required for P53 binding and degradation perfectly overlap with those required for overcoming damage-induced G_1 arrest.[77] Of interest is the observation that E6 from HPV-6 (a low-risk nontransforming viral type) binds to P53 but does not lead to its degradation,[78] which suggests that it is the ability to downregulate P53 protein levels that is important in HPV-associated tumorigenesis. Besides allowing the virus to escape the shutdown of DNA synthesis machinery, this function of E6 contributes to genomic instability. Forced expression of E6 results in the accumulation of mutations allowing escape from drug toxicity.[61] E6 also bypasses several checkpoints that regulate both entry to and exit from mitosis.[76] These functions of E6 ultimately lead to cells with an abnormal chromosome number and profound nuclear atypia.[65]

Another important function of E6 is its ability to immortalize primary human mammary epithelial cells[79] and to collaborate with E7 to immortalize primary human keratinocytes.[19,80] Immortalization of cells in culture may be thought of as an in vitro surrogate for the unregulated growth of cells seen in the development of malignancy. Intriguingly, mutational analysis of E6 revealed that the P53-binding domain is not essential for immortalization,[81] indicating an additional function of E6 in addition to P53 binding/degradation. This function has been identified as the ability of E6 to activate the expression of telomerase, an enzyme that adds hexamer repeats to the telomeric ends of chromosomes. This enzyme is normally active only during embryogenesis and in stem cells. Serial divisions of somatic cells result in a shortening of the telomere ends and in eventual senescence. Cancer cells usually demonstrate reactivated telomerase, resulting in stabilized chromosome ends and a prolonged cell life span. It is this function of E6 that is required for cell immortalization in vitro.

E6 binds to other cellular proteins and has numerous other effects on cell physiology. For example, E6 can bind to the PDZ family of proteins, which are involved in cell-cell contact and in signaling pathways. The PDZ-binding domain of E6 is located in the C-terminal of the protein; deletion of this domain has no effect on P53 binding but results in the loss of the ability to cause epidermal hyperplasia in E6 transgenic mice.[82] E6 binds to paxillin,[83–85] a cytoskeletal protein found in the focal adhesion plaque that integrates signaling pathways from the exterior of the cell; paxillin's function is targeted by other oncogenes, presumably as a means to overcome growth-inhibitory signals from neighboring cells and the extracellular matrix.[84] E6 also binds to the transcriptional activator p300/CBP, resulting in downregulation of p53 transcriptional activity.[86–88]

In summary, E6 functions to overcome the p53 checkpoint, allowing DNA replication of the viral genome and blocking cell death in the host cell. In addition, it interacts with other cellular proteins to alter transcription, activate telomerase, and alter signaling from the cell exterior, all of which are presumably important in allowing and maintaining viral episomal replication but which also contribute to the malignant potential of HPV. Viral genes also contribute to the interaction between the epithelium and the host defense response against the virus (discussed below).

Stromal and Immune Influences

Angiogenesis

Vascularity has long been associated with CIN lesions because of punctate and mosaic patterns on the surface of dysplastic lesions, detectable by colposcopy.[89] In addition, colposcopic detection of atypical vessels is associated with microinvasion of CIN lesions.[90] Thus, angiogenesis has been associated clinically with the progression of CIN to invasion. CIN lesions demonstrate a profuse microvasculature at the stromal-epithelial junction, characterized by increased vessel density as well as closer apposition of the vessels to the base of the epithelium.[91–97]

Several investigative groups have shown that angiogenesis is accompanied by upregulated expression of an important angiogenic factor, vascular endothelial growth factor (VEGF).[92,94,96] VEGF expression is regulated through several mechanisms. One mechanism of regulation is hypoxia owing to a hypoxia-inducible element in the gene promoter. Presumably as a result of the high metabolic activity in dysplastic epithelium, oxygen tension is reduced, resulting in the activation of the transcription factor hypoxia inducible factor (HIF). Genes with HIF promoter elements, such as VEGF, are upregulated in conditions of low oxygen tension.[98] Another mechanism of VEGF regulation in the cervix is through direct effects of the HPV genes. Overexpression of the HPV-16 *E6* and *E7* genes in primary human keratinocytes results in the up-regulation of VEGF expression,[99] and HPV-16 E6 can transactivate the VEGF prompter independently of P53.[100] Therefore, the HPV oncogenes contribute to the recruitment of a neovasculature, presumably to maintain host cell homeostasis in the face of increased metabolic expenditure due to viral replication. In addition to the up-regulation of angiogenic factors, HPV-positive cell lines demonstrate down-regulation of a family of potent inhibitors of angiogenesis, namely, thrombospondin 1 (TSP-1) and thrombospondin 2 (TSP-2)[101]; TSP-1 levels are inversely correlated with microvessel count and prognosis in cervical cancer.[102,103] This effect again may be directly mediated by the HPV oncogenes as expression of E6 and E7 in primary keratinocytes results in a reduction in levels of the antiangiogenic proteins TSP-1 and maspin.[99] Because angiogenesis is required for premalignant progression and for tumor growth and development,[104,105] the role of HPV oncogenes in promoting angiogenesis through altered expression of angiogenic regulators is likely important for carcinogenesis. Indeed, this ability of the HPV oncogenes to alter the expression of angiogenic factors is another example of a gene function that is important in the physiologic regulation of viral life cycle but that is co-opted into contributing to a neoplastic phenotype in certain contexts.

Role of the Immune Response: Protection Against Viral Infection

Protection against foreign pathogens such as viruses occurs primarily at respiratory, intestinal, and genital mucosal surfaces. Mechanisms governing local mucosal immune responses to viruses are complex and involve the infected epithelium, the stroma, and the host immune system. HPV infection is the most common sexually acquired infection in the United States, yet little is known about local mucosal immune responses to HPV or about the overall properties of cervical mucosa–associated lymphoid tissue (MALT). The majority of HPV infections are innocuous, resulting in no obvious clinical disease. However, HPV infection infrequently results in CIN and rarely results in invasive cervical cancer. The immune response is important in clearing the virus and results in protection from subsequent infection by the same viral type. The importance of the immune response in the outcome of HPV infection is evident from a vast body of literature indicating that immunocompromised individuals are more likely to have persistent HPV infections, to have recurrent disease after treatment, and (possibly) to develop invasive cancer.[106–109] Both the innate and acquired immune responses are implicated in the clearance of HPV infection.[110] Much examination of cytotoxic response to HPV has focused on cells isolated from peripheral blood. However, we also know that at the site of HPV infection, cervical stroma of CIN lesions contain significantly increased numbers of germinal centers and lymphoid follicles when compared with the normal cervix.[111] The presence of cervical lymphoid aggregates was not due to chlamydial infection (an association made by others in the past) but appeared to be due at least partly to HPV as based on the detection of E6 and E7 antigens on follicular dendritic cells in a subset of aggregates. Cervical stromal cells focally produce a chemokine implicated in germinal-center formation (B cell–attracting chemokine [BCA1]). Therefore, a complex interaction between the viral infection in the epithelium and the cells and chemokines in the stroma results in the formation of a local inductive immune response at least partly directed against HPV antigens. These surprising results clearly implicate the cervix as a site of MALT.

In addition to lymphoid follicles, the local microenvironment of CIN contains significantly increased numbers of cells from both the innate and the acquired immune responses.[112–120] Compared with the normal cervical stroma, a CIN-associated stroma contains increased numbers of CD4[+] and CD8[+] T cells, macrophages, mast cells, B cells, neutrophils, and natural killer (NK) cells, and dysplastic epithelium contains increased numbers of CD4[+] T cells, macrophages, and NK cells (Table 12–2). Lymphocytes in the stroma of CIN lesion express interleukin-2 receptor (IL-2R), an activation marker, and a transcription factor (T bet) whose expression is restricted to Th1 CD4[+] T cells.[120] The production of interferon (IFN)-γ is significantly upregulated in CIN lesions (see Table 12–2), and IFN-γ is expressed by CD4[+] and CD8[+] T cells as well as by NK cells.[120] These data indicate an adaptive Th1 response in CIN 2 and 3 in comparison with the normal cervix.

Nevertheless, the presence of CIN and cervical cancer indicates that the immune response may not be adequate to reverse HPV-induced carcinogenesis. Certainly, the fact that greater than 95% of CIN lesions and cervical cancers contain HPV DNA indicates an apparent immunologic failure of the body to rid itself of a cancer-causing virus. HPV typically does not elicit strong local or systemic immune responses because of various mechanisms of immune evasion[121–123]; these include (1) the relative paucity of antigen-presenting cells in the transformation zone (the site of CIN development) as compared with the exocervix[124] and (2) the low expression of CD3 zeta chain in the T cells of women with CIN and cervical cancer.[125,126] In addition, the viral genes *E6* and *E7* have direct effects on the suppression of the immune response. E7 blocks the transcription of genes within keratinocytes induced by inflammatory mediators such as tumor necrosis factor-α, thus protecting against the local killing of keratinocytes.[127,128] E7 can also block the effects of IFN-α produced by innate immune cells, allowing continued cell growth despite the presence of this cytokine.[129] In addition, E7 can inhibit the activation of the IFN-β promoter by binding to IFN-regulatory factor 1.[130] E6 binds to IFN-regulatory factor 3 and has a similar inhibitory effect on cytotoxic responses to local cytokines,[131] which again protects the cell from antiviral host defense mechanisms.

There are other mechanisms by which HPV evades the immune response. There is emerging evi-

Table 12–2. DENSITIES OF IMMUNE CELL TYPES IN NORMAL CERVIX AND IN CERVICAL INTRAEPITHELIAL NEOPLASIA 2 AND 3

		Normal Cervix	CIN2 and 3
CD4[+] T cells	Epithelium	$N = 11$ 62 ± 51*	$N = 14$ 167 ± 161 $p = .02$
	Stroma	$N = 10$ 215 ± 157	$N = 14$ 1083 ± 689 $p = .002$
CD8[+] T cells	Epithelium	$N = 11$ 408 ± 560	$N = 13$ 434 ± 321 NS
	Stroma	$N = 10$ 330 ± 264	$N = 13$ 850 ± 577 $p = .04$
B cells	Epithelium	$N = 11$ 4 ± 9	$N = 13$ 10 ± 21 NS
	Stroma	$N = 10$ $26 + 38$	$N = 14$ 206 ± 242 $p = .01$
Macrophages	Epithelium	$N = 11$ 64 ± 101	$N = 14$ 483 ± 325 $p = .0002$
	Stroma	$N = 9$ 277 ± 204	$N = 14$ 550 ± 273 $p = .04$
Neutrophils[†]	Stroma	$N = 10$ 48 ± 83	$N = 11$ 351 ± 250 $p = .001$
NK cells	Epithelium	$N = 8$ 27 ± 37	$N = 11$ 103 ± 100
	Stroma	$N = 8$ 8 ± 13	$N = 11$ 116 ± 102 $p = .0007$
IFN-γ[+] cells	Stroma	$N = 9$ 34 ± 42	$N = 15$ 426 ± 338 $p = .002$

CIN - cervical intraepithelial neoplasia; IFNγ – interferon γ; N - sample size; NK - natural killer; NS - not significant.
*Cell densities are expressed by cell number/mm^2 ± standard deviation.
N represents the number of samples counted for each cell. Counting was performed as described in Kobayashi A et al.[120]
†Neutrophils were essentially absent from normal and CIN epithelium.

dence that HPV can induce immune tolerance.[121] In addition, HPV replicates in terminally differentiated keratinocytes in the outer layers of stratified squamous epithelium and may thereby avoid immune detection during the replicative phase of the viral life cycle. But the situation is more complex than the direct effects of HPV blocking the immune response. There is emerging evidence that infiltrating immune cells recruited to CIN lesions can contribute directly to angiogenesis and cancer development (as elaborated below).

Role of Stromal Inflammatory Cells in Angiogenesis and Carcinogenesis

Researchers have developed a genetically engineered mouse model of HPV-induced disease, in which the promoter/enhancer of the keratin 14 gene (expressed in basal keratinocytes of squamous epithelia) is fused to the HPV-16 early region containing the known oncogenes E6 and E7. Transgenic mice carrying this hybrid oncogene (K14/HPV-16 transgenic mice) develop spontaneous squamous carcinomas of the skin; female mice can develop cervical carcinomas.[21] When females that are 1 month of age are treated with subcutaneous time-release estrogen pellets to mimic estrus (HPV-16/E2 transgenic mice), invasive cervical cancers develop with a high penetrance (90% by 7 months of age).[20,22] Tumors occur at the cervical transformation zone, the same site targeted by HPV in human cervical cancer.[132] In younger mice, a series of preinvasive lesions develop, mimicking the multistage progression of CIN lesions seen in the human cervix: hyperplasia appears at 2 months of age, and dysplasias appear at 3 to 4 months of age. A dense network of new blood vessels analogous to those seen in human lesions appears at the stromal-epithelial junction during the premalignant stages of carcinogenesis in both the skin of K14/HPV-16 mice[92] and the cervices of E2/HPV-16 mice.[133] Thus, the animal model reliably mimics the human disease in its mechanism (HPV-16 oncogenes), its multistage progression, and the appearance of neovascularization in premalignant stages.

This model and related animal models have demonstrated a novel role for stromal immune cells in angiogenesis and in the development of cancer. In early work using the K14/HPV-16 skin model, hyperplastic and dysplastic lesions showed a progressive up-regulation of enzymatically active matrix metalloprotease 9 (MMP9).[134] When K14/HPV-16 mice were crossed into an MMP9-null (MMP$^{-/-}$) background, the occurrence of skin dysplasias and invasive cancers was significantly retarded. In addition, the occurrence of angiogenesis was markedly delayed; intense neovasculature appeared at 5 months in K14/HPV-16 MMP9$^{+/+}$ mice but not until 11 months in mice in the MMP9$^{-/-}$ background.[135] These data argue that MMP9 plays a role in angiogenesis and thus in carcinogenic progression. It was intriguing that MMP9 was contributed by infiltrating inflammatory cells, not by the dysplastic epithelium; the angiogenic phenotype and the development of invasive tumors were restored when MMP9$^{+/+}$ cells derived from bone marrow were adoptively transferred into lethally irradiated K14/HPV-16 MMP9$^{-/-}$ mice.[135] Similar observations were made in a genetically engineered model of pancreatic islet cell cancer.[136] These findings have resulted in an increased focus on immune cells as important contributors to angiogenesis and hence to carcinogenesis.

Because of the potential pathogenic significance of angiogenesis in the development of cervical cancer, preclinical trials were designed to test the effect of antiangiogenic agents in the HPV-16/E2 model as a platform for human trials. A known MMP9 inhibitor, BB94, was shown to inhibit the occurrence of angiogenesis and tumors,[133] but this agent is not available for trials in humans. Therefore, another preclinical trial used zoledronic acid (ZA), an aminobisphosphonate approved by the Food and Drug Administration for the treatment of bone pain secondary to cancer metastasis. ZA acts systemically to reduce vessel recruitment into subcutaneous implants[137]; in addition, it sensitizes endothelial cells to apoptotic signals.[138] Cancer patients treated with ZA have reduced circulating levels of VEGF.[139] On the basis of these promising data indicating that ZA is antiangiogenic, HPV-16/E2 animals were treated from the age of 3.5 to 5 months to determine the effect of ZA on the progression of CIN lesions to tumors. Provocative data from these trials indicate that ZA has therapeutic activity in the HPV-16/E2 model of cervical cancer.[133] Female HPV-16 mice that were treated with ZA from the age of 3.5 to 5 months showed a significant reduction in the numbers of tumors and a shift to lower-grade CIN lesions when compared with mice treated with placebo. Neovascularization at the stromal-epithelial interface was dramatically reduced in ZA-treated animals. While the mitotic rate in dysplastic epithelium was not affected by ZA, the rate of cell death was increased both in the dysplastic epithelium and in stromal endothelial cells. The formation of VEGF complexes with its receptor was inhibited in ZA-treated mice. MMP9 activity (as measured by zymography) and expression levels were significantly decreased in ZA-treated mice. A pivotal role for MMP9 was confirmed by studying carcinogenesis in MMP9$^{-/-}$ mice crossed onto the HPV-16/E2 background. As in ZA-treated mice, angiogenesis was impaired and the appearance of tumors was inhibited in MMP9$^{-/-}$ mice.[133] These data indicate that MMP9 plays an important role in the angiogenesis seen during cervical carcinogenesis. It is intriguing that the mechanism of action of ZA appears to be the inhibition of MMP9 production by stroma-infiltrating macrophages, again underscoring the importance of stromal contributions. ZA also demonstrated direct antitumor activity: treatment of animals from 5 to 6 months of age resulted in smaller tumor volumes. Therefore, through modulation of MMP9 production by stromal macrophages, ZA was antiangiogenic and inhibited the development and growth of cervical tumors. Of interest in this regard is the recent finding that expression and enzymatic activity of MMP9 are upregulated in more than 80% of human CIN3 cases and more than 90% of cervical cancers and correlate with subsequent metastasis and recurrence.[140–142]

Direct Role of Inflammation

Recent advances in our understanding of cancer biology indicate that contrary to our expectations that it will be protective, the local immune environment may potentiate cancer development and progression. This model is based on many convergent findings stemming from Virchow's observations in 1863 regarding the "lymphoreticular infiltrate" in tumors, linking

cancer to inflammation.[143] Many cancers have been linked to inflammatory agents or processes; such cancers include bladder cancer (schistosomiasis), gastric cancer and MALT lymphomas (*Helicobacter pylori*), hepatocellular cancer (hepatitis B and C viruses), colorectal cancer (inflammatory bowel disease), and, of course, cervical cancer (HPV). Mechanisms governing this relationship include the production of growth-promoting cytokines, chemokines, angiogenic factors, and proteases by tumor-associated inflammatory cells.[144–146] An appreciation of the link between inflammation and cancer underlies the recent interest in using immunomodulators to prevent cancer. For example, cyclooxygenase made by inflammatory cells fuels angiogenesis and metastasis and can be targeted by nonsteroidal antiinflammatory agents, which have been shown to be protective against cancer in certain instances.[147–149]

In the case of HPV-induced cervical cancer, a direct role for the immune response in enhancing the malignant potential of HPV has been described above; MMP9 contributed by stromal macrophages fuels angiogenesis and hence malignant progression in the cervices of HPV-16/E2 transgenic mice, and inhibition of MMP9 production with ZA blocks the progression of CIN to cancer.[133] In addition, in a related model of HPV-16–induced skin cancer, CD4$^+$ T cells were found to be important in malignant progression; mice lacking CD4$^+$ T cells exhibited delayed tumor development and smaller tumors than mice with CD4$^+$ T cells showed.[150] In tumors from animals lacking CD4$^+$ T cells, there were fewer neutrophils and lower amounts of MMP9 than there were in animals with CD4$^+$ T cells. The model developed from these data is one of dysplastic epidermis allowing the entry of usually absent skin organisms owing to disruption of the normal epidermal barrier; local inflammatory responses elicited to these microorganisms contribute procarcinogenic factors such as MMP9. Finally, another contributor to the carcinogenic process in the cervix might be cyclooxygenase, which displays angiogenic activity and is overexpressed in cervical cancer.[151–154] Thus, inflammatory processes are implicated in the angiogenesis and pathogenesis of cervical cancer.

A critical factor in local response to microorganisms is tumor necrosis factor-α (TNF-α).

Although its name suggests that it would be tumoricidal in action, a large body of literature suggests that TNF-α can act as a tumor promoter.[155] Recent research has implicated NF-κB induction by TNF-α as the critical link between inflammation and carcinogenesis.[156,157] The proposed role of TNF-α in tumor promotion has resulted in the use of TNF-α inhibitors in cancer patients in clinical trials.

What is known about the role of TNF-α in HPV-induced carcinogenesis? HPV-infected cells are protected against TNF-α–induced apoptosis by direct effects of E7.[128] In addition, TNF-α results in increased expression of E6 and E7 in cultures of HPV-immortalized keratinocytes enhancing the malignant potential of HPV.[158] TNF-α levels are higher in cervical mucus from women with cervical cancer than in that from women with a normal cervix and CIN.[159] Information regarding the expression of TNF-α by stromal inflammatory cells in CIN and cervical cancer is limited but would be important for understanding the potential role of TNF-α in cervical carcinogenesis.

New Insights into the Role of Immunologic Suppression

Recent discoveries in the field of mucosal immunity indicate another potential mechanism for immune evasion by HPV. In the gut, the innate immune system is geared to suppress local responses against commensal gut flora and dietary antigens.[160] Immunosuppression is mediated by the expression of interleukin (IL)-10 and transforming growth factor-β (TGF-β). These suppressive cytokines are made by a subset of CD4+ T cells (called regulatory T cells) that constitutively express IL-2R on their surfaces (CD25+); these cells protect against autoimmune disease.[161] In addition, genetic ablation of this cell type in mice results in lethal inflammatory bowel disease, underscoring the importance of these cells in suppressing potentially harmful immune responses against nonpathogenic organisms in the local environment.[161] A specific transcription factor, foxp3, is necessary for the development of regulatory T cells. Genetic loss of this factor in mice or humans results in lethal autoimmune disease.[162] Therefore, understanding of the workings of the acquired immune response is now being expanded to include a specific cell type (CD4+ CD25+ foxp3+) whose role is suppression of recognition of self-antigens as well as innocuous antigens such as non-pathogenic organisms at mucosal surfaces.

Dendritic cells (DCs) play a critical role in determining the polarity of the immune response at mucosal sites (Figure 12–2). In acute inflammation, toll-like receptors are engaged, and DCs mature into antigen-presenting cells and are activated to produce proinflammatory cytokines such as IL-1, TNF-α, and IL-12. These cytokines activate a Th1 or Th2 response by stimulating the differentiation of effector CD4+ T cells. In sites of chronic infection, however (perhaps such as the cervix in women with chronic HPV infection), dendritic cells fail to mature, and they produce immunosuppressive cytokines such as TGF-β and IL-10. In this environment, CD4+ T cells are induced to differentiate into regulatory cells that themselves secrete TGF-β and IL-10. The interaction between the B7 receptor on DCs and cytotoxic T-lymphocyte antigen 4 (CTLA4) causes DCs to produce an enzyme called indolamine 2,3-dioxygenase (IDO).[163,164] IDO is an important enzyme in the suppression of immune responses by depriving cells of the essential amino acid tryptophan. Proliferation of T cells is inhibited by IDO, owing to a tryptophan-

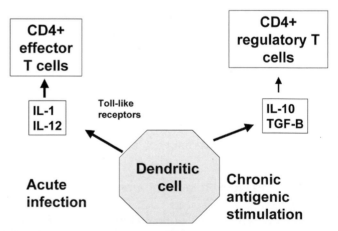

Figure 12–2.   Dendritic cells (DCs) bridge the innate and acquired immune responses and play a pivotal role in determining the type of acquired immune response elicited by specific antigens. DCs either mature to antigen-presenting cells and induce CD4+ cell differentiation to an effector phenotype (Th1 or Th2) or remain immature and induce T-regulatory-cell differentiation. Distinct cytokines made by DCs contribute to CD4+ T-cell differentiation. IL = interleukin; TGF-β = transforming growth factor-β.

sensitive G_1 checkpoint and the induction of apoptosis by IDO-mediated tryptophan catabolism and release of metabolites (eg, kynurenines).[165] IDO-arrested T cells adopt a regulatory phenotype.[166–168] Thus, IDO is an important mediator of local immunosuppression.

Accumulating data indicate an important role for immunosuppression in the development of cancer. Potent cytotoxic responses are not always induced in tumors; regulatory T cells within the tumor microenvironment have been implicated in this phenomenon. Subsets of $CD25^+$ regulatory T cells induced by IL-10 have been shown to block antitumor immunoreactivity.[169] In addition, the depletion of regulatory T cells has an antitumor effect in numerous mouse models.[170,171] The contributions of DCs in cancer are also being increasingly recognized, and efforts have been made to use autologous DCs to prime tumor-specific immune responses. IDO made by DCs has important antitumor effects.[167] The importance of IDO production is highlighted by findings in malignant melanoma that IDO detection in draining lymph nodes correlates with a significantly worse clinical outcome.[172] Therefore, the suppressive environment exists not only locally within the tumor environment but also regionally in the draining lymph nodes, where an effector immune response against tumor antigens is also suppressed.

Do these findings have relevance for the understanding of the role of HPV in carcinogenesis? Data from an E7 transgenic mouse model indicate that E7 induces immunologic tolerance; transplants of E7 transgenic skin to syngeneic hosts were not rejected unless the host was exposed to a strong inflammatory signal such as endotoxin.[173] E7 in transgenic mice downregulates the activity of $CD8^+$ T cells directly not only against E7, which again implies that E7 generates an immunosuppressive environment.[174] In humans, high levels of IL-10 have been detected in CIN cases and have led to the conclusion that the cervix may be a site of active immunosuppression.[175] The presence of TGF-β expressing $CD4^+$ $CD25^+$ cells in the stroma of CIN2 and CIN3 lesions and cancer suggests that regulatory T cells are recruited to areas of CIN.[120] Indeed, these cells also express $foxp3^+$ cells (a marker for T regulatory cells) (Figure 12–3 A) (Kobayashi and Smith-McCune, unpub-

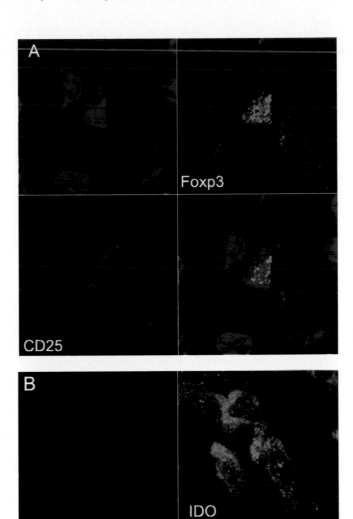

Figure 12–3. Immunosuppressive cytokines and indolamine 2,3-dioxygenase (IDO) in cervical cancer. *A*, Foxp3 (*green*) and CD25 (*red*) proteins colocalize in $CD4^+$ lymphocytes in cervical cancer, indicating a regulatory phenotype. These cells also express transforming growth factor-β.[120] (Nuclei are stained with DAPI blue fluorescent dye) *B*, IDO (*green*) localizes (*yellow*) to $CD1a^+$ (*red*) human leukocyte antigen (HLA-DR)–positive cells (not shown). IDO^+ cells also express IL10 (*not shown*), indicating two immunosuppressive factors made by cervical dendritic cells.

lished data) The densities of these cells show significant increases from the normal cervix to one with CIN2 or CIN3 and from CIN2 or CIN3 to cancer. In addition, the stroma of CIN lesions and cervical cancer contain increased numbers (compared with those of a normal cervix) of IDO^+ $IL-10^+$ cells (see Figure 12–3, B) with expression of the DC marker CD1a, suggesting that immature immunosuppressive DCs may contribute to the immune response against HPV in the cervix.

The presence of immunosuppressive cytokines and enzymes in cervical disease induced by HPV suggests that, as in the gut, a mechanism to protect host tissues from a potentially harmful immune response to normal flora exists but may impair the ability of the host to clear the infection. In addition, the presence of an inflammatory response contributes factors (such as MMP9) that are permissive of neoplastic growth. Clearly, the immune response to HPV is a two-way street with important protective effects but also with significant potential to contribute to carcinogenesis. Improved understanding of both sides of the immune response will be important in the development of effective immunomodulatory therapeutic strategies for treating CIN and cancer.

REFERENCES

1. Munoz N, Bosch FX, Shah KV, Meheus A, editors. The epidemiology of human papillomavirus and cervical cancer. Oxford: Oxford University Press; 1992.
2. Lorincz AT, Reid R, Jenson AB, et al. Human papillomavirus infection of the cervix: relative risk associations of 15 common anogenital types. Obstet Gynecol 1992;79:328–37.
3. Doorbar J. The papillomavirus life cycle. J Clin Virol 2005; 32 Suppl 1:S7–15.
4. Ostor AG. Natural history of cervical intraepithelial neoplasia: a critical review. Int J Gynecol Pathol 1993;12:186–92.
5. Parkin DM, Pisani P, Ferlay J. Estimates of the worldwide incidence of eighteen major cancers in 1985. Int J Cancer 1993;54:594–606.
6. Waggoner SE. Cervical cancer. Lancet 2003;361:2217–25.
7. Gissmann L, Boshart M, Durst M, et al. Presence of human papillomavirus in genital tumors. J Invest Dermatol 1984; 83(1 Suppl):26–8.
8. Durst M, Gissmann L, Ikenberg H, et al. A papillomavirus DNA from a cervical carcinoma and its prevalence in cancer biopsy samples from different geographic regions. Proc Natl Acad Sci U S A 1983;80:3812–5.
9. Boshart M, Gissmann L, Ikenberg H, et al. A new type of papillomavirus DNA, its presence in genital cancer biopsies and in cell lines derived from cervical cancer. Embo J 1984;3:1151–7.
10. Munoz N, Bosch FX, de Sanjose S, et al. Epidemiologic classification of human papillomavirus types associated with cervical cancer. N Engl J Med 2003;348:518–27.
11. Bosch FX, Munoz N, de Sanjose S, et al. Risk factors for cer-
12. Munoz N, Franceschi S, Bosetti C, et al. Role of parity and human papillomavirus in cervical cancer: the IARC multicentric case-control study. Lancet 2002;359:1093–101.
13. Moreno V, Bosch FX, Munoz N, et al. Effect of oral contraceptives on risk of cervical cancer in women with human papillomavirus infection: the IARC multicentric case-control study. Lancet 2002;359:1085–92.
14. Smith JS, Bosetti C, Munoz N, et al. Chlamydia trachomatis and invasive cervical cancer: a pooled analysis of the IARC multicentric case-control study. Int J Cancer 2004; 111:431–9.
15. Koskela P, Anttila T, Bjorge T, et al. Chlamydia trachomatis infection as a risk factor for invasive cervical cancer. Int J Cancer 2000;85:35–9.
16. Smith JS, Munoz N, Herrero R, et al. Evidence for Chlamydia trachomatis as a human papillomavirus cofactor in the etiology of invasive cervical cancer in Brazil and the Philippines. J Infect Dis 2002;185:324–31.
17. Castellsague X, Bosch FX, Munoz N, et al. Male circumcision, penile human papillomavirus infection, and cervical cancer in female partners. N Engl J Med 2002;346:1105–12.
18. Barbosa MS, Schlegel R. The E6 and E7 genes of HPV-18 are sufficient for inducing two-stage in vitro transformation of human keratinocytes. Oncogene 1989;4:1529–32.
19. Munger K, Phelps WC, Bubb V, et al. The E6 and E7 genes of the human papillomavirus type 16 together are necessary and sufficient for transformation of primary human keratinocytes. J Virol 1989;63:4417–21.
20. Elson DA, Riley RR, Lacey A, et al. Sensitivity of the cervical transformation zone to estrogen-induced squamous carcinogenesis. Cancer Res 2000;60:1267–75.
21. Arbeit JM, Munger K, Howley PM, et al. Progressive squamous epithelial neoplasia in K14-human papillomavirus type 16 transgenic mice. J Virol 1994;68:4358–68.
22. Arbeit JM, Howley PM, Hanahan D. Chronic estrogen-induced cervical and vaginal squamous carcinogenesis in human papillomavirus type 16 transgenic mice. Proc Natl Acad Sci U S A 1996;93:2930–5.
23. Lambert PF, Pan H, Pitot HC, et al. Epidermal cancer associated with expression of human papillomavirus type 16 E6 and E7 oncogenes in the skin of transgenic mice. Proc Natl Acad Sci U S A 1993;90:5583–7.
24. Riley RR, Duensing S, Brake T, et al. Dissection of human papillomavirus E6 and E7 function in transgenic mouse models of cervical carcinogenesis. Cancer Res 2003;63: 4862–71.
25. Goodwin EC, Yang E, Lee CJ, et al. Rapid induction of senescence in human cervical carcinoma cells. Proc Natl Acad Sci U S A 2000;97:10978–83.
26. Alazawi W, Pett M, Arch B, et al. Changes in cervical keratinocyte gene expression associated with integration of human papillomavirus 16. Cancer Res 2002;62:6959–65.
27. Wentzensen N, Vinokurova S, von Knebel Doeberitz M. Systematic review of genomic integration sites of human papillomavirus genomes in epithelial dysplasia and invasive cancer of the female lower genital tract. Cancer Res 2004;64:3878–84.
28. Pett MR, Alazawi WO, Roberts I, et al. Acquisition of high-

level chromosomal instability is associated with integration of human papillomavirus type 16 in cervical keratinocytes. Cancer Res 2004;64:1359–68.

29. Melsheimer P, Vinokurova S, Wentzensen N, et al. DNA aneuploidy and integration of human papillomavirus type 16 E6/E7 oncogenes in intraepithelial neoplasia and invasive squamous cell carcinoma of the cervix uteri. Clin Cancer Res 2004;10:3059–63.

30. von Knebel Doeberitz M. New markers for cervical dysplasia to visualise the genomic chaos created by aberrant oncogenic papillomavirus infections. Eur J Cancer 2002; 38:2229–42.

31. Steenbergen RD, de Wilde J, Wilting SM, et al. HPV-mediated transformation of the anogenital tract. J Clin Virol 2005; 32 Suppl 1:S25–33.

32. Duensing S, Munger K. Human papillomaviruses and centrosome duplication errors: modeling the origins of genomic instability. Oncogene 2002;21:6241–8.

33. Barbosa MS, Lowy DR, Schiller JT. Papillomavirus polypeptides E6 and E7 are zinc-binding proteins. J Virol 1989; 63:1404–7.

34. Longworth MS, Laimins LA. The binding of histone deacetylases and the integrity of zinc finger-like motifs of the E7 protein are essential for the life cycle of human papillomavirus type 31. J Virol 2004;78:3533–41.

35. Barbosa MS, Edmonds C, Fisher C, et al. The region of the HPV E7 oncoprotein homologous to adenovirus E1a and Sv40 large T antigen contains separate domains for Rb binding and casein kinase II phosphorylation. Embo J 1990;9:153–60.

36. Massimi P, Banks L. Differential phosphorylation of the HPV-16 E7 oncoprotein during the cell cycle. Virology 2000;276:388–94.

37. Angeline M, Merle E, Moroianu J. The E7 oncoprotein of high-risk human papillomavirus type 16 enters the nucleus via a nonclassical Ran-dependent pathway. Virology 2003;317:13–23.

38. Davies R, Hicks R, Crook T, et al. Human papillomavirus type 16 E7 associates with a histone H1 kinase and with p107 through sequences necessary for transformation. J Virol 1993;67:2521–8.

39. Smith-McCune K, Kalman D, Robbins C, et al. Intranuclear localization of human papillomavirus 16 E7 during transformation and preferential binding of E7 to the Rb family member p130. Proc Natl Acad Sci U S A 1999;96:6999–7004.

40. Dyson N. The regulation of E2F by pRB-family proteins. Genes Dev 1998;12:2245–62.

41. Morris JD, Crook T, Bandara LR, et al. Human papillomavirus type 16 E7 regulates E2F and contributes to mitogenic signalling. Oncogene 1993;8:893–8.

42. Brooks LA, Sullivan A, O'Nions J, et al. E7 proteins from oncogenic human papillomavirus types transactivate p73: role in cervical intraepithelial neoplasia. Br J Cancer 2002;86:263–8.

43. Thierry F, Benotmane MA, Demeret C, et al. A genomic approach reveals a novel mitotic pathway in papillomavirus carcinogenesis. Cancer Res 2004;64:895–903.

44. Motoyama S, Ladines-Llave CA, Luis Villanueva S, et al. The role of human papilloma virus in the molecular biology of cervical carcinogenesis. Kobe J Med Sci 2004;50:9–19.

45. Helt AM, Galloway DA. Destabilization of the retinoblastoma tumor suppressor by human papillomavirus type 16 E7 is not sufficient to overcome cell cycle arrest in human keratinocytes. J Virol 2001;75:6737–47.

46. Heck DV, Yee CL, Howley PM, et al. Efficiency of binding the retinoblastoma protein correlates with the transforming capacity of the E7 oncoproteins of the human papillomaviruses. Proc Natl Acad Sci U S A 1992;89:4442–6.

47. Schmitt A, Harry JB, Rapp B, et al. Comparison of the properties of the E6 and E7 genes of low- and high-risk cutaneous papillomaviruses reveals strongly transforming and high Rb-binding activity for the E7 protein of the low-risk human papillomavirus type 1. J Virol 1994;68:7051–9.

48. Ciccolini F, Di Pasquale G, Carlotti F, et al. Functional studies of E7 proteins from different HPV types. Oncogene 1994;9:2633–8.

49. Psyrri A, DeFilippis RA, Edwards AP, et al. Role of the retinoblastoma pathway in senescence triggered by repression of the human papillomavirus E7 protein in cervical carcinoma cells. Cancer Res 2004;64:3079–86.

50. Bischof O, Nacerddine K, Dejean A. Human papillomavirus oncoprotein E7 targets the promyelocytic leukemia protein and circumvents cellular senescence via the Rb and p53 tumor suppressor pathways. Mol Cell Biol 2005;25: 1013–24.

51. Funk JO, Waga S, Harry JB, et al. Inhibition of CDK activity and PCNA-dependent DNA replication by p21 is blocked by interaction with the HPV-16 E7 oncoprotein. Genes Dev 1997;11:2090–100.

52. Jones DL, Alani RM, Munger K. The human papillomavirus E7 oncoprotein can uncouple cellular differentiation and proliferation in human keratinocytes by abrogating p21Cip1-mediated inhibition of cdk2. Genes Dev 1997;11:2101–11.

53. Zerfass-Thome K, Zwerschke W, Mannhardt B, et al. Inactivation of the cdk inhibitor p27KIP1 by the human papillomavirus type 16 E7 oncoprotein. Oncogene 1996;13: 2323–30.

54. Vousden KH, Vojtesek B, Fisher C, et al. HPV-16 E7 or adenovirus E1A can overcome the growth arrest of cells immortalized with a temperature-sensitive p53. Oncogene 1993;8:1697–702.

55. Massimi P, Pim D, Banks L. Human papillomavirus type 16 E7 binds to the conserved carboxy-terminal region of the TATA box binding protein and this contributes to E7 transforming activity. J Gen Virol 1997;78(Pt 10):2607–13.

56. Phillips AC, Vousden KH. Analysis of the interaction between human papillomavirus type 16 E7 and the TATA-binding protein, TBP. J Gen Virol 1997;78(Pt 4):905–9.

57. Zwerschke W, Jansen-Durr P. Cell transformation by the E7 oncoprotein of human papillomavirus type 16: interactions with nuclear and cytoplasmic target proteins. Adv Cancer Res 2000;78:1–29.

58. Mazurek S, Grimm H, Boschek CB, et al. Pyruvate kinase type M2: a crossroad in the tumor metabolome. Br J Nutr 2002;87 Suppl 1:S23–9.

59. Zwerschke W, Mazurek S, Massimi P, et al. Modulation of type M2 pyruvate kinase activity by the human papillomavirus type 16 E7 oncoprotein. Proc Natl Acad Sci U S A 1999;96:1291–6.

60. Shim JH, Cho KJ, Lee KA, et al. E7-expressing HaCaT ker-

atinocyte cells are resistant to oxidative stress-induced cell death via the induction of catalase. Proteomics 2005;5:2112–22.

61. White AE, Livanos EM, Tlsty TD. Differential disruption of genomic integrity and cell cycle regulation in normal human fibroblasts by the HPV oncoproteins. Genes Dev 1994;8:666–77.

62. Thomas JT, Laimins LA. Human papillomavirus oncoproteins E6 and E7 independently abrogate the mitotic spindle checkpoint. J Virol 1998;72:1131–7.

63. Duensing S, Duensing A, Crum CP, et al. Human papillomavirus type 16 E7 oncoprotein-induced abnormal centrosome synthesis is an early event in the evolving malignant phenotype. Cancer Res 2001;61:2356–60.

64. Southern SA, Lewis MH, Herrington CS. Induction of tetrasomy by human papillomavirus type 16 E7 protein is independent of pRb binding and disruption of differentiation. Br J Cancer 2004;90:1949–54.

65. Duensing S, Munger K. The human papillomavirus type 16E6 and E7 oncoproteins independently induce numerical and structural chromosome instability. Cancer Res 2002;62:7075–82.

66. He W, Staples D, C. Smith, et al. Direct activation of cyclin-dependent kinase 2 by human papillomavirus E7. J Virol 2003;77:10566–74.

67. Longworth MS, Laimins LA. Pathogenesis of human papillomaviruses in differentiating epithelia. Microbiol Mol Biol Rev 2004;68:362–72.

68. zur Hausen H. Papillomaviruses and cancer: from basic studies to clinical application. Nat Rev Cancer 2002;2:342–50.

69. Munger K, Basile JR, Duensing S, et al. Biological activities and molecular targets of the human papillomavirus E7 oncoprotein. Oncogene 2001;20:7888–98.

70. Scheffner M, Werness BA, Huibregtse JM, et al. The E6 oncoprotein encoded by human papillomavirus types 16 and 18 promotes the degradation of p53. Cell 1990;63:1129–36.

71. Sedman SA, Hubbert NL, Vass WC, et al. Mutant p53 can substitute for human papillomavirus type 16 E6 in immortalization of human keratinocytes but does not have E6-associated trans-activation or transforming activity. J Virol 1992;66:4201–8.

72. Huibregtse JM, Scheffner M, Howley PM. A cellular protein mediates association of p53 with the E6 oncoprotein of human papillomavirus types 16 or 18. Embo J 1991;10:4129–35.

73. Huibregtse JM, Scheffner M, Howley PM. Cloning and expression of the cDNA for E6-AP, a protein that mediates the interaction of the human papillomavirus E6 oncoprotein with p53. Mol Cell Biol 1993;13:775–84.

74. Scheffner M, Huibregtse JM, Vierstra RD, et al. The HPV-16 E6 and E6-AP complex functions as a ubiquitin-protein ligase in the ubiquitination of p53. Cell 1993;75:495–505.

75. Kessis TD, Slebos RJ, Nelson WG, et al. Human papillomavirus 16 E6 expression disrupts the p53-mediated cellular response to DNA damage. Proc Natl Acad Sci U S A 1993;90:3988–92.

76. Thompson DA, Belinsky G, Chang TH, et al. The human papillomavirus-16 E6 oncoprotein decreases the vigilance of mitotic checkpoints. Oncogene 1997;15:3025–35.

77. Foster S, Demers GW, Etscheid BG, et al. The ability of human papillomavirus E6 proteins to target p53 for degradation in vivo correlates with their ability to abrogate actinomycin D-induced growth arrest. J Virol 1994;68:5698–705

78. Crook T, Tidy JA, Vousden KH. Degradation of p53 can be targeted by HPV E6 sequences distinct from those required for p53 binding and trans-activation. Cell 1991;67:547–56.

79. Band V, De Caprio JA, Delmolino L, et al. Loss of p53 protein in human papillomavirus type 16 E6-immortalized human mammary epithelial cells. J Virol 1991;65:6671–6.

80. Hawley-Nelson P, Vousden KH, Hubbert NL, et al. HPV16 E6 and E7 proteins cooperate to immortalize human foreskin keratinocytes. Embo J 1989;8:3905–10.

81. Kiyono T, Foster SA, Koop JI, et al. Both Rb/p16INK4a inactivation and telomerase activity are required to immortalize human epithelial cells. Nature 1998;396:84–8.

82. Nguyen ML, Nguyen MM, Lee D, et al. The PDZ ligand domain of the human papillomavirus type 16 E6 protein is required for E6's induction of epithelial hyperplasia in vivo. J Virol 2003;77:6957–64.

83. Tong X, Howley PM. The bovine papillomavirus E6 oncoprotein interacts with paxillin and disrupts the actin cytoskeleton. Proc Natl Acad Sci U S A 1997;94:4412–7.

84. Sattler M, Pisick E, Morrison PT, et al. Role of the cytoskeletal protein paxillin in oncogenesis. Crit Rev Oncog 2000;11:63–76.

85. Vande Pol SB, Brown MC, Turner CE. Association of bovine papillomavirus type 1 E6 oncoprotein with the focal adhesion protein paxillin through a conserved protein interaction motif. Oncogene 1998;16:43–52.

86. Patel D, Huang SM, Baglia LA, et al. The E6 protein of human papillomavirus type 16 binds to and inhibits co-activation by CBP and p300. Embo J 1999;18:5061–72.

87. Zimmermann H, Degenkolbe R, Bernard HU, et al. The human papillomavirus type 16 E6 oncoprotein can down-regulate p53 activity by targeting the transcriptional coactivator CBP/p300. J Virol 1999;73:6209–19.

88. O'Connor MJ. Targeting of transcriptional cofactors by the HPV E6 protein: another tale of David and Goliath. Trends Microbiol 2000;8:45–7.

89. Stafl A, Mattingly RF. Angiogenesis of cervical neoplasia. Am J Obstet Gynecol 1975;121:845–52.

90. Sillman F, Boyce J, Fruchter R. The significance of atypical vessels and neovascularization in cervical neoplasia. Am J Obstet Gynecol 1981;139:154–9.

91. Smith-McCune KK, Weidner N. Demonstration and characterization of the angiogenic properties of cervical dysplasia. Cancer Res 1994;54:800–4.

92. Smith-McCune K, Zhu YH, Hanahan D, et al. Cross-species comparison of angiogenesis during the premalignant stages of squamous carcinogenesis in the human cervix and K14-HPV16 transgenic mice. Cancer Res 1997;57:1294–300.

93. Smith-McCune KK, Zhu Y, Darragh T. Angiogenesis in histologically benign squamous mucosa is a sensitive marker for nearby cervical intraepithelial neoplasia. Angiogenesis 1998;2:135–42.

94. Guidi AJ, Abu-Jawdeh G, Berse B, et al. Vascular permeability factor (vascular endothelial growth factor) expression and angiogenesis in cervical neoplasia. J Natl Cancer Inst 1995;87:1237–45.

95. Dellas A, Moch H, Schultheiss E, et al. Angiogenesis in cer-

vical neoplasia: microvessel quantitation in precancerous lesions and invasive carcinomas with clinicopathological correlations. Gynecol Oncol 1997;67:27–33.

96. Dobbs SP, Hewett PW, Johnson IR, et al. Angiogenesis is associated with vascular endothelial growth factor expression in cervical intraepithelial neoplasia. Br J Cancer 1997;76:1410–5.

97. Maxwell G, Sosson A, Oster C, et al. Subepithelial angiogenesis in cervical intraepithelial neoplasia. J Low Genit Tract 1998;2:191–4.

98. Mukhopadhyay D, Datta K. Multiple regulatory pathways of vascular permeability factor/vascular endothelial growth factor (VPF/VEGF) expression in tumors. Semin Cancer Biol 2004;14:123–30.

99. Toussaint-Smith E, Donner DB, Roman A. Expression of human papillomavirus type 16 E6 and E7 oncoproteins in primary foreskin keratinocytes is sufficient to alter the expression of angiogenic factors. Oncogene 2004;23:2988–95.

100. Lopez-Ocejo O, Viloria-Petit A, Bequet-Romero M, et al. Oncogenes and tumor angiogenesis: the HPV-16 E6 oncoprotein activates the vascular endothelial growth factor (VEGF) gene promoter in a p53 independent manner. Oncogene 2000;19:4611–20.

101. Bequet-Romero M, Lopez-Ocejo O. Angiogenesis modulators expression in culture cell lines positives for HPV-16 oncoproteins. Biochem Biophys Res Commun 2000;277:55–61.

102. Wu MP, Tzeng CC, Wu LW, et al. Thrombospondin-1 acts as a fence to inhibit angiogenesis that occurs during cervical carcinogenesis. Cancer J 2004;10:27–32.

103. Kodama J, Hashimoto I, Seki N, et al. Thrombospondin-1 and -2 messenger RNA expression in invasive cervical cancer: correlation with angiogenesis and prognosis. Clin Cancer Res 2001;7:2826–31.

104. Hanahan D, Weinberg RA. The hallmarks of cancer. Cell 2000;100:57–70.

105. Hanahan D, Folkman J. Patterns and emerging mechanisms of the angiogenic switch during tumorigenesis. Cell 1996;86:353–64.

106. Maiman M. Management of cervical neoplasia in human immunodeficiency virus-infected women. J Natl Cancer Inst Monogr 1998;:43–9.

107. Penn I. Cancers of the anogenital region in renal transplant recipients. Analysis of 65 cases. Cancer 1986;58:611–6.

108. Fruchter RG, Maiman M, Sedlis A, et al. Multiple recurrences of cervical intraepithclial neoplasia in women with the human immunodeficiency virus. Obstet Gynecol 1996;87:338–44.

109. Ahdieh L, Munoz A, Vlahov D, et al. Cervical neoplasia and repeated positivity of human papillomavirus infection in human immunodeficiency virus-seropositive and -seronegative women. Am J Epidemiol 2000;151:1148–57.

110. Scott M, Nakagawa M, Moscicki AB. Cell-mediated immune response to human papillomavirus infection. Clin Diagn Lab Immunol 2001;8:209–20.

111. Kobayashi A, Darragh T, Herndier B, et al. Lymphoid follicles are generated in high-grade cervical dysplasia and have differing characteristics depending on HIV status. Am J Pathol 2002;160:151–64.

112. Bontkes HJ, de Gruijl TD, Walboomers JM, et al. Assessment of cytotoxic T-lymphocyte phenotype using the specific markers granzyme B and TIA-1 in cervical neoplastic lesions. Br J Cancer 1997;76:1353–60.

113. Bell MC, Edwards RP, Partridge EE, et al. CD8+ T lymphocytes are recruited to neoplastic cervix. J Clin Immunol 1995;15:130–6.

114. Edwards RP, Pitts A, Crowley-Nowick P, et al. Immunoglobulin-containing plasma cells recruited to cervical neoplasia. Obstet Gynecol 1996;87:520–6.

115. Edwards RP, Kuykendall K, Crowley-Nowick P, et al. T lymphocytes infiltrating advanced grades of cervical neoplasia. CD8-positive cells are recruited to invasion. Cancer 1995;76:1411–5.

116. Bell MC, Schmidt-Grimminger D, Turbat-Herrera E, et al. HIV+ patients have increased lymphocyte infiltrates in CIN lesions. Gynecol Oncol 2000;76:315–9.

117. Bethwaite PB, Holloway LJ, Thornton A, et al. Infiltration by immunocompetent cells in early stage invasive carcinoma of the uterine cervix: a prognostic study. Pathology 1996;28:321–7.

118. Cromme FV, Walboomers JM, Van Oostveen JW, et al. Lack of granzyme expression in T lymphocytes indicates poor cytotoxic T lymphocyte activation in human papillomavirus-associated cervical carcinomas. Int J Gynecol Cancer 1995;5:366–73.

119. Nicol AF, Fernandes AT, Grinsztejn B, et al. Distribution of immune cell subsets and cytokine-producing cells in the uterine cervix of human papillomavirus (HPV)-infected women: influence of HIV-1 coinfection. Diagn Mol Pathol 2005;14:39–47.

120. Kobayashi A, Greenblatt RM, Anastos K, et al. Functional attributes of mucosal immunity in cervical intraepithelial neoplasia and effects of HIV infection. Cancer Res 2004;64:6766–74.

121. Tindle RW. Immune evasion in human papillomavirus-associated cervical cancer. Nat Rev Cancer 2002;2:59–65.

122. Frazer IH, Thomas R, Zhou J, et al. Potential strategies utilised by papillomavirus to evade host immunity. Immunol Rev 1999;168:131–42.

123. Man S, Fiander A. Immunology of human papillomavirus infection in lower genital tract neoplasia. Best Pract Res Clin Obstet Gynaecol 2001;15:701–14.

124. Giannini SL, Hubert P, Doyen J, et al. Influence of the mucosal epithelium microenvironment on Langerhans cells: implications for the development of squamous intraepithelial lesions of the cervix. Int J Cancer 2002;97:654–9.

125. Kono K, Ressing ME, Brandt RM, et al. Decreased expression of signal-transducing zeta chain in peripheral T cells and natural killer cells in patients with cervical cancer. Clin Cancer Res 1996;2:1825–8.

126. de Gruijl TD, Bontkes HJ, Peccatori F, et al. Expression of CD3-zeta on T-cells in primary cervical carcinoma and in metastasis-positive and -negative pelvic lymph nodes. Br J Cancer 1999;79:1127–32.

127. Bachmann A, Hanke B, Zawatzky R, et al. Disturbance of tumor necrosis factor alpha-mediated beta interferon signaling in cervical carcinoma cells. J Virol 2002;76:280–91.

128. Thompson DA, Zacny V, Belinsky GS, et al. The HPV E7 oncoprotein inhibits tumor necrosis factor alpha-

mediated apoptosis in normal human fibroblasts. Oncogene 2001;20:3629–40.

129. Barnard P, Payne E, McMillan NA. The human papillomavirus E7 protein is able to inhibit the antiviral and anti-growth functions of interferon-alpha. Virology 2000;277:411–9.

130. Park JS, Kim EJ, Kwon HJ, et al. Inactivation of interferon regulatory factor-1 tumor suppressor protein by HPV E7 oncoprotein. Implication for the E7-mediated immune evasion mechanism in cervical carcinogenesis. J Biol Chem 2000;275:6764–9.

131. Ronco LV, Karpova AY, Vidal M, et al. Human papillomavirus 16 E6 oncoprotein binds to interferon regulatory factor-3 and inhibits its transcriptional activity. Genes Dev 1998;12:2061–72.

132. Wright T, Ferenczy A, Kurman R. Pre-cancerous lesions of the cervix. In: Kurman R, editor. Blaustein's pathology of the female genital tract. New York: Springer-Verlag; 1994. p. 229–77.

133. Giraudo E, Inoue M, Hanahan D. An amino-bisphosphonate targets MMP-9-expressing macrophages and angiogenesis to impair cervical carcinogenesis. J Clin Invest 2004; 114:623–33.

134. Coussens LM, Raymond WW, Bergers G, et al. Inflammatory mast cells up-regulate angiogenesis during squamous epithelial carcinogenesis. Genes Dev 1999;13:1382–97.

135. Coussens LM, Tinkle CL, Hanahan D, et al. MMP-9 supplied by bone marrow-derived cells contributes to skin carcinogenesis. Cell 2000;103:481–90.

136. Bergers G, Brekken R, McMahon G, et al. Matrix metalloproteinase-9 triggers the angiogenic switch during carcinogenesis. Nat Cell Biol 2000;2:737–44.

137. Wood J, Bonjean K, Ruetz S, et al. Novel antiangiogenic effects of the bisphosphonate compound zoledronic acid. J Pharmacol Exp Ther 2002;302:1055–61.

138. Bezzi M, Hasmim M, Bieler G, et al. Zoledronate sensitizes endothelial cells to tumor necrosis factor-induced programmed cell death: evidence for the suppression of sustained activation of focal adhesion kinase and protein kinase B/Akt. J Biol Chem, 2003;278:43603–14.

139. Santini, D., B. Vincenzi, G. Dicuonzo, et al., Zoledronic acid induces significant and long-lasting modifications of circulating angiogenic factors in cancer patients. Clin Cancer Res 2003;9:2893–7.

140. Davidson B, Goldberg I, Kopolovic J, et al. Expression of matrix metalloproteinase-9 in squamous cell carcinoma of the uterine cervix-clinicopathologic study using immunohistochemistry and mRNA in situ hybridization. Gynecol Oncol 1999;72:380–6.

141. Asha Nair S, Karunagaran D, Nair MB, et al. Changes in matrix metalloproteinases and their endogenous inhibitors during tumor progression in the uterine cervix. J Cancer Res Clin Oncol 2003;129:123–31.

142. Sheu BC, Lien HC, Ho HN, et al. Increased expression and activation of gelatinolytic matrix metalloproteinases is associated with the progression and recurrence of human cervical cancer. Cancer Res 2003;63:6537–42.

143. Balkwill F, Mantovani A. Inflammation and cancer: back to Virchow? Lancet 2001;357:539–45.

144. Coussens LM, Werb Z. Inflammation and cancer. Nature 2002;420:860–7.

145. Balkwill F, Coussens LM. Cancer: an inflammatory link. Nature 2004;431:405–6.

146. Balkwill F. Cancer and the chemokine network. Nat Rev Cancer 2004;4:540–50.

147. Jones MK, Wang H, Peskar BM, et al. Inhibition of angiogenesis by nonsteroidal anti-inflammatory drugs: insight into mechanisms and implications for cancer growth and ulcer healing. Nat Med 1999;5:1418–23.

148. Li G, Yang T, Yan J. Cyclooxygenase-2 increased the angiogenic and metastatic potential of tumor cells. Biochem Biophys Res Commun 2002;299:886–90.

149. Oshima M, Murai N, Kargman S, et al. Chemoprevention of intestinal polyposis in the Apcdelta716 mouse by rofecoxib, a specific cyclooxygenase-2 inhibitor. Cancer Res 2001;61:1733–40.

150. Daniel D, Meyer-Morse N, Bergsland EK, et al. Immune enhancement of skin carcinogenesis by CD4+ T cells. J Exp Med 2003;197:1017–28.

151. Kulkarni S, Rader JS, Zhang F, et al. Cyclooxygenase-2 is overexpressed in human cervical cancer. Clin Cancer Res 2001;7:429–34.

152. Ryu HS, Chang KH, Yang HW, et al. High cyclooxygenase-2 expression in stage IB cervical cancer with lymph node metastasis or parametrial invasion. Gynecol Oncol 2000;76:320–5.

153. Sales KJ, Katz AA, Davis M, et al. Cyclooxygenase-2 expression and prostaglandin E synthesis are up-regulated in carcinomas of the cervix: a possible autocrine/paracrine regulation of neoplastic cell function via EP2/EP4 receptors. J Clin Endocrinol Metab 2001;86:2243–9.

154. Sales KJ, Katz AA, Howard B, et al. Cyclooxygenase-1 is up-regulated in cervical carcinomas: autocrine/paracrine regulation of cyclooxygenase-2, prostaglandin e receptors, and angiogenic factors by cyclooxygenase-1. Cancer Res 2002;62:424–32.

155. Szlosarek PW, Balkwill FR. Tumor necrosis factor alpha: a potential target for the therapy of solid tumours. Lancet Oncol 2003;4:565–73.

156. Pikarsky E, Porat RM, Stein I, et al. NF-kappaB functions as a tumour promoter in inflammation-associated cancer. Nature 2004;431:461–6.

157. Greten FR, Eckmann L, Greten TF, et al. IKKbeta links inflammation and tumorigenesis in a mouse model of colitis-associated cancer. Cell 2004;118:285–96.

158. Gaiotti D, Chung J, Iglesias M, et al. Tumor necrosis factor-alpha promotes human papillomavirus (HPV) E6/E7 RNA expression and cyclin-dependent kinase activity in HPV-immortalized keratinocytes by a ras-dependent pathway. Mol Carcinog 2000;27:97–109.

159. Tjiong MY, van der Vange N, ter Schegget JS, et al. Cytokines in cervicovaginal washing fluid from patients with cervical neoplasia. Cytokine 2001;14:357–60.

160. Allez M, Mayer L. Regulatory T cells: peace keepers in the gut. Inflamm Bowel Dis 2004;10:666–76.

161. Sakaguchi S, Sakaguchi N, Shimizu J, et al. Immunologic tolerance maintained by CD25+ CD4+ regulatory T cells: their common role in controlling autoimmunity, tumor immunity, and transplantation tolerance. Immunol Rev 2001;182:18–32.

162. Ochs HD, Ziegler SF, Torgerson TR. FOXP3 acts as a rheo-

stat of the immune response. Immunol Rev 2005;203: 156–64.

163. Uyttenhove C, Pilotte L, Theate I, et al. Evidence for a tumoral immune resistance mechanism based on tryptophan degradation by indoleamine 2,3-dioxygenase. Nat Med 2003;9:1269–74.

164. Fallarino F, Grohmann U, Hwang KW, et al. Modulation of tryptophan catabolism by regulatory T cells. Nat Immunol 2003;4:1206–12.

165. Grohmann U, Fallarino F, Puccetti P. Tolerance, DCs and tryptophan: much ado about IDO. Trends Immunol 2003;24:242–8.

166. Wakkach A, Fournier N, Brun V, et al. Characterization of dendritic cells that induce tolerance and T regulatory 1 cell differentiation in vivo. Immunity 2003;18:605–17.

167. Munn DH, Mellor AL. IDO and tolerance to tumors. Trends Mol Med 2004;10:15–8.

168. Mellor AL, Munn DH. IDO expression by dendritic cells: tolerance and tryptophan catabolism. Nat Rev Immunol 2004;4:762–74.

169. Seo N, Hayakawa S, Takigawa M, et al. Interleukin-10 expressed at early tumour sites induces subsequent generation of CD4(+) T-regulatory cells and systemic collapse of antitumour immunity. Immunology 2001;103:449–57.

170. Shimizu J, Yamazaki S, Sakaguchi S. Induction of tumor immunity by removing CD25+CD4+ T cells: a common basis between tumor immunity and autoimmunity. J Immunol 1999;163:5211–8.

171. Onizuka S, Tawara I, Shimizu J, et al. Tumor rejection by in vivo administration of anti-CD25 (interleukin-2 receptor alpha) monoclonal antibody. Cancer Res 1999;59:3128–33.

172. Munn DH, Sharma MD, Hou D, et al. Expression of indoleamine 2,3-dioxygenase by plasmacytoid dendritic cells in tumor-draining lymph nodes. J Clin Invest 2004; 114:280–90.

173. Frazer IH, De Kluyver R, Leggatt GR, et al. Tolerance or immunity to a tumor antigen expressed in somatic cells can be determined by systemic proinflammatory signals at the time of first antigen exposure. J Immunol 2001; 167:6180–7.

174. Tindle RW, Herd K, Doan T, et al. Nonspecific down-regulation of CD8+ T-cell responses in mice expressing human papillomavirus type 16 E7 oncoprotein from the keratin-14 promoter. J Virol 2001;75:5985–97.

175. Giannini SL, Al-Saleh W, Piron H, et al. Cytokine expression in squamous intraepithelial lesions of the uterine cervix: implications for the generation of local immunosuppression. Clin Exp Immunol 1998;113:183–9.

13

Human Papillomavirus–Related Malignancies With and Without HIV: Epidemiology, Diagnosis, and Management

PETER V. CHIN-HONG

JOEL M. PALEFSKY

Human papillomavirus (HPV) is one of the most common sexually transmitted infections and an important cause of anogenital and other malignancies. HPV-associated cervical cancer is the most common cancer in women in developing countries and the second most common cancer in women worldwide. Anal cancer is also strongly linked to HPV infection. Although anal cancer is a rare disease in the general population, its incidence is increasing and is especially high among human immunodeficiency virus (HIV)-positive women and men who have sex with men. More common than invasive cancer are HPV-associated cancer precursor lesions, such as cervical intraepithelial neoplasia (CIN) and anal intraepithelial neoplasia (AIN). HPV is also linked to other malignancies (such as squamous cell cancers of the oropharynx, larynx, and skin) as well as a wide array of nonmalignant lesions such as common cutaneous warts and recurrent respiratory papillomatosis. The spectrum of HPV-associated disease in the HIV-positive individual is similar, but these patients have a higher prevalence and incidence of intraepithelial neoplasia and invasive cancer compared with HIV-negative individuals. It is controversial how the widespread use of highly active anti-retroviral therapy (HAART) is changing the epidemiology of HPV-associated disease in HIV-positive women and men, with several studies showing a benefit of HAART in regression of CIN and AIN, and others showing no

difference. This chapter will focus on HPV-related anogenital malignancies in HIV-positive and HIV-negative individuals, although extragenital HPV malignancies will also be briefly reviewed.

EPIDEMIOLOGY

Cervical Cancer

Prevalence and Incidence

The incidence of cervical cancer was estimated to be 40 to 50 cases per 100,000 person-years in the United States prior to the widespread institution of cervical cancer cytology screening.[1] Currently, the incidence of cervical cancer is 8 to 10 cases per 100,000 person-years, now accounting for 1.4% of cancer deaths in women and attesting to the impact of effective screening programs in disease control.[2-4] In the nondeveloped world, the statistics are more sobering. It is estimated that cervical cancer is the most common malignancy in women in developing countries, accounting for almost a quarter of a million deaths annually. Most of this discrepancy is thought to be due to few, if any, programs for cervical cancer screening in many of these countries.[5]

In HIV-positive patients, the incidence of cervical cancer is higher than that in HIV-negative women. One study early in the HIV epidemic showed a 100%

mortality associated with cervical cancer in HIV-positive women.[6] This and similar studies resulted in the designation of cervical cancer as an acquired immune deficiency syndrome (AIDS)-defining condition.[6,7] Cervical cancer may occur at a younger age compared with HIV-uninfected women.[8] The progression of CIN to invasive cancer has also been found to be shorter in HIV-positive women compared with HIV-negative women.[8] "Invasive cervical cancer" is listed under 1993 CDC guidelines as an AIDS-defining illness. However, its association with HIV infection is confounded by HPV, and the strength of association with HIV varies widely depending on the geographic location and risk factor for HIV infection. The International Agency for Research on Cancer concluded in 1996 that there was no evidence for a significant increase in invasive cervical cancer among HIV-positive women.[9] Other reports have different findings, with some showing an increased incidence of cervical cancer in HIV-positive women in South Africa and in Europe.[10,11]

Risk Factors

Human papillomavirus is universally accepted as the causative agent for invasive cervical cancer, based on rigorous investigation and review.[12,13] HPV DNA has been isolated in 90 to 100% of cervical cancer specimens compared with 5 to 20% of HPV DNA in cervical specimens from women without cervical cancer.[14] In one recent study pooling data from 11 case-control studies conducted in nine countries, HPV DNA was detected in 91% of women with cervical cancer compared with 13% of women without cervical cancer, with odds ratios in most countries being over 100.[15] Of the more than 100 HPV types isolated, 15 (types 16, 18, 31, 33, 35, 39, 45, 51, 52, 56, 58, 59, 68, 73, and 82) have been designated as high-risk types based on their association with invasive cervical cancer.[15] HPV type 16 alone accounts for about 50% of cervical cancers, and types 16, 18, 31, 33, and 45 together account for about 90% of the cases of cervical cancer worldwide.[15,16]

Although HPV infection is seen as being necessary for the development of invasive cervical cancer, it may not be sufficient, and several cofactors that influence the development of cervical cancer have

been determined.[13] These can be grouped into three categories: (1) environmental cofactors, (2) viral cofactors, and (3) host cofactors.[17] Environmental cofactors have been extensively studied. Those that have been demonstrated to increase the risk of cervical cancer include the use of oral contraceptives, tobacco smoking, low socioeconomic status, and coinfection with HIV and other sexually transmitted infections such as *Chlamydia trachomatis*.[18–22] Viral cofactors include specific HPV type, infection with multiple types, HPV type variant, and HPV viral load.[15,23–27] Host cofactors include host genetic factors and immunosuppression.[28,29] Many of the other risk factors that have been associated with cervical cancer, such as early onset of sexual activity and the number of sexual partners, may reflect acquisition of HPV infection.[14]

Cervical Intraepithelial Neoplasia

Nomenclature

CIN is a treatable and identifiable precursor lesion of cervical cancer. The grading schema CIN I to III (Figure 13–1) reflect the degree of histologic abnormality observed on biopsy. CIN I is not thought to

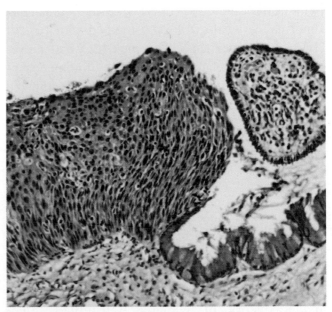

Figure 13–1. Cervical intraepithelial neoplasia III. Most of the epithelium is replaced by immature cells with large nuclear-to-cytoplasmic ratios. Courtesy of Dr. Teresa Darragh, University of California at San Francisco, USA.

progress to cervical cancer. However, CIN II and III are likely the true cervical cancer precursor lesions. Cytologic abnormalities detected on cervical Papanicolaou (Pap) tests are classified using the Bethesda system.[30] Low-grade squamous intraepithelial lesions (LSIL) are equivalent to condylomata and CIN I, and high-grade SIL (HSIL) is equivalent to CIN II and III. Atypical squamous cells (ASC) do not have all of the features of HSIL or LSIL but are not benign; they may be of undetermined significance (ASC-US) or suspicious for HSIL (ASC-H).

Prevalence and Incidence

The prevalence of CIN varies with the population sampled. This varies from 1% in some populations to 14% in sexually transmitted disease clinics in the United States.[31] A cross-sectional study including 482 at-risk HIV-negative women enrolled in the Women's Interagency HIV Study (WIHS) demonstrated that 16% of women had abnormal cervical cytology.[32] In general, approximately 5% of cervical Pap tests performed each year in the United States are abnormal.[33]

The prevalence of CIN in HIV-positive women is higher than that in HIV-negative women. In one cross-sectional study of 755 women, 20% of HIV-positive women were diagnosed with CIN, compared with 4% of at-risk HIV-negative women.[34] In the WIHS study, 38% of HIV-positive women had abnormal cervical cytology compared with 16% of HIV-negative women.[32] The incidence and prevalence of CIN is related to the degree of immunosuppression. In a multisite European study, compared with women who had CD4 > 500 cells/μL[3], women with CD4 < 200 cells/μL had a twofold increase in CIN prevalence and incidence.[35]

Risk Factors

Infection with HPV is one of the most powerful determinants of CIN. Sexual activity has been consistently demonstrated to be a risk factor for CIN in all women. Specific behavioral determinants include age at first sexual activity, multiple sexual partners, and a history of sexually transmitted infections.[14,17,36] These sexual risk factors likely reflect risk factors for HPV infection. In one case-control study of 1,000 women examining potential risk factors for CIN, the odds ratios of many behavioral and sociodemographic factors were substantially diminished after HPV infection was adjusted for in the analysis.[37] The role of cigarette smoking was thought to be related to the exposure of tobacco-related carcinogens on HPV-infected cervical epithelial cells as well as promoting local immunosuppression through its effect on number and function of Langerhans cells. However, when data were adjusted for HPV infection in some studies, cigarette smoking was no longer an independent risk factor for the development of CIN. Other risk factors include immunosuppression and multiparity.[29,34,38] The role of oral contraceptives and other dietary determinants such as β-carotene and folate with CIN is more controversial.[14,17]

Natural History of CIN and Cervical Cancer

Understanding the natural history of CIN is important for cervical cancer prevention strategies. Young sexually active women have a disproportionately high prevalence of HPV infection. After the age of 30 years, the prevalence of cervical HPV infection decreases substantially.[39,40] A fraction of women have persistent HPV infection, and it is these women who are thought to be at the highest risk for the development of invasive cervical cancer. Similarly, a large proportion of low-grade CIN eventually spontaneously regresses to normal. Moscicki and colleagues studied 187 young women (median age, 20 years) with incident CIN I.[41] They found that the probability of regression for the entire cohort was 61% at 12 months, and 91% at 36 months of follow-up.[41] Using population-based sampling, Herrero and colleagues reported that the prevalence of LSIL peaked under the age of 25 years, decreased significantly by age 25 to 34 years, and then continued to fall in women over 65 years of age.[39,40] The prevalence of HSIL peaked later at ages 25 to 34 years, followed by a decline at ages 35 to 44 years and a smaller rise in prevalence in women older than 65 years of age. If undetected, more than 10% of cervical HSIL has been estimated to progress to invasive cervical cancer in 9 to 10 years.[5,42]

In vitro studies have shown that HIV infection can increase HPV gene expression.[43] However, whether this translates into accelerated progression of clinical disease to invasive cancer has not been conclusively proven (see "Pathogenesis of CIN and AIN in HIV-Positive Individuals and the Role of HAART," below).

Anal Cancer

Prevalence and Incidence

Anal cancer is an uncommon cancer of the digestive tract that is increasing in incidence in women and men, from about 10 cases per million to 20 cases per million from 1973 to 2000.[44] This increase is seen most dramatically in urban areas with large proportions of at-risk populations, such as men who have sex with men (MSM). Before the HIV epidemic, it was estimated that the incidence of anal cancer was estimated to be as high as 37 per 100,000 person-years in MSM, a comparable figure to the incidence of invasive cervical cancer in women prior to the introduction of cervical cytology screening.[45] In San Francisco, the incidence of anal cancer was reported to have increased in men aged 40 to 64 years, from 3.7 per 100,000 in 1973 to 1978, to 20.6 per 100,000 in 1996 to 1999.[46]

Studies suggest that the incidence of anal cancer is even higher among HIV-positive women and men. Data from matching cancer and AIDS registries show that the relative risk of invasive anal cancer was 6.8 in HIV-positive women and 37 in HIV-positive men compared with the general population.[8] Anal and cervical cancers are similar in histologic appearance and are often associated with adjacent AIN II or III and CIN II or III, respectively. Both anal and cervical cancers usually arise in the transformation zone, the junction between the columnar epithelium of the rectum or endocervix, and the squamous epithelium of the anus or exocervix.[1]

Risk Factors

Similar to cervical cancer, HPV infection is one of the most important risk factors for anal cancer. HPV DNA has been associated with up to 100% of squamous cell cancers of the anal canal.[47–49] Frisch and colleagues demonstrated in a case-control study that 88% of individuals with anal cancer had HPV DNA isolated compared with none of 20 control patients with rectal adenocarcinoma.[47] HPV type 16 is the most common HPV type isolated in anal cancer. Although sexual activity was shown in early studies to be a risk factor for anal cancer, this may be confounded with the role of anal HPV infection, which is commonly sexually transmitted. In a Scandinavian population-based case-control study, strong independent risk factors for anal cancer in women and men included higher numbers of sexual partners and a history of other sexually transmitted infections.[47] Using the Surveillance, Epidemiology and End Results (SEER) program in the United States, the relative risk of anal cancer in women following a diagnosis of invasive cervical cancer was 4.6, attesting to shared risk factors for these two cancers, the most important of which is likely to be HPV infection.[50] Cigarette smoking is another risk factor for anal cancer. One case-control study showed that the relative risks of anal cancer were 1.9 for 20-pack-year smokers and 5.2 for 50-pack-year smokers.[51] Apart from MSM and HIV-infected men and women, other immunocompromised patients such as transplant recipients are at increased risk of anal cancer.[52,53]

Anal Intraepithelial Neoplasia

Nomenclature

Like CIN, AIN is a precursor to invasive cancer. After HPV infection, the anus may demonstrate disease ranging from AIN I to III. The grading system reflects the degree of histologic abnormality observed. AIN I is not likely to progress to anal cancer whereas AIN II and III are believed to be the true anal cancer precursors. Like the cervical cytologic classification, the findings of anal cytologic examination are considered either "normal" or "abnormal." The abnormal category comprises LSIL (Figure 13–2), which is equivalent to condylomata and AIN I, and HSIL (Figure 13–3A), which is equivalent to AIN II and III (Figure 13–3B). Similar to cervical cytologic terminology, ASCs of undetermined significance (ASC-US) or ASC suspicious for HSIL (ASC-H) do not have all of the features of HSIL or LSIL but are not benign.

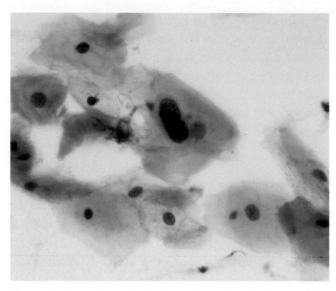

Figure 13–2. Anal cytologic changes consistent with low-grade squamous intraepithelial lesions. Compared with unaffected epithelial cells, the affected cells have denser chromatin and an increased nuclear to cytoplasmic ratio. Courtesy of Dr. Teresa Darragh, University of California at San Francisco, USA.

Prevalence and Incidence

The prevalence of AIN is highest in subpopulations such as MSM, HIV-infected men and women, women with HPV-associated vulvar disease, and transplant recipients. In one study of 1,262 HIV-negative MSM from four US cities, 20% of participants were found to have AIN. AIN II or III was found in 5%.[54] This is likely an underestimate, since only cytologic analysis was performed. The prevalence of AIN is higher in HIV-positive individuals compared with HIV-negative individuals. This is true of both men and women. One cross-sectional study of MSM demonstrated a higher prevalence of AIN in HIV-positive men (36 %) compared with HIV-negative men (7 %).[55] In another cross-sectional study, 26% of HIV-positive women had AIN diagnosed, compared with 8% of HIV-negative women.[56]

HIV-positive men are still at risk for AIN in the absence of anal intercourse. One study showed that 46% of heterosexual injection drug users had anal HPV infection, 16% had AIN I, and 18% had AIN II or III.[57] Even if there was no AIN found at baseline, the incidence of AIN in at-risk populations is high. One study showed that the incidence of AIN II or III was 49% over 4 years in HIV-positive men and 17% in HIV-negative men.[55]

Risk Factors

Anal HPV infection is the most significant risk factor for the development of AIN. In the Explore study of AIN in HIV-negative MSM, risk factors identified included number of receptive anal sex partners and injection drug use; however, HPV infection, and a higher number of HPV types detected, were the

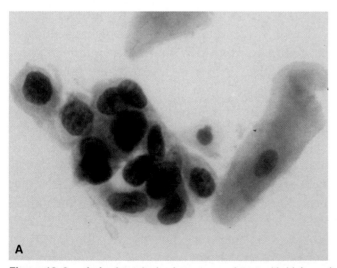

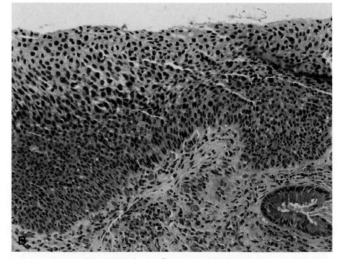

Figure 13–3. *A,* Anal cytologic changes consistent with high-grade squamous intraepithelial lesions. Compared with the low-grade squamous intraepithelial lesion seen in Figure 13–2, the affected cells have a larger nucleus with dense chromatin and very little cytoplasm. *B,* Anal intraepithelial neoplasia III. There is replacement of most of the epithelium by immature cells with large nuclear to cytoplasmic ratios. Courtesy of Dr. Teresa Darragh, University of California at San Francisco, USA.

strongest risk factors for AIN.[54] In women, additional risk factors include a history of CIN II or III, and cervical and vulvar cancers.[58–60] In HIV-positive men and women, lower CD4 cell count is found to correlate with AIN.[61,62]

Natural History of AIN and Anal Cancer

There has been only limited information about age-associated changes in AIN in affected subgroups. One cross-sectional study of sexually active HIV-negative MSM aged 18 to 89 years demonstrated that there was no change in AIN prevalence with age.[54] Another cross-sectional analysis using the same cohort showed that these MSM had a stable prevalence of HPV infection across all age groups.[63] Because the overall prevalence of HPV and the number of HPV types did not increase with age, it implied that newly acquired HPV infections were transient.

Pathogenesis of CIN and AIN in HIV-Positive Individuals and the Role of HAART

It is thought that HPV infection is acquired early after the initiation of sexual activity. Individuals may subsequently acquire HIV infection. With ongoing sexual activity, individuals may acquire more HPV types (Figure 13–4). In early HIV disease, the immune system is relatively intact; there is a low prevalence of HPV and little CIN or AIN. With more advanced HIV disease and declining CD4 cell counts, HPV-specific immunity may be attenuated and more HPV types can be detected, perhaps because of reactivation of old HPV types. This may lead to the development of CIN I or AIN I, and progression to CIN II and III or AIN II and III.

Observational studies suggest that immunosuppression is linked to the development of CIN and AIN. However, the role of immunosuppression in the progression to invasive cancer is unclear. Unlike other HIV-related malignancies such as Kaposi's sarcoma and non-Hodgkin's lymphoma, there is no significant increase in invasive cervical or anal cancer after an AIDS diagnosis.[64,65] Other factors such as host genomic mutations, not intrinsic immunosuppression, may be more important in the progression to invasive cancer.[66] HIV-associated immunosuppression may permit the continued high-level expression of oncogenic proteins such as E6 and E7 by HPV-infected epithelial cells, which in turn may lead to genetic instability.[67] It is speculated that it is this instability, rather than the immunosuppression per se, that results in the subsequent progression of disease from CIN II or III and AIN II or III to invasive cervical and anal cancers, respectively. If this is true, then we would expect HAART to have only a limited impact on the incidence of cervical and anal cancer.

Several reports have been published that have examined the role of HAART on the natural history

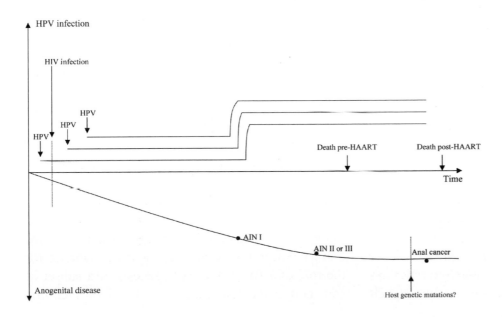

Figure 13–4. Pathogenesis of human papillomavirus–related anal intraepithelial neoplasia (AIN) and anal cancer, before and after the introduction of highly active anti-retroviral therapy (HAART).

HPV is first acquired after the initiation of sexual activity, followed by AIN. After HIV infection and the attenuation of HIV-specific immunity, there is high-level expression of HPV proteins resulting in genomic instability. Genomic instability may lead to anal cancer which may increase in prevalence given the longer survival conferred by HAART.

of CIN and AIN. Heard and colleagues reported the experience of 168 HIV-positive women with CIN.[68] Of these, 96 women received HAART during the study period. Women with CIN II or III were more likely to regress (either to CIN I or normal) compared with women with CIN I, and multivariate analysis showed that regression was related to HAART. However, only 6 women (7.5 %) with CIN II or III regressed to normal, and it is debatable whether the regression from CIN II or III to CIN I was a clinically meaningful event. Ahdieh-Grant and colleagues used data collected from the WIHS to demonstrate that HAART was associated with increased regression of CIN.[69] Women who had higher CD4 cell counts were more likely to have CIN regression. However, even in women on HAART, the majority of lesions did not regress to normal. One study by Palefsky and colleagues compared anal HPV infection and AIN in 98 HIV-positive men, 6 months prior to the initiation of HAART, to the time period 6 months after HAART was started.[70] Of 38 men who were diagnosed with AIN I or ASC prior to the initiation of HAART, 18% progressed to AIN II or III, and 21% regressed 6 months after starting HAART. Only 1 of 28 men with pre-HAART AIN II or III regressed to normal 6 months after HAART was started. There was no change in the proportion of participants who were found to have anal HPV infection before and after HAART was introduced. In one French cross-sectional study, 64% of men who had received HAART for a median of 32 months had AIN and 80% had anal HPV infection.[71] The proportion of anal HPV infection and AIN was similar, whether or not patients had a HAART-associated increase in CD4 cell count. Overall, these studies show that HAART has little impact on regression of AIN or CIN to normal. Moreover, there is no evidence that rates of cervical and anal cancers have declined since the introduction of HAART.[46,72]

Vulvar Cancer and Vulvar Intraepithelial Neoplasia

The incidence of HPV-associated vulvar cancer (squamous cell cancer, classic or solenoid type) has remained stable. Risks for vulvar squamous cell carcinoma include cigarette smoking, a history of cervical cancer, older age, vulvar HPV infection, vulvar intraepithelial neoplasia (VIN), and HIV disease.[73] Unlike anal or cervical cancers, a high proportion of vulvar cancer (about 50%) is not associated with HPV and may have a different disease pathogenesis than cancers linked to HPV infection.[74,75] The incidence of VIN has been increasing, even prior to the HIV epidemic.[76] This may be because of increased detection or it could also be because of a different disease pathogenesis. The prevalence of VIN is higher in HIV-positive women, particularly with lower CD4 cell count.[77,78] HIV-positive women with VIN also have high rates of recurrent disease. Risk factors for VIN mirror those for invasive vulvar carcinoma, and also include injection drug use.[77]

Penile Cancer and Penile Intraepithelial Neoplasia

Penile squamous cell carcinoma is an HPV-associated malignancy that is more common in the developed world. Risk factors for penile cancer include psoralen plus ultraviolet A (PU VA) photochemotherapy, a higher number of sexual partners, and penile trauma.[79] Infection with HPV is also a risk factor, but unlike anal and cervical cancers, HPV is only responsible for about 70% of all penile cancers.[80] Although penile cancer is not an AIDS-defining cancer, Frisch and colleagues linked AIDS and cancer registries to demonstrate that the relative risk of penile cancer was 3.9 in HIV-positive men compared with the general population.[65] However, because penile cancer is a rare disease, it is unclear how HIV disease precisely modulates the natural history of penile intraepithelial neoplasia (PIN) and invasive penile cancer.

Extragenital HPV-Related Malignancies

The role of HPV infection in the pathogenesis of extragenital malignancies has also been investigated (Table 13–1). Apart from anogenital malignancies that have been reviewed, there is some evidence for the role of HPV in the pathogenesis of a subset of squamous cell carcinomas (SCC) of the oropharynx,

	Table 13–1. EXTRAGENITAL HUMAN PAPILLOMAVIRUS–RELATED MALIGNANCIES	
Site	**Role of HPV**	**Evidence**
Oropharynx	Subset of SCC linked to HPV, especially tonsils (most oropharyngeal SCCs attributable to alcohol and tobacco use).	High-risk HPV types (mainly 16, 31, 33) isolated.[106] Cases have higher prevalence of HPV types 16 and 18 E6 and E7 antibodies.[107] HIV-positive men have increased risk of tonsillar cancer.[8]
Larynx	Subset of SCC linked to HPV (most laryngeal SCCs attributable to alcohol and tobacco use).	High-risk HPV types detected in malignancies.[108] HPV type 16 E6 expression detected in cases.[108] Increased risk of laryngeal cancer if HPV type 16 L1-seropositive.[109]
Skin	HPV-associated epidermodysplasia verruciformis (EV) is a rare hereditary disease notable for disseminated cutaneous warts, macules, and plaques that arise in childhood. Nonmelanoma skin cancer (NMSC) includes SCC and basal cell carcinoma. Possible role of HPV in non-EV NMSC.	High risk of later SCC in sun-exposed areas.[110] HPV types 5 and 8 mainly isolated in SCC.[111] HPV DNA isolated in up to 50% of NMSC in immunocompetent patients, up to 90% of SCC in immunocompromised patients.[110]
Conjunctiva	Likely role of HPV in subset of conjunctival SCC.	HPV detected in dysplastic lesions and in invasive SCC.[81] HIV-positive individuals have a 13-fold risk of conjunctival SCC compared with HIV-negative individuals.[112] HPV types 16 and 18 E6 and E7 transcripts demonstrated in SCC.[113]
Esophagus	Possible role of HPV in esophageal SCC.	HPV isolated in esophageal carcinomas.[114] HPV type 16 capsid protein antibodies were associated with a fivefold risk of esophageal cancer in one study.[115] Not replicated in other studies.[81]

HPV = human papillomavirus; SCC = squamous cell carcinoma.

larynx, skin, and conjunctiva. There is limited evidence for the role of HPV in esophageal SCC. HPV has been investigated in, and is unlikely to play a role in, the etiology of retinoblastoma, and cancers of the prostate, breast, lung, bladder, ovary, endometrium, and colon.[81]

SCREENING AND DIAGNOSIS

General Principles

The diagnosis of HPV-related disease in each patient begins with a thorough physical examination. Even if the physical examination is normal, cervical cancer and—in the opinion of these authors—anal cancer screening, should be offered to at-risk populations. For cervical cancer screening, this includes all sexually active women. Anal cancer screening should be offered to all HIV-positive women and men, MSM, women with a history of vulvar or cervical cancer, and possibly organ transplant recipients. Given that CIN II and III as well as AIN II and III are the likely precursors of cervical and anal cancers, respectively, screening programs that have been developed incorporate the identification and removal of these lesions. Screening programs have not been developed for other HPV-associated malignancies at present. The Pap cytologic test (see Figure 13–3A) followed by histologic confirmation (see Figure 13–3B) is the common strategy employed by most cervical and anal cancers screening programs.

Physical Examination

Examination of the external genitalia is performed in women and men using a magnifying glass and a bright light source. Because genital warts can coexist with CIN and AIN, we recommend further investigation in these individuals. Women who present with genital warts should be considered for colposcopy, and women and men presenting with perianal or perineal warts should be considered for high-resolution anoscopy (HRA).

Cervical Cancer and CIN Screening

Because cervical cancer has a long preinvasive state (ie, CIN) and CIN can be successfully treated using a variety of methods once identified, cervical cancer screening has been very successful where it has been implemented. There have been no randomized controlled trials showing that cervical cancer screening reduces cervical cancer incidence and mortality. However, several observational studies demonstrated that incident cervical cancer and cervical cancer-related mortality declined after the introduction of cervical Pap testing.[4] The American Cancer Society and the American College of Obstetrics and Gynecologists have recommended initiation of cervical Pap testing in sexually active women approximately 3 years after the initiation of vaginal intercourse, and no later than 21 years of age.[82,83] The recommended screening interval depends on previous test results (Figure 13–5) and the type of testing performed. The American College of Obstetrics and Gynecology recommends that cervical Pap testing be offered annually if younger than 30 years old. Older women who have had three consecutive negative Pap tests, who are not immunocompromised, and who have no history of CIN II or III may extend the screening interval to every 2 to 3 years. The American Cancer Society has issued similar guidelines that vary depending on whether liquid-based cytology is performed (routine screening can be performed every 2 years

instead of annually) and whether there is concomitant HPV DNA testing (screening interval can be increased to every 3 years if both negative for cytology and negative for HPV DNA testing for high-risk HPV types). The US Preventative Services Task Force recommends that the screening interval be extended to every 3 years in women of any age with three consecutively negative Pap tests. Because of increased incident CIN in HIV-positive women compared with HIV-negative women, an increased periodicity of Pap testing is recommended for HIV-positive women. The US Centers for Disease Control and the Agency for Health Care Policy and Research recommend that a cervical Pap test be performed at baseline for all HIV-positive women. Cervical Pap testing should be repeated at 6-month intervals, which can be changed to annual Pap testing for patients with normal cervical cytology.

Cervical cytologic findings are classified as abnormal or normal (see Figure 13–5). The abnormal category comprises ASC-US, ASC-H, LSIL, HSIL, and invasive carcinoma. In general, women are referred to colposcopy (Figures 13–6, 13–7, and 13–8) and/or biopsy (see Figure 13–1) if ASC-H, LSIL, or HSIL is diagnosed on cytology.[84] HIV-positive women are managed in a similar fashion, except that some specialists recommend referral to colposcopy if there is any cytologic abnormality seen (including ASC-US). The rationale for this is that there is a higher underlying prevalence of CIN

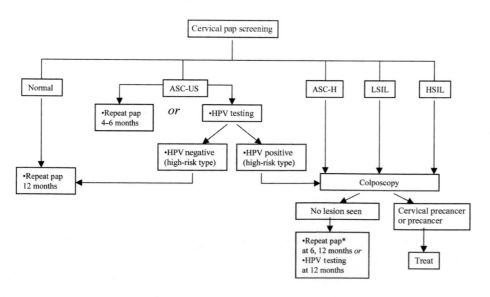

Figure 13–5. Protocol for screening cervical intraepithelial neoplasia. *If high-grade squamous intraepithelial lesion identified on cytology, and no lesions are seen on colposcopy, most guidelines recommend a diagnostic excisional procedure.

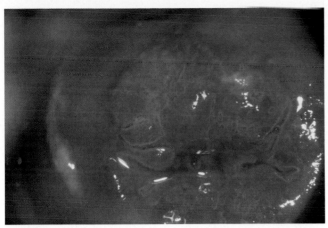

Figure 13–6. Normal cervix with transformation zone seen on colposcopy. Courtesy of Mary Rubin, NP, University of California at San Francisco, USA.

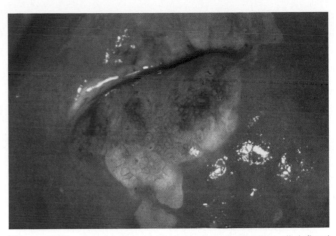

Figure 13–7. Cervical intraepithelial neoplasia III with well-defined borders, acetowhitening, and atypical vessels. Courtesy of Mary Rubin, NP, University of California at San Francisco, USA.

in HIV-positive women compared with HIV-negative women.[34]

Although the sensitivity of Pap tests to detect high-grade cervical lesions is only 55 to 80%, the specificity is over 90%.[85] HPV testing has been evaluated as alternative method for cervical cancer screening.[83] The sensitivity of HPV DNA testing to detect CIN is 84 to 100% and is generally higher than cervical Pap testing to detect CIN. However, when compared with Pap smears to detect CIN, the specificity for HPV DNA testing is lower (64 to 95%).[86,87] Given these characteristics, HPV DNA testing has been approved by the US Food and Drug Administration to triage women who have ASC-US on Pap testing.[84] Colposcopy is recommended for women who have ASC-US Pap test results and found to have high-risk HPV types on DNA testing. A repeat Pap test in 1 year is recommended for women with ASC-US and no high-risk HPV types identified. One other area where HPV testing may be indicated is in combination with Pap testing in women 30 years of age and older. In this population, the periodicity of cervical cancer screening may be increased to every 2 to 3 years if the Pap test is normal and the HPV DNA test is negative for high-risk HPV types.[83]

Anal Cancer and AIN Screening

Given the similarity between anal and cervical cancers, and because cervical Pap testing has been successful in cervical cancer screening, Chin-Hong and Palefsky have proposed an anal cancer screening program that incorporates many of the principles of cervical cancer screening.[88] Anal cancer screening is recommended for populations at high risk of anal cancer. These include all HIV-positive women and men, MSM, women with a history of vulvar or cervical cancer, and organ transplant recipients. Anal Pap testing every year to 2 years has been projected to be a cost-effective intervention to prevent anal cancer in HIV-positive and HIV-negative MSM.[89,90] To date, there have been no comparable analyses in other groups such as HIV-positive women and transplant recipients.

To perform an anal Pap test, a water-moistened Dacron swab (Baxter Healthcare Corporation,

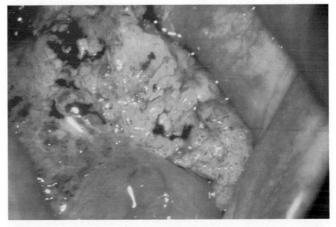

Figure 13–8. Invasive cervical cancer. Courtesy of Mary Rubin, NP, University of California at San Francisco, USA.

McGraw Park, IL, USA) is inserted in the anal canal. Dacron is used because cells cling to cotton and may decrease the yield of the Pap test. The Dacron swab is then withdrawn slowly, while rotating the swab and maintaining some pressure against the anal canal. The goal is to obtain exfoliated cells from the lower rectum, the squamocolumnar junction, and the anal canal. A traditional glass slide or liquid-based media can be used as for cervical Pap tests.

Similar to the classification system used in cervical cancer screening, anal cytology is classified as normal, ASC-US, ASC-H, LSIL (see Figure 13–2), HSIL (see Figure 13–3A), and invasive carcinoma. Individuals who are found to have abnormal cytology (including ASC-US and ASC-H) are referred to HRA (Figures 13–9 through 13–12) and biopsy. The sensitivity of anal cytology to detect biopsy-proven AIN is 50 to 80%, similar to the sensitivity of cervical Pap tests to detect biopsy-proven CIN.[85,91] In general, anal Pap tests are more sensitive in HIV-positive men compared with HIV-negative men in detecting AIN. This is likely due to the presence of more extensive HIV-associated disease in the HIV-positive population.

HRA is similar to cervical colposcopy and uses identical equipment (a powerful light source and binocular lenses). Using HRA, lesions that have contributed to abnormal cytologic findings can be identified and biopsied. As in cervical colposcopy, acetic acid (3% acetic acid in the anal canal, 5%

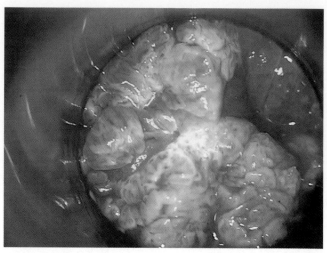

Figure 13–10.   Internal anal condylomata. Courtesy of Dr. Michael Berry, University of California at San Francisco, USA.

acetic acid in the cervix) can be used to assist in the visualization of abnormal tissue by a change known as "acetowhitening," where HPV-infected lesions turn white in contrast to surrounding normal tissue. Other tools used by clinicians can increase the specificity of HRA. These include the physical appearance of abnormal vasculature with features such as punctation, mosaicism, and atypical vessels. The application of Lugol's (iodine) solution can also increase specificity. Abnormal tissue remains unstained or appears light yellow, unlike adjacent normal tissue that stains dark brown or mahogany.

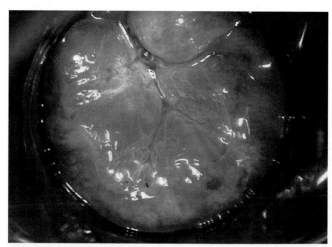

Figure 13–9.   Normal anal canal with transformation zone visualized using high-resolution anoscopy. Courtesy of Dr. Michael Berry, University of California at San Francisco, USA.

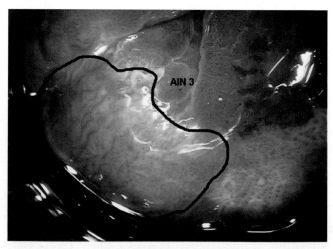

Figure 13–11.   Anal intraepithelial neoplasia III with atypical vessels and acetowhitening. Courtesy of Dr. Michael Berry, University of California at San Francisco, USA.

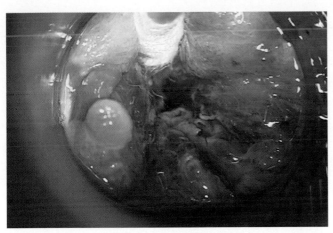

Figure 13–12.   Invasive anal cancer. Courtesy of Dr. Michael Berry, University of California at San Francisco, USA.

MANAGEMENT

General Principles

There are several goals in the treatment of HPV-associated malignant and premalignant disease, depending on the size, location, and grade of the particular lesion. CIN I and AIN I have very low malignant potential. Most cases of CIN 1 are treated if they are persistent. AIN 1 is treated if patients are symptomatic, to reduce the risk of progression to higher-grade lesions and to reduce patient anxiety. Some health care providers may treat CIN I or AIN I in HIV-positive individuals because of the rapid progression to higher-grade disease observed in clinical studies.[92,93] We treat CIN II and III, and AIN II and III to prevent cancer.

Treatment of Cervical Cancer

Management of invasive cervical cancer depends on whether the disease is early staged or locally advanced. For early-stage cervical squamous cell carcinoma (up to stage IIa disease), patients may be treated either surgically (radical hysterectomy with para-aortic and pelvic lymphectomy) or nonsurgically (primary radiotherapy [RT] with chemotherapy). One randomized controlled trial compared RT alone to hysterectomy and RT in women with early-stage cervical cancer.[94] Survival was similar at 5 years (74% versus 83%, respectively). Surgery alone has the advantage of maintaining functional ovaries, but surgery followed by RT with chemotherapy may be necessary in bulky early-stage disease. Conization is another option that may be offered to young women who desire to maintain fertility in early-stage microinvasive (< 3 mm) disease.[95] Women with locally advanced disease are best treated with primary RT together with cisplatin-based chemotherapy.[96] For women with metastatic disease, chemotherapy alone can provide a palliative benefit.

Treatment of CIN

The decision to treat CIN is based on histology obtained from biopsy of lesions seen on colposcopy, as well as HIV status. CIN I is considered to be of low malignant potential. Since many of these lesions regress, clinicians usually only follow CIN I without treatment in HIV-negative women.[97] However, the natural history of CIN is more unpredictable in HIV-infected women and some clinicians have a lower threshold to treat, particularly if the patient has a low likelihood of follow-up. CIN II and III lesions are treated in all women to prevent cancer. Excision or ablative therapies are employed. These include excision, the loop electrosurgical excision procedure (LEEP), cryotherapy, laser therapy, cold-knife conization, and hysterectomy. The simplest method may be local excisional biopsy, but this may be challenging if the lesion extends into the endocervical canal. LEEP is generally the treatment of choice for CIN II and III. The procedure uses an adjustable electric wire loop to diathermically excise lesions of various dimensions. The advantages of this procedure are its low complication rate, ease of use, and the ability to obtain relatively well-preserved tissue for pathologic assessment.

Cryotherapy involves the direct application of a supercooled probe to the affected cervical area using multiple freeze-thaw cycles. Adverse effects are mild cramping and persistent vaginal discharge. The advantages of this approach are low cost and complication rate, and ease of use. The disadvantage is the higher failure rate compared with LEEP and the inability to obtain tissue for histopathology, so tissue margins cannot be assessed. Laser therapy uses carbon dioxide under colposcopy to precisely vaporize lesions to an adequate depth. There is minimal bleeding and the surrounding tissues are only minimally damaged with little scarring. The disadvantages of this approach are the cost and specialized training needed and the inability to obtain tissue for pathologic assessment. Cold-knife conization uses a scalpel to excise a cone-shaped portion of the cervix. This is typically done if the patient cannot be treated with laser therapy or LEEP. The advantage is the higher quality of tissue obtained (no thermal damage) for histology. The disadvantages are the need for general anesthesia, and a higher complication rate compared with the other procedures, including bleeding, infection, cervical stenosis, cervical incompetence, and scarring. Finally, hysterectomy can be performed if disease is intractable.

Treatment of Anal Cancer

The standard of care for the treatment of invasive anal cancer is currently combined-modality therapy (CMT) with both RT and chemotherapy (5-fluorouracil and mitomycin used together). CMT avoids the morbidity of abdominoperineal resection, which involves removal of the anorectum and necessitates a permanent colostomy. CMT has also been successfully employed in HIV-positive men.[98] HIV-positive men with CD4 counts > 200 cells/μL have been observed to tolerate standard doses of CMT well. Compared with HIV-negative men, a higher proportion of patients with CD4 counts < 200 cells/μL may experience CMT-related toxicity.[99] For this population, CMT may be individualized with lower doses of RT and/or alternative chemotherapeutic agents such as cisplatin instead of mitomycin.[98] Nevertheless, these patients may eventually require salvage therapy with abdominoperineal resection.

Treatment of AIN

Because of anatomic challenges, it can be more difficult to treat AIN compared with CIN. Recent guidelines were published by Chin-Hong and Palefsky.[88] As in cervical disease, the histology and HIV status are important determinants that may influence treatment modalities and treatment goals. We treat AIN I to reduce the risk of enlargement, which may

preclude the use of topical agents, to decrease the risk of progression to AIN II or III, and for symptomatic or psychological relief. We treat AIN II and III to prevent cancer. We have a lower threshold to treat HIV-positive men with minimal AIN I because there is a faster rate of progression to AIN II or III compared with HIV-negative men.

The size and location of AIN may also influence our treatment strategy. Smaller lesions are generally easier to treat than larger lesions. We have had success in using only topical therapy for relatively flat intra-anal (85% trichloroacetic acid, liquid nitrogen) or perianal (imiquimod, podophyllotoxin, 85 % trichloroacetic acid, liquid nitrogen) lesions of < 1 cm^2 at the base. At the other extreme, large circumferential intra-anal lesions, particularly in HIV-positive men, have a high recurrence rate if removed. Because treatment of extensive intra-anal lesions may require multiple-staged procedures and is associated with a high morbidity (postoperative pain) and complications (anal stenosis or anal incontinence), we sometimes elect to follow these individuals closely without treatment. We may sometimes surgically remove large circumferential intra-anal lesions if patients are symptomatic or if the goal is to rule out anal carcinoma, in which case we need to define the extent of disease. Lesions in the middle category (too big for topical therapy) have been traditionally referred for intraoperative fulguration with HRA guidance. Alternatively, our group has begun to use an infrared coagulator (Redfield Corporation, Rochelle Park, NJ, USA), which has been licensed for treatment of condylomata acuminata and tattoo removal.[100] After local anesthesia with 1% lidocaine with epinephrine, the infrared coagulator is used to destroy the lesion by generating intense heat at the tip of the probe. Coagulative necrosis occurs without a smoke plume. The lesions are then debrided using a forceps down to the submucosal vessels. This procedure is very well tolerated with fewer complications compared with surgery, with only mild to moderate postprocedure discomfort that lasts for a few days. Goldstone and colleagues recently showed that with repeated infrared coagulation, 72% of high-grade AIN lesions could be successfully treated.[100]

In terms of the location of disease, perianal condyloma may be amenable to local patient-applied therapy such as imiquimod or podophyllotoxin, which are not recommended for intra-anal use. Although there has been some anecdotal success after several months of use inside the anal canal, there have been no controlled trials reporting the efficacy of imiquimod for high-grade perianal disease. Perianal high-grade disease may be treated with trichloroacetic acid, infrared coagulation, or surgery.

VACCINES

Preventative and therapeutic immunizations directed at HPV-infected cells are promising new options. Therapeutic immunizations augment the host cell-mediated immunologic response in an already HPV-infected individual. There are a variety of methods, but most use HPV E6 and E7 peptides of oncogenic HPV types to activate host T cells.[101] Thus far, however, therapeutic vaccines have not been demonstrated to be effective to induce regression of high-grade CIN or AIN, except for women under the age of 25 years with CIN, as shown in one recent study.[102]

Prophylactic immunizations use components of the major HPV capsid proteins (L1 alone or in combination with L2). These self-assemble into virus-like particles (VLP) that contain no HPV DNA and so are not infectious, but induce neutralizing antibodies before the host becomes exposed to HPV infection. The first large randomized controlled proof-of-concept trial of a HPV prophylactic vaccine was published in 2002.[103] More than 2,000 women were randomized to receive HPV-16 vaccine demonstrating 100% efficacy in the prevention of HPV-16-related cervical dysplasia. In another study, investigators used a bivalent HPV-16/-18 L1 VLP vaccine.[104] They demonstrated over 90% efficacy against HPV-16 and HPV-18 incident and persistent infections. One recently completed randomized controlled trial reported the efficacy of a quadrivalent (HPV types 6, 11, 16, and 18) HPV L1 VLP vaccine. Investigators demonstrated that women assigned to treatment had 90% less HPV disease related to HPV types 6, 11, 16, and 18,

compared with those receiving placebo, over 36 months of observation.[105] Ongoing and future trials will test the efficacy of combined vaccines for additional HPV subtypes and will evaluate the impact of prophylactic vaccines on other HPV-associated disease states such as anal disease.

CONCLUSION

Infection with human papillomavirus plays an etiologic role in a large proportion of malignancies worldwide. Cervical cancer is the second most common cancer in women in developed countries, and the most common cause of cancer in women in some developing countries. The incidence of anal cancer is increasing in women and men, and is particularly common in populations such as men who have sex with men, where the incidence in the United States is as high as the incidence of cervical cancer was prior to the adoption of cervical Pap tests. Other HPV-associated anogenital malignancies include squamous cell carcinomas of the vulva and penis. HPV has also been implicated in extragenital malignancies such as cancers of the oropharynx, larynx, skin (in patients with epidermodysplasia verruciformis), and conjunctiva. There is also some evidence for the role of HPV in esophageal cancer and nonmelanoma skin cancers (in patients with no history of epidermodysplasia verruciformis), and this is still an area of active investigation. Apart from infection with HPV—a necessary step for most of these malignancies—risk factors have been best established for cervical cancer and include environmental factors such as smoking, use of oral contraceptives, higher parity, and sexual behavior. Coinfection with HIV is associated with higher prevalence, incidence, and progression of many of these HPV-related malignancies, particularly cervical and anal squamous cell cancers. It is still controversial whether HAART is associated with higher rates of regression of precancerous lesions, and it is unknown how HAART will affect the incidence of HPV-associated malignancies.

Many of these malignancies are preventable because of a long preinvasive state, such as CIN for cervical cancer. We are able to successfully intervene and treat these preinvasive lesions, leading to a reduction in cancer incidence and mortality. The cornerstone of many of these successful screening programs is the Pap test, followed by histologic confirmation using colposcopically aided biopsies. Similarly, anal Pap screening is recommended by some experts for all HIV-positive individuals (including MSM and women) with a history of cervical or vulvar cancers. However, more clinicians need to be trained to identify and treat AIN using high-resolution anoscopy. Preventative vaccines are promising for future disease control strategies.

REFERENCES

1. Palefsky JM. Anogenital squamous cell cancer and its precursors. In: Goedert JJ, editor. Infectious causes of cancer: targets for intervention. Totawa (NJ): Humana Press Inc.; 2000. p. 263–87.

2. Jemal A, Murray T, Ward E, et al. Cancer statistics, 2005. CA Cancer J Clin 2005;55:10–30.

3. Peto J, Gilham C, Fletcher O, Matthews FE. The cervical cancer epidemic that screening has prevented in the UK. Lancet 2004;364:249–56.

4. Eddy DM. Screening for cervical cancer. Ann Intern Med 1990;113:214–26.

5. Ponten J, Adami HO, Bergstrom R, et al. Strategies for global control of cervical cancer. Int J Cancer 1995;60:1–26.

6. Maiman M, Fruchter RG, Serur E, et al. Human immunodeficiency virus infection and cervical neoplasia. Gynecol Oncol 1990;38:377–82.

7. Maiman M, Fruchter RG, Serur E, Boyce JG. Prevalence of human immunodeficiency virus in a colposcopy clinic. JAMA 1988;260:2214–5.

8. Frisch M, Biggar RJ, Goedert JJ. Human papillomavirus-associated cancers in patients with human immunodeficiency virus infection and acquired immunodeficiency syndrome. J Natl Cancer Inst 2000;92:1500–10.

9. IARC Working Group on the Evaluation of Carcinogenic Risks to Humans. Human immunodeficiency viruses and human T-cell lymphotropic viruses. 1996 June 1–18; Lyon, France. IARC Monogr Eval Carcinog Risks Hum 1996;67:1–424.

10. Sitas F, Pacella-Norman R, Carrara H, et al. The spectrum of HIV-1 related cancers in South Africa. Int J Cancer 2000;88:489–92.

11. Serraino D, Dal Maso L, La Vecchia C, Franceschi S. Invasive cervical cancer as an AIDS-defining illness in Europe. AIDS 2002;16:781–6.

12. Bosch FX, Lorincz A, Munoz N, et al. The causal relation between human papillomavirus and cervical cancer. J Clin Pathol 2002;55:244–65.

13. International Agency for Research on Cancer. Human Papillomaviruses. IARC Monogr Eval Carcinog Risks Hum 2005;90.

14. Bosch FX, de Sanjose S. Chapter 1: Human papillomavirus and cervical cancer—burden and assessment of causality. J Natl Cancer Inst Monogr 2003:3–13.

15. Munoz N, Bosch FX, de Sanjose S, et al. Epidemiologic classification of human papillomavirus types associated with cervical cancer. N Engl J Med 2003;348:518–27.

16. Shah KV. Human papillomaviruses and anogenital cancers. N Engl J Med 1997;337:1386–8.

17. Castellsague X, Munoz N. Chapter 3: Cofactors in human papillomavirus carcinogenesis—role of parity, oral contraceptives, and tobacco smoking. J Natl Cancer Inst Monogr 2003:20–8.

18. Moreno V, Bosch FX, Munoz N, et al. Effect of oral contraceptives on risk of cervical cancer in women with human papillomavirus infection: the IARC multicentric case-control study. Lancet 2002;359:1085–92.

19. Hildesheim A, Herrero R, Castle PE, et al. HPV co-factors related to the development of cervical cancer: results from a population-based study in Costa Rica. Br J Cancer 2001;84:1219–26.

20. Lacey JV Jr, Brinton LA, Abbas FM, et al. Oral contraceptives as risk factors for cervical adenocarcinomas and squamous cell carcinomas. Cancer Epidemiol Biomarkers Prev 1999;8:1079–85.

21. IARC Tobacco smoke and involuntary smoking. IARC Monogr Eval Carcinog Risks Hum 2004;83:1–1438.

22. Smith JS, Munoz N, Herrero R, et al. Evidence for *Chlamydia trachomatis* as a human papillomavirus cofactor in the etiology of invasive cervical cancer in Brazil and the Philippines. J Infect Dis 2002;185:324–31.

23. Palefsky JM, Minkoff H, Kalish LA, et al. Cervicovaginal human papillomavirus infection in human immunodeficiency virus-1 (HIV)-positive and high-risk HIV-negative women. J Natl Cancer Inst 1999;91:226–36.

24. Xi LF, Carter JJ, Galloway DA, et al. Acquisition and natural history of human papillomavirus type 16 variant infection among a cohort of female university students. Cancer Epidemiol Biomarkers Prev 2002;11:343–51.

25. Josefsson AM, Magnusson PK, Ylitalo N, et al. Viral load of human papilloma virus 16 as a determinant for development of cervical carcinoma in situ: a nested case-control study. Lancet 2000;355:2189–93.

26. Ylitalo N, Sorensen P, Josefsson AM, et al. Consistent high viral load of human papillomavirus 16 and risk of cervical carcinoma in situ: a nested case-control study. Lancet 2000;355:2194–8.

27. Moberg M, Gustavsson I, Wilander E, Gyllensten U. High viral loads of human papillomavirus predict risk of invasive cervical carcinoma. Br J Cancer 2005;92:891–4.

28. Storey A, Thomas M, Kalita A, et al. Role of a p53 polymorphism in the development of human papillomavirus-associated cancer. Nature 1998;393:229–34.

29. Palefsky JM, Holly EA. Chapter 6: Immunosuppression and coinfection with HIV. J Natl Cancer Inst Monogr 2003:41–6.

30. Solomon D, Davey D, Kurman R, et al. The 2001 Bethesda System: terminology for reporting results of cervical cytology. JAMA 2002;287:2114–9.

31. Mitchell MF, Tortolero-Luna G, Wright T, et al. Cervical human papillomavirus infection and intraepithelial neoplasia: a review. J Natl Cancer Inst Monogr 1996:17–25.

32. Massad LS, Riester KA, Anastos KM, et al. Prevalence and predictors of squamous cell abnormalities in Papanicolaou smears from women infected with HIV-1. J Acquir Immune Defic Syndr 1999;21:33–41.

33. Jones BA, Davey DD. Quality management in gynecologic cytology using interlaboratory comparison. Arch Pathol Lab Med 2000;124:672–81.

34. Wright TC Jr, Ellerbrock TV, Chiasson MA, et al. Cervical intraepithelial neoplasia in women infected with human immunodeficiency virus: prevalence, risk factors, and validity of Papanicolaou smears. New York Cervical Disease Study. Obstet Gynecol 1994;84:591–7.

35. Delmas MC, Larsen C, van Benthem B, et al. Cervical squamous intraepithelial lesions in HIV-infected women: prevalence, incidence and regression. European Study Group on Natural History of HIV Infection in Women. AIDS 2000;14:1775–84.

36. Shepherd J, Weston R, Peersman G, Napuli IZ. Interventions for encouraging sexual lifestyles and behaviours intended to prevent cervical cancer. Cochrane Database Syst Rev 2000:CD001035.

37. Schiffman MH, Bauer HM, Hoover RN, et al. Epidemiologic evidence showing that human papillomavirus infection causes most cervical intraepithelial neoplasia. J Natl Cancer Inst 1993;85:958–64.

38. Munoz N, Franceschi S, Bosetti C, et al. Role of parity and human papillomavirus in cervical cancer: the IARC multicentric case-control study. Lancet 2002;359:1093–101.

39. Herrero R, Hildesheim A, Bratti C, et al. Population-based study of human papillomavirus infection and cervical neoplasia in rural Costa Rica. J Natl Cancer Inst 2000;92:464–74.

40. Herrero R, Schiffman MH, Bratti C, et al. Design and methods of a population-based natural history study of cervical neoplasia in a rural province of Costa Rica: the Guanacaste Project. Rev Panam Salud Publica 1997;1:362–75.

41. Moscicki AB, Shiboski S, Hills NK, et al. Regression of low-grade squamous intra-epithelial lesions in young women. Lancet 2004;364:1678–83.

42. Arends MJ, Buckley CH, Wells M. Aetiology, pathogenesis, and pathology of cervical neoplasia. J Clin Pathol 1998;51:96–103.

43. Vernon S, Hart C, Reeves W, et al. The HIV-1 tat protein enhances E2-dependent human papillomavirus 16. Virus Res 1993;27:133–45.

44. Johnson LG, Madeleine MM, Newcomer LM, et al. Anal cancer incidence and survival: the surveillance, epidemiology, and end results experience, 1973–2000. Cancer 2004;101:281–8.

45. Palefsky JM. Perspectives: anal cancer in HIV infection. Top HIV Med 2000;8:14–7.

46. Cress RD, Holly EA. Incidence of anal cancer in California: increased incidence among men in San Francisco, 1973–1999. Prev Med 2003;36:555–60.

47. Frisch M, Glimelius B, van den Brule A, et al. Sexually transmitted infection as a cause of anal cancer. N Engl J Med 1997;337:1350–8.

48. Ryan DP, Compton CC, Mayer RJ. Carcinoma of the anal canal. N Engl J Med 2000;342:792–800.

49. Daling JR, Madeleine MM, Johnson LG, et al. Human papillomavirus, smoking, and sexual practices in the etiology of anal cancer. Cancer 2004;101:270–80.

50. Rabkin CS, Biggar RJ, Melbye M, et al. Second primary cancers following anal and cervical carcinoma: evidence of shared etiologic factors. Am J Epidemiol 1992;136:54–8.

51. Holly EA, Whittemore AS, Aston DA, et al. Anal cancer incidence: genital warts, anal fissure or fistula, hemorrhoids, and smoking. J Natl Cancer Inst 1989;81:1726–31.

52. Penn I. Cancers of the anogenital region in renal transplant recipients. Analysis of 65 cases. Cancer 1986;58:611–6.

53. Adami J, Gabel H, Lindelof B, et al. Cancer risk following organ transplantation: a nationwide cohort study in Sweden. Br J Cancer 2003;89:1221–7.

54. Chin-Hong PV, Vittinghoff E, Cranston RD, et al. Age-related prevalence of anal cancer precursors in homosexual men: the EXPLORE study. J Natl Cancer Inst 2005;97:896–905.

55. Palefsky JM, Holly E, Ralston MR, et al. Prevalence and risk factors for human papillomavirus infection of the anal canal in human immunodeficiency virus (HIV)-positive and HIV-negative homosexual men. J Infect Dis 1998;177:361–7.

56. Holly E, Ralston MR, Darragh TM, et al. Prevalence and risk factors for anal squamous intraepithelial lesions in women. J Natl Cancer Inst 2001;93:943–9.

57. Piketty C, Darragh TM, Costa MD, et al. High prevalence of anal human papillomavirus infection and anal cancer precursors among HIV-infected persons in the absence of anal intercourse. Ann Intern Med 2003;138:453–9.

58. Williams AB, Darragh TM, Vranizan K, et al. Anal and cervical human papillomavirus infection and risk of anal and cervical epithelial abnormalities in human immunodeficiency virus-infected women. Obstet Gynecol 1994;83:205–11.

59. Melbye M, Sprogel P. Aetiological parallel between anal cancer and cervical cancer. Lancet 1991;338:657–9.

60. Ogunbiyi OA, Scholefield JH, Raftery AT, et al. Prevalence of anal human papillomavirus infection and intraepithelial neoplasia in renal allograft recipients. Br J Surg 1994;81:365–7.

61. Palefsky JM. Cervical human papillomavirus infection and cervical intraepithelial neoplasia in women positive for human immunodeficiency virus in the era of highly active antiretroviral therapy. Curr Opin Oncol 2003;15:382–8.

62. Palefsky JM, Holly EA, Ralston ML, et al. Anal squamous intraepithelial lesions in HIV-positive and HIV-negative homosexual and bisexual men: prevalence and risk factors. J Acquir Immune Defic Syndr Hum Retrovirol 1998;17:320 6.

63. Chin-Hong PV, Vittinghoff E, Cranston RD, et al. Age-specific prevalence of anal human papillomavirus infection in HIV-negative sexually active men who have sex with men: the EXPLORE study. J Infect Dis 2004;190:2070–6.

64. Goedert JJ, Cote TR, Virgo P, et al. Spectrum of AIDS-associated malignant disorders. Lancet 1998;351:1833–9.

65. Frisch M, Biggar RJ, Engels EA, Goedert JJ. Association of cancer with AIDS-related immunosuppression in adults. JAMA 2001;285:1736–45.

66. Haga T, Kim S-H, Jensen R, et al. Detection of genetic changes in anal intraepithelial neoplasia (AIN) of HIV-positive and HIV-negative men. J Acquir Immune Defic Syndr 2001;26:256–62.

67. Palefsky JM, Holly EA. Molecular virology and epidemiology of human papillomavirus and cervical cancer. Cancer Epidemiol Biomarkers Prev 1995;4:415–28.

68. Heard I, Schmitz V, Costagliola D, et al. Early regression of cervical lesions in HIV-seropositive women receiving highly active antiretroviral therapy. AIDS 1998;12:1459–64.

69. Ahdieh-Grant L, Li R, Levine AM, et al. Highly active antiretroviral therapy and cervical squamous intraepithelial lesions in human immunodeficiency virus-positive women. J Natl Cancer Inst 2004;96:1070–6.

70. Palefsky JM, Holly EA, Ralston ML, et al. Effect of highly active antiretroviral therapy on the natural history of anal squamous intraepithelial lesions and anal human papillomavirus infection. J Acquir Immune Defic Syndr 2001;28:422–8.

71. Piketty C, Darragh TM, Heard I, et al. High prevalence of anal squamous intraepithelial lesions in HIV-positive men despite the use of highly active antiretroviral therapy. Sex Transm Dis 2004;31:96–9.

72. Bower M, Powles T, Newsom-Davis T, et al. HIV-associated anal cancer: has highly active antiretroviral therapy reduced the incidence or improved the outcome? J Acquir Immune Defic Syndr 2004;37:1563–5.

73. Ansink A. Vulvar squamous cell carcinoma. Semin Dermatol 1996;15:51–9.

74. Ansink AC, Heintz AP. Epidemiology and etiology of squamous cell carcinoma of the vulva. Eur J Obstet Gynecol Reprod Biol 1993;48:111–5.

75. Crum CP. Carcinoma of the vulva: epidemiology and pathogenesis. Obstet Gynecol 1992;79:448–54.

76. Sturgeon SR, Brinton LA, Devesa SS, Kurman RJ. In situ and invasive vulvar cancer incidence trends (1973 to 1987). Am J Obstet Gynecol 1992;166:1482–5.

77. Conley LJ, Ellerbrock TV, Bush TJ, et al. HIV-1 infection and risk of vulvovaginal and perianal condylomata acuminata and intraepithelial neoplasia: a prospective cohort study. Lancet 2002;359:108–13.

78. Baldwin P, Sterling J. HIV-1 infection and intraepithelial neoplasia of lower genital tract. Lancet 2002;359:2040.

79. Misra S, Chaturvedi A, Misra NC. Penile carcinoma: a challenge for the developing world. Lancet Oncol 2004;5:240–7.

80. Picconi MA, Eijan AM, Distefano AL, et al. Human papillomavirus (HPV) DNA in penile carcinomas in Argentina: analysis of primary tumors and lymph nodes. J Med Virol 2000;61:65–9.

81. Gillison ML, Shah KV. Chapter 9: Role of mucosal human papillomavirus in nongenital cancers. J Natl Cancer Inst Monogr 2003:57–65.

82. ACOG practice bulletin. Cervical cytology screening. Number 45, August 2003. Int J Gynaecol Obstet 2003;83:237–47.

83. Saslow D, Runowicz CD, Solomon D, et al. American Cancer Society guideline for the early detection of cervical neoplasia and cancer. CA Cancer J Clin 2002;52:342–62.

84. Wright TC Jr, Cox JT, Massad LS, et al. 2001 Consensus guidelines for the management of women with cervical cytological abnormalities. JAMA 2002;287:2120–9.

85. Soost HJ, Lange HJ, Lehmacher W, Ruffing-Kullmann B. The validation of cervical cytology. Sensitivity, specificity and predictive values. Acta Cytol 1991;35:8–14.

86. Kulasingam SL, Hughes JP, Kiviat NB, et al. Evaluation of human papillomavirus testing in primary screening for cervical abnormalities: comparison of sensitivity, specificity, and frequency of referral. JAMA 2002;288:1749–57.

87. Ratnam S, Franco EL, Ferenczy A. Human papillomavirus testing for primary screening of cervical cancer precursors. Cancer Epidemiol Biomarkers Prev 2000;9:945–51.

88. Chin-Hong PV, Palefsky JM. Natural history and clinical management of anal human papillomavirus disease in men and women infected with human immunodeficiency virus. Clin Infect Dis 2002;35:1127–34.

89. Goldie SJ, Kuntz KM, Weinstein MC, et al. The clinical effectiveness and cost-effectiveness of screening for anal squamous intraepithelial lesions in homosexual and bisexual HIV-positive men. JAMA 1999;281:1822–9.

90. Goldie SJ, Kuntz KM, Weinstein MC, et al. Cost-effectiveness of screening for anal squamous intraepithelial lesions and anal cancer in human immunodeficiency virus-negative homosexual and bisexual men. Am J Med 2000;108:634–41.

91. Palefsky JM, Holly EA, Hogeboom CJ, et al. Anal cytology as a screening tool for anal squamous intraepithelial lesions. J Acquir Immune Defic Syndr Hum Retrovirol 1997;14:415–22.

92. Ellerbrock TV, Chiasson MA, Bush TJ, et al. Incidence of cervical squamous intraepithelial lesions in HIV-infected women. JAMA 2000;283:1031–7.

93. Palefsky JM, Holly EA, Ralston ML, et al. High incidence of anal high-grade squamous intra-epithelial lesions among HIV-positive and HIV-negative homosexual and bisexual men. AIDS 1998;12:495–503.

94. Landoni F, Maneo A, Colombo A, et al. Randomised study of radical surgery versus radiotherapy for stage Ib–IIa cervical cancer. Lancet 1997;350:535–40.

95. Schorge JO, Lee KR, Sheets EE. Prospective management of stage IA(1) cervical adenocarcinoma by conization alone to preserve fertility: a preliminary report. Gynecol Oncol 2000;78:217–20.

96. Committee on Practice B-G. ACOG practice bulletin. Diagnosis and treatment of cervical carcinomas. Number 35, May 2002. Obstet Gynecol 2002;99:855–67.

97. Holowaty P, Miller AB, Rohan T, To T. Natural history of dysplasia of the uterine cervix. J Natl Cancer Inst 1999;91:252–8.

98. Berry JM, Palefsky JM, Welton ML. Anal cancer and its precursors in HIV-positive patients: perspectives and management. Surg Oncol Clin N Am 2004;13:355–73.

99. Hoffman R, Welton ML, Klencke B, et al. The significance of pretreatment CD4 count on the outcome and treatment tolerance of HIV-positive patients with anal cancer. Int J Radiat Oncol Biol Phys 1999;44:127–31.

100. Goldstone SE, Kawalek AZ, Huyett JW. Infrared coagulator: a useful tool for treating anal squamous intraepithelial lesions. Dis Colon Rectum 2005;48:1042–54.

101. Roden RB, Ling M, Wu TC. Vaccination to prevent and treat cervical cancer. Hum Pathol 2004;35:971–82.

102. Garcia F, Petry KU, Muderspach L, et al. ZYC101a for treatment of high-grade cervical intraepithelial neoplasia: a randomized controlled trial. Obstet Gynecol 2004;103:317–26.

103. Koutsky LA, Ault KA, Wheeler CM, et al. A controlled trial of a human papillomavirus type 16 vaccine. N Engl J Med 2002;347:1645–51.

104. Harper DM, Franco EL, Wheeler C, et al. Efficacy of a bivalent L1 virus-like particle vaccine in prevention of infection with human papillomavirus types 16 and 18 in young women: a randomised controlled trial. Lancet 2004;364:1757–65.

105. Villa LL, Costa RL, Petta CA, et al. Prophylactic quadrivalent human papillomavirus (types 6, 11, 16, and 18) L1 virus-like particle vaccine in young women: a randomised double-blind placebo-controlled multicentre phase II efficacy trial. Lancet Oncol 2005;6:271–8.

106. Gillison ML, Koch WM, Capone RB, et al. Evidence for a causal association between human papillomavirus and a subset of head and neck cancers. J Natl Cancer Inst 2000;92:709–20.

107. Zumbach K, Hoffmann M, Kahn T, et al. Antibodies against oncoproteins E6 and E7 of human papillomavirus types 16 and 18 in patients with head-and-neck squamous-cell carcinoma. Int J Cancer 2000;85:815–8.

108. Venuti A, Manni V, Morello R, et al. Physical state and expression of human papillomavirus in laryngeal carcinoma and surrounding normal mucosa. J Med Virol 2000;60:396–402.

109. Mork J, Lie AK, Glattre E, et al. Human papillomavirus infection as a risk factor for squamous-cell carcinoma of the head and neck. N Engl J Med 2001;344:1125–31.

110. Pfister H. Chapter 8: Human papillomavirus and skin cancer. J Natl Cancer Inst Monogr 2003:52–6.

111. Pfister H, Ter Schegget J. Role of HPV in cutaneous premalignant and malignant tumors. Clin Dermatol 1997;15:335–47.

112. Waddell KM, Lewallen S, Lucas SB, et al. Carcinoma of the conjunctiva and HIV infection in Uganda and Malawi. Br J Ophthalmol 1996;80:503–8.

113. Scott IU, Karp CL, Nuovo GJ. Human papillomavirus 16 and 18 expression in conjunctival intraepithelial neoplasia. Ophthalmology 2002;109:542–7.

114. Syrjanen KJ. HPV infections and oesophageal cancer. J Clin Pathol 2002;55:721–8.

115. Han C, Qiao G, Hubbert NL, et al. Serologic association between human papillomavirus type 16 infection and esophageal cancer in Shaanxi Province, China. J Natl Cancer Inst 1996;88:1467–71.

14

Viral Hepatitis and Hepatocarcinogenesis

ANNETTE Y. KWON
RAYMOND T. CHUNG

Hepatocellular carcinoma (HCC) is the most serious and dreaded complication of chronic liver disease that affects approximately half a million persons worldwide. In the United States, it constitutes 84% of primary liver cancer, with intrahepatic cholangiocarcinoma (15%) and fibrolamellar carcinoma (< 1%) comprising the rest.[1] The incidence of HCC has increased markedly over the last two decades. Until the mid-1980s, rates had been stable and relatively low, but it is currently estimated that 8,500 to 11,500 new cases of HCC occur annually in the United States alone, and that there are approximately 560,000 cases worldwide. The age-adjusted incidence rates of HCC increased approximately twofold between 1985 and 1998, from 1.3 per 100,000 persons during 1978 to 1980 to 3.0 per 100,000 persons during 1996 to 1998.[2]

Some studies indicate that hepatitis C virus (HCV) infection acquired two to four decades ago can explain at least half of the observed increase in HCC incidence. The annual incidence of acute HCV infection peaked in the mid-1980s and has declined since then. However, because of the natural history of HCV infection and the time for progression of acute infection to chronic liver disease and cirrhosis, it is estimated that the incidence of HCC will continue to increase, with the peak incidence projected between 2015 and 2019.

HCC is a common cause of death among patients with compensated cirrhosis, irrespective of etiology. Recent epidemiologic data indicate that the mortality rate from HCC is increasing.[3–5] According to European cohort studies, among persons who died of a liver-related cause, HCC was the cause of death in 54 to 70% for all-cause cirrhosis and, more specifically, in 50% of patients with HCV-related cirrhosis.[6] Conversely, cirrhosis-related mortality not due to HCC is declining. A possible explanation for these trends is that improvements in management of complications of cirrhosis, such as variceal bleeding and ascites, have led to longer survival of these patients, who in turn are at increasing risk of developing HCC.

The prevalence of cirrhosis in persons with HCC is about 80 to 90% in autopsy series.[7] Cirrhosis of all etiologies can predispose patients to the development of HCC, but chronic hepatitis B virus (HBV) or HCV infection account for over 80% of HCC cases worldwide.[8] Among HCC cases with cirrhosis, HCV infection was identified in 27 to 73%, HBV infection in 12 to 55%, heavy alcohol intake in 4 to 38%, hemochromatosis and other causes in 2 to 6%, and 4 to 6% had no identifiable cause. Among persons with HCC but without cirrhosis, HCV infection was identified in 3 to 54%, HBV infection in 4 to 29%, and heavy alcohol intake in 0 to 28%.[9–12] Although HCC nearly always occurs in the setting of cirrhosis, studies in noncirrhotics have shown that HCC nearly always occurs in a histologically abnormal liver with some degree of fibrosis and inflammation due to chronic liver disease or infection.[13]

Older age and male gender have also been found to be associated with increased risk of HCC among persons with cirrhosis.[14–17] Older age is likely to be reflective of a longer duration of cirrhosis. Males have an approximate relative risk of 2 for developing HCC, compared with females with cirrhosis. The mechanism is unclear but possible explanations include higher frequency of alcohol abuse in males as well as potential carcinogenic effects of androgens. The stage of cirrhosis based on Child-Pugh classification has also been shown to be an independent prognostic factor for HCC, with a threefold and eightfold increased risk for class B and C cirrhotics, respectively.[18] Activity of liver disease, as defined by persistent elevation of alanine aminotransferase (ALT) levels, is associated with higher risk and more rapid development of HCC.[19,20] Meanwhile, studies assessing histologic characteristics, such as the presence of large cell change, irregular regeneration, or hepatocytes and macroregenerative nodules, have not clearly demonstrated an association with increased risk of HCC.[21,22] Although nonviral causes of HCC can be identified, this chapter will focus on our current understanding of the pathogenesis of HBV- and HCV-related HCC.

HEPATITIS B VIRUS INFECTION

Hepatitis B virus is a major pathogen that has infected 2 billion people worldwide and chronically infects more than 350 million people, who in turn are at significant risk for death from cirrhosis and HCC (Figure 14–1). In the United States, approximately 200,000 people are infected annually, of whom 50,000 develop clinical symptoms of acute hepatitis, 10,000 become hospitalized, and 250 die of fulminant hepatic failure. Approximately 1 to 6% and 29 to 40% of infected adults and children develop chronic HBV infection, respectively. Individuals chronically positive for hepatitis B surface antigen (HBsAg) have a relative risk of 10 for developing HCC. They carry an annual risk of 0.3 to 6.6%, if cirrhosis is also present.[23–25]

Virology

HBV is a 3.2 kb, partially double-stranded circular DNA virus, consisting of an outer envelope and an inner core. The core contains DNA, hepatitis B core antigen, DNA-dependent polymerase, and hepatitis B e antigen (HBeAg). The envelope contains HBsAg, which can be present alone as noninfectious incomplete viral particles.

The HBV virion binds to a receptor at the surface of the hepatocyte. A number of candidate receptors have been identified, including the transferrin receptor, the asialoglycoprotein receptor molecule, and human liver endonexin. The mechanism by which HBsAg binds a specific receptor to enter cells has not been clearly established. Viral nucleocapsids enter the cell and deliver the viral genome to the nucleus where second-strand DNA synthesis is completed and the gaps in both strands are repaired to yield a covalently closed circular supercoiled

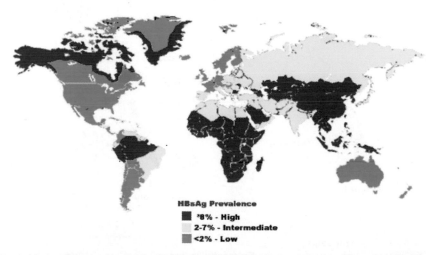

Figure 14–1. Geographic distribution of chronic hepatitis B virus infection. Reproduced with permission from World Health Organization. Hepatitis B. Available at: <http://www.who.int/csr/disease/hepatitis/HepatitisB_whocdscsrlyo2002_2.pdf> p 39. Accessed November 8, 2005.

DNA (cccDNA) molecule that serves as a template for transcription and subsequent translation into viral nucleocapsid and precore antigen (C, pre-C), polymerase, envelope L (large), M (medium), S (small), and transcriptional transactivating proteins (X). The envelope proteins insert themselves as integral membrane proteins into the lipid membrane of the endoplasmic reticulum (ER). The RNA coding the C and pre-C viral products is packaged together with HBV polymerase and a protein kinase into core particles, where it serves as a template for reverse transcription of negative-strand DNA within the particles. The new mature viral nucleocapsids can then follow two different intracellular pathways: one that leads to the formation and secretion of new virions, and the other that leads to amplification of the viral genome inside the cell nucleus. In the virion assembly pathway, the nucleocapsids reach the ER, where they associate with the envelope proteins and bud into the lumen of the ER from which they are secreted via the Golgi apparatus out of the cell. In the genome amplification pathway, the nucleocapsids deliver their genome to amplify the intranuclear pool of cccDNA. The precore polypeptide is transported into the ER lumen where its amino and carboxy termini are trimmed and the resulted HBeAg is secreted. Protein X (HBx) contributes to the efficiency of HBV replication by interacting with various transcription factors involved in cell proliferation and cell death (Figure 14–2).

Mechanisms of Hepatocarcinogenesis in Chronic HBV Infection

DNA Insertional Mutagenesis

HBV DNA integration into cellular DNA is not necessary for viral replication but allows for persistence of the viral genome as well as abnormalities of cellular DNA at a chromosomal level.[26,27] Long-term chronic inflammation associated with increased hepatocyte proliferation and repair induces rearrangements of the integrated viral sequences. It can induce chromosomal deletions at the integration sites as well as transpositions from one chromosome to another of viral sequences with flanking cellular sequences, resulting in chromosomal instability.[28,29]

Insertion of viral DNA into cellular genes is another potential consequence of HBV DNA integration. In woodchuck hepatitis virus (WHV)-related HCC models, insertion of WHV DNA into the c-*myc* or predominantly N-*myc* oncogenes has been a frequent finding.[30] However, integration of the HBV genome directly into known oncogenes has been found to be a relatively rare event. Meanwhile, more recent studies have shown that the HBV insertion

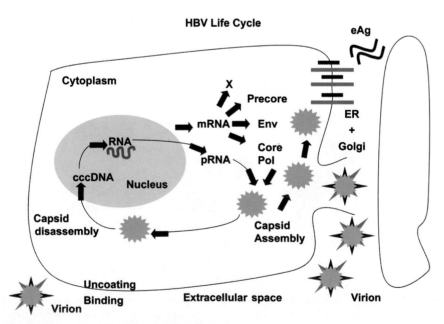

Figure 14–2. Hepatitis B virus (HBV) life cycle.

into cellular genes is indeed relatively frequent, and in that setting, HBV integration can occur in genes that are important in the control of cell signaling, proliferation, and viability. For example, studies suggest that the telomerase gene is targeted for integration in different HBV-related HCCs.[31] Other cell signaling pathways including genes regulating calcium homeostasis and MAP kinase-dependent signaling have been implicated as possible targets for integration leading to development of HCC.[32–34]

Direct Effects of HBV Proteins

In addition to direct or random insertional mutagenesis, direct hepatocarcinogenic effects by HBV proteins have been implicated. Examination of viral DNA sequences present in HBV-related HCC has shown that both RNA sequences encoding for HBx and truncated envelope preS2/S viral protein are retained in a significant proportion of HCC tumor cells.[27] In addition, antibodies to HBx (anti-HBx) are not only detectable in the serum of HBV-infected patients, as some studies have demonstrated that anti-HBx is more frequent among patients with HCC than those with chronic hepatitis B without cancer.[35,36] Although the mechanism by which HBx causes or contributes to hepatocarcinogenesis has not been clearly elucidated, the biologic actions of

HBx have been investigated in detail, and it has the following properties:

1. HBx transactivates a number of cellular promoters by acting on *cis*-acting regulatory elements. These interactions lead to activating cellular signaling pathways, which in turn regulate target gene expression and modulate apoptosis, cell proliferation, and response to DNA damage. HBx has been shown to inhibit *p53* gene function in vitro via its transactivation mechanism.
2. HBx regulates proteasome function and thus controls degradation of cellular proteins, which may include oncoproteins.
3. HBx protein may modulate calcium homeostasis, leading to altered calcium-dependent cell signaling events, including growth pathways.
4. HBx interacts with mitochondria and may influence the mitochondrial transmembrane potential.[27,37–40]

Figure 14–3 schematically summarizes putative HBx protein function.

Recent studies have demonstrated the presence of a spliced HBV transcript, which can be reverse transcribed and encapsidated in defective HBV particles or expressed as a new HBV protein, referred to as HBV spliced protein (HBSP). HBSP has been shown to induce apoptosis without cell cycle block

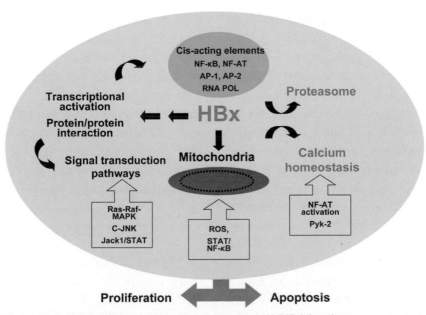

Figure 14–3. Schematic representation of the protein X (HBx) functions.

and to modulate transforming growth factor β-dependent signaling.[41] Collectively, these studies suggest that HBV proteins may participate directly in the progression of hepatocarcinogenesis and may at least in part explain cases of HBV-related HCC in noncirrhotic individuals.

Immunopathogenesis

Previous studies of transgenic mice that produce hepatotoxic quantities of the HBV large envelope protein demonstrated hepatocellular injury, regenerative hyperplasia, chronic inflammation, Kupffer cell hyperplasia, oxygen radical production, glutathione depletion, oxidative DNA damage, transcriptional deregulation, and aneuploidy that inevitably progress to HCC.[42–48] Although these studies suggested the possible role of HBV-specific immune response causing hepatocellular injury and subsequent steps toward development of HCC, the large excess of toxic viral protein expressed was a confounding factor.

Therefore, in order to more specifically assess the effects of immune response in HBV-associated hepatocarcinogenesis, adoptive transfer of cellular immunity in HbsAg-tolerant transgenic mice expressing a lower, more physiologic level of HBV envelope protein was investigated.[49] Two groups of 8- to 10-week-old male transgenic mice were thymectomized, irradiated, and reconstituted with either syngeneic HbsAg-immunized nontransgenic (group 1) or nonimmunized transgenic T-cell depleted (group 2) donor bone marrow and splenocytes. Consistent with the transfer of HBsAg-specific B cells, HBsAg disappeared from the serum of group 1 mice within 3 days after adoptive transfer. Furthermore, consistent with the transfer of HBsAg-specific transfer of cytotoxic T lymphocytes, ALT activity increased from pre-injection levels of 20 to 40 U/L to approximately 4,000 U/L in group 1 recipients, within 7 days after adoptive transfer, with subsequent decrease thereafter until 17 months, at which time increases in both groups were observed. Of note, ALT levels never returned to baseline in the group 1 animals, remaining at least 2 to 3 times above normal, reflecting ongoing hepatocyte injury and immune response. Meanwhile, serum HBsAg levels did not fall in group 2, consistent with the absence of anti-HBs in their serum. Similarly, ALT levels remained within normal range throughout most of the study.

The differential ALT activities observed was supported by gross and histologic appearance of the mice livers at various times after adoptive transfer, in which group 1 animals showed subacute inflammatory liver disease just 3 weeks after bone marrow and splenocyte reconstitution. At 3 months, the mice displayed multiple portal and intralobular inflammatory infiltrates and moderate lobular disarray indicative of chronic hepatitis. By 8 months, pathologic changes were more severe with portal inflammatory infiltrate, piecemeal necrosis, and development of preneoplastic foci. When all the animals were sacrificed at 17 months, all displayed multiple liver tumors with 8 of 9 having HCCs and the remaining animal having hepatocellular adenoma. Group 2 animals displayed much less severe necroinflammatory changes and resulted in only 1 of 9 animals developing hepatocellular adenoma. Finally, nonirradiated or nontransfer controls (group 3) had grossly and histologically normal livers and no development of either benign or malignant tumors during the study period.

In summary, HBV hepatocarcinogenesis appears to occur at multiple levels. Insertional mutagenesis by viral DNA genome and direct viral protein mechanisms such as transactivation by HBx seem to occur as secondary events in the setting of chronic inflammation, injury, and repair, with eventual progression to HCC. In addition, transgenic mice data suggest that overexpression of viral proteins under certain conditions may be oncogenic, and more importantly, that introduction of the virus-specific cellular immune response may be sufficient to initiate and sustain malignant transformation in the absence of the virally induced mutagenic and transactivating mechanisms discussed previously. Figure 14–4 demonstrates a model for HBV-associated HCC.

HEPATITIS C VIRUS INFECTION

HCV is an important cause of morbidity and mortality worldwide as a major cause of chronic liver disease, including liver cancer. Globally, it is estimated that 170 million persons are chronically

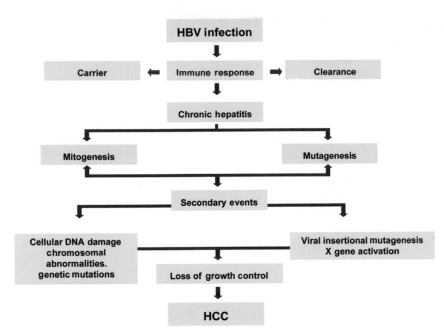

Figure 14–4. Schematic representation of hepatitis B virus–associated hepatocellular carcinoma. Among those who develop chronic hepatitis after an acute infection (1 to 6% and 29 to 40% in adults and children, respectively), immune responses leading to chronic inflammation, injury, and repair results in increased mitogenesis and mutagenesis. In that setting, cellular DNA damage, chromosomal abnormalities, and genetic mutations occur. In addition, direct viral effects including insertional mutagenesis and multiple direct mechanisms by HBx protein ultimately results in loss of cell growth control and sets the stage for malignant transformation.

infected and that 3 to 4 million persons are newly infected each year (Figures 14–5 and 14–6). The incidence of acute HCV infection in the United States has declined since its peak in 1989, but is currently approximately 35,000 cases a year. About 80% of newly infected patients progress to develop chronic infection. Cirrhosis develops in about 10 to 20% of persons with chronic infection, and liver cancer develops in 1 to 5% of persons with cirrhosis

over a period of 20 to 30 years.[6] Chronic HCV infection is remarkably common in the United States, with a current prevalence rate of nearly 4 million people. It is the most common reason for liver transplantation in the United States and worldwide, and claims 8,000 to 10,000 lives annually. Although preventive measures aimed at decreasing the rates of HCV acquisition may eventually prove effective, it is highly likely that HCV-related HCC will continue

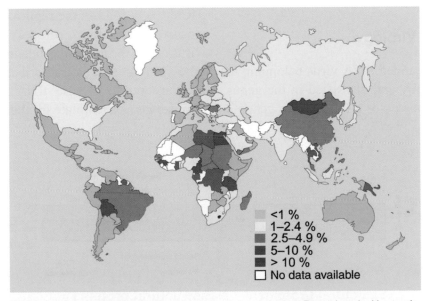

Figure 14–5.   Global prevalence of hepatitis C virus infection. Reproduced with permission from World Health Organization.

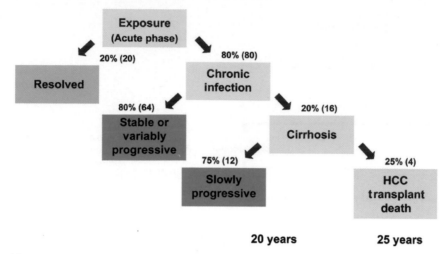

Figure 14–6. Natural history of hepatitis C virus infection.

to increase in frequency in the future, especially for the large cohort of persons infected in the 1970s and 1980s. HCV-related HCC is expected to contribute significantly to the projected increase in HCV-related mortality of twofold to threefold over the next 10 to 20 years. A recent study examining the records of 1,605 veterans diagnosed with HCC between 1993 and 1998 showed a threefold increase in the age-adjusted rate of HCV-associated HCC between the periods from 1993 to 1995 and 1996 to 1998. In contrast, the relative risk for HCC in patients with other risk factors for HCC, such as hepatitis B or alcohol abuse, remained constant throughout this period.[50]

Virology

HCV is a positive-stranded RNA virus belonging to the *Flaviviridae* family and classified in the genus *Hepacivirus*. HCV possesses a long 9.4 kb genome that is translated into a 3,011 amino acid polyprotein, which is processed into N-terminal structural proteins and C-terminal nonstructural proteins. The structural genes include nucleocapsid (core) and envelope (*E1* and *E2*) genes, and the nonstructural genes include *P7*, *NS2*, *NS3*, *NS4A*, *NS4B*, *NS5A*, and *NS5B* (Figure 14–7). The functions of each gene product have not been elucidated completely, but various putative pleiotropic functions besides their roles in the viral life cycle have been described and are summarized in Table 14–1.

There are limited data on the replication cycle of HCV because there is no in vitro cell culture system that is permissive for virus replication. However, HCV likely follows the replication strategy of other positive-strand RNA viruses (Figure 14–8). The virus enters the cell and is uncoated in the cytoplasm. The viral genome is transcribed to form a complementary negative-sense RNA molecule, which in turn serves as a template for the synthesis of progeny

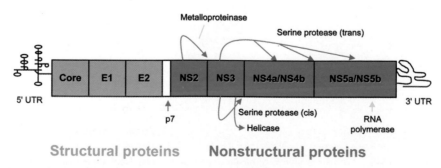

Figure 14–7. Hepatitis C virus (HCV) genomic organization.

Table 14–1. SOME OF THE PUTATIVE PLEIOTROPIC FUNCTIONS OF HEPATITIS C VIRUS GENE PRODUCTS[53,57,70–83]

Protein	Function
Core	Apoptosis Reactive oxygen species Signal transduction Transcription Transformation Immune suppression Inhibition of IFN signal transduction
E1–E2	Endoplasmic reticulum stress
E2	Interference with actions of interferon
NS3/4A	Signal transduction Transformation Inhibition of interferon regulatory factor 3-mediated induction of type 1 interferon
NS4B	Membranous web
NS5A	Apoptosis Reactive oxygen species Signal transduction Transactivation Transformation Interference with actions of interferon (PKR)

E1, E2 = envelope proteins; NS = nonstructural proteins; PKR = protein kinase R.

positive-strand RNA molecules. The newly translated polyprotein is cleaved by a host-cell signal peptidase as well as virus-specific proteases, NS2 and NS3. The enzyme capable of performing both steps of RNA synthesis is the virally encoded RNA-dependent RNA polymerase NS5B. The NS3 of HCV also has helicase activity. The glycosylated E1 and E2 molecules are anchored inside the lumen of the ER while the C protein remains on the cytosol side. NS proteins have been localized to the membrane of the ER, suggesting that it is the site of polyprotein maturation and viral particle assembly.

Mechanisms of Hepatocarcinogenesis in Chronic HCV Infection

The Viral Contribution to Hepatocarcinogenesis

Unlike HBV, a DNA virus, the HCV RNA genome is not integrated into the host chromosome and is therefore unlikely to cause transformation through direct disruption of host genes. Most studies examining the association of HCV with HCC have found that the majority of HCV-related tumors arise in the setting of chronic inflammation and cirrhosis, implying that tumorigenesis is associated with derangements in the chronic cycle of inflammation, injury, and repair. Chronic injury invariably results in ongoing regeneration and proliferation of hepatocytes. With increased turnover of hepatocytes, frequent genetic mutations and/or instability likely result in various procarcinogenic events that set the stage for subsequent malignant transformation.[51–53] Figure 14–9 shows a schematic

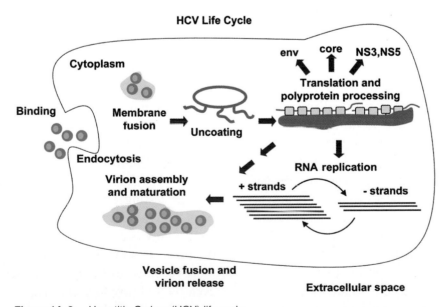

Figure 14–8. Hepatitis C virus (HCV) life cycle.

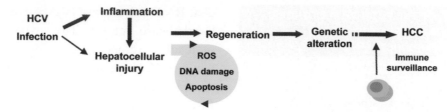

Figure 14–9. A model of hepatocellular carcinoma (HCC) due to chronic inflammation and injury from hepatitis C virus (HCV).

for the inflammation or injury model of HCV-associated HCC. As plausible as this hypothesis appears to be, however, it does not explain the paucity of HCC in other nonviral chronic inflammatory diseases of the liver, such as primary biliary cirrhosis or autoimmune chronic active hepatitis. Similarly, it cannot account for the reports of HCC in noncirrhotic or near-normal livers in chronically HCV-infected individuals. Even if the chronic injury model did explain the appearance of some cases of HCC, it still does not exclude the possibility of a direct immune response-independent link between HCV infection and malignant transformation.

Under such a model, viral proteins may directly alter the function of products of host oncogenes, tumor suppressor genes, or proteins related to apoptosis, to produce the transformed phenotype. Experimental evidence suggests that the HCV core protein interacts with oncogenes and tumor suppressor genes at the cellular level, cooperates with *ras* to transform primary rat embryo fibroblasts, and suppresses apoptosis in cultured cells.[54] Furthermore, the core protein has also been shown to interact with the cytoplasmic tail of the lymphotoxic receptor, a member of the tumor necrosis factor-α (TNF-α) receptor family that participates in the apoptotic pathway, raising the distinct possibility that perturbations of TNF-α-induced cell death signals underlie hepatocyte transformation.[55,56]

Other data exist to support a role for the HCV nonstructural proteins in transformation. A provocative report recently demonstrated that the N-terminal (or serine protease-containing) portion of the NS3 protein is capable of transforming fibroblasts in tissue culture.[57] Moreover, NIH3T3 cells that express a carboxy terminally truncated NS3 are more resistant to actinomycin D-induced apoptosis than are con-

trols. This may be mediated by decreased expression of p53.[58] Indeed, subsequent studies showed that the N-terminus of NS3 possesses a nuclear localization signal and that wild type, but not mutant p53 enhances nuclear accumulation of NS3, suggesting a direct interaction between NS3 and p53. It is tempting to speculate that NS3 binding sequesters p53 from its role in mediating apoptosis induced by genotoxic insult. Whether such a dynamic interplay between HCV NS3 and cellular p53 underlies the development of the transformed phenotype in hepatocytes awaits further study. NS5A is another nonstructural protein with regulatory effects on cell proliferation and viability. An inhibitory effect on cell apoptosis as well as a transforming effect on NIH3T3 cell lines has been reported.[59-61]

Tissue Culture Models of HCV

Historically, culture approaches have been severely limited by the lack of cell lines supportive of HCV replication. As a result, most early work focused on expression-based systems characterizing enzymatic function These approaches have been successful in gaining an understanding of virus-specific protein effects in vitro, but have not been able to shed light on the cellular effects of viral replication. The development by several groups of a self-replicating system ("replicon") using stable RNA transfection has provided a significant boost to studies aimed at elucidating mechanisms of RNA strand replication as well as testing of antiviral compounds. These systems, which lead to autonomous generation of high copy numbers of HCV RNA per cell, have employed the nonstructural portion of the HCV genome and, more recently, full-length viral sequences.[62,63] However, their ability to yield insights about viral pathogenesis is limited by the unusually high levels of viral replication, the need for constant selection, and by the adaptive mutations for high-level replication.

Animal Models of HCV

Unlike replicon systems, transgenic mouse models offer the advantage of viral protein expression in the whole animal and permit study of pathogenesis. However, mice constitutively expressing viral structural proteins have until recently failed to reveal significant pathology. For example, a study of transgenic expression of HCV structural proteins in FVB mice using two liver-specific promoters, the major urinary protein and albumin promoter provide constitutive high-level expression of transgenes in the liver. Immunohistochemical analysis revealed an authentic intracellular localization of core and E2. However, at 6 months of age, the livers of all transgenic lineages remained histologically normal, without evidence of steatosis or inflammation.[64] This failure to develop a significant phenotype likely reflects the limitations of using constitutive promoters to drive the expression of the HCV transgene. Constitutive gene expression in utero often results in adaptive or compensatory mechanisms in global gene expression, and typically induces tolerance to the transgene. Induction of tolerance would therefore preclude demonstration of viral protein effects in the setting of a host immune response, which clearly appears to play a role in HCV-related hepatocarcinogenesis.

However, in contrast, an important recent finding suggested that HCV core protein alone may be sufficient to produce HCC in transgenic mice. In a study from Japan, Moriya and colleagues prepared a transgenic construct expressing genotype 1b HCV core protein alone, downstream of a transcriptional regulatory region corresponding to the hepatitis B virus X protein.[65] Following introduction of this construct into C57BL/6 mice, these animals were found to develop hepatic steatosis as early as 3 months of age. This steatosis progressed as the mice grew to 12 months. No inflammation was seen in these animals. However, after the age of 16 months, gross hepatic nodules were noted, which compressed neighboring parenchyma and were identified as trabecular, well-differentiated HCC. These tumors

developed in two independent lines, and were found in 26% and 31% of male mice from each line compared with 0% of controls. The core protein was found to localize in the nuclei and mitochondria of affected livers, and was concentrated in tumors relative to surrounding nontumorous tissue, suggesting that the protein product is directly toxic and, in the absence of a host inflammatory response, sufficient to produce HCC. Of additional interest, the same group also found that transgenic mice expressing the envelope glycoproteins E1 and E2 alone under the same promoter do not develop hepatic pathology, suggesting that the property of malignant transformation is confined to core rather than envelope proteins.

A major concern raised by this model is that expressed core protein levels, under the control of a highly active HBV promoter element, may be substantially higher than those described in other models. Indeed, the readily detectable immunostaining of core protein in the livers of these mice is at considerable odds with the observation that core immunostaining of the livers from infected humans is highly insensitive and that levels of core seen in other transgenic mouse models are also sparse. The discordance in findings from the various transgenic studies may also be partly explained by the possible modulation of effects of core protein by other viral proteins such as E1 and E2, which were included in the construct by Kawamura and colleagues.[64] The genetic background of the host mice may also play a role, again raising the distinct possibility that an endogenous host predisposition to malignancy may play a key role in hepatocarcinogenesis.

The effects of viral proteins other than core protein have also been investigated in transgenic mice. Lerat and colleagues constructed transgenic C57BL/6 mice with liver-specific expression of RNA encoding the complete viral polyprotein (FL-N transgene) or viral structural proteins (S-N), and these were compared with nontransgenic littermates for altered liver morphology and function.[66] There was no inflammation in transgenic livers, but mice expressing either transgene developed age-related hepatic steatosis that was more severe in males. Hepatocellular adenoma or carcinoma developed in older males expressing either transgene, but their incidence reached statistical significance only in FL-N animals, suggesting expression of nonstructural proteins may increase the risk of developing HCC.

In order to explore the basis for the discrepant findings between models, HCV core-E1-E2 transgenic and HCV core transgenic mice inbred on the FVBxC57BL/6 background were bred.[67] The mice were treated with either (1) diethylnitrosamine (DEN) and sacrificed at 16, 24, and 32 weeks of age, or (2) saline and sacrificed at 32 weeks of age. No HCCs were identified in any of the saline-treated animals, suggesting that the FVB background has a dominant suppressive effect on tumor formation. HCCs were identified at 32 weeks of age in all of the DEN-treated core-E1-E2 transgenic, core transgenic, and nontransgenic mice. There was microscopically mild steatosis and no inflammation in all mice studied, suggesting that in this model, steatosis is not a required precursor to HCC. Although the mean number of HCCs was not significantly different among the three groups of mice, the mean size of HCCS were significantly larger in core-E1-E2 compared with core transgenic and nontransgenic mice, which was attributable to suppression of apoptosis rather than enhanced proliferation. These data implicate HCV E1 and/or E2 as tumor accelerator proteins and, consistent with the findings from Lerat and colleagues discussed above, that noncore HCV gene products may modify risk of developing cancer. The data also raise the concept of a "second hit" contributing to hepatocarcinogenesis in the setting of HCV infection.

How might core protein lead to HCC? One possible mechanism may be through its production of steatosis. A model of HCV core-induced steatosis was proposed by Perlemuter and colleagues, based on an investigation using HCV core transgenic mice.[68] Core expression led to significant reduction in microsomal triglyceride transfer protein (MTP) activity, a major regulator of the assembly and secretion of triglyceride (TG)-rich very low-density lipoprotein (VLDL) particles from the liver. Thus, with decreased MTP activity, fewer VLDL particles formed and more cytoplasmic TGs were retained, producing steatosis.

Another study investigating possible direct toxic effects of HCV core found that core expression increased the reactive oxygen species (ROS) content of three independent cell lines by two- to four-fold.[69] There was a similarly significant increase in lipid peroxide products. These resultant ROS would then be postulated to increase the risk of genotoxic injury, triggering the early events in hepatocarcinogenesis.

Review of current data regarding HCV-associated hepatocarcinogenesis can be summarized as follows:

1. Genetic background is an important determinant, as shown by the suggestion of C57BL/6 transgenic mice background being permissive for steatosis.
2. HCV core protein causes steatosis by inhibiting MTP, leading to impaired secretion of VLDL particles, and induces ROS and lipid peroxidation by manipulating the mitochondrial electron transport or cytochrome c pathway (Figure 14–10).
3. Other HCV structural or nonstructural proteins may play a role in accelerating progression to HCC.
4. Immune response occurs in the setting of chronic inflammation, injury, and repair, resulting in genomic instability, which predisposes hepatocytes to the progression of carcinogenesis.

The Host Genetic Contribution to Hepatocarcinogenesis

Because not all patients with HCV infection go on to develop HCC, efforts have been made to identify other factors that contribute to the observed increased cancer risk. The observed high rates of HCV-related HCC in some countries raises the distinct possibility that there is an endogenous (genetic) host predisposition to malignancy, especially given the observation that no particular HCV genotype appears to be overrepresented in cases of HCC. The observation of HCCs arising usually after typically long periods of chronic infection suggests the accumulation of serial "hits" to key genes responsible for growth regulation or cell death. Classical candidate genes include cellular proto-oncogenes or tumor suppressor genes. Experimental evidence has emerged, demonstrating alterations in several of these genes in human hepatocellular carcinoma, with or without the cooperation of hepatotropic viral infection. These include *p53*, *Rb*, the c-*met* oncogene, c-*myc*, *p16*, *ras*, and cyclin D1. Additional associations with human HCC have been made for chromosomal locations whose gene products are not yet known, including deletions of loci in chromosome 4q, 16q, and loss of heterozygosity (LOH) of 8p, 17p, 22q, and at an early-stage 1p. The observation of allelic loss or LOH in these chromosomal regions implies that they are likely to correspond to tumor suppressor genes. Indeed, the 17p region and the 22q region correspond to the chromosomal loci of the known suppressor genes *p53* and *Nf2*.

Chronic HBV infection, as well as aflatoxin exposure, has been associated most frequently with mutations or deletions in *p53* and *Rb*, as well as c-*myc* gene amplification. However, these would not appear to be the direct consequence of insertional mutagenesis associated with viral genomic integration, but rather are an indirect effect of chronic infection. The genetic alterations associated with HCV-related HCC are even less well worked out, but it appears that the prevalence of *p53* mutations in these tumors approximates the frequency seen in HBV-related HCC. Nonetheless, the finding of *p53* mutations in fewer than half of the HCV-related HCCs suggests that other pathways must also be operative in HCV-related hepatocarcinogenesis. Furthermore, since *p53* alterations have been identified as late events in the tumorigenesis of other solid cancers, the identity of earlier genetic events in the multistep pathway to HCC in HCV infection remains to be elucidated.

A Unified Model for Viral HCC

Various steps appear to lead to a common pathway of increased ROS production and genomic instability that ultimately result in procarcinogenic events toward developing HCC. Contributing factors include the following:

1. Viral-specific proteins, such as HCV core and HBx proteins, modulate cellular proteins, mitochondria, and/or various cell signaling pathways, resulting in increased ROS and genomic instability. ROS can subsequently increase expression of antiapoptotic genes such as *NFκB*.
2. The immune response has also been shown to play a key role in induction of malignant transformation, as demonstrated by development of HCC in the setting of adoptive cellular transfer in transgenic mice.
3. Direct insertional mutagenesis by HBV DNA also leads to chromosomal and genomic instability.
4. Exogenous mutagens may also contribute to the development of DNA damage.
5. Finally, direct effects by other viral proteins, such as HCV E1 and E2, may play a role in accelerating malignant transformation (Figure 14–11).

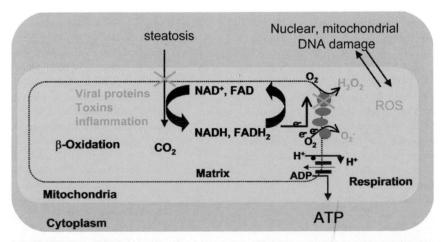

Figure 14–10. Schematic model for the role of mitochondria in hepatocellular carcinoma-induced oxidative injury.

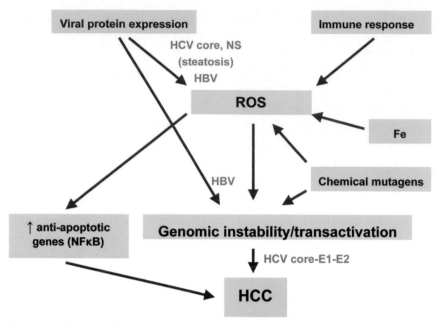

Figure 14–11. A unified model for viral hepatocellular carcinoma (HCC).

REFERENCES

1. Hankey BF, Ries LA, Edwards BK. The surveillance, epidemiology, and end results program: a national resource. Cancer Epidemiol Biomarkers Prev 1999;8:1117–21.
2. El-Serag HB. Hepatocellular carcinoma: recent trends in the United States. Gastroenterology 2004;127(5Suppl1): S27–34.
3. Deuffic S, Poynard T, Buffat L, Valleron AJ. Trends in primary liver cancer. Lancet 1998;351:214–5.
4. El-Serag HB, Mason AC. Rising incidence of hepatocellular carcinoma in the United States. N Engl J Med 1999; 340:745–50.
5. La Vecchia C, Lucchini F, Franceschi S, et al. Trends in mortality from primary liver cancer in Europe. Eur J Cancer 2000;36:909–15.
6. Fattovich G, Pantalena M, Zagni I, et al. Effect of hepatitis B and C virus infections on the natural history of compensated cirrhosis: a cohort study of 297 patients. Am J Gastroenterol 2002;97:2886–95.
7. Simonetti RG, Camma C, Fiorello F, et al. Hepatocellular carcinoma. A worldwide problem and the major risk factors. Dig Dis Sci 1991;36:962–72.
8. Bosch FX, Ribes J, Borras J. Epidemiology of primary liver cancer. Semin Liver Dis 1999;19:271–85.
9. Trevisani F, D'Intino PE, Caraceni P, et al. Etiologic factors and clinical presentation of hepatocellular carcinoma. Differences between cirrhotic and noncirrhotic Italian patients. Cancer 1995;75:2220–32.
10. Stroffolini T, Andreone P, Andriulli A, et al. Characteristics of hepatocellular carcinoma in Italy. J Hepatol 1998;29: 944–52.
11. Van Roey G, Fevery J, Van Steenbergen W. Hepatocellular carcinoma in Belgium: clinical and virological characteristics of 154 consecutive cirrhotic and non-cirrhotic patients. Eur J Gastroenterol Hepatol 2000;12:61–6.
12. Bralet MP, Regimbeau JM, Pineau P, et al. Hepatocellular carcinoma occurring in nonfibrotic liver: epidemiologic and histopathologic analysis of 80 French cases. Hepatology 2000;32:200–4.
13. De Mitri MS, Poussin K, Baccarini P, et al. HCV-associated liver cancer without cirrhosis. Lancet 1995;345:413–5.
14. Sangiovanni A, Del Ninno E, Fasani P, et al. Increased survival of cirrhotic patients with a hepatocellular carcinoma detected during surveillance. Gastroenterology 2004;126: 1005–14.
15. Benvegnu L, Chemello L, Noventa F, et al. Retrospective analysis of the effect of interferon therapy on the clinical outcome of patients with viral cirrhosis. Cancer 1998; 83:901–9.
16. Bolondi L, Sofia S, Siringo S, et al. Surveillance programme of cirrhotic patients for early diagnosis and treatment of hepatocellular carcinoma: a cost effectiveness analysis. Gut 2001;48:251–9.
17. Zaman SN, Melia WM, Johnson RD, et al. Risk factors in development of hepatocellular carcinoma in cirrhosis: prospective study of 613 patients. Lancet 1985;1:1357–60.
18. Zaman SN, Melia WM, Johnson RD, et al. Effects of hepatitis C and B viruses infection on the development of hepatocellular carcinoma. J Med Virol 1994;44:92–5.
19. Tarao K, Rino Y, Ohkawa S, et al. Association between high serum alanine aminotransferase levels and more rapid development and higher rate of incidence of hepatocellular carcinoma in patients with hepatitis C virus-associated cirrhosis. Cancer 1999;86:589–95.
20. Benvegnu L, Fattovich G, Noventa F, et al. Concurrent hepatitis B and C virus infection and risk of hepatocellular carcinoma in cirrhosis. A prospective study. Cancer 1994;74:2442–8.
21. Borzio M, Bruno S, Roncalli M, et al. Liver cell dysplasia is a major risk factor for hepatocellular carcinoma in cirrhosis: a prospective study. Gastroenterology 1995;108:812–7.

22. Degos F, Christidis C, Ganne-Carrie N, et al. Hepatitis C virus related cirrhosis: time to occurrence of hepatocellular carcinoma and death. Gut 2000;47:131–6.

23. Befeler AS, Di Bisceglie AM. Hepatitis B. Infect Dis Clin North Am 2000;14:617–32.

24. Goldstein ST, Alter MJ, Williams IT, et al. Incidence and risk factors for acute hepatitis B in the United States, 1982–1998: implications for vaccination programs. J Infect Dis 2002;185:713–9.

25. Groseclose SL, Brathwaite WS, Hall PA, et al. Summary of notifiable diseases—United States, 2002. MMWR Morb Mortal Wkly Rep 2004;51:1–84.

26. Brechot C, et al. Persistent hepatitis B virus infection in subjects without hepatitis B surface antigen: clinically significant or purely "occult"? Hepatology 2001;34:194–203.

27. Brechot C. Pathogenesis of hepatitis B virus-related hepatocellular carcinoma: old and new paradigms. Gastroenterology 2004;127(5 Suppl 1):S56–61.

28. Dandri M, Burda MR, Burkle A, et al. Increase in de novo HBV DNA integrations in response to oxidative DNA damage or inhibition of poly(ADP-ribosyl)ation. Hepatology 2002;35:217–23.

29. Wang XW, Forrester K, Yeh H, et al. Hepatitis B virus X protein inhibits p53 sequence-specific DNA binding, transcriptional activity, and association with transcription factor ERCC3. Proc Natl Acad Sci USA 1994;91:2230–4.

30. Jacob JR, Sterczer A, Toshkov IA, et al. Integration of woodchuck hepatitis and N-myc rearrangement determine size and histologic grade of hepatic tumors. Hepatology 2004;39:1008–16.

31. Chisari FV, Klopchin K, Moriyama T, et al. Molecular pathogenesis of hepatocellular carcinoma in hepatitis B virus transgenic mice. Cell 1989;59:1145–56.

32. Paterlini-Brechot P, Saigo K, Murakami Y, et al. Hepatitis B virus-related insertional mutagenesis occurs frequently in human liver cancers and recurrently targets human telomerase gene. Oncogene 2003;22:3911–6.

33. Horikawa I, Barrett JC. cis-Activation of the human telomerase gene (hTERT) by the hepatitis B virus genome. J Natl Cancer Inst 2001;93:1171–3.

34. Ferber MJ, Thorland EC, Brink AA, et al. Preferential integration of human papillomavirus type 18 near the c-myc locus in cervical carcinoma. Oncogene 2003;22:7233–42.

35. Moriarty AM, Alexander H, Lerner RA, Thornton GB. Antibodies to peptides detect new hepatitis B antigen: serological correlation with hepatocellular carcinoma. Science 1985;227:429–33.

36. Hwang GY, Lin CY, Huang LM, et al. Detection of the hepatitis B virus X protein (HBx) antigen and anti-HBx antibodies in cases of human hepatocellular carcinoma. J Clin Microbiol 2003;41:5598–603.

37. Yen TS. Hepadnaviral X protein: review of recent progress. J Biomed Sci 1996;3:20–30.

38. Rahmani Z, Huh KW, Lasher R, Siddiqui A. Hepatitis B virus X protein colocalizes to mitochondria with a human voltage-dependent anion channel, HVDAC3, and alters its transmembrane potential. J Virol 2000;74:2840–6.

39. Chami M, Ferrari D, Nicotera P, et al. Caspase-dependent alterations of Ca2+ signaling in the induction of apoptosis by hepatitis B virus X protein. J Biol Chem 2003;278:31745–55.

40. Bouchard MJ, Wang LH, Schneider RJ. Calcium signaling by HBx protein in hepatitis B virus DNA replication. Science 2001;294:2376–8.

41. Soussan P, Garreau F, Zylberberg H, et al. In vivo expression of a new hepatitis B virus protein encoded by a spliced RNA. J Clin Invest 2000;105:55–60.

42. Chisari FV, Pinkert CA, Milich DR, et al. A transgenic mouse model of the chronic hepatitis B surface antigen carrier state. Science 1985;230:1157–60.

43. Chisari FV, Filippi P, McLachlan A, et al. Expression of hepatitis B virus large envelope polypeptide inhibits hepatitis B surface antigen secretion in transgenic mice. J Virol 1986;60:880–7.

44. Chisari FV, Filippi P, Buras J, et al. Structural and pathological effects of synthesis of hepatitis B virus large envelope polypeptide in transgenic mice. Proc Natl Acad Sci USA 1987;84:6909–13.

45. Dunsford HA, Sell S, Chisari FV. Hepatocarcinogenesis due to chronic liver cell injury in hepatitis B virus transgenic mice. Cancer Res 1990;50:3400–7.

46. Hagen TM, Huang S, Curnutte J, et al. Extensive oxidative DNA damage in hepatocytes of transgenic mice with chronic active hepatitis destined to develop hepatocellular carcinoma. Proc Natl Acad Sci USA 1994;91:12808–12.

47. Huang SN, Chisari FV. Strong, sustained hepatocellular proliferation precedes hepatocarcinogenesis in hepatitis B surface antigen transgenic mice. Hepatology 1995;21:620–6.

48. Pasquinelli C, Bhavani K, Chisari FV. Multiple oncogenes and tumor suppressor genes are structurally and functionally intact during hepatocarcinogenesis in hepatitis B virus transgenic mice. Cancer Res 1992;52:2823–9.

49. Nakamoto Y, Guidotti LG, Kuhlen CV, et al. Immune pathogenesis of hepatocellular carcinoma. J Exp Med 1998;188:341–50.

50. El-Serag HB, Mason AC. Risk factors for the rising rates of primary liver cancer in the United States. Arch Intern Med 2000;160:3227–30.

51. Lauer GM, Walker BD. Hepatitis C virus infection. N Engl J Med 2001;345:41–52.

52. Liang TJ, Rehermann B, Seeff LB, Hoofnagle JH. Pathogenesis, natural history, treatment, and prevention of hepatitis C. Ann Intern Med 2000;132:296–305.

53. Liang TJ, Heller T. Pathogenesis of hepatitis C-associated hepatocellular carcinoma. Gastroenterology 2004;127(5 Suppl 1):S62–71.

54. Ray RB, Meyer K, Ray R. Suppression of apoptotic cell death by hepatitis C virus core protein. Virology 1996;226:176–82.

55. You LR, Chen CM, Lee YH. Hepatitis C virus core protein enhances NF-kappaB signal pathway triggering by lymphotoxin-beta receptor ligand and tumor necrosis factor alpha. J Virol 1999;73:1672–81.

56. Zhu N, Khoshnan A, Schneider R, et al. Hepatitis C virus core protein binds to the cytoplasmic domain of tumor necrosis factor (TNF) receptor 1 and enhances TNF-induced apoptosis. J Virol 1998;72:3691–7.

57. Sakamuro D, Furukawa T, Takegami T. Hepatitis C virus nonstructural protein NS3 transforms NIH 3T3 cells. J Virol 1995;69:3893–6.

58. Kwun HJ, Jung EY, Ahn JY, et al. p53-dependent transcrip-

tional repression of p21(waf1) by hepatitis C virus NS3. J Gen Virol 2001;82(Pt 9):2235–41.

59.   Gale M Jr, Blakely CM, Kwieciszewski B, et al. Control of PKR protein kinase by hepatitis C virus nonstructural 5A protein: molecular mechanisms of kinase regulation. Mol Cell Biol 1998;18:5208–18.

60.   Gale M Jr, Kwieciszewski B, Dossett M, et al. Antiapoptotic and oncogenic potentials of hepatitis C virus are linked to interferon resistance by viral repression of the PKR protein kinase. J Virol 1999;73:6506–16.

61.   Ghosh AK, Steele R, Meyer K, et al. Hepatitis C virus NS5A protein modulates cell cycle regulatory genes and promotes cell growth. J Gen Virol 1999;80(Pt 5):1178–83.

62.   Blight KJ, Kolykhalov AA, Rice CM. Efficient initiation of HCV RNA replication in cell culture. Science 2000; 290:1972–4.

63.   Lohmann V, Korner F, Koch J, et al. Replication of subgenomic hepatitis C virus RNAs in a hepatoma cell line. Science 1999;285:110–3.

64.   Kawamura T, Furusaka A, Koziel MJ, et al. Transgenic expression of hepatitis C virus structural proteins in the mouse. Hepatology 1997;25:1014–21.

65.   Moriya K, Fujie H, Shintani Y, et al. The core protein of hepatitis C virus induces hepatocellular carcinoma in transgenic mice. Nat Med 1998;4:1065–7.

66.   Lerat H, Honda M, Beard MR, et al. Steatosis and liver cancer in transgenic mice expressing the structural and nonstructural proteins of hepatitis C virus. Gastroenterology 2002;122:352–65.

67.   Kamegaya Y, Hiasa Y, Zukerberg L, et al. Hepatitis C virus (HCV) acts as a tumor accelerator by blocking apoptosis in a mouse model of hepatocarcinogenesis. Hepatology 2005.[In press]

68.   Perlemuter G, Sabile A, Letteron P, et al. Hepatitis C virus core protein inhibits microsomal triglyceride transfer protein activity and very low density lipoprotein secretion: a model of viral-related steatosis. FASEB J 2002;16:185–94.

69.   Okuda M, Li K, Beard MR, et al. Mitochondrial injury, oxidative stress, and antioxidant gene expression are induced by hepatitis C virus core protein. Gastroenterology 2002;122:366–75.

70.   Kittlesen DJ, Chianese-Bullock KA, Yao ZQ, et al. Interaction between complement receptor gC1qR and hepatitis C virus core protein inhibits T-lymphocyte proliferation. J Clin Invest 2000;106:1239–49.

71.   Lai MM, Ware CF. Hepatitis C virus core protein: possible roles in viral pathogenesis. Curr Top Microbiol Immunol 2000;242:117–34.

72.   Gale MJ Jr, Korth MJ, Tang NM, et al. Evidence that hepatitis C virus resistance to interferon is mediated through repression of the PKR protein kinase by the nonstructural 5A protein. Virology 1997;230:217–27.

73.   Gong G, Waris G, Tanveer R, Siddiqui A. Human hepatitis C virus NS5A protein alters intracellular calcium levels, induces oxidative stress, and activates STAT-3 and NF-kappa B. Proc Natl Acad Sci USA 2001;98:9599–604.

74.   Pavio N, Romano PR, Graczyk TM, et al. Protein synthesis and endoplasmic reticulum stress can be modulated by the hepatitis C virus envelope protein E2 through the eukaryotic initiation factor 2alpha kinase PERK. J Virol 2003;77:3578–85.

75.   Lundin M, Monne M, Widell A, et al. Topology of the membrane-associated hepatitis C virus protein NS4B. J Virol 2003;77:5428–38.

76.   Gao L, Aizaki H, He JW, Lai MM. Interactions between viral nonstructural proteins and host protein hVAP-33 mediate the formation of hepatitis C virus RNA replication complex on lipid raft. J Virol 2004;78:3480–8.

77.   Khabar KS, Polyak SJ. Hepatitis C virus-host interactions: the NS5A protein and the interferon/chemokine systems. J Interferon Cytokine Res 2002;22:1005–12.

78.   He Y, Nakao H, Tan SL, et al. Subversion of cell signaling pathways by hepatitis C virus nonstructural 5A protein via interaction with Grb2 and P85 phosphatidylinositol 3-kinase. J Virol 2002;76:9207–17.

79.   Chung KM, Song OK, Jang SK. Hepatitis C virus nonstructural protein 5A contains potential transcriptional activator domains. Mol Cells 1997;7:661–7.

80.   Lan KH, Sheu ML, Hwang SJ, et al. HCV NS5A interacts with p53 and inhibits p53-mediated apoptosis. Oncogene 2002;21:4801–11.

81.   Taylor DR, Shi ST, Romano PR, et al. Inhibition of the interferon-inducible protein kinase PKR by HCV E2 protein. Science 1999;285:107–10.

82.   Tseng CT, Klimpel GR. Binding of the hepatitis C virus envelope protein E2 to CD81 inhibits natural killer cell functions. J Exp Med 2002;195:43–9.

83.   Crotta S, Stilla A, Wack A, et al. Inhibition of natural killer cells through engagement of CD81 by the major hepatitis C virus envelope protein. J Exp Med 2002;195:35–41.

15

Screening for Hepatocellular Cancer: Current Strategies and Controversies

NATALIE LEE

JEFF KOHLWES

Hepatocellular carcinoma (HCC) is the third leading cause of cancer death and the fifth leading cause of cancer worldwide. It causes nearly 1 million deaths annually, and unlike many other cancers, its incidence and mortality rate is rising.[1] HCC's high death rate clearly demonstrates its virulence as well as our inability to reliably detect it at an early and potentially curative stage. HCC has long been recognized as an important cause of cancer death in Asia, but the increasing rates of HCC in the Western World are bringing this disease to the forefront internationally.

Hepatocellular carcinoma has all the characteristics of a disease that should be amenable to cancer screening (Table 15–1). It has a well-defined "at-risk" population, significant morbidity and mortality, effective early treatment (liver transplantation), and there is a presymptomatic, potentially treatable stage. Unfortunately, there are significant limitations of the screening modalities used for HCC surveillance that have made widespread screening controversial. This chapter will review HCC epidemiology, touch briefly on its pathogenesis, review the test characteristics of screening tests in general, and finally, discuss the efficacy of the whole range of screening tests for HCC that clinicians have at their disposal today.

HCC RISK FACTORS

Eighty percent of HCC develops in already cirrhotic livers.[2] Noncirrhotic HCC is usually associated with vertical transmission of hepatitis B virus (HBV) and is more common in developing countries. Incident cancers have different etiologies in different parts of the world. Asia and sub-Saharan Africa are areas hyperendemic for HBV infection. In fact, in one study, vertically infected hepatitis B carriers had a 100 times increase in relative risk of HCC compared with noncarriers.[3]

These patients tend to be the youngest patients with HCC and the most common group to develop HCC without preexisting cirrhosis. This high rate is exacerbated by exposure to the fungal toxin, aflatoxin B, which is found in foodstuffs contaminated by *Aspergillus flavus* or *parasiticus* and known to be a major risk factor in the multifactorial etiology of human HCC. A synergistic interaction between the carcinogenic effects of hepadnavirus infection and aflatoxin ingestion offers a plausible explanation for

Table 16–1. CHARACTERISTICS OF DISEASES APPROPRIATE FOR SCREENING

Disease Characteristics

Has significant associated morbidity or mortality
High prevalence in screened population
Long asymptomatic period that is detectable
Early detection offers a treatment or survival advantage
Relatively cost effective to screen

Screening Test Characteristics

Morbidity of screening test acceptable
Adequate test sensitivity to reliably detect disease when present
Reasonably high predictive value to prevent further testing

the very high incidence of the tumor in younger patients in these regions.[4]

A nationwide pediatric vaccination program implemented as a public health measure in Taiwan has reduced the carriage state of hepatitis B virus from 15 to 1%. This has been associated with a dramatic 60% reduction in incident rates of HCC development when compared with nonimmunized children.[2,5]

In the developed world, hepatitis C infection has overtaken hepatitis B as the most common etiology associated with cirrhosis and the development of HCC. This is likely multifactorial and due to public health efforts such as widespread hepatitis B immunization, education, and routine screening of the blood supply in most developed nations. The American Cancer Society statistics show that in 2003 there were 17,300 new cases of, and 14,400 deaths from, HCC in the United States.[6] Hepatitis C–related cirrhosis is thought to be the main cause of the recent increase in incidence and mortality due to HCC. Approximately 2.7 million individuals are actively infected with hepatitis C virus (HCV) in the United States, and up to 186,000 of these persons could develop HCC over the next 20 years.[7,8] The rate of development of HCC in hepatitis C–infected patients with cirrhosis in the United States is between 3 and 5% per year.[9]

In this highly selective population, HCC is even more common than other cancers for which screening tests to detect for cancer are routinely applied.

It is estimated that HBV and HCV infections account for 70 to 85% of HCC cases worldwide.[10] Other factors are also associated with HCC development, however. These other risk factors may be independent risks or serve as cofactors for HCC exacerbating viral tumorigenesis in hepatitis-infected individuals. Most factors that are associated with cirrhosis are also associated with HCC. Recently, Marrero and colleagues presented a case-controlled study demonstrating that heavy alcohol consumption, body mass index > 30, and tobacco smoking > 15 pack-years were significant independent predictors of HCC. This is controversial, however, and like most epidemiologic studies, this study demonstrates association, but does not prove causality. Thus, we must await larger prospective studies to better describe the degree of risk from each of these hepatotoxins.[8,11]

Other risk factors associated with the development of HCC are hemochromatosis, tyrosinemia, alpha$_1$-antitrypsin deficiency, and glycogen storage disease.[10] It is difficult to measure the degree of risk that these factors pose individually for HCC, since they are so rare. Our discussion of screening tests for HCC should be applied to the populations who are hepatitis B and C infected and at risk for HCC development.

REVIEW OF EPIDEMIOLOGY AND TEST CHARACTERISTICS

When applying a screening test to a disease, it is important to have a test that will capture all patients with disease in a population. This is the concept of test sensitivity. Sensitivity is the proportion of patients who *have* a disease and will have a *positive* test. This can be remembered by the mnemonic "PID is sensitive" where PID stands for "positivity in disease." It can also be represented numerically (as in the 2 × 2 Figure 15–1) as follows:

A/A+C

Unfortunately, tests with a sensitivity that is high enough for use as a screening test comes at the cost of being certain that a person with a positive test will actually have the disease. Setting a diagnostic test threshold at a low value enables one to capture

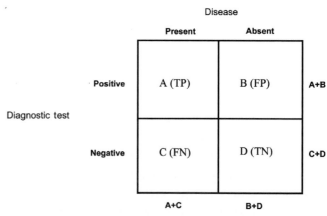

Figure 15–1. 2 x 2 Table for calculating screening test characteristics. A+C = all patients with disease; A+B = All patients with a positive test; A+B+C+D = All patients being tested; B+D = All patients without disease; C+D = All patients with a negative test; FN = false negative test; FP = false positive test; TN = true negative test; TP = true positive test; negative predictive value = D (TN)/C+D; positive predictive value = A (TP)/A+B; sensitivity = A (TP)/A+C; specificity = D (TN)/B+D.

everyone with disease, but it will also capture many people without disease who just have a positive test. This can lead to significant patient anxiety as well as added cost for additional work-up. Adding sensitivity, or lowering the threshold for a positive test, inevitably affects the test's specificity, or those individuals who will have true negative tests. This is the description of test specificity.

Specificity is the proportion of patients who do *not* have disease, who have a *negative* test. The mnemonic for specificity is "NIH" or "negativity in health," and can be shown numerically as follows (see Figure 15–1):

D/B+D

Confirmatory tests should have a very high test specificity so that a negative test truly *rules out* having that disease. An example of this kind of test is a Western blot for HIV disease. This test has an incredibly high specificity, thus a positive (or equivocal) sensitive screening test for HIV disease is always confirmed with a Western blot. This is because if blot testing is negative, then there is an incredibly high certainty that the individual does not have HIV disease. The sensitivity and specificity of tests are fixed characteristics of the test and are therefore *not* affected by disease prevalence in a community. Although a high sensitivity and specificity is useful for a clinician to feel reassured with a test result, they do not address what the posttest probability is for an individual patient to have a disease with a positive test. To take a test result to "the bedside," a clinician must be able to understand the concept of positive and negative predictive values.

The positive predictive value (A/A+B) and the negative predictive value (D/C+D) enable a clinician to complete Bayes' theorem. This theorem, simply stated, is that the clinician's prior probability of encountering a disease, plus a test result, leads to a refined posttest probability of disease. Positive predictive value can also be called the posttest probability of disease. The negative predictive value can also be thought of as the posttest probability of health. These terms are useful when thinking about diagnostic tests, because they are dependent upon the disease prevalence in a population. For example, a positive thick smear for malaria infection has good sensitivity and outstanding specificity for malaria infection in an experienced laboratory. When these test characteristics are applied to a patient with a very low pretest probability of having malaria, such as an Eskimo who had never traveled away from his or her home in Northern Alaska, then a positive malaria smear would still lead to a very low posttest probability for malaria despite the outstanding test characteristics of the malaria blood smear.

To best understand the problems associated with screening tests for HCC, one has to remember that sensitivity and specificity are fixed characteristics of the screening test. Thus, they are independent of the disease prevalence in a population. In the remainder of this chapter, the flaws of the current diagnostic tests available for detecting and diagnosing HCC will be examined.

GOALS OF SCREENING

Screening is defined as a one-time application of a diagnostic test to detect disease at an early stage, whereas surveillance is the repetition of a screening test over a period of time. However, most studies on HCC do not make this distinction, and use the term "screening" to cover both initial screening and subsequent surveillance. The criteria for an effective screening program rests on several factors: the importance or prevalence of the disease; a well-defined population at risk; the availability of noninvasive, low-cost screening tests that can detect disease at an early stage; and curative treatments resulting in long-term survival. HCC meets many of these criteria.

The goals of screening are to detect cancer early enough such that curative resection, liver transplant, or other treatments will be possible in patients who are healthy enough to withstand treatment. Several cohort studies have shown increased survival in screened patients. However, in cohort studies, the problems of lead-time and length-time bias arise. Lead-time bias occurs when the tumors are detected earlier because of screening, but overall survival is not increased compared with nonscreened patients. Length bias occurs because screening procedures tend to detect slow-growing tumors, whereas rapidly growing tumors may present symptomatically in between screening procedures.

Unfortunately, there are no randomized controlled studies of screening and mortality from HCC. Controversy remains over whether screening results in decreased mortality, which patients should undergo screening, the best methods for screening, and the timing of testing. Despite the lack of evidence from randomized controlled studies, most physicians have implemented screening into their practices. In a survey of members of the American Association for the Study of Liver Diseases, 84% indicated that they were routinely screening cirrhotic patients with alpha fetoprotein (AFP) and ultrasonography.[12] Since screening has become so widespread, at this point, it is unlikely that a randomized controlled trial will be feasible. Physicians may also believe that omitting screening may lead to malpractice liability. Therefore, the question has shifted from whether or not to screen, to which patients should receive screening and by what methods.

DEFINING THE HIGH-RISK POPULATION FOR SCREENING

Eighty percent of HCC cases develop in patients with cirrhosis. Although there are cases of HCC in chronic hepatitis B carriers without cirrhosis, this is a relatively rare occurrence outside of Asia, where the incidence of hepatitis B is high and infection often occurs at a young age. Patients with hepatitis C rarely develop HCC unless the patient has cirrhosis, although the rate of development of HCC in hepatitis C–infected patients with cirrhosis in the United States is between 3 and 5% per year.[9]

The general consensus is that all patients with cirrhosis from any etiology should undergo screening. Patients awaiting liver transplantation routinely undergo screening, as detection of HCC can either lead to status upgrade or, occasionally, removal from the list. Finally, surveillance posttransplant is important, as recurrent hepatitis is nearly universal and progression to cirrhosis occurs at a more rapid rate in posttransplant patients.[13] Thus the ideal patient for HCC screening at this time is a patient with Child-Pugh class A cirrhosis who would be a suitable candidate for partial hepatectomy, or any patient with well-compensated cirrhosis who would be a suitable candidate for liver transplantation or percutaneous therapies.

SERUM MARKERS

The most common serum marker used in screening for HCC is AFP, a glycosylated protein secreted by the fetal liver and which is elevated in many patients with HCC. Normal levels are < 20 μg/L, and levels above 500 μg/L are considered diagnostic of HCC. Serum levels of AFP do not correlate with the size or stage of tumor, although up to 40% of small tumors have normal or only mildly elevated AFP levels.[14] A steadily increasing AFP is highly suggestive of HCC, even in the absence of a visible tumor. However, AFP levels can be elevated in chronic viral hepatitis without HCC. In one study of 357 patients with hepatitis C but without HCC, 23% had an AFP > 10 mg/mL.[15]

In a recent systematic review of five studies, the sensitivity of AFP using a cut-off of 20 μg/L or greater was 41 to 65% and the specificity was 80 to 94% (Table 15–2).[16] At a 5% prevalence of HCC, an AFP level of 20 μg/mL or higher corresponds to a positive predictive value of only 25%. When the cut-off was raised from 20 μg/L to 200 μg/L, the specificity increased to 99 to 100% but the sensitivity fell to 20 to 45%. In addition, the quality of the evidence was limited, as three of the five studies used a case-

Table 15–2. ABSTRACTED TEST CHARACTERISTICS OF AFP LEVELS HIGHER THAN 20 OR 200 μG/L FOR DETECTING HEPATOCELLULAR CARCINOMA				
	Cut-Off Level for AFP			
(μg/L)	Sensitivity (95% CI)	Specificity (95% CI)	Positive Likelihood Ratio (95% CI)	Negative Likelihood Ratio (95% CI)
20	41–65	80–94	3.1–6.8	0.4–0.6
200	20–45	99–100	29–37	0.6–0.8

AFP = alpha fetoprotein; CI = confidence interval.
Adapted from Gupta S et al.[16]

control design that may overestimate diagnostic accuracy. Therefore, AFP as a single test has limited use for screening for HCC.

Other tumor markers for HCC have been evaluated for use alone or together with AFP. However, none of these markers are in wide clinical use.

Lectins are proteins that bind to specific sugars, and the specific sugar-chain structures have been shown to vary among AFPs from different sources. For example, in one study, three isoforms of AFP (+I, +II, and +III) were identified that correlated with chronic liver disease, HCC, and nonseminomatous germ-cell tumors, respectively.[17] Other lectins with increased specificity for AFP from HCC include concanavalin A lectin and lentil lectin.[18]

Hepatoma cells fail to express prothrombin carboxylase, which leads to increased levels of des-gamma-carboxy prothrombin, also known as protein induced by vitamin K absence or antagonism II (PIVKA-II). In one study, PIVKA-II was elevated in 69 of 76 patients with HCC, with a mean concentration of 900 µg/L compared with 10 µg/L in patients with chronic active hepatitis, 42 µg/L in patients with metastatic disease to the liver, and undetectable in normal patients.[19] However, PIVKA-II tends to be elevated mainly in larger tumors; in one study, this marker was elevated in only 20% of tumors < 3 cm.[20] This would limit its use as a screening tool to detect early tumors.

Serum α-L-fucosidase activity may have increased specificity compared with AFP, but it has been shown to have low sensitivity.[21] Other HCC markers include urinary transforming growth factor β-1, tumor-associated isoenzymes of γ-glutamyl transpeptidase, and serum circulating intercellular adhesion molecule-1.[22–24]

Because of the poor sensitivity and specificity of AFP, many use AFP in combination with ultrasound. The evidence for this will be discussed below in the ultrasound section.

RADIOLOGIC IMAGING

With rapid improvements in technology, radiologic imaging is playing an increased role in screening for HCC. However, there is no clear consensus on which imaging modalities are the best.

A recent systematic review examined the best method for radiologic imaging of HCC in patients with cirrhosis. Twenty-nine studies met inclusion criteria and 10 used the explanted liver as the "gold standard." However, all except one of the studies found no significant difference or did not directly compare sensitivities among imaging modalities. Therefore, no imaging technique was clearly shown to be superior.[25] Care in the evaluation of the literature regarding the radiologic evaluation of HCC is needed, given the rapid changes in imaging technology that make the imaging studies of the previous 10 years quite different from the studies of today.

Ultrasonography

Ultrasound is the most widely used modality for screening because it is readily available and noninvasive. In addition, ultrasonography can assess the patency of the hepatic arteries and veins and detect tumor invasion of these vessels. Small HCC lesions are usually hypoechoic, and may be indistinguishable from regenerative nodules (Figure 15–2). Larger tumors may become isoechoic or hyperechoic because of coagulation necrosis, and tend to have a mosaic pattern with peripheral sonolucency. The presence of a pseudocapsule is characteristic of HCC. Posterior acoustic enhancement is uncommon. More advanced cases of HCC may show por-

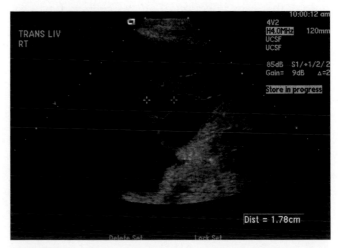

Figure 15–2. Transabdominal ultrasound of the right upper quadrant in the transverse plane demonstrates a small coarsely echogenic nodular cirrhotic liver with abundant ascites. Anterior to the gallbladder is a hypoechoic mass, representing a hepatocellular carcinoma.

tal vein thrombosis, hepatic or portal vein invasion, or biliary obstruction.[26]

The sensitivity of ultrasound in detecting HCC ranges from 35 to 85% in various studies, with lower sensitivities shown in studies using explanted livers or autopsy specimens as diagnostic confirmation.[27–29] In a large prospective study of noncirrhotic hepatitis B carriers, the sensitivity was 71%, the specificity was 93%, and the positive predictive value was 15%.[30] Because of the low positive predictive value, tumors detected by ultrasound generally require additional confirmatory studies for diagnosis and staging, and ultrasonography is frequently used as a means of guiding percutaneous needle biopsy of hepatic masses.

Many methods have been developed to improve the quality of sonographic imaging, such as harmonic imaging, color Doppler, and contrast-enhanced ultrasonography. Harmonic imaging detects second harmonic signals generated by the tissue during the nonlinear propagation of the acoustic signal. This results in improved resolution, decreased artifact, and increased signal-to-noise ratio. There are several types of harmonic imaging, including tissue harmonic imaging, pulse inversion harmonic imaging, and coded harmonic imaging.[31] Color Doppler ultrasonography can show fine vessels around a tumor nodule and pulsatile flow in more advanced HCC. It also can measure portal venous flow in portal hypertension and evaluate portosystemic shunts.[32] Contrast-enhanced ultrasonography is an emerging technology that uses injection of agents such as Levovist, which contains microbubbles that allow enhanced visualization of tumors.[33] One study suggested that contrast-enhanced Doppler ultrasonography had a similar diagnostic accuracy compared to helical computed tomography (CT); however, ultrasound contrast agents are not yet in widespread use.[34]

The optimal screening interval with abdominal ultrasonography is not established, with common intervals ranging from 3 to 12 months, but in general, ultrasonography is performed every 6 months. This is estimated to represent the average doubling time of a hepatic tumor.[35] However, some advocate for more frequent screening (every 3 months) in high-risk patients.[36]

Ultrasonography in combination with AFP screening has been shown to increase sensitivity over AFP alone. One study evaluated AFP and ultrasonography in 1,125 patients infected with hepatitis B and/or C for at least 5 years. Sensitivity of AFP alone was 75%, ultrasonography alone was 87%, and the combination was 100% sensitive.[37]

Computed Tomography

Computed tomography is often used as a confirmatory test for lesions detected by ultrasound. In some centers, it is now used as a primary screening test in lieu of ultrasonography. Improvements in technology have allowed for increased diagnostic accuracy and its use is growing.

Helical (spiral) CT is the diagnostic standard for hepatic imaging. In clinical use since the early 1990s, helical CT improves acquisition time over conventional axial CT imaging by obtaining images continuously as the patient moves through the gantry. The imaging is faster and obtained as volumetric data. This improves image quality, studies can frequently be done during a single-breath hold, and three-dimensional reconstruction is easier. The most recent advance in helical CT imaging is the introduction of the multidetector (multislice) helical CT, in which a bank of several detectors (typical present-day scanners have 4 to 16 detectors) is used to simultaneously capture imaging data, allowing even faster patient imaging, frequently with slice collimation of 1 mm or less.[38]

Hepatic lesions are generally lower in attenuation on unenhanced CT than the surrounding hepatic parenchyma. HCC may present as a solitary mass, a dominant mass with surrounding satellite lesions, multifocal lesions, or diffusely infiltrating tumor.[32] Small well-differentiated lesions, however, may not show low attenuation and are more difficult to detect. Contrast-enhanced CT is the standard for evaluation of liver masses, including HCC. In particular, the use of dynamic, or multiphasic, helical CT increases diagnostic accuracy by imaging the liver in different stages of enhancement after the bolus administration of intravenous contrast agent (typically divided into precontrast, hepatic arterial, portal venous, and delayed phases). Because HCC generally obtains its blood supply from the hepatic artery, the lesion appears hypervascular during the arterial phase, and relatively hypodense on the portal venous and delayed phases due to early washout of contrast by the arterial blood (Figure 15–3). Some lesions are isoattenuating in both arterial and venous phases, and therefore, delayed imaging is useful for detecting these tumors.[39] The speed of multidetector-row helical CT allows for two arterial-phase (early and late) imagings with portal venous phase imaging, all within a single breath-hold, which can additionally improve tumor detection.[40,41]

The accuracy of conventional CT scans was studied in a prospective study of 200 patients with cirrhosis prior to liver transplantation. The sensitivity of CT was 68% and specificity was 81% compared with the histologic examination of the explanted livers.[42] Nodular cirrhotic lesions, often found in advanced cirrhosis, reduce specificity. Triple-phase multidetector-row helical CT had a sensitivity of 88.5% and specificity of 93.4% in one study, although the authors found that the dual arterial-phase imaging did significantly increase sensitivity and specificity compared with late arterial-phase imaging.[43]

Other techniques have been combined with CT imaging in efforts to enhance tumor detection. Lipiodol, an iodized oil, can be injected directly into the

hepatic artery and is retained for long periods within HCC lesions. Lipiodol-enhanced CT has a sensitivity of 93% or more.[44] However, the need for intra-arterial injection of lipiodol has limited its clinical use.

Magnetic Resonance Imaging

Thought to hold great promise, magnetic resonance imaging (MRI) is presently used largely as a problem-solving modality for evaluation of lesions found at initial screening. MRI has similar sensitivity for diagnosing HCC compared to helical CT.[45] On MRI, HCC presents as a high-intensity lesion on T2-weighted images, and a low-intensity pattern on T1-weighted images. With the development of faster MRI techniques, dynamic multiphasic MRI is becoming more commonly used (Figures 15–4 A and B). MRI angiography using arterial, portal-venous, and late-venous phases was found to have higher sensitivity for HCC than triphasic CT in a study with pathologic confirmation from explanted livers.[46] Newer tissue-specific MR contrast agents are also being developed for use in hepatic imaging.[47] One benefit of MRI is the avoidance of use of contrast in patients with renal insufficiency or contrast allergy. MRI is also more sensitive than CT and ultrasonography in the case of extremely nodular livers, and can improve differentiation of small HCCs from dysplastic nodules.[48,49]

Angiography

Although previously used as a diagnostic modality for evaluation of hepatic lesions prior to more recent advancements in cross-sectional imaging, angiography is not considered a screening modality for HCC. Angiography, however, continues to play an important role in the operative evaluation of patients with HCC, and there is active interest in using intravascular techniques to palliate and treat patients with the disease, by control of bleeding from ruptured HCC and chemoembolization of tumors.

POSITRON EMISSION TOMOGRAPHY

The use of positron emission tomography (PET) for detection of HCC is still relatively uncommon.

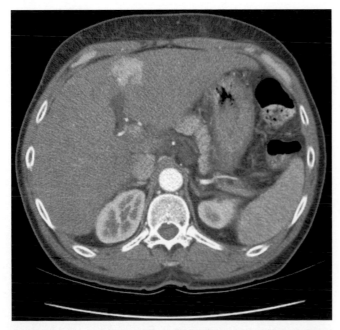

Figure 15–3. A CT scan obtained in the early arterial phase of intravenous contrast administration demonstrates an enhancing hepatocellular carcinoma in the left lobe of the liver. Subsequent delayed images through this region showed rapid washout of contrast material from the lesion.

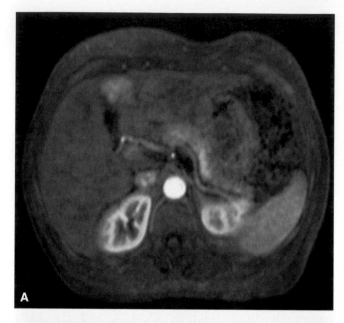

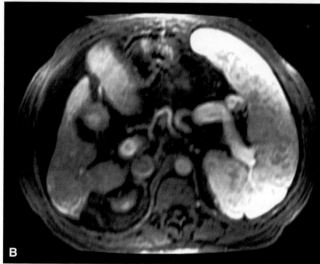

Figure 15–4. *A,* Dynamic hepatic MRI obtained immediately following gadolinium administration demonstrates an enhancing hepatocellular carcinoma in the left lobe of the liver. *B,* Dynamic hepatic MRI obtained immediately following gadolinium administration demonstrates enhancement of the lesion anterior to the gallbladder. A second larger enhancing mass is present in the posterior inferior liver. This patient had multifocal hepatocellular carcinoma. Note the enlarged spleen and splenic vein consistent with portal hypertension.

2-[Fluorine-18]fluoro-2-deoxy-D-glucose (FDG) is a glucose analog that competes with glucose at the cell membrane and intracellular transport pathways. Although of generally lower spatial resolution than CT or ultrasound, it is theorized that small tumors undetectable on routine CT or ultrasonography could still be sufficiently functionally active to be seen on PET, as malignant tumors have increased glucose metabolism.

Clinical results with PET as a screening modality for HCC are mixed. One study performed PET scanning on eight hepatitis C cirrhotic patients awaiting liver transplantation with AFP > 100 µg/mL but no detectable lesions on abdominal CT. Two patients had evidence of HCC on explant and lipiodol-enhanced CT, but these lesions were not detected by PET; thus, the authors concluded that PET has no role in HCC detection.[50]

Others have reported an overall 50% in the sensitivity of PET in detection of HCC, in part because well-differentiated tumors tend to have lower FDG uptake.[51] Other types of radiolabels such as carbon-11-labeled acetate have shown improved sensitivity and specificity for HCC compared with FDG, and oxygen-15 PET has been used to measure hepatic and tumor blood flow.[52] However, these radiolabels are more difficult to produce and are not readily available in many areas.

The role of PET is still being defined, and will be weighted against the relatively high cost of obtaining these studies. PET has been advocated as a sensitive method for detecting suspected extrahepatic metastases.[53] PET may also find increased use with the ongoing clinical introduction of combined PET-CT scanners that fuse data between the anatomic imaging of CT and the functional imaging of PET.

BIOPSY

The role of biopsy in the screening process is controversial. With improvement in radiologic technology, the sensitivity of detecting lesions has increased. However, in cirrhotic livers, many focal lesions, especially small lesions, are benign regenerative nodules or dysplastic nodules rather than HCC. The questions of whether and when diagnostic biopsy should be performed are still being debated. The risks of complications such as bleeding and needle tract seeding should also be taken into consideration.

The 2000 European Association for the Study of the Liver (EASL) conference recommended imaging-guided biopsy for lesions of 1 to 2 cm detected with ultrasound screening. For lesions < 1 cm, a "watch and wait" approach of repeating the ultrasonography at 3 months was recommended. For lesions > 2 cm with AFP > 400 ng/L and confirmed by CT, MRI, or angiography, the diagnosis of HCC was presumed without the need for biopsy (see Figures 15–2, 3, and 4).

A recent study of 4,581 patients with cirrhosis looked at screening with ultrasound-guided biopsy. Patients who had no focal lesions at initial ultrasonography were followed with AFP and ultrasound every 4 to 6 months. If a lesion was detected and AFP was < 400 ng/L, then a biopsy was performed. Of the lesions < 2 cm, 87.6% were diagnosed as HCC (69% of lesions < 1 cm, and 91% of lesions 1 to 2 cm). The rate of false-negatives was 10%. Therefore, in a screening population of cirrhotics, more than two-thirds of small nodules proved to be HCC, with ultrasound-guided biopsy able to detect 90% of these lesions. This study would seem to advocate biopsying all lesions, no matter their size, in contrast to the EASL recommendations.[54]

As HCC lesions are often hypervascular, bleeding risk can be greater when biopsy is performed. In one series of 159 HCC patients undergoing fine-needle aspiration biopsy, four patients developed significant bleeding (2.5%), and one patient died.[55]

Tumor seeding is another potential complication of fine-needle biopsy. In one series of 137 patients who underwent ultrasound-guided biopsy prior to resection or transplant for HCC, needle tract seeding occurred in two patients (1.6%).[56] Another study of 59 patients undergoing biopsy had needle tract seeding in three patients (5.1%).[57] The patients in both studies were without recurrences after local excision.

COST-EFFECTIVENESS ANALYSES

There are several analyses of the cost-effectiveness of screening for HCC. One study of surveillance of hepatitis B carriers showed that yearly AFP and ultrasound screening would detect 90% of tumors early, at a cost of $11,800 (US) per tumor detected.[58] Lin and colleagues used a Markov model to evaluate the cost-effectiveness of screening with AFP and ultrasonography.[59] They compared screening strategies of biannual AFP/annual ultrasonography with biannual AFP/biannual ultrasonography and biannual AFP/annual CT, and found that biannual AFP/annual ultrasonography gave the highest quality-adjusted life-year (QALY) gain for the least additional cost, at

$33,000 (US)/QALY. Another model estimated that $285,000 (US) was required per cured case.[60] With an assumed 75 to 85% 10-year survival (likely less for HCV carriers), this results in about $35,000 to $45,000 (US) per QALY, a figure slightly higher than that for breast cancer screening.[61]

Conclusions about the cost-effectiveness of screening forHCC must take into account the prevalence of HCC. In countries with lower prevalence of HCC such as the United States and Europe, the cost-effectiveness of screening is controversial. For example, an Italian study concluded that screening was not cost-effective, with the cost of screening each treatable HCC at $17,934 (US) and the cost per year of life saved at $112,993 (US). Other studies in Southeast Asia and Africa, where the prevalence of hepatitis B is high, show that screening is much more cost-effective. For example, in Hong Kong, the annual cost for detecting a treatable case of HCC was only $1,667 (US), and 61% of HCC cases were discovered at a treatable stage.[62] Therefore, the prevalence of the disease and the resources available should be considered when deciding whether or not screening is cost-effective.

GUIDELINES

Guidelines from major organizations on screening for HCC are fairly limited. The National Cancer Institute states that there is insufficient evidence to establish that screening by AFP and/or imaging such as CT or ultrasonography would result in decreased mortality from HCC.

The American Association for the Study of Liver Disease recommends that hepatitis B carriers at high risk for HCC, such as men over 45 years, cirrhotics, and people with a family history of HCC, should be screened periodically (optimally every 6 months) with AFP and ultrasonography, and that periodic screening with AFP for low-risk HBV-infected patients from endemic areas should be considered. However, it is not known at what age screening should begin and what the role of screening is in nonendemic populations, such as Caucasian carriers in developed countries.[63] No specific recommendation has been made about screening patients with hepatitis C for HCC.[64]

CONCLUSIONS

The goals of screening are to detect cancer early enough such that curative resection, liver transplant, or other treatments will be possible in patients who are healthy enough to withstand treatment. Screening for HCC has become commonplace, despite lack of clear evidence that screening decreases mortality from HCC. Since 80% of HCC arises in cirrhotic livers, screening protocols that focus on well-compensated cirrhotic patients who are candidates for treatment or transplantation will generally have increased diagnostic accuracy and cost-effectiveness. In patients with chronic hepatitis B infection without cirrhosis, especially older patients or those from endemic areas, screening should also be considered. There are many diagnostic modalities for detecting HCC. Screening tests such as AFP or ultrasonography alone suffer from low sensitivity, specificity, and positive predictive value, so they are often done in combination. The most common screening method in use is biannual AFP and annual ultrasonography, which has been shown to be a cost-effective combination. However, improvements in radiologic imaging, such as multidetector or multiphasic CT and MRI and newer contrast agents, may lead to changes in screening protocols in the future. There are few guidelines from major organizations that discuss screening protocols. Therefore, screening recommendations should take into consideration the prevalence of the disease and the resources available for screening.

REFERENCES

1. Burroughs A, Hochhauser D, Meyer T. Systemic treatment and liver transplantation for hepatocellular carcinoma: two ends of the therapeutic spectrum. Lancet Oncol 2004;5:409–18.
2. Llovet JM, Burroughs A, Bruix J. Hepatocellular carcinoma. Lancet 2003;362:1907–17.
3. Beasley RP, Hwang LY, Lin CC, Chien CS. HCC and hepatitis B virus; a prospective study of 22,707 men in Taiwan. Lancet 1981;2:1129–33.
4. Kew MC. Synergistic interaction between aflatoxin B1 and hepatitis B virus in hepatocarcinogenesis. Liver Int 2003; 23:405–9.
5. Chang MH, Shau WY, Chen CJ, et al. The Taiwan Childhood Hepatoma Study Group: hepatitis B vaccination and hepatocellular carcinoma rates in boys and girls. JAMA 2000;284:3040–2.
6. Jemal A, Murray T, Samuels A, et al. Cancer statistics, 2003. CA Cancer J Clin 2003;53:5–26.
7. Befeler AS, Di Bisceglie AM. Hepatocellular carcinoma: diagnosis and treatment. Gastroenterology 2002;122:1609–19.
8. Befeler, AS. New developments in hepatocellular carcinoma. Available at: http://www.medscape.com/viewarticle/464173?src=search. (accessed July 20, 2005).
9. Bruno S, Silini E, Crosignani A, et al. Hepatitis C virus genotypes and the risk of hepatocellular carcinoma in cirrhosis: a prospective study. Hepatology 1997;25:754–8.
10. Szabo E, Paska C, Kaposi Novak P, et al. Similarities and differences in hepatitis B and C virus induced hepatocarcinogenesis. Pathol Oncol Res 2004;10:5–11.
11. Marrero JA, Banegura A, Fu S, et al. Smoking, obesity and alcohol are important risk factors in American patients with hepatocellular carcinoma: a case control study. Hepatology 2003;38:278A.
12. Chalasani N, Said A, Ness R, et al. Screening for hepatocellular carcinoma in patients with cirrhosis in the United States: results of a national survey. Am J Gastroenterol 1999;94:2224–9.
13. Gane EJ, Portmann BC, Naoumov NV, et al. Long-term outcome of hepatitis C infection after liver transplantation. N Engl J Med 1996;334:815–20.
14. Chen D, Sung J, Shen J, et al. Serum alpha-fetoprotein in early stages of human hepatocellular carcinoma. Gastroenterology 1984;86:1404.
15. Hu KG, Kyulo NL, Lim N, et al. Clinical significance of elevated alpha-fetoprotein in patients with chronic hepatitis C, but not hepatocellular carcinoma. Am J Gastroenterol 2004;99:860.
16. Gupta S, Bent S, Kohlwes J. Test characteristics of alpha-fetoprotein for detecting hepatocellular carcinoma in patients with hepatitis C. Ann Intern Med 2003;139:46–50.
17. Ho S, Cheng P, Yuen J, et al. Isoelectric focusing of alpha-fetoprotein in patients with hepatocellular carcinoma: frequency of specific binding patterns at non-diagnostic serum levels. Br J Cancer 1996;73:985–8.
18. Sato Y, Nakata K, Kato Y, et al. Early recognition of hepatocellular carcinoma based on altered profiles of alpha-fetoprotein. N Engl J Med 1993;328:1802–6.
19. Liebman HA, Furie BC, Tong MJ, et al. Des-gamma-carboxy (abnormal) prothrombin as a serum marker of primary hepatocellular carcinoma. N Engl J Med 1984;310:1427.
20. Weitz IC, Liebman HA. Des-gamma-carboxy (abnormal) prothrombin and hepatocellular carcinoma: a critical review. Hepatology 1993;18:990.
21. Takahashi H, Saiabara T, Iwamura S, et al. Serum alpha-L-fucosidase activity and tumor size in hepatocellular carcinoma. Hepatology 1994;19:1414.
22. Tsai FJ, Jeng JE, Chuang LY, et al. Clinical evaluation of urinary transforming growth factor-beta1 and serum alpha-fetoprotein as tumor markers of hepatocellular carcinoma. Br J Cancer 1997;75:1460.
23. Kew MC, Wolf P, Whittaker D, et al. Tumor associated isoenzymes of gamma-glutamyl transferase in the serum of patients with hepatocellular carcinoma. Br J Cancer 1984; 50:451.
24. Hamazaki K, Gochi A, Shimamura H, et al. Serum levels of circulating intercellular adhesion molecule 1 in hepatocellular carcinoma. Hepatogastroenterology 1996;43:229.
25. Fung KTT, Li FTW, Raimondo ML, et al. Systematic review of radiological imaging for hepatocellular carcinoma in cirrhotic patients. Br J Radiol 2004;77:633–40.
26. Yu SCH, Yeung DTK, So NMC. Imaging features of hepatocellular carcinoma. Clin Radiol 2004;59:145–56.
27. Dodd GD, Miller WJ, Barol RL, et al. Detection of malignant tumors in end-stage cirrhotic livers: efficacy of sonogra-

phy as a screening technique. AJR Am J Roentgenol 1992;159:727.

28. Takayasu K, Moriyama N, Muramatsu Y, et al. The diagnosis of small hepatocellular carcinomas: efficacy of various imaging procedures in 100 patients. AJR Am J Roentgenol 1990;155:49–54.

29. Larcos G, Sorokopud H, Berry G, et al. Sonographic screening for hepatocellular carcinoma in patients with chronic hepatitis or cirrhosis: an evaluation. AJR Am J Roentgenol 1998;171:433.

30. Sherman M, Peltekian KM, Lee C. Screening for hepatocellular carcinoma in a North American urban population. Hepatology 1995;22:432.

31. Choi BI. The current status of imaging diagnosis of hepatocellular carcinoma. Liver Transpl 2004;10:S20–5.

32. Kamel IR, Bluemke DA. Imaging evaluation of hepatocellular carcinoma J Vasc Intervent Radiol 2002; 13(9 part 2): S173–83.

33. Choi BI, Kim AY, Lee JY, et al. Hepatocellular carcinoma contrast enhancement with Levovist. J Ultrasound Med 2002;21:77–84.

34. Francanzani AL, Burdick L, Borzio M, et al. Contrast-enhanced Doppler ultrasonography in the diagnosis of hepatocellular carcinoma and premalignant lesions in patients with cirrhosis. Hepatology 2001;34:1109–27.

35. Sheu JC, Sung JL, Chen DS, et al. Growth rate of asymptomatic hepatocellular carcinoma and its clinical implications. Gastroenterology 1985;89:259–66.

36. Colombo M. Screening for cancer in viral hepatitis. Clin Liver Dis 2001;5:109–22.

37. Izzo F, Cremona F, Ruffolo F, et al. Outcome of 67 patients with hepatocellular cancer detected during screening of 1125 patients with chronic hepatitis. Ann Surg 1998;277: 513–8.

38. Hu H, He HD, Foley WD, et al. Four multidetector-row helical CT: image quality and volume coverage speed. Radiology 2000;215:55–62.

39. Lim JH, Choi D, Kim SH, et al. Detection of hepatocellular carcinoma: value of adding delayed phase imaging to dual-phase helical CT. AJR Am J Roentgenol 2002;179:67.

40. Kopp AF, Heuschmid M, Claussen CD. Multidetector helical CT of the liver for tumor detection and characterization. Eur Radiol 2002;12:745–52.

41. Murakami T, Kim T, Takahasi S, et al. Hepatocellular carcinoma: multidetector row helical CT. Abdom Imaging 2002;27:139–46.

42. Miller WJ, Baron RL, Dodd GD, et al. Malignancies in patients with cirrhosis: CT sensitivity and specificity in 200 consecutive transplant patients. Radiology 1994; 193:645.

43. Laghi A, Iannaccone R, Rossi P, et al. Hepatocellular carcinoma: detection with triple-phase multi-detector row helical CT in patients with chronic hepatitis. Radiology 2003; 226:543–9.

44. Ngan H. Lipiodol computerized tomography: how sensitive and specific is the technique in the diagnosis of hepatocellular carcinoma? Br J Radiol 1990;63:771.

45. Szklaruk J, Silverman PM, Charnsangavej C. Imaging in the diagnosis, staging, treatment and surveillance of hepatocellular carcinoma. AJR Am J Roentgenol 2003;180:441.

46. Burrel M, Llovet JM, Ayuso C, et al. MRI angiography is superior to helical CT for detection of HCC prior to liver transplantation: an explant correlation. Hepatology 2003; 38:1034.

47. Yu JS, Kim MJ. Hepatocellular carcinoma: contrast-enhanced MRI. Abdom Imaging 2002;27:157–67.

48. Libbrect L, Bielen D, Verslype C, et al. Focal lesions in cirrhotic explant livers: pathological evaluation and accuracy of pretransplantation imaging examinations. Liver Transpl 2002;8:749.

49. Ito K, Fujita T, Shimizu A, et al. Multiarterial phase dynamic MRI of small early enhancing hepatic lesions in cirrhosis or chronic hepatitis: differentiating between hypervascular hepatocellular carcinomas and pseudolesions. AJR Am J Roentgenol 2004;183:699–705.

50. Liangpunsakul S, Agarwal D, Horlander JC, et al. Positron emission tomography for detecting occult hepatocellular carcinoma in hepatitis C cirrhotics awaiting for liver transplantation. Transplant Proc 2003;35:2995–7.

51. Khan MA, Combs CS, Brunt EM, et al. Positron emission tomography scanning in the evaluation of hepatocellular carcinoma. J Hepatol 2000;32:792–7.

52. Gharib AM, Thomasson D, Li KC. Molecular imaging of hepatocellular carcinoma. Gastroenterology 2004; 127(5 Suppl 1):S153–8.

53. Sugiyama M, Sakahara H, Torizuka T, et al. 18F-FDG PET in the detection of extrahepatic metastases from hepatocellular carcinoma. J Gastroenterol 2004;39:961–8.

54. Caturelli E, Solmi L, Anti M, et al. Ultrasound guided fine needle biopsy of early hepatocellular carcinoma complicating liver cirrhosis: a multicentre study. Gut 2004;53:1356–62.

55. Bret PM, Labadie M, Bretagnolle M, et al. Hepatocellular carcinoma: diagnosis by percutaneous fine needle biopsy. Gastrointest Radiol 1988;13:253–5.

56. Durand F, Regimbeau JM, Belghiti J, et al. Assessment of the benefits and risks of percutaneous biopsy before surgical resection of hepatocellular carcinoma. J Hepatol 2001;35: 254–8.

57. Takamori R, Wong LL, Dang C, et al. Needle-tract implantation from hepatocellular cancer: is needle biopsy of the liver always necessary? Liver Transpl 2000;6:67–72.

58. Kang JY, Lee TP, Yap I, Lun KC. Analysis of cost-effectiveness of different strategies for hepatocellular carcinoma screening in hepatitis B virus carriers. J Gastroenterol Hepatol 1992;7:463–8.

59. Lin OS, Keeffe EB, Sanders GD, et al. Cost-effectiveness of screening for hepatocellular carcinoma with cirrhosis due to chronic hepatitis C. Aliment Pharmacol Ther 2004;19: 1159–72.

60. Sarasin FP, Giostra E, Hadengue A. Cost-effeciveness of sceening for detection of small hepatocellular carcinoma in western patients with Child-Pugh class A cirrhosis. Am J Med 1996;101:422–34.

61. Everson GT. Increasing incidence and pretransplantation screening of hepatocellular carcinoma. Liver Transpl 2000;6 Suppl 2):S2–10.

62. Yuen MF, Cheng CC, Lauder IJ, et al. Early detection of hepatocellular carcinoma increases the chance of treatment: Hong Kong experience. Hepatology 2000;31:330–5.

63. Lok AS, McMahon BJ. AASLD practice guidelines: chronic hepatitis B. Hepatology 2001;34:1225–41.

64. Strader DB, Wright T, Thomas DL, et al. AASLD practice guideline. Diagnosis, management and treatment of hepatitis C. Hepatology 2004;39:1147–71.

16

Hepatocellular Cancer: Diagnosis and Management

KENNETH HIRSCH

Hepatocellular carcinoma (HCC) is a primary cancer of the liver that is frequently associated with the presence of cirrhosis. It is an important worldwide cause of cancer morbidity and mortality. HCC is the fifth most common solid malignancy and the fourth leading cause of cancer-related death worldwide.[1] In 1990, there were 437,000 new cases of HCC globally and 427,000 deaths attributable to HCC. Historically, HCC has primarily been a health issue of the developing world, and 80% of new cases occur in sub-Saharan Africa and Southeast Asia even today. However, over the last several decades, the incidence has been markedly increasing in economically advantaged countries such as Japan, the United States, and those of Western Europe.[2] The incidence of HCC doubled in the United States between 1975 and 1995, and it continued to increase through 1998.[3] It is predicted that approximately 18,000 new cases of HCC will occur in the United States in 2005.[4]

Most cases of HCC occur in patients infected with hepatitis B virus (HBV) or hepatitis C virus (HCV). It is estimated that worldwide, approximately 60% of HCC cases are etiologically related to HBV infection and approximately 25% are related to HCV infection.[5] The variation in the international distribution of HBV and HCV infection largely explains the geographic heterogeneity of HCC prevalence. The high rates of HCC in Africa and Asia are at least partly due to the endemic presence of HBV in these areas. Increases in HCC rates in North America and Western Europe over the past two decades have largely been attributed to increases

in the prevalence of HCV infection.[6] In Japan, the incidence of HCC has doubled in the last decade, and HCC is the third leading cause of cancer death in that country.[7] Of interest, despite the fact that the prevalence of HCV infection is comparable in Japan and the United States, the incidence of HCC is eight times higher in Japan. Because of the long period from initial infection with HCV to manifestation of HCC, it is postulated that this observed difference represents a lead-time bias caused by an earlier spread of HCV infection in Japan. If this is true, the United States can reasonably anticipate further substantial increases in HCC cases as the HCV-positive population continues to age.[8]

NATURAL HISTORY

HCC occurs almost exclusively in the context of chronic liver disease. The majority of cases develop in patients with preexisting cirrhosis[9]; the most common exceptions to this rule are noncirrhotic patients with HBV infection. Cirrhosis is a final common pathway for most chronic liver diseases whether viral (HBV, HCV), metabolic (hemachromatosis, fatty liver disease), toxic (alcoholic liver disease), or autoimmune. In cirrhosis, the liver becomes diffusely fibrotic because of the long-standing inflammation of chronic hepatitis (Figure 16–1). The normal hepatic architecture is replaced by fibrous septa that circumscribe nodules of regenerating hepatocytes. Thus, the normally continuous and compliant hepatic parenchyma is transformed

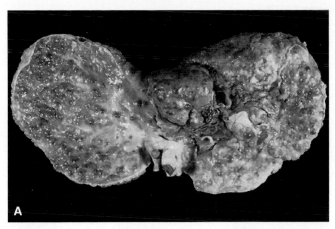
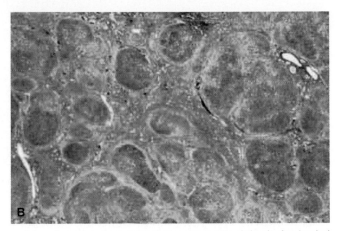

Figure 16–1. Macronodular cirrhosis. *A,* Photograph showing irregular nodules of varying sizes, typical of postnecrotic cirrhosis due to viral hepatitis. *B,* High-power photomicrograph showing regenerative nodules of hepatocytes surrounded by fibrous septa. (Hematoxylin-eosin; ×100 original magnification)

into a more rigid and segregated aggregate of regenerative nodules. The functional consequences of cirrhosis are the result of altered blood flow through the hepatic parenchyma, caused by progressive fibrosis and progressively decreasing viable hepatocyte mass. In cirrhosis, the fibrous septa interrupt the normal flow of blood through the hepatic sinusoids and lead to the development of shunts from the portal triads to the central veins. This shunting leads to poor perfusion of hepatocytes and resultant progressive hepatic dysfunction (Table 16–1). Furthermore, the shunts have a lower capacitance than the native hepatic vasculature has, and the regenerative nodules tend to impinge on the hepatic veins. This results in portal hypertension and its associated complications, including gastroesophageal varices, splenomegaly, and ascites (Figure 16–2).

Consequently, patients with cirrhosis tend to be demonstrably ill from the premalignant condition well in advance of actual oncogenesis. Thus, in contrast to other malignancies such as colon or prostate cancer, the clinical outcome of a patient with a hepatoma is strongly influenced not only by tumor stage but also by the degree of hepatic impairment.

In the current era of pervasive HCC screening of high-risk patients and increasingly effective curative therapies for early disease, it is difficult to define the untreated natural history of early HCC. The most optimistic outcome for patients with untreated single tumors and Child A cirrhosis has been reported as 65% survival at 3 years.[10] This contrasts with the 1- and 2-year survival rates (derived from the con-

trol arms of multiple randomized controlled trials) of 10 to 72% and 8 to 50%, respectively, for patients with advanced HCC.[11]

SCREENING

According to National Cancer Institute guidelines, there are at least two requirements for a useful cancer screening program. First, there must be a test or procedure that will detect the cancer earlier than the cancer will be detected as a result of the development of symptoms. Second, there must be evidence that treatment initiated earlier as a consequence of screening results in an improved outcome. Of course, common sense and economic reality also require that any screening test be safe, minimally invasive, and reasonably inexpensive. Finally, the discriminatory capacity (ie, the positive and negative predictive value) of any screening test is highly dependent on the prevalence of the disease in the screened popula-

Table 16–1. CHILD-PUGH CLASSIFICATION			
	Points*		
	1	2	3
Total bilirubin (mg/dL)	< 2	2–3	>3
Albumin (g/dL)	> 3.5	3.0–3.5	< 3
Ascites	–	+	++
Encephalopathy	–	+	++
Prothrombin time†	< 4 s	4–6 s	> 6 s

*Total points determine Child stage, as follows: Child A < 8 points, Child B = 8–10 points, Child C > 10 points. Prognosis declines as Child-Pugh score increases.
†Seconds prolonged.

tion. All other test characteristics—such as sensitivity and specificity—being equal, the predictive value of a screening test improves as the prevalence of disease in the screened population increases.

Because HCC almost always arises in the context of chronic liver disease and because all curative therapies are applicable only to relatively healthy patients with early-stage disease, screening this high-risk population seems logical. Because of this compelling line of reasoning, HCC screening of patients with cirrhosis has become the standard of care among hepatologists worldwide. However, no proven survival benefit of any screening program has been found in a large randomized trial. To answer the question of whether periodic screening is effective at detecting HCC at an early stage and prolongs survival, a randomized controlled trial with many thousands of high-risk subjects and a follow-up period of a decade would be necessary. The long period of follow-up would be necessary to eliminate the lead-time bias that would be introduced by early detection in the screened group. Unfortunately, the ubiquity of HCC screening in standard clinical practice and the enormous expense and technical difficulty of performing such a trial essentially preclude the possibility of such a randomized trial ever being undertaken.[12]

Despite the absence of incontrovertible evidence of utility, the current standard of care in HCC screening relies on the long-standing practices of periodic measurements of serum alpha fetoprotein (AFP) and/or liver ultrasonography. First described in 1956, AFP is a fetal glycoprotein produced by the yolk sac and the fetal liver. Serum levels of AFP fall to < 10 ng/mL soon after birth, but there are a number of diseases that can lead to elevated AFP levels in adults; these diseases include germ cell tumors, active hepatitis, cirrhosis, and HCC. Many different forms of chronic liver disease can lead to transitory, intermittent, or persistent elevations of serum AFP, and this has substantial implications for this test's usefulness as a screening modality. Used alone as an HCC screening test, AFP measurement has a sensitivity of 39 to 64%, a specificity of 76 to 91%, and a positive predictive value of 9 to 32%, depending on the screened population.[13] These test characteristics can be somewhat optimized by adjusting the level of AFP considered to be abnormal, but even

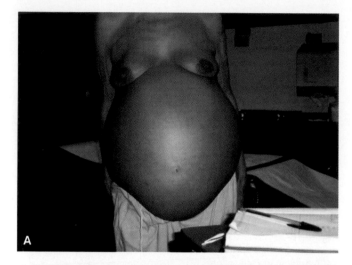

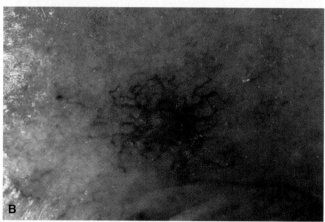

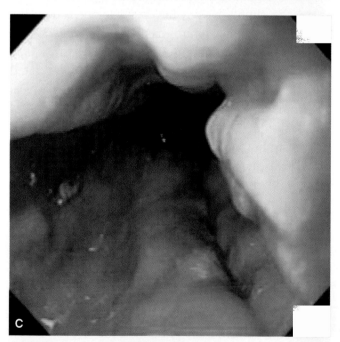

Figure 16–2. Clinical manifestations of cirrhosis. *A*, A male patient with massive ascites and gynecomastia. *B*, Spider angioma, a dermatologic manifestation of the elevated estrogens in cirrhotic patients. *C*, Endoscopic view of esophageal varices.

with such manipulation, the sensitivity of AFP measurement does not substantially exceed 50%.[14] Additionally, the test characteristics of AFP measurement in African Americans have been shown to be even poorer than those of AFP measurement in a Caucasian population, and this casts further aspersions upon its usefulness as a screening tool.

The test characteristics of hepatic ultrasonography as an independent screening test differ throughout the literature. The sensitivity of ultrasonography for the detection of HCC varies between 11% and 99%, with a specificity of 95 to 100%.[15] This wide variation is due to the subjectivity of ultrasonographic interpretation, to interobserver variability, and to the heterogeneity of definitions of "true" cases. This last limitation was addressed in a 2001 study from San Francisco in which different imaging techniques were compared against pathologic findings in explanted livers.[16] The authors demonstrated a sensitivity of 79.4% for ultrasonography, but detection of satellite lesions was poor, with a sensitivity of between 27% and 43%.

A report of a large randomized controlled trial that examined HCC screening in 17,920 hepatitis B surface antigen (HBsAg)–positive patients was published in 1997.[17] In this study, 8,109 patients were assigned to be screened with AFP and liver ultrasonography every 6 months, and 9,711 patients were randomized to no screening. During a mean follow-up of 1.2 years, 38 persons with HCC were identified in the screening group and 18 HCC cases were found in the control group. Of the HCC patients in the screening group, 77% were asymptomatic at the time of diagnosis, and 71% of those patients underwent surgical resection of their tumors. All patients in the control arm were symptomatic at the time of diagnosis, and none of their tumors were amenable to surgical resection. The 1- and 2-year survival rates of patients who underwent resection were 88% and 78%, respectively, compared with no survival in the HCC-positive patients in the control group. However, because of the short follow-up period, lead-time bias compromises the statistical interpretation of the survival results. Despite that necessary interpretive caveat, this study does appear to support the usefulness of AFP measurement and ultrasonographic screening in the high-risk population of HBsAg-positive patients.

In a cohort study, 1,487 HBsAg-positive patients from Alaska were observed while undergoing routine AFP and ultrasonographic testing for 16 years.[18] This investigation demonstrated detection of HCC at a surgically resectable stage in 83% of cases. Furthermore, an improvement in 5- and 10-year tumor-free survival among screened patients was shown when compared to historical controls. Although these data were not derived in the context of a randomized controlled trial and involved relatively few patients, they nonetheless further bolster the argument in favor of screening and provide further evidence of the survival benefit of screening.

DIAGNOSIS

Role of Imaging Modalities

Unlike diagnosis of most other forms of cancer, diagnosis of HCC does not necessarily require histologic confirmation. HCC develops in approximately 4% of cirrhotic patients each year,[19] so new focal lesions in cirrhotic livers that have typical imaging characteristics have a high probability of being HCCs. Therefore, noninvasive criteria for the diagnosis of HCC in cirrhotic patients were proposed during a European Association for the Study of the Liver (EASL) conference on HCC in 2000.[12] The EASL criteria include the presence of a focal lesion of > 2 cm with characteristic arterial enhancement as seen by two different imaging modalities or by a single imaging modality but with an AFP level > 400 ng/mL. The application of these criteria obviates the need to perform a biopsy on many lesions, thus accelerating access to therapy and eliminating the risk of tumor seeding of a biopsy tract.[20]

Increased use of surveillance programs in high-risk cirrhotic patients has led to the increased detection of focal liver lesions < 2 cm in diameter.[21] Unfortunately, the noninvasive EASL criteria are not applicable to the diagnosis of lesions of < 2 cm, and these are potentially the earliest lesions that would be expected to be most amenable to curative therapy. For example, investigators in a recent Italian study found that application of the EASL criteria alone would have missed HCC in 38% of their cases.[22] In such cases, liver biopsy is typically indicated. However, depending on the method used to obtain the biopsy specimen (radiographically guided percutaneous needle biopsy versus a laparoscopic or open surgical approach) and the experience of the interpreting pathologist, there may be false-negative results for up to 40% of small nodules.[20] A Japanese study compared magnetic resonance imaging (MRI), digital subtraction angiography, and ultrasonography (US)-guided biopsy for the diagnosis of 180 HCC nodules with a diameter of < 2 cm.[23] This investigation demonstrated that only 68% of lesions measuring 1.1 to 2 cm in diameter and only 45% of lesions of < 1 cm in diameter could be diagnosed by imaging methods alone whereas the balance required biopsy for proper identification. Conversely, there are substantial morbidities and mortality risks associated with a false-positive diagnosis of HCC as well. In a study of 160 HCC patients, 2.5% were misdiagnosed when only radiographic criteria were used, and those patients ultimately underwent surgery for nonmalignant lesions.[24]

Role of Liver Biopsy

A biopsy of a hepatoma may be performed by several different approaches. Frequently, a needle biopsy is performed under ultrasonographic or computed tomography (CT) guidance. In some cases, however, a percutaneous approach is not feasible owing to a disadvantageous anatomy or an absence of local expertise. A laparoscopic approach is another option, but it is frequently limited by the fact that HCC often develops deep within a cirrhotic liver, making it difficult to visualize from the surface. If those other less invasive approaches are inapplicable, then laparotomy may be required to accurately identify and perform a biopsy of a mass within the liver.

There are several significant risks associated with any attempt to obtain a tissue sample of an HCC. First, the risk of bleeding from a biopsy of a hepatoma is significantly higher than that from a biopsy of nonmalignant liver tissue.[25] This is due to the hypervascular nature of these tumors. Another risk of biopsy is the possibility of tumor seeding. There have been numerous reported cases of this occurring in the context of needle biopsies.[26,27]

Many authors consider this to be rare phenomenon (incidence of < 0.01%)[28,29] although several small published series have reported rates of seeding as high as 1.6 to 5%.[30,31] Neither the exact frequency with which this serious complication occurs nor the context in which it is more likely to occur are clearly understood. A number of other rare but serious potential complications are associated with liver biopsy, including sepsis, pancreatitis, local infections, pneumothorax, and shock. Given these possible adverse outcomes, it is vital that liver biopsy be used in a judicious manner to minimize the patient's exposure to excess morbidity and mortality.

PATHOLOGY

There are three major anatomic pathologic patterns of HCC development: expanding, infiltrating, and multifocal (Figures 16–3 and 16–4). The expanding pattern is characterized by a solitary and frequently large mass that compresses and displaces the surrounding hepatic parenchyma. Expanding HCC may or may not be encapsulated. Infiltrating HCC is defined by the absence of distinct margins between neoplastic and non-neoplastic tissues; this type causes significantly less compression of the neighboring liver tissue. Multifocal HCC is present when several discrete tumor foci are present.

Macroscopically, an HCC may be homogeneous or may have necrotic, hemorrhagic, or fibrotic areas. Vascular invasion of portal and hepatic veins is com-

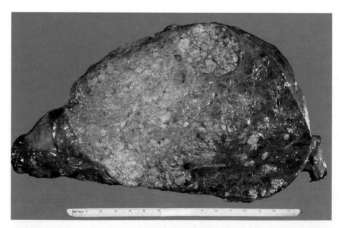

Figure 16–3. Gross pathology specimen of cirrhotic liver with a massive expansive hepatocellular carcinoma. The tumor has a visible fibrous capsule; also, note the presence of numerous satellite lesions.

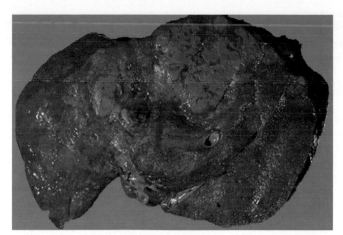

Figure 16–4. Gross pathology specimen of a cirrhotic liver with an infiltrative irregularly shaped hepatocellular carcinoma (yellow/beige area). Tumor margins are indistinct and appear to interdigitate with cirrhotic parenchyma.

mon. Microscopically, the cells of HCC frequently resemble normal liver cells, and it can therefore be very difficult to differentiate malignant HCC cells from normal hepatocytes (Figure 16–5).

Pathologic diagnosis of HCC may not be straightforward. As with most malignancies, HCC has a wide spectrum of possible histologic features ranging from well-differentiated to poorly differentiated forms. In a situation analogous to what has occurred with HCC staging (described below), the precursor lesions and the histologic features of HCC have been defined in a variety of ways by different authors. For example, the apparently same precursor lesions have been described as macroregenerative nodules types 1 and 2, ordinary adenomatous hyperplasia, atypical adenomatous hyperplasia, very well-differentiated HCC, and dysplastic nodules. In an effort to consolidate nomenclature and clarify definitions, the International Working Party (IWP) of the World Congresses of Gastroenterology proposed a system in which all presumably premalignant histologies were consolidated under the categories of low-grade and high-grade dysplastic nodules.[32] The IWP described 16 distinct histologic features and categorized lesions as nondysplastic regenerative nodules, regenerative nodules, or HCCs, according to the number of characteristics present (Table 16–2).

Unfortunately, although these definitions facilitated improved communication regarding HCC specimens, there remained substantial variation in rendered diagnoses when these criteria were applied to a collection of representative samples by a consensus group of 18 international expert hepatopathologists.[33] This led to the convening of the International Consensus Group for Hepatic Neoplasia, which proposed a new set of criteria for the description of HCCs, known as the Laennec classification of hepatocellular neoplasia. This system defines three criteria: nuclear atypia, nucleus-to-cytoplasmic ratio, and architectural atypia. Each of these components is assigned a numeric score based on comparison with a set of standards for each parameter. The individual scores are then summed, which produces the Laennec score. There are a number of features of this system that appear to offer improvements over previous iterations of pathologic HCC descriptions. However, the practical utility and reproducibility of this classification remain to be proven in clinical studies.

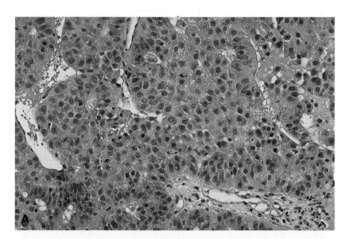

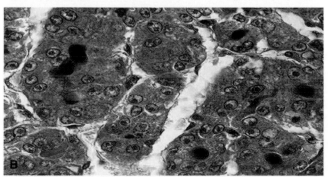

Figure 16–5. Photomicrographs of hepatocellular carcinoma (HCC). *A*, Tumor composed of liver cords that are much wider than the normal two-cell-thick liver plate. There is no discernable normal lobular architecture. *B*, Malignant cells with some nuclear atypia. Dark pigment is intracellular bile, which indicates that this is a well-differentiated HCC. (Hemotoxylin-eosin; ×100 original magnification)

Table 16–2. INTERNATIONAL WORKING PARTY CRITERIA FOR DIAGNOSIS OF HEPATIC NEOPLASIA: DELINEATION OF HISTOLOGIC CHANGES ASSOCIATED WITH HEPATOCARCINOGENESIS

Histologic Feature	Large Regenerative Nodule	Dysplastic Nodule, Low Grade	Dysplastic Nodule, High Grade	Well-Differentiated HCC	Moderately Differentiated HCC
Clone-like population	−	+	+	+	+
Plates > 3 cells wide	−	−	−	−	+
Mitotic figures > 5/10 HPF	−	−	−	−	+
Cell density > 2 × normal	−	−	−	+	+
Invasion of stroma or portal tracts	−	−	−	+	+
Irregular nuclear contour, moderate	−	−	−	+	+
Absence of portal tracts (arterial supply)	−	−	+	+	+
Mitotic figures 1–5/10 HPF	−	−	+	+	+
Cell density > 1.3 × normal	−	−	+	+	+
Nuclear hyperchromasia	−	−	+	+	+
Irregular nuclear contour, mild	−	−	+	+	+
Pseudogland formation	+	−	+	+	+
Cytoplasmic basophilia	−	−	+	+	+
Cytoplasmic clear cell change	−	−	−	−	+
Reticulin less than normal	−	−	−	−	+
Resistance to iron accumulation	−	+	+	+	+

HCC = hepatocellular carcinoma; HPF = high powered field.
Adapted from International Working Party of World Congresses of Gastroenterology.[32]

IMAGING

A variety of imaging technologies can be used in the diagnosis of HCC. The diagnostic resolution of most of these methods relies on both the anatomy altered by the presence of the neoplasm and the skewed vascular supply of these tumors. Normal hepatic parenchyma receives the majority of its blood supply from the portal vein, with only a small contribution from the hepatic artery. HCCs are hypervascular tumors that typically receive most of their blood supply from branches of the hepatic artery. Therefore, imaging modalities that can exploit and enhance these differences between cancerous and noncancerous liver tissues are of enormous value in the diagnosis and surveillance of HCC. Imaging modalities commonly used in the diagnosis of HCC include US, triple-phase CT, and MRI. The choice of a particular diagnostic imaging technology is very much dependent on the availability of local resources and expertise.

Modern advancements in imaging methodology have increased the capacity of clinicians to detect HCC. Simultaneously, it has increased the detection of a large number of pseudolesions (such as aberrantly enhancing cirrhotic nodules) as well as benign tumors (some of which mimic the appearance of HCC).[34] These false-positive imaging diagnoses subject patients to radical morbid therapies for no benefit. Conversely, if HCC is actually present but imaging incorrectly identifies additional liver nodules as suspicious or as diagnostic of multifocal disease, then a patient who is eligible for a curative therapy would be denied that opportunity. These facts emphasize the importance of a clear understanding of the characteristics of HCC as seen by all of the common imaging methodologies and a recognition that there are significant overlaps between the imaging findings of benign lesions and malignant lesions in cirrhotic livers.

Clear assessment of the blood supply in a liver nodule is vital to the proper characterization of the lesion. This is because there are sequential changes to a nodule's feeding vessels and blood flow as hepatocarcinogenesis occurs. Regenerative nodules and low-grade dysplastic nodules are typically fed by normal portal veins and hepatic arteries. As a dysplastic nodule becomes increasingly high grade, it loses the normal portal vascular architecture and begins to develop neovascular branches from the hepatic artery. By the time a lesion has become a high-grade HCC, it is essentially exclusively fed by those abnormal arteries, and normal portal tracts are almost completely absent. Confusion can arise when distinguishing between a high-grade dysplastic nodule and a well-differentiated HCC. Both of these conditions demonstrate some increased arterial neovascularization and diminution in normal portal vascular supply, but there is no characteristic vascular signature that differentiates these neighbors on the hepatocarcinogenesis continuum.[35]

As HCCs grow in the cirrhotic liver, they typically demonstrate an expansive growth pattern, an infiltrative growth pattern, or a mixture of these two growth patterns. Expansive HCCs are well demarcated on imaging, nodular in appearance, and frequently encapsulated. Infiltrative HCCs are characterized by irregular and indistinct boundaries and are frequently accompanied by vascular invasion. Extrahepatic metastases of HCCs may be found anywhere in the body. Intraperitoneal metastasis is uncommon, occurring only with tumor rupture or external manipulation such as percutaneous biopsy, local ablation, or surgery.[36] With improvements in technology and with the routine use of imaging for HCC screening in high-risk populations, there has been a marked increase in the frequency of the identification of small HCCs.[7] However, despite technologic advancements, it remains difficult and sometimes impossible to definitively characterize small nodules found in a cirrhotic liver.

Ultrasonography

HCC may grow as solitary or multiple discrete nodules, or it may appear as a poorly demarcated infiltrative mass (Figure 16–6). There is not a single characteristic echo texture for HCCs on conventional US. Small tumors without fatty metamorphosis are usually hypoechoic; however, the echo pattern may change as the tumor grows. A hepatoma with an expansive growth pattern is typically seen as a discrete nodule with a heterogenous echo. It may have a thin hypoechoic rim corresponding to its fibrous capsule.[37] An infiltrative HCC is difficult to see clearly on standard gray-scale US, typically appearing as a poorly demarcated area with heterogenous echogenicity. However, this type of tumor is frequently associated with portal vein invasion; therefore, color Doppler ultrasonographic evaluation of the portal vasculature is a critical component of

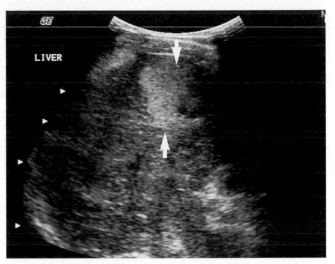

Figure 16–6. Standard gray-scale ultrasonographic image of a right hepatic lobe, showing a 4.5 × 2.0 cm mass of mixed echogenicity (*arrows*).

any ultrasonographic evaluation concerned with the diagnosis of HCC (Figure 16–7). Additionally, Doppler US can be used to demonstrate the presence of arterial hypervascularity within the mass and the typical morphology of intratumoral and peritumoral vessels (known as a "basket" pattern).[38]

Although US has traditionally played an important role in screening for HCC, the limited capacity of conventional US to define the vascular characteristics of a lesion limits its usefulness in establishing a diagnosis. There are a number of centers that are attempting to enhance the diagnostic capabilities of US with the use of a variety of contrast agents, and some of these agents are available for clinical use overseas. However, these technologies are not cur-

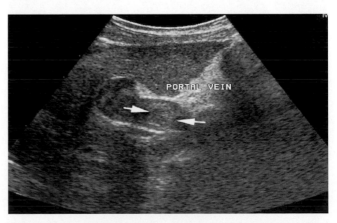

Figure 16–7. Harmonic ultrasonographic image demonstrating low-level echoes within a dilated portal vein. This finding is highly suggestive of the presence of a tumor thrombus.

rently available in the United States, and they have not been studied as extensively as have the more established techniques.

Computed Tomography

Multiphasic CT has become the most common imaging modality used for both diagnosis and management of HCC. With typical triple-phase CT, liver images are obtained from precontrast arterial and portal venous phases by using intravenous contrast agents combined with rapid multislice scanning (Figure 16–8). HCC lesions usually demonstrate hyperdense enhancement in the arterial phase, followed by rapid washout of contrast in the portal venous phase, leaving them hypoattenuated as compared with the surrounding contrast-enhanced hepatic parenchyma.[39] In the context of cirrhosis, the presence of a hypervascular mass during the arterial phase of CT scanning is highly predictive of the presence of HCC.[40] The portal venous phase is useful for detecting small hypovascular local metastases; these can be overlooked during the arterial phase because of the lack of hepatic parenchymal enhancement. In the portal venous phase, the nonneoplastic liver tissue takes up contrast, becoming hyperdense, while the tumor's contrast (acquired during the arterial phase) washes out, making the tumor iso- or hypodense. Hypovascular small tumors will also appear iso- or hypodense during this phase, but their identification is facilitated by the enhancement of the surrounding hepatic parenchyma. In addition to identifying the presence and number of HCCs present, CT can provide additional information in regard to overall prognosis and treatment eligibility. For example, CT can provide information on the feasibility of tumor resection, the presence of portal hypertension, the patency of the surrounding vasculature, and the presence of vascular invasion.[41]

It is difficult to assess accurately the true sensitivity of CT for the diagnosis of HCC because such sensitivity is highly dependent on the size and differentiation of the lesions, the type of machine and protocol used, and the diagnostic standard used to define true cases. In a 1990 Japanese unblinded retrospective study, CT detected 84% of tumors smaller than 3 cm.[42] However, the scanner used was a low-speed low-resolution scanner, and the diagnostic standard in this study was a combination of serum AFP measurements or other imaging studies, which limited the applicability of these results. A small Korean study using modern helical CT equipment demonstrated a sensitivity of 80%, compared to histologic examination of explanted livers. However, sensitivity was 60% for lesions smaller than

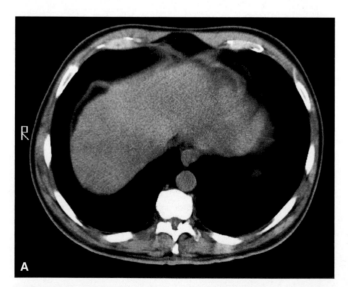
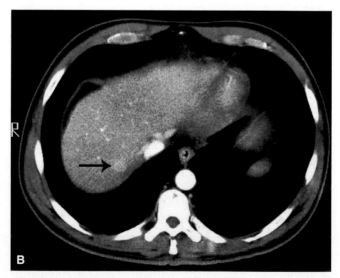

Figure 16–8.   Multiphase contrast computed tomography scans. *A,* Dome of the liver prior to the injection of contrast. *B,* The same area of the liver after the injection of contrast, now highlighting the presence of a 1.5-cm nodule in the right lobe, which enhances preferentially during the arterial phase (*arrow*).

2 cm.[43] A larger study in the United States, involving 430 patients who were undergoing liver transplantation, found triphasic helical CT to have a prospective sensitivity of 59% and a retrospective sensitivity of 68% for the diagnosis of HCC.[44]

Several modifications to CT protocols are available to enhance CT's sensitivity for the detection of hepatomas. In CT portography with CT hepatic angiography, helical CT is performed after the infusion of contrast into the superior mesenteric artery and the hepatic artery via catheters inserted through the femoral artery. A decade ago, this technique was shown to be more sensitive than MRI for detecting multiple lesions in a cirrhotic liver,[45] but modern improvements in imaging technology and the invasive nature of this procedure have led most authors to abandon it as part of the initial diagnostic work-up for HCC.

Lipiodol-CT was also proposed as an improvement over conventional triple-phase CT.[46] Lipiodol is an iodized poppy seed oil that is taken up by hepatocytes but is selectively retained by HCC cells over time. Despite its theoretic attractiveness and despite initial enthusiasm, subsequent pathologic studies found lipiodol-CT to be less sensitive than conventional multiphasic CT.[47]

Magnetic Resonance Imaging

MRI has a number of potential advantages over CT for the diagnosis and management of HCC. These include the absence of ionizing radiation exposure, increased image detail, and an enhanced capacity to differentiate dysplastic nodules from actual HCCs. The appearance of a hepatoma on an MRI image varies depending on the histology of the tumor, the degree of hepatic fibrosis, and even local variations in biochemical composition. For example, on T1-weighted images, advanced HCCs typically demonstrate a hypointense signal whereas well-differentiated HCCs and borderline lesions routinely manifest a hyperintense signal.[48] On T2-weighted images, the presence of hyperintensity in a nodule within a cirrhotic liver is very suggestive of the presence of malignancy. However, a well-differentiated HCC can appear as isointense or hypointense on T2-weighted images as well.[49] If present, the tumor's fibrous capsule is seen as a hypointense rim on both T1- and T2-weighted images.

The variable appearance of HCC on unenhanced MRI scans has prompted the use of contrast agents to distinguish between malignant and benign tissues (Figure 16–9). These agents include standard MRI contrast agents, such as gadolinium, as well as some tissue-specific agents, such as ferumoxide, or superparamagnetic iron oxide (SPIO). SPIO is taken up by Kupffer cells, and it has been shown that the number of Kupffer cells in a liver nodule decreases as the grade of malignancy increases. A small Japanese study demonstrated that SPIO-enhanced MRI is useful for estimating the histologic grade of some HCCs.[50] Multiphasic gadolinium-enhanced T1-weighted imaging yields results similar to those seen with multiphasic contrast-enhanced CT.[51]

The literature varies in regard to the sensitivity of MRI for the detection of HCC. The reasons for this variability are similar to those for the variability in regard to CT. In a study of 34 transplantation patients, MRI was found to have a sensitivity of 74% for lesions larger than 1 cm but only 27% for those smaller than 1 cm.[52] Another small study of transplantation patients found sensitivities of 100% for lesions larger than 2 cm in diameter, 52% for lesions between 1 cm and 2 cm, and 4% for lesions smaller than 1 cm in diameter.[53]

Studies comparing CT and MRI for diagnosis of HCC are limited. One group examined 34 patients

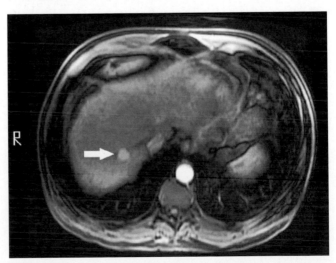

Figure 16–9. Gadolinium-enhanced T1-weighted magnetic resonance imaging scan of the patient of Figure 16–8. The identical 1.5 cm arterially enhancing mass (*arrow*) is seen here as well.

prior to transplantation and found the sensitivities of the two modalities to be similar (50–60%) for the diagnosis of HCC. They did note that MRI was better than helical CT for the diagnosis of dysplastic nodules although its sensitivity for these lesions was nonetheless quite low (27%). Another study compared MRI with magnetic resonance angiography (MRA) to triple-phase CT in 50 cirrhotic patients undergoing liver transplantation.[54] In this investigation, all HCC lesions > 2 cm in diameter were detected by both imaging techniques, but MRI/MRA was superior to helical CT for proper identification of nodules 1 to 2 cm in diameter (89% versus 65%). The published studies are limited by the number of patients studied, the number of sites included, and the state of the technology. In routine clinical care, the choice between multiphasic CT and MRI will be dictated by available equipment and local expertise.

STAGING

Clinical staging of cancers is necessary to assess prognosis and to guide the choice of appropriate therapeutic intervention. There are numerous well-defined and widely applied prognostic staging systems for most solid tumors, including cancers of the breast, colon,[55] and prostate.[56] Application of these staging systems has been useful in the design of surveillance and therapeutic programs. A good staging system (1) is simple and easy to apply in clinical scenarios, (2) is reproducible in various situations, (3) allows for accurate predictions of the disease's natural history, and (4) permits classification of patients into specific treatment groups.

In the case of HCC, determining a prognosis is uniquely complicated and poorly standardized. This is because there are two serious diseases in most patients with HCC: cirrhosis and the cancer. Both of these pathologic processes have numerous incompletely understood variables that influence the prognosis when they occur alone, and the interaction of these variables further complicates the accurate prediction of outcome. Furthermore, the progression of one disease can have a profound impact on the behavior of the other.

The prognostic complexity is evidenced by the fact that there are at least 10 different staging systems that have been developed for HCC. Unlike the situation with most other malignancies, no single system is acknowledged as the "gold standard." The sometimes competing and sometimes complementary systems have been explored and debated extensively in the literature, but the fact remains that there is no ideal system for classifying the clinical behavior of HCC. One obstacle to standardization is the confusion regarding the diagnostic criteria for HCC. Some authors rely on noninvasive criteria[57] whereas others use pretreatment histologic confirmation, postsurgical pathologic evaluation, or a combination of these. Unfortunately, even histologic diagnosis of HCC is a potentially gray area. Up to 40% of biopsies of small nodules return a false-negative result.[20] Furthermore, as already noted, there can be disagreement on the pathologic definition of HCC; the same small lesion may be termed a well-differentiated HCC in Japan whereas American pathologists may define it as a regenerative nodule.[58] Other impediments to a standardized universally applicable staging system for HCC include variations in the severity of underlying liver disease, heterogeneity in the availability or effectiveness of therapy, and a lack of standardization of the tests required to determine tumor burden and extent of disease.

The HCC staging systems described below were developed with different patient populations, inclusion criteria, pathologic tumor characteristics, and available therapies. Therefore, side-by-side comparisons of many of these systems are impractical and inappropriate. Furthermore, some of the systems described are applicable only to patients in particular clinical situations, such as after resection[59,60] or after liver transplantation.[61]

Tumor-Node-Metastasis Staging System

The tumor-node-metastasis (TNM) classification of the anatomic extent of malignant disease was initially proposed in the 1940s and was subsequently developed by L'Union Internationale Contre le Cancer (UICC). This system classifies cancers according to the depth of the primary tumor (T), the presence of lymph node spread (N), and/or the presence of distant metastasis (M). These various independent criteria are then aggregated into a stage assignation between I and IV. The American Joint Committee on Cancer (AJCC)/UICC staging system for HCC was proposed in 1988 (Table 16–3). It uses a TNM classification system to predict patient survival following resection of HCC.[62] When used alone, this system is of limited value for evaluating HCC patients because it does not address underlying liver function, nor does it predict recurrence or survival. Furthermore, some commentators felt that the T classification (based on the number and location of tumor nodules, the size of the largest nodule, and the presence of vascular or adjacent organ invasion) was unwieldy.

Vauthey Modification

A retrospective multicenter study of 557 patients who underwent resection of HCC evaluated the ability of the AJCC/UICC staging system to stratify patients with regard to survival.[59] The independent predictors of survival identified in this study included the presence of major vascular invasion, microvascular invasion, advanced fibrosis in the adjacent liver, and multiple tumors or tumors larger than 5 cm. These independent survival predictors were used to construct a simplified T classification and a revised staging system. The simplified T classification categorized cases of single tumors and no vascular invasion as sT1. Those with single tumors with microvascular invasion or multiple tumors (none > 5 cm) were classified as sT2, and cases of tumors manifesting major vascular invasion were classified as sT3. This Vauthey modification of the AJCC/UICC system also considered the effect of

fibrosis stage on survival. Patients were segregated into two groups, those with advanced fibrosis or cirrhosis and those without. Members of the former group had increased mortality in all TNM stages. One major deficiency of the Vauthey staging system is its use of microvascular invasion as a stratification criterion. That this phenomenon can only be identified on pathologic specimens limits the applicability of this system to only those patients undergoing surgical resection.

Izumi Modification

An alternative modification to the TNM system was proposed by Izumi and colleagues.[60] This system was developed from a retrospective study of 104 patients undergoing surgical resection of HCC, and the main end points were overall survival and disease-free survival. This study found that the standard TNM system was unable to provide prognostic resolution between stages I and II or between stages III and IVA. The authors therefore proposed a modified staging classification that applied a number of clinicopathologic findings such as portal vein invasion. The capability of the Izumi modified system to predict differences in survival between stages was confirmed in several studies.[63,64]

Okuda Staging System

The first HCC staging system to integrate both tumor characteristics and clinical measurements of hepatic dysfunction was published in 1985 by Okuda and colleagues.[65] Based on a retrospective review of 850 patients, the scheme classifies cases on the basis of tumor size, serum bilirubin, serum albumin, and the presence or absence of ascites; it then groups them into three stages (Table 16–4). This system has demonstrable prognostic capability for patients with HCC and advanced cirrhosis, but that is probably mostly explained by the high mortality associated with advanced cirrhosis alone. The Okuda system has limited capacity to stratify asymptomatic HCC patients, and it is further limited by its inability to account for other significant tumor characteristics, such as vascular invasion or metastasis.

Table 16–3. TUMOR-NODE-METASTASIS CLASSIFICATION FOR HEPATOCELLULAR CARCINOMA, 2002

Stage	Tumor*	Node	Metastasis
I	T1	N0	M0
II	T2	N0	M0
IIIA	T3	N0	M0
IIIB	T4	N0	M0
IIIC	Any T	N1	M0
IV	Any T	Any N	M1

*T definitions: T1, solitary tumor without vascular invasion; T2, solitary tumor with vascular invasion or multinodular (< 5 cm); T3: multinodular (> 5 cm) or tumor with major vascular invasion; T4: tumor with invasion of adjacent organs.

Table 16–4. OKUDA STAGING SYSTEM*		
	Score	
Parameter	0	1
Bilirubin (mg/dL)	< 3	> 3
Albumin (g/dL)	> 3	< 3
Ascites	Absent	Present
Tumor size	< 50% of liver	> 50% of liver

*Staging is by score, as follows: stage I = 0, stage II = 1–2, stage III = 3–4.

Cancer of the Liver Italian Program Score

As previously described, HCC is a cancer that typically occurs in a host who is compromised by varying degrees of hepatic dysfunction. The Cancer of the Liver Italian Program (CLIP) score was designed to surmount the deficiencies of the various TNM-based systems by integrating a number of clinical parameters with tumor morphology in an effort to produce a staging system with greater sensitivity and discriminatory capability than prior staging systems had shown.[66] This classification schema was based on a retrospective analysis of 435 patients, only 2.8% of whom underwent surgical therapy for their HCCs. The CLIP score includes a description of tumor morphology, Child-Pugh classification, serum AFP level, and the presence or absence of portal vein thrombosis (Table 16–5). The point values for each variable are summed, and this produces the CLIP score. Higher scores are associated with decreased median survival rates (Table 16–6).

Table 16–5. CANCER OF THE LIVER ITALIAN PROGRAM SCORING SYSTEM	
Parameter	Score
Child-Pugh class	
A	0
B	1
C	2
Tumor morphology	
Uninodular and ≤ 50% extension	0
Multinodular and ≥ 50% extension	1
Massive or ≥ 50% extension	2
Alpha fetoprotein (ng/dL)	
< 400	0
≥ 400	1
Portal vein thrombosis	
No	0
Yes	1

Subsequent prospective validation of the CLIP score demonstrated that this system had greater power to predict survival than the earlier Okuda system had.[67] In that study, survival rates at 1 and 5 years, respectively, were 84% and 65% for patients with a CLIP score of 0; 66% and 45% for those with a score of 1; 45% and 17% for those with a score of 2; 36% and 12% for those with a score of 3; and 9% and 0% for those with a score of 4 to 6. The improved capacity of the CLIP score to stratify patients and predict survival has been confirmed in a number of other studies from numerous international sites. The utility of the CLIP score has been demonstrated in patient populations undergoing both surgical and conservative therapy,[68] transarterial chemoembolization,[69] and surgical resection for early disease.[70]

The CLIP score has clear advantages over its predecessors, including improved predictive capacity and applicability to a more diverse group of patients receiving a variety of therapeutic interventions, but there are some notable limitations. First, the tumor morphology described in the best prognostic group (single nodule and tumor extent < 50% of liver) actually describes a potentially heterogeneous group with very different tumor characteristics. For example, included in this group would be a patient with a malignancy of < 1 cm found at resection as well as a patient with a 6-cm irregularly bordered malignancy. This heterogeneity limits the ability of the CLIP score to accurately determine outcomes in the best-prognosis category. Second, the majority of cases in these studies were classified with CLIP scores of 0 to 2. This suggests that the system lacks stratification capability. Also highlighting this weak stratification capability is Cillo and colleagues' finding of overlapping survival

Table 16–6. STRATIFICATION OF SURVIVAL, BASED ON CANCER OF THE LIVER ITALIAN PROGRAM SCORE	
CLIP Score	Median Survival (mo)
0	42.5
1	32.0
2	16.5
3	4.5
4	2.5
5, 6	1.0

CLIP = Cancer of the Liver Italian Program.

curves for patients with CLIP scores of 2 and 3.[71] Finally, the CLIP score is unable to discriminate survival differences in patients with advanced disease (CLIP scores 4–6).

Japan Integrated Staging

Japan Integrated Staging (JIS) is another system that both modifies the pathologic classifications of the TNM system and further integrates clinical parameters in an attempt to enhance prognostic capacity.[72] The modified Japanese TNM system identifies three tumor characteristics that constitute the basis of T grading: single tumor, tumor size < 2 cm, and lack of vascular involvement. The fewer of these criteria that are satisfied, the higher the T grade that is assigned (Table 16–7). The JIS score is calculated by adding points for modified TNM staging to points assigned for Child-Pugh stage (Table 16–8). The authors of the JIS system analyzed 722 consecutive Japanese HCC patients with both JIS scores and CLIP scores. They determined that a JIS score of 0 signified a 10-year survival rate of 65% whereas a CLIP score of 0 signified a 10-year survival rate of 23%. Based on these data, they concluded that the JIS score stratified mortality risk of early HCC better than the CLIP score did. However, these results have not been reproduced in different patient populations; this may represent a difference in the biologic or clinical characteristics of the Japanese patients, or it may represent heterogeneity in screening and treatment practices in different geographic areas.

Groupe d'Etude et de Traitement du Carcinome Hepatocellulaire Score

In 1999, the Groupe d'Etude et de Traitement du Carcinome Hepatocellulaire (GRETCH) consortium proposed another classification system designed to predict HCC patient survival.[73] This system was developed with data from 779 HCC patients prospectively recruited in 24 centers in France, Belgium, and Canada. The cohort used to derive this system received a variety of therapies ranging from resection to symptomatic palliation. To develop an easily applicable system, the authors of the GRETCH score system considered only characteris-

tics that could be assessed without invasive or highly technologic methodologies. By multivariate analysis of their data, they identified five prognostic factors associated with survival. These were Karnofsky index, serum bilirubin, alkaline phosphatase, AFP, and ultrasonographic evidence of portal obstruction (Table 16–9). Each factor was assigned a score, and the resultant sums were divided into three risk groups. The 1-year survival rates for risk groups A, B, and C were 79%, 31%, and 4%, respectively. Although this system is attractive for its simplicity and apparent good discriminatory capacity, it is important to note that the GRETCH scoring system has not been externally validated.

Chinese University Prognostic Index

In 2002, a research group in Hong Kong analyzed a database of 926 Chinese HCC patients seen at a single center.[74] This analysis identified AFP, serum bilirubin, alkaline phosphatase, ascites, and asymptomatic disease on presentation as independent prognostic variables (Table 16–10). These variables were combined with the TNM stage, and each component was assigned a numeric value. The individual values were summed, and the result was the patient's prognostic score. Patients were divided into three risk groups based upon their score. In the original study,

Table 16–7. JAPANESE MODIFICATION OF TUMOR-NODE-METASTASIS STAGING SYSTEM

Stage	Tumor*	Node	Metastasis
I	T1	N0	M0
II	T2	N0	M0
III	T3	N0	M0
IVA	T4	N0	M0
IVB	Any T	Any N	M1

*T criteria are (1) single tumor, (2) tumor < 2 cm, (3) no vascular invasion. T definitions are as follow: T1, all criteria are met; T2, 2 of 3 criteria are met; T3, 1 of 3 criteria is met; T4, no criteria are met.

Table 16–8. JAPANESE INTEGRATED STAGING SCORE

	Score			
	0	1	2	3
Japanese TNM stage	I	II	III	IV
Child-Pugh classification	A	B	C	

TNM = tumor-node-metastasis.

Table 16–9. GROUPE D'ETUDE ET DE TRAITEMENT DU CARCINOME HEPATOCELLULAIRE CLASSIFICATION

Parameter	Score			
	0	1	2	3
Karnofsky index (%)	≥ 80	—	—	< 80
Serum bilirubin (μmol/L)	< 50	—	—	≥ 50
Serum alkaline phosphatase (× ULN)	< 2	—	≥ 2	—
Serum AFP	< 35	—	≥ 35	—
Portal vein thrombosis	No	Yes	—	—
Group A (low mortality risk): score, 0				
Group B (intermediate mortality risk): score, 1–5				
Group C (high mortality risk): score, > 5				

AFP = alpha fetoprotein; ULN = upper limit of normal.

this score, the Chinese University Prognostic Index (CUPI) score, was found to have better discriminatory capabilities than the TNM system, the Okuda system, and the CLIP score. Several caveats need to be considered in the interpretation of these results. First, 80% of the cases used in deriving this system were HBV-related, which indicates a population significantly different from that seen in the West. Second, the majority of these patients had advanced-stage disease with the expected associated short survival; therefore, there is considerable question regarding this system's capacity to accurately stratify individuals with early-stage disease. Finally, CUPI scoring has not yet been prospectively validated nor properly investigated in other cohorts of patients.

Barcelona Clinic Liver Cancer Staging System

The Barcelona Clinic Liver Cancer (BCLC) system differs from previously published staging systems because it divides, a priori, patients into those with early-, intermediate-, or late-stage disease and constructs prognostic models for each stage.[75] Rather than yield a prognostic index as the previously described systems have done, the BCLC system provides a treatment algorithm based on anticipated survival. The authors of this system suggested that prior classification systems offered useful information only for patients with advanced disease and that a pragmatically applicable system for classifying early-stage HCC was lacking. There is a compelling need for effective discrimination in this group of patients, given the curative potential of radical therapies in early-stage disease. The BCLC schema characterizes patient performance status, tumor characteristics, and assessments of liver function to assign patients into one of four risk groups (Table 16–11). Patients with stage A HCC are candidates for radical therapies such as resection, transplantation, or percutaneous ablative techniques. The authors assign patients with stage B and stage C disease to palliative or experimental treatments. Patients with stage D lesions (end-stage disease as defined by Child-Pugh class C or poor performance status) are considered for only symptomatic therapies because of their abysmal prognoses irrespective of treatment modality.

The 1-, 3-, and 5-year survival rates for patients with stage A disease were 85%, 62%, and 51%, respectively. Patients with stage B and C disease had

Table 16–10. CHINESE UNIVERSITY PROGNOSTIC INDEX SCORING

Parameter	Score*
TNM stage	
I and II	–3
IIIa and IIIb	–1
IVa and IVb	0
Total bilirubin (μmol/L)	
< 34	0
34–51	3
≥ 52	4
Alkaline phosphatase ≥ 200 units/L	3
Alpha fetoprotein ≥ 500 ng/mL	2
Absence of symptoms	–4

*Patients are stratified by total score as low risk (≤ 1), intermediate risk (2–7), and high risk (> 8).

Table 16–11. BARCELONA CLINIC LIVER CANCER STAGING CLASSIFICATION

Stage*	Performance Status	Tumor Stage	Okuda Stage	Liver Function
A1	0	Single < 5 cm	I	No portal HTN, nl bilirubin
A2	0	Single < 5 cm	I	Portal HTN, nl bilirubin
A3	0	Single < 5 cm	I	Portal HTN, elevated bilirubin
A4	0	3 tumors < 3 cm	I–II	Child stage A/B
B	0	Multinodular	I–II	Child stage A/B
C	1–2	Vascular invasion or extrahepatic spread	I–II	Child stage A/B
D	3–4	Any	III	Child stage C

HTN = hypertension; nl = normal-level.
*Definitions: stage A = early hepatocellular carcinoma (HCC), stage B = intermediate HCC, stage C = advanced HCC, stage D = end-stage HCC.

1-, 3-, and 5-year survival rates of 54%, 28%, and 7%, respectively, whereas those with stage D disease had only a 10% rate of survival at 1 and 3 years and no survival at 5 years. Unsurprisingly, the survival rate for stage A patients was significantly influenced by the degree of hepatic functional perturbation before resection. Stage A patients without elevated portal venous pressure and elevated serum bilirubin had a significantly better 3-year survival when compared with patients who had elevations in both of these parameters.

Summary of Staging Systems

The consequent confusion reminiscent of the story of the tower of Babel that ensued in an attempt to properly classify prognosis and determine appropriate treatment assignment for patients with HCC, is clear testimony of the disease's wide spectrum of presentation, natural history, and treatment options. Although some of the systems described above have been discarded for independent use (ie, TNM and Okuda staging), the diversity of the remaining competing systems is an indication of the reality that no single system has been shown to be ideal for broad application. Further complicating the HCC landscape is the increasing number of serologic tests and genetic markers that are purported to contribute to prognosis and that have not yet been integrated into any staging system.

Despite the clear absence of an ideal system, guidelines for clinical practice are necessary. Therefore, a 2002 American Hepato-Pancreato-Biliary Association (AHPBA)/AJCC consensus panel made the following recommendations[76]:

1. The primary staging should be clinical staging, and the CLIP system should be the clinical staging system of choice because it is generally applicable to most patients and includes easily collected variables.
2. A secondary staging system for patients undergoing resection or liver transplantation is needed; the AJCC version of the modified TNM system should be used because it has been internally validated (although external and prospective validation is still lacking).
3. Because neither of the systems mentioned above are free of limitations, other factors that might be included in assessing prognosis are treatment-directed variables (according to the BCLC system), the etiology of the underlying liver disease, and newly discovered factors affecting tumor biology.
4. Further studies on the validation of staging systems and the harmonization of the different systems are urgently needed to clarify prognosis and provide optimal treatment options to patients.

MANAGEMENT

There is no single optimal therapeutic approach to the treatment of HCC. The choice of available therapies is dependent on the size, location, number, and invasiveness of the tumors as well as on the severity of the underlying liver disease. Wide application of screening programs has lead to the increasingly early detection of HCC. This has expanded the applicability of potentially curative therapies such as surgical resection, liver transplantation, and percutaneous ablation. However, there is marked international heterogeneity in the proportion of cases in which these curative modalities are appropriate. In Japan, 50 to 70% of cases are eligible for curative treatments whereas only 25 to 40% of cases in Europe and the United States and fewer than 10% of cases in Africa have this option.[77] Even if a patient is eligible for a potentially curative therapy, there are no randomized controlled trials comparing the various options, and there are no widely applicable guidelines to facilitate this decision. Surgical resection and liver transplantation result in a 5-year survival rate of 60 to 70% for well-selected patients, and these are probably the first-choice therapies when feasible. Percutaneous ablative therapies appear to be inferior to surgical options in terms of outcome, having an average 5-year survival rate of 40 to 50%. However, these therapies are potentially available to patients with tumor or cirrhosis characteristics that might otherwise disqualify them for a surgical intervention.

Patients with vascular invasion of the tumor, extrahepatic spread, or cancer-related symptoms are defined as having advanced HCC. There is no clearly defined therapeutic algorithm for this scenario. Some authors advocate ablative interventions, chemoembolization, or irradiation for control of symptoms or to potentially down-stage the extent of disease. Numerous systemic therapies have been investigated for treatment of advanced disease; these include systemic chemotherapy, immunotherapy, internal radiation, anti-androgenic drugs, and a variety of modern biologic agents. Unfortunately, none of these therapies have yet demonstrated significant antitumor activity or survival benefit.

Surgical Resection

Surgery is a reasonable curative option for the limited number of patients with small solitary tumors and well-preserved hepatic function.[78] A major concern when performing this procedure in a cirrhotic patient is the possibility of precipitating acute liver failure owing to a lack of adequate functional reserve in the remaining liver. Therefore, surgery is typically restricted to patients with well-compensated liver disease and no significant comorbidities. Several clinical variables have been associated with increased

risk of liver failure after resection; these include splenomegaly, esophageal varices, platelet counts of $< 100,000/mm^3$, and a hepatic vein pressure gradient of > 10 mm Hg.[79] Absolute contraindications to liver resection include markedly impaired performance status, Child C cirrhosis, uncontrolled ascites, tumor invasion of the main portal vein, and extrahepatic tumor spread. Relative contraindications include clinically relevant portal hypertension, a serum bilirubin level > 2 mg/dL, a predicted postresection liver volume of < 450 cc, and an anticipated inability (for technical or anatomic reasons) to achieve a complete resection of the tumor.

There are a number of formal tests for measuring hepatic function and for estimating postsurgical reserve; these include the indocyanine green (ICG) retention test, a variety of carbon-13 breath tests (including aminopyrine and caffeine),[80] and a number of liver metabolism–based scintigraphic modalities.[81] The ICG retention test involves the intravenous injection of ICG and the determination of the retention of this pigment in plasma 15 minutes after injection. Typically, an ICG retention rate of $< 15\%$ indicates hepatic function adequate to tolerate resection.[82] Some Japanese centers routinely perform the ICG retention test preoperatively[83]; however, this evaluation has not become part of standard practice in the West. In the United States, surgeons tend to estimate adequate postoperative residual liver function on the basis of serum bilirubin level, evidence of portal hypertension, and radiographic volumetric measurements. Although no formal guidelines exist to guide this decision, experts tend to resect no more than 40% of the preoperative liver volume when liver disease is present and no more than 75% of liver volume when the liver is normal. With careful patient selection, operative mortality in most surgical centers is less than 3 to 5%.[84]

Long-term survival after liver resection depends on tumor size, the presence of vascular invasion, and the severity of underlying liver disease. The optimal candidates with small tumors and excellent liver function have a 5-year survival rate of 50 to 70%.[85] However, the oncogenic milieu of the cirrhotic liver persists after HCC resection, with ongoing hepatocyte damage and regeneration. Therefore, both local recurrence and de novo tumor formation are common, and the 5-year cumulative recurrence rate approaches 75%.[86]

Owing to this dramatic recurrence rate, much research has been devoted to identifying effective forms of adjuvant therapy to be administered either before or after surgery. Neither systemic nor intra-arterial chemotherapy has shown significant efficacy for improving long-term survival.[87,88] Similarly, preoperative chemoembolization has been shown to be ineffective.[89] A small randomized controlled trial investigating the use of adjuvant intra-arterial I-131 lipiodol did demonstrate a significant improvement in disease-free survival for patients so treated, in comparison with controls.[90] Investigators found that after a median follow-up period of 36 months, the recurrence rate in the irradiated group was 28.5%, compared with a 59% recurrence rate in the untreated group (*p* = .04), and this salutary effect of internal irradiation was reproduced in a subsequent small case-control study.[91] Also, several Japanese studies have been looking at the utility of postoperative therapy with interferon-α[92] or interferon-β.[93] These studies did show improved survival for treated patients; however, the studies were very small and the follow-up periods were relatively short.

Liver Transplantation

Prior to 1995, orthotopic liver transplantation (OLT) was not considered to be a viable treatment option for patients with HCC. During the early years of liver transplantation (the 1980s and early 1990s), most centers used resection as the preferred treatment of early HCC. Because of this, there was a bias toward transplanting patients with "unresectable" tumors, and overall survival rates were poor.[94] However, a review of the United Network for Organ Sharing (UNOS) database from that period revealed that patients who underwent transplantation and were found to have incidental small HCCs in the explanted liver tended to have a reasonable disease-free survival.[95] This led to a prospective trial of OLT for early-stage HCC (defined as a single tumor < 5 cm in diameter or as no more than 3 tumors, each < 3 cm in diameter). Using these rules, which became known as the Milan criteria, the investigators demonstrated a 75% survival rate at 4 years,

which was not different from the expected survival of patients without HCC but undergoing OLT.[96] Outcomes using these criteria were confirmed by several other investigators, and the criteria have since been adopted as a fundamental component of the pretransplantation evaluation of patients with HCC.

A major difficulty faced by clinicians when treating HCC is the presence of cirrhosis and its associated sequelae. Liver transplantation obviates this concern by replacing the diseased liver and treating the malignancy concurrently. This raises issues regarding prognosis and staging that are unique to this treatment modality. Whereas most modern staging systems consider tumor characteristics and degree of hepatic dysfunction, the latter is significantly less important in patients undergoing liver transplantation. When HCC is treated with OLT, cancer characteristics such as tumor size, number, and grade; macroscopic and microscopic vascular invasion; lymph node metastasis; distant metastasis; and expression of oncogene products have been shown to be the major risk factors for recurrence and poor overall survival.[97,98] It is difficult to accurately establish all of these characteristics prior to transplantation; therefore, tumor number, macroscopic vascular invasion, and extrahepatic disease are used to establish the best estimate of overall tumor biology. These proxies are typically ascertained via multiphasic CT or MRI. Further complicating prognostic matters, these radiologic staging methodologies can both over- and underestimate tumor size and number. This was highlighted in a review of 666 explanted livers culled from the UNOS database.[99] This review demonstrated that at least 30% of all HCC patients who underwent transplantation were understaged and would not have met the Milan criteria to qualify for transplantation. Furthermore, 23% of those patients' extent of tumor had been overestimated by radiographic analysis.

The widespread application of the Milan criteria opened the door for OLT for patients with HCC, but an additional obstacle quickly became apparent. Although patients who met the Milan criteria were eligible for transplantation, many of them became ineligible owing to tumor progression on account of long waiting times for available organs. In 2001, an HCC patient had a 25%-per-year probability of tumor progression beyond limits acceptable for transplantation.[100] At that time, prioritization for organ allocation was based primarily on the patient's Child-Pugh score and time accrued on the waiting list, and this led to a significant bias against successful transplantation in patients with HCC. In February 2002, a new system for liver allocation, known as the model for end-stage liver disease (MELD)–based prioritization system, went into effect in the United States. The MELD score is calculated by using several laboratory values and was initially designed for predicting mortality after transhepatic portal systemic shunt placement.[101] Subsequently, it was recognized that the MELD score was also effective at predicting 3-month mortality while patients awaited OLT. Although the raw MELD score does not account for the presence of HCC, the final allocation system provides additional points to patients with HCC, thus facilitating the prioritization of these patients during organ assignment.

Although adoption of the MELD score has improved the availability of OLT for HCC patients, disqualification due to tumor progression remains a substantial problem. This has led to consideration of several strategies for slowing or reversing tumor progression while the patient awaits transplantation. Various adjuvant therapies, including percutaneous ablation, chemoembolization, and systemic chemotherapy while patients are on the waiting list, have been examined in a number of observational studies.[102,103] These therapies have failed to definitively demonstrate a survival benefit; however, many centers nonetheless offer ablative and/or embolic interventions on an empiric basis to patients who are awaiting transplantation. Another tactic advocated by some authors for addressing the dropout problem is expansion of the Milan criteria. This remains a controversial and actively debated possibility. Finally, there has been some enthusiasm for undertaking living donor liver transplantation (LDLT) in HCC patients whose tumor characteristics exceed the Milan criteria. A single-center series in the United States demonstrated a 48% posttransplantation recurrence-free survival at 5 years for LDLT patients whose tumors were larger than 5 cm, an outcome that some authors argue justifies wider application of this therapeutic alternative.[104] However, there remain many controversial issues regarding this option, including

risk to the donor, increased risk of primary graft non-function, and biologic heterogeneity of the larger tumors. These issues are currently under investigation in a multicenter prospective study exploring LDLT in HCC patients.[105]

Local Ablative Therapies

HCC tends to occur as anatomically discrete nodules, and this fact has been exploited with a variety of treatment modalities aimed at destroying the tumor cells while sparing the adjacent non-neoplastic liver parenchyma. These therapies are generally less expensive and better tolerated than surgical resection, but they tend to have lower rates of complete lesion eradication and higher rates of tumor recurrence. Currently, percutaneous ablation techniques are considered to be first-choice therapeutic interventions for patients with early-stage HCC who are not candidates for either surgical resection or OLT.[106] Local ablative therapies can be divided into those that use chemical ablation (ethanol, acetic acid, hot saline) and those that rely on thermal ablation (radiofrequency, microwave, laser).

Percutaneous Ethanol Injection

First described in 1983, Percutaneous Ethanol Injection (PEI) is the most widely used (and was the first) local ablative methodology targeting HCC. The procedure is performed by injecting pure ethanol into the tumor with imaging guidance while the patient is under local anesthesia. Ethanol induces coagulative necrosis as a result of cellular dehydration, protein denaturation, and chemical occlusion of small tumor vessels. Patients are usually treated during four to six sessions weekly. PEI results in complete ablation of approximately 70% of tumors that are < 3 cm in diameter.[107] Although generally well tolerated, PEI has been associated with complications that include local pain, fever, bleeding, alcohol intoxication, and abscess formation.[108] In a report on 1,066 patients undergoing PEI at 11 centers in Italy, one death, seven occurrences of tumor seeding, and 27 other symptomatic complications were described.[109]

There are no published prospective randomized trials comparing PEI to surgical resection, OLT, or supportive care. However, there is a substantial retrospective literature that supports the contention that PEI improves the natural history of HCC. As with other potentially curative therapies for HCC, the prognosis of a patient treated with PEI is very dependent on the size and number of tumors as well as on the severity of the underlying liver disease. A number of retrospective studies showed that the 5-year survival rate of Child A patients with early-stage tumors was 41 to 53%, a mortality comparable to that reported in surgical series.[110,111] In an Italian retrospective comparative study involving 391 patients with uninodular HCCs < 5 cm, the cumulative 3-year survival rates after surgical resection, PEI, or no treatment were 79%, 71%, and 26%, respectively, for Child A patients and 40%, 41%, and 13%, respectively, for Child B patients.[112] These results are in agreement with other studies suggesting that both surgery and PEI improve survival for early-stage HCC patients with Child A or B cirrhosis. Unfortunately, tumor recurrence in the PEI group was high, ranging from 74 to 98% at 5 years. Similar improvements in survival were seen in a Japanese series of PEI patients with three or fewer tumors of up to 3 cm in diameter. This study reported 1-, 3-, and 5-year survival rates of 93%, 76%, and 50%, respectively, for patients treated with PEI.[113]

Other Chemical Ablation Techniques

Percutaneous administration of both acetic acid and hot saline have been proposed as alternatives to PEI in the treatment of HCC. Two studies have investigated the efficacy of acetic acid injection compared with that of PEI,[114,115] and one published study has looked at outcomes in patients who received hot saline injections.[116] All of these studies were small, and the two acetic acid studies produced conflicting results. Although these techniques may be shown to have some usefulness in the future, there is at present neither data nor significant clinical enthusiasm to support their use over the well-established PEI therapy.

Radiofrequency Ablation

Radiofrequency ablation (RFA) seeks to inflict thermal injury to specific targeted tissues through the deposition of electromagnetic energy. In RFA, an electrode is inserted into the tumor under imaging guidance, and the patient becomes part of a closed-loop circuit that includes a radiofrequency generator, the electrode needle, and a grounding pad (Figure 16–10). As current is passed into the electrode tip, an alternating electric field is created within the tumor. High electrical resistance within biologic tissues relative to the electrode leads to the conversion of the current to heat, and specific design elements of the electrodes, current configuration, and ground pads allow reasonably precise focusing of the thermal injury. The generated heat causes coagulative necrosis of the surrounding tissue, leading to a uniform area of ablation that is not impeded by the tumor capsule or the fibrous septa of the cirrhotic liver. The goal of RFA is to destroy both the tumor and a rim of normal tissue immediately adjacent to it, thus approximating a surgical margin without the need for surgery.

The conventional monopolar electrodes used during the early experience with RFA were only capable of producing cylindric areas of necrosis up to 1.6 cm in diameter.[117] Therefore, numerous electrode insertions were necessary to treat most lesions, and this increased both the technical difficulty of the procedure and the risk to the patient. However, the broad application of RFA was facilitated by the advent of modified electrodes, including cooled-tip electrode needles[118] and expandable electrode needles with multiple retractable lateral-exit prongs on the tip.[119] Cooling the electrode tip prevents the

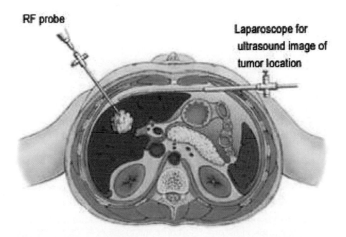

Figure 16–10. Cross-sectional illustration of the radiofrequency (RF) ablation procedure.

overheating of tissues closest to the electrode, thereby eliminating charring that would limit propagation of the radiofrequency waves. Expandable needles with geometrically diverse tips allow for variation in the length of electrode deployment, which results in the production of a predictably enlarged volume of necrosis with a single needle insertion (Figure 16–11).

The safety of RFA is comparable to that of PEI. In a multicenter study of 2,320 patients, 6 deaths were noted, giving a procedural mortality rate of 0.3%.[120] Other major complications, including tumor seeding, massive hemorrhage, and acute liver failure, occurred in 2.2% of patients in this study. A review of other complications reported in the literature reveals that ablation of superficial lesions that are adjacent to any part of the gastrointestinal tract increases the risk of thermal injury to the nearby viscera.[121]

One randomized study of 104 Child A or B cirrhosis patients with early-stage HCC compared treatment with RFA to treatment with PEI and then observed patients for about 2 years afterwards.[122] The

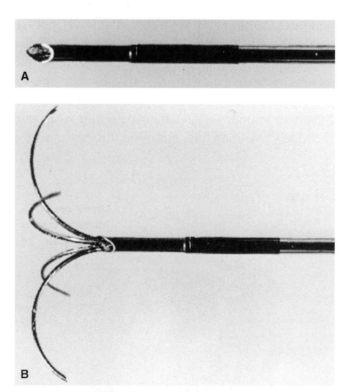

Figure 16–11. Multipronged electrode for radiofrequency ablation. *A*, The electrode in its pre-insertion configuration. *B*, Once inserted into the tumor, hook-shaped tips are deployed to permit the ablation of larger tissue volumes.

overall survival rates at 1 and 2 years were greater than 90% and did not differ for either treatment group. However, recurrence-free survival rates were higher for the RFA group than for the PEI group. The discrepancy between overall survival and recurrence-free survival in this trial may be explained by the relatively short follow-up period. In a subsequent study, 206 patients with early-stage HCC who were not candidates for resection or transplantation were enrolled in a prospective trial examining the outcome of local ablative therapy.[123] More than 90% of these patients were treated with RFA, and the overall survival rate in this group was 71% at 3 years and 48% at 5 years. Survival in this study was primarily linked to tumor number and severity of cirrhosis. Child A patients had 3- and 5-year survival rates of 76% and 51%, respectively, whereas the respective rates for Child B patients were 46% and 31%.

Although compelling data demonstrating its superiority to other ablative technologies are lacking, RFA has become the preferred form of ablative therapy at many centers. The extant studies do establish the safety and efficacy of the treatment, and many clinicians prefer RFA because of its optimizable capacity for tumor necrosis and the convenience of completing therapy in relatively few sessions.

Microwave Ablation

Microwave ablation is a set of technologies that facilitate tumor destruction through the application of electromagnetic energy at frequencies of 900 kHz or greater. Penetration of microwaves into any water-containing material induces the rotation of individual molecules. The resultant rapid molecular motion generates and uniformly distributes heat that is instantaneous and continuous until the microwave bombardment is stopped. Microwave irradiation creates an ablation area around the needle in a columnar or round shape, depending on the type of needle used and the amount of power applied.[124]

Several uncontrolled studies of HCC patients who received microwave ablation demonstrated 3-year survival rates of 68 to 73%.[125,126] A small retrospective study examined microwave ablation and PEI for the treatment of small HCCs.[127] Investigators found no difference in the overall 5-year survival of patients with well-differentiated HCC. However, a subgroup analysis of those patients with less well-differentiated tumors suggested improved survival with microwave ablation. One randomized trial compared microwave ablation with RFA in 72 patients.[128] Investigators found no significant differences in efficacy or morbidity between the two methodologies although the number of required treatment sessions was significantly lower for the RFA group.

Palliative Therapies

Despite the widespread adoption of HCC screening and surveillance programs, only about 30% of patients diagnosed with this malignancy are candidates for potentially curative therapies such as surgical resection, OLT, or local ablation.[129] Patients are deemed ineligible for curative therapy either because of advanced tumor characteristics (such as a single tumor larger than 5 cm or the presence of more than three tumor nodules) or because of clinically advanced liver failure (Child B or C cirrhosis). This large group of patients is therefore considered for one or more of the available palliative therapeutic alternatives, which include chemoembolization, bland embolization, systemic chemotherapy, hormonal therapy, and internal radiotherapy. Prior to symptomatic terminal phases of disease, the main goal of a palliative therapy is to prolong the patient's life expectancy despite the inability to completely arrest the underlying pathologic process. Of the palliative strategies routinely considered for HCC patients, only chemoembolization has been clearly shown to provide this benefit.

Transarterial Chemoembolization

The purpose of embolization therapy is to disrupt the blood supply to the HCC while limiting collateral damage to the nontumorous liver. This is a practical undertaking because the blood supply to most HCCs is provided through vessels arising from branches of the hepatic artery whereas the bulk of perfusion for the nonmalignant hepatic parenchyma is provided by the portal vein. The principle underlying embolic therapy is that selective occlusion of hepatic artery branches will cause ischemia and resultant tumor

necrosis, which may be augmented with simultaneous local administration of chemotherapy. When used, a chemotherapeutic drug tends to be compounded into an emulsion with lipiodol. This facilitates the concentration of the therapeutic agent within the HCC and leads to levels of drug in the tumor that are 10 to 100 times higher than would be achieved if chemotherapy were given systemically.[130]

Embolization procedures are generally performed in an angiography suite. Initially, visceral angiography is performed to identify the hepatic arterial anatomy, the location of the tumor(s), and the tumors' associated feeding vessels. A catheter is then advanced into an appropriate arterial branch, and the therapeutic agent is infused through the catheter (Figure 16–12). Compounds that can be used to achieve embolization include a variety of gelatin products, polyvinyl alcohol particles, glass microspheres, and metallic coils. The most common chemotherapeutic agents used in transarterial chemoembolization (TACE) include doxorubicin, cisplatin, mitomycin, and epirubicin.[131] There is no compelling evidence indicating the superiority of any one of these agents for this indication, and there is no clear consensus on optimal dosing. TACE treatments are typically repeated either on the basis of tumor response as measured by imaging or on a preset schedule (although, as discussed below, this is a source of controversy). Most patients undergoing TACE experience a postembolization syndrome including fever, abdominal pain, vomiting, and elevations of serum transaminases.[132] Other rare complications include worsening ascites, variceal hemorrhage, acute liver failure, ischemic hepatitis, hepatic abscess, and renal failure.

A recently published meta-analysis examined the survival benefits of embolic therapy compared with those of conservative management.[133] This systematic review involved seven small randomized controlled trials with a total of 516 patients. Only two of the original studies identified survival benefits for embolized patients[134,135]; however, the meta-analysis found embolic therapy to have a salutary effect on survival. The two positive randomized controlled trials administered three to four treatment sessions per year; one trial used doxorubicin, and the other used cisplatin. However, as previously noted,

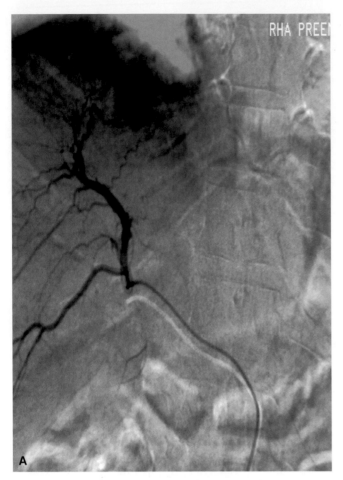
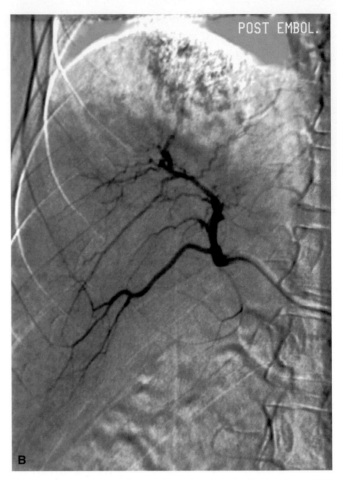

Figure 16–12.   Visceral angiograms made before and after transarterial chemoembolization (TACE). *A,* Selective catheterization of the right hepatic artery and contrast enhancement of the tumor vessel web. *B,* Post-TACE angiogram shows occlusion of the feeding arterial branch and the presence of lipiodol in the tumor distribution. (RHA PREEM-right hepatic artery, before embolization; POST EMBOL-post embolization.)

there is no reliable evidence to support any particular treatment schedule or chemotherapeutic agent.

A number of different radiographic modalities are used to evaluate the effectiveness of TACE, including CT, MRI, US, and nuclear medicine imaging. Because most patients who undergo TACE do not eventually undergo surgery, there is little evidence that radiographic findings truly reflect pathologic changes. Lipiodol is radiopaque and hepatomatropic; therefore, noncontrast CT has frequently been used to assess the technical success of chemoembolization by demonstrating lipiodol deposition in the desired areas of the liver. Lipiodol deposition has been associated with increased tumor necrosis and decreased tumor vascularity.[136] However, lipiodol distribution has not correlated well with changes in tumor size, suggesting that the absence of tumor shrinkage does not necessarily

mean that a particular TACE session was unsuccessful. Contrast-enhanced CT has limited usefulness following TACE because the lipiodol obscures the area of interest, namely, enhancing areas within the tumor. Conventional MRI is also of limited usefulness for monitoring the effectiveness of embolic intervention because it does not easily distinguish viable areas from necrotic or granulation tissue after treatment. A number of advanced imaging technologies are being explored for monitoring response to TACE. These include functional MRI, contrast-enhanced harmonic gray-scale ultrasonography,[137] and fluorodeoxyglucose positron emission tomography.[138] However, the current situation is one in which TACE is recognized as an effective therapy but in which there are no established posttreatment parameters that predict response to this therapy or predict survival.

Systemic Chemotherapy

HCC responds poorly to chemotherapy for a variety of reasons. First, HCC cells, like their progenitor hepatocytes, express numerous genes concerned with drug metabolism and inactivation. Second, genetic analysis of HCCs has demonstrated frequent overexpression of the multidrug-resistance protein and loss of the p53 tumor suppressor gene.[139] These and other genetic alterations that develop in the course of oncogenesis contribute to the tumor's resistance to antineoplastic agents. Finally, it is reasonable to predict that HCC patients with impaired hepatic function will be more susceptible to the varied toxicities associated with systemic chemotherapy.

There have been many studies investigating a panoply of systemic chemotherapeutic agents. These studies have been typically unsuccessful, and the chemotherapy frequently results in the anticipated profound toxicities in cirrhotic patients. Systemic chemotherapy trials demonstrate an overall response rate of < 20%.[140] The most commonly used drug is doxorubicin, but in the only prospective randomized controlled trial to investigate this drug as monotherapy, efficacy was marginal and fatal complications occurred in 25% of the patients.[141] Combination chemotherapy trials also have not yielded improved response rates although some preliminary studies using chemotherapy to augment another salvage therapy such as internal irradiation[142] or interferon therapy[143] have shown some promise. Several studies have examined chemotherapy as adjuvant treatment after resection, but these showed either no benefit or a worsened prognosis.[87] Because of the poor responsiveness of HCC to any known chemotherapeutic regimen and the substantial toxicity risk from these agents, the use of systemic chemotherapy should be avoided in the routine management of these patients. The only setting in which its use is justified is that of a clinical trial involving patients who have advanced disease and who are not eligible for other therapies.

Hormonal Therapy

Experimental models of hepatic carcinogenesis and several human epidemiologic investigations have sug-gested a possible relationship between sex hormones and hepatocarcinogenesis.[144] Early molecular studies demonstrated the presence of cell surface estrogen receptors in advanced HCC. This led to the investigation of antiestrogenic therapy with tamoxifen. Despite early enthusiasm and promising results from some small trials,[145] a recent meta-analysis of seven randomized controlled trials that compared tamoxifen with conservative therapy demonstrated neither tumor diminution nor a survival benefit in the treated groups.[11] There have been several small studies suggesting that use of the progestational steroid megestrol acetate is associated with an improved quality of life and with prolonged survival for selected HCC patients.[146,147] These results require confirmation in larger and more methodologically rigorous studies before megestrol acetate can be considered for application in clinical practice. Androgen receptors are also frequently detected in malignant hepatocytes, and this has led to studies looking at flutamide (a pure antiandrogen) and triptorelin (a luteinizing hormone–releasing hormone). These studies have failed to demonstrate any survival benefit.[148]

Somatostatin receptors have been found on HCC cells, and this has led to interest in treatment with somatostatin analogues. One small study of 58 patients compared twice-daily subcutaneous octreotide with supportive care in patients with advanced HCC.[149] The study demonstrated a substantial increase in median survival. Unfortunately, this finding was not replicated in a subsequent investigation that used a longer-acting octreotide preparation.[150] Both studies suffered from methodologic deficiencies, and further studies are currently under way to address the usefulness of this treatment strategy.

CONCLUSION

Hepatocellular carcinoma is a major worldwide cause of substantial morbidity and mortality. It tends to present insidiously in patients who are already burdened with significant preexisting disease. Two decades ago, a diagnosis of this malignancy was essentially synonymous with a sentence of incipient death from HCC. Early detection, improvements in diagnostic and therapeutic technology, and careful selection of patients for potentially curative therapies have significantly improved survival. Numerous challenges remain. Improved classification of disease stage is necessary. Which histology is malignant versus dysplastic, and what are the clinical implications of that distinction? Which imaging modalities are best for diagnosis and surveillance of HCC? Is there a staging system that can be applied broadly, or will there be regional staging systems based on local epidemiologic characteristics? Although improvements in diagnosis and treatment have made HCC a "treatable" malignancy, it is important to bear in mind that it remains curable in only a minority of patients. Future investigation needs to explore improved therapeutic options for the large fraction of HCC patients who are not eligible for radical therapies but are nonetheless typically the sickest patients in this group.

REFERENCES

1. Parkin DM, Pissani P, Ferlay J. Estimates of the worldwide incidence of 25 major cancers in 1990. Int J Cancer 1999;80:827–41.
2. Taylor-Robinson SD, Foster GR, Arora S, et al. Trends in primary liver cancer. Lancet 1997;350:1142–3.
3. El-Serag HB, Davila JA, Petersen NJ, et al. The continuing increase in the incidence of hepatocellular carcinoma in the United States: an update. Ann Intern Med 2003; 139:817–23.
4. Jemal AT, Murray T, Ward E, et al. Cancer Statistics 2005. CA Cancer J Clin 2005;55:8–29.
5. Pisani P, Bray F, Parkin DM. Estimates of the world-wide prevalence of cancer for 25 sites in the adult population. Int J Cancer 2002;97:72–81.
6. El-Serag HB. Hepatocellular carcinoma and hepatitis C in the United States. Hepatology 2002;36:S74–83.
7. Toyoda H, Kumada T, Kiriyama S, et al. Changes in the characteristics and survival rate of hepatocellular carcinoma from 1976 to 2000: analysis of 1365 patients in a single institution in Japan. Cancer 2004;100:2415–21.
8. Yoshizawa H. Hepatocellular carcinoma associated with hepatitis C virus infection in Japan: projection to other countries in the foreseeable future. Oncology 2002;62 Suppl 1:8–17.
9. Johnson PJ, Williams R. Cirrhosis and the aetiology of hepatocellular carcinoma. J Hepatol 1987;4:140–7.
10. Llovet JM, Burroughs A, Bruix J. Hepatocellular carcinoma. Lancet 2003;362:1907–17.
11. Llovet JM, Bruix J. Systematic review of randomized trials for unresectable hepatocellular carcinoma: chemoembolization improves survival. Hepatology 2003;37:429–42.
12. Bruix J, Sherman M, Llovet JM, et al. Clinical management of hepatocellular carcinoma. Conclusions of the Barcelona-2000 EASL conference. European Association for the Study of the Liver. J Hepatol 2001;35:421–30.
13. Sherman M. Alphafetoprotein: an obituary. J Hepatol 2001; 34:603–5.
14. Nguyen MH, Garcia RT, Simpson PW, et al. Racial differences in effectiveness of alpha-fetoprotein for diagnosis of hepatocellular carcinoma in hepatitis C virus cirrhosis. Hepatology 2002;36:410–7.
15. Gebo KA, Chander G, Jenckes MW, et al. Screening tests for hepatocellular carcinoma in patients with chronic hepatitis C: a systematic review. Hepatology 2002;36:S84–92.
16. Yao FY, Ferrell L, Bass NM, et al. Liver transplantation for hepatocellular carcinoma: expansion of the tumor size limits does not adversely impact survival. Hepatology 2001;33:1394–403
17. Yang B, Zhang B, Xu Y, et al. Prospective study of early detection for primary liver cancer. J Cancer Res Clin Oncol 1997;123:357–60.
18. McMahon BJ, Bulkow L, Harpster A, et al. Screening for hepatocellular carcinoma in Alaska Natives infected with chronic hepatitis B: a 16-year population-based study. Hepatology 2000;32:842–6.
19. Bolondi L, Sofia S, Siringo S, et al. Surveillance programme of cirrhotic patients for early diagnosis and treatment of hepatocellular carcinoma: a cost effectiveness analysis. Gut 2001;48:251–9.
20. Durand F, Regimbeau JM, Belghiti J, et al. Assessment of the benefits and risks of percutaneous biopsy before surgical resection of hepatocellular carcinoma. J Hepatol 2001; 35:254–8.
21. Collier J, Sherman M. Screening for hepatocellular carcinoma. Hepatology 1998;27:273–8.
22. Bolondi L, Gaiani S, Celli N, et al. Characterization of small nodules in cirrhosis by assessment of vascularity: the problem of hypovascular hepatocellular carcinoma. Hepatology 2005;42:27–34.
23. Horigome H, Nomura T, Saso K, et al. Limitations of imaging diagnosis for small hepatocellular carcinoma: comparison with histological findings. J Gastroenterol Hepatol 1999;14:559–65.
24. Torzilli G, Minagawa M, Takayama T, et al. Accurate preoperative evaluation of liver mass lesions without fine-needle biopsy. Hepatology 1999;30:889–93.
25. McGill DB, Rakela J, Zinsmeister AR, Ott BJ. A 21-year experience with major hemorrhage after percutaneous liver biopsy. Gastroenterology 1990;99:1396–400.
26. Yamada N, Shinzawa H, Ukai K, et al. Subcutaneous seeding of small hepatocellular carcinoma after fine needle aspiration biopsy. J Gastroenterol Hepatol 1993;8:195–8.
27. Takamori R, Wong LL, Dang C, Wong L. Needle-tract implantation from hepatocellular cancer: is needle biopsy of the liver always necessary? Liver Transpl 2000;6:67–72.
28. Smith EH. Complications of percutaneous abdominal fine-needle biopsy. Radiology 1991;178:253–8.
29. Giorgio A, Tarantino L, De Stefano G, et al. Complications after interventional sonography of focal liver lesions: a 22-year single-center experience. J Ultrasound Med 1997; 22:193–205.
30. Kim SH, Lim HK, Lee WJ, et al. Needle-tract implantation in hepatocellular carcinoma: frequency and CT findings after biopsy with a 19.5-gauge automated biopsy gun. Abdom Imaging 2000;25:246–50.

31. Huang GT, Sheu JC, Yang PM, et al. Ultrasound-guided cutting biopsy for the diagnosis of hepatocellular carcinoma—a study based on 420 patients. J Hepatol 1996;25:334–8.

32. International Working Party of World Congresses of Gastroenterology. Terminology of nodular lesions of the liver. Hepatology 1995;22:983–93.

33. Wanless IR. Pathology and nomenclature of early hepatocellular neoplasia. J Gastroenterol Hepatol 2004;19:S361–3.

34. Kim TK, Choi BI, Han JK, et al. Nontumorous arterioportal shunt mimicking hypervascular tumor in cirrhotic liver: two-phase spiral CT findings. Radiology 1998;208: 597–603.

35. Hayashi M, Matsui O, Ueda K, et al. Correlation between the blood supply and grade of malignancy of hepatocellular nodules associated with liver cirrhosis: evaluation by CT during intraarterial injection of contrast medium. Am J Roentgenol 1999;172:969–76.

36. Kim TK, Han JK, Chung JW, et al. Intraperitoneal drop metastases from hepatocellular carcinoma: CT and angiographic findings. J Comput Assist Tomogr 1996;20:638–42.

37. Choi BI, Kim CW, Han MC, et al. Sonographic characteristics of small hepatocellular carcinoma. Gastrointest Radiol 1989;14:255–61.

38. Tanaka S, Kitamura T, Fujita M, et al. Color Doppler flow imaging of liver tumors. AJM Am J Roentgenol 1990;154: 509–14.

39. Paul SB, Gulati MS. Spectrum of hepatocellular carcinoma on triple phase helical CT: a pictorial essay. Clin Imaging 2002;26:270–9.

40. Lee HM, Lud DSK, Krasny RM, et al. Hepatic lesion characterization in cirrhosis: significance of arterial hypervascularity on dual-phase helical CT. AJM Am J Roentgenol 1997;169:125–30.

41. Kamel IR, Bluemke DA. Imaging evaluation of hepatocellular carcinoma. J Vasc Interv Radiol 2002;13:S173–84.

42. Takayasu K, Moriyama N, Muramatsu Y, et al. The diagnosis of small hepatocellular carcinomas: efficacy of various imaging procedures in 100 patients. AJM Am J Roentgenol 1990;155:49–54.

43. Lim JH, Kim CK, Lee WJ, et al. Detection of hepatocellular carcinomas and dysplastic nodules in cirrhotic livers. AJM Am J Roentgenol 2000;175:693–8.

44. Peterson MS, Baron RL, Marsh, JW, et al. Pretransplantation surveillance for possible hepatocellular carcinoma in patients with cirrhosis: epidemiology and CT-based tumor detection rate in 430 cases with surgical pathologic correlation. Radiology 2000;217:743–9.

45. Kanematsu M, Hoshi H, Murakami T, et al. Detection of hepatocellular carcinoma in patients with cirrhosis: MR imaging versus angiographically assisted helical CT. AJM Am J Roentgenol 1997;169:1507–15.

46. Choi BI, Park JH, Kim BH, et al. Small hepatocellular carcinoma: detection with sonography, computed tomography (CT), angiography, and Lipiodol-CT. Br J Radiol 1989;62:897–903.

47. Bizollon T, Rode A, Bancel B, et al. Diagnostic value and tolerance of lipiodol-computed tomography for the detection of small hepatocellular carcinoma: correlation with pathologic examination of explanted livers. J Hepatol 1998;28:491–6.

48. Bartolozzi C, Lencioni R, Donati F, Cioni D. Abdominal MR: liver and pancreas. Eur Radiol 1999;9:1496–512.

49. Kadoya M, Matsui O, Takashima T, et al. Hepatocellular carcinoma: correlation of MR imaging and histopathologic findings. Radiology 1992;183:819–25.

50. Imai Y, Murakami T, Yoshida S, et al. Superparamagnetic iron oxide-enhanced magnetic resonance images of hepatocellular carcinoma: correlation with histological grading. Hepatology 2000;32:205–12.

51. Pauleit D, Textor J, Bachmann, R, et al. Hepatocellular carcinoma: detection with gadolinium- and ferumoxides-enhanced MR imaging of the liver. Radiology 2002; 222:73–80.

52. de Ledinghen V, Laharie D, Lecesne R, et al. Detection of nodules in liver cirrhosis: spiral computed tomography or magnetic resonance imaging? A prospective study of 88 nodules in 34 patients. Eur J Gastroenterol Hepatol 2002;14:159–65.

53. Krinsky G, Lee VS, Theise ND, et al. Transplantation for hepatocellular carcinoma and cirrhosis: sensitivity of magnetic resonance imaging. Liver Transpl 2002;8:1156–64.

54. Burrel M, Llovet JM, Ayuso C, et al. MRI angiography is superior to helical CT for detection of HCC prior to liver transplantation: an explant correlation. Hepatology 2003;38:1034–42.

55. Compton CC, Fielding LP, Burgart LJ, et al. Prognostic factors in colorectal cancer. College of American Pathologists Consensus Statement 1999. Arch Pathol Lab Med 2000;124:979–94.

56. Gleason DF, Veterans Administration Cooperative Urological Research Group. Histologic grading and staging of prostatic carcinoma. In: Tannenbaum M, editor. Urologic pathology: the prostate. Philadelphia: Lea & Febiger; 1977. p. 171–87.

57. Bruix J, Sherman M, Llovet JM, et al. Clinical management of hepatocellular carcinoma. Conclusions of the Barcelona-2000 EASL conference. European Association for the Study of the Liver. J Hepatol 2001;35:421–30.

58. Sakamoto M, Hiroshashi S, Shimosato Y. Early stages of multistep hepatocarcinogenesis: adenomatous hyperplasia and early hepatocellular carcinoma. Hum Pathol 1999;22:172–8.

59. Vauthey JN, Lauwers GY, Esnaola NF, et al. Simplified staging system for hepatocellular carcinoma. J Clin Oncol 2002;20:1527–36.

60. Izumi R, Shimizu K, Ii T, et al. Prognostic factors of hepatocellular carcinoma in patients undergoing hepatic resection. Gastroenterology 1994;106:720–7.

61. Yao FY, Ferrell L, Bass NM, et al. Liver transplantation for hepatocellular carcinoma: comparison of the proposed UCSF criteria with the Milan criteria and the Pittsburgh modified TNM criteria. Liver Transpl 2002;8:765–74.

62. Fleming ID, Cooper JS, Henson DE, et al. AJCC cancer staging manual. Philadelphia: Lippincott-Raven; 1997.

63. Staudacher C, Chiappa A, Biella F. Validation of the modified TNM-Izumi classification for hepatocellular carcinoma. Tumori 2000;86:8–11.

64. Marsh JW, Dvorchik I, Bonham CA, Iwatsuki S. Is the pathologic TNM staging system for patients with hepatoma predictive of outcome? Cancer 2000;88:538–43.

65. Okuda K, Ohtsuki T, Obata H, et al. Natural history of hepatocellular carcinoma and prognosis in relation to treatment. Cancer 1985;56:918–28.

66. The Cancer of the Liver Italian Program (CLIP) Investigators. A new prognostic system for hepatocellular carcinoma: a retrospective study of 435 patients. Hepatology 1998;28:751–5.

67. The Cancer of the Liver Italian Program (CLIP) Investigators. Prospective validation of the CLIP score: a new prognostic system for patients with cirrhosis and hepatocellular carcinoma. Hepatology 2000;31:840–5.

68. Levy I, Sherman M, the Liver Cancer Study Group of the University of Toronto. Staging of hepatocellular carcinoma: assessment of the CLIP, Okuda, and Child-Pugh staging systems in a cohort of 257 patients in Toronto. Gut 2002;50:881–5.

69. Farinati F, Rinaldi M, Gianni S, et al. How should patients with hepatocellular carcinoma be staged? Validation of a new prognostic system. Cancer 2000;89:2266–73.

70. Zhao WH, Ma ZM, Zhou XR, et al. Prediction of recurrence and prognosis in patients with hepatocellular carcinoma after resection by use of CLIP score. World J Gastroenterol 2002;8:237–42.

71. Cillo U, Bassanello M, Vitale A, et al. The critical issue of hepatocellular carcinoma prognostic classification: which is the best tool available? J Hepatol 2004;40:124–31.

72. Kudo M, Chung H, Osaki Y. Prognostic staging system for hepatocellular carcinoma (CLIP score): its value and limitations and a proposal for a new staging system, the Japan Integrated Staging score (JIS score). J Gastroenterol 2003;38:207–15.

73. Chevret S, Trinchet JC, Mathieu D, et al. A new prognostic classification for predicting survival in patients with hepatocellular carcinoma. J Hepatol 1999;31:133–41.

74. Leung TW, Tang AM, Zee B, et al. Construction of the Chinese University Prognostic Index for hepatocellular carcinoma and comparison with the TNM staging system, the Okuda staging system, and the Cancer of the Liver Italian Program staging system: a study based on 926 patients. Cancer 2002;94:1760–9.

75. Llovet JM, Bru C, Bruix J. Prognosis of hepatocellular carcinoma: the BCLC staging classification. Semin Liver Dis 1999;19:329–38.

76. Henderson JM, Sherman M, Tavill A, et al. AHPBA/AJCC consensus conference on staging of hepatocellular carcinoma: consensus statement. HPB 2003;5:243–50.

77. Llovet JM. Updated treatment approach to hepatocellular carcinoma. J Gastroenterol 2005;40:225–35.

78. Arii S, Yamaoka Y, Futagawa S, et al. Results of surgical and nonsurgical treatment for small-sized hepatocellular carcinomas: a retrospective and nationwide survey in Japan. Hepatology 2000;32:1224–9.

79. Bruix J, Castells A, Bosch J, et al. Surgical resection of hepatocellular carcinoma in cirrhotic patients: prognostic value of preoperative portal pressure. Gastroenterology 1996;111:1018–22.

80. Villeneuve JP, Arsene D, Huet PM. Assessment of liver function by the aminopyrine breath test. Clin Invest Med 1983;6:5–9.

81. Onodera Y, Takahashi K, Togashi T, et al. Clinical assessment of hepatic functional reserve using 99mTc DTPA galactosyl human serum albumin SPECT to prognosticate chronic hepatic diseases—validation of the use of SPECT and a new indicator. Ann Nucl Med 2003;17:181–8.

82. Fan ST, Lai EC, Lo CM, et al. Hospital mortality of major hepatectomy for hepatocellular carcinoma associated with cirrhosis. Arch Surg 1995;130:198–203.

83. Takayama T, Makuuchi S, Hirohashi S, et al. Early hepatocellular carcinoma as an entity with high rate of surgical cure. Hepatology 1998;28:1241–6.

84. Choti MA. Surgical management of hepatocellular carcinoma: resection and ablation. J Vasc Interv Radiol 2002;13:S197–203.

85. Llovet JM, Fuster J, Bruix J. Intention to treat analysis of surgical treatment for early hepatocellular carcinoma: resection versus transplantation. Hepatology 1999;30:1434–40.

86. Grazi GL, Cescon M, Ravaioli M, et al. Liver resection for hepatocellular carcinoma in cirrhotics and noncirrhotics. Evaluation of clinicopathologic features and comparison of risk factors for long-term survival and tumor recurrence in a single centre. Aliment Pharmacol Ther 2003;17 Suppl 2:119–29.

87. Ono T, Yamanoi A, Nazmy El Assal O, et al. Adjuvant chemotherapy after resection of hepatocellular carcinoma causes deterioration of long-term prognosis in cirrhotic patients: metaanalysis of three randomized controlled trials. Cancer 2001;91:2378–85.

88. Kwok PC, Lam TW, Lam PW, et al. Randomized controlled trial to compare the dose of adjuvant chemotherapy after curative resection of hepatocellular carcinoma. J Gastroenterol Hepatol 2003;18:450–5.

89. Wu CC, Ho YZ, Ho WL, et al. Preoperative transcatheter arterial chemoembolization for respectable large hepatocellular carcinoma: a reappraisal. Br J Surg 1995;82:122–6.

90. Lau WY, Leung TW, Ho SK, et al. Adjuvant intra-arterial iodine-131-labelled lipiodol for respectable hepatocellular carcinoma: a prospective randomized trial. Lancet 1999;353:797–801.

91. Boucher E, Corbinais S, Rolland Y, et al. Adjuvant intra-arterial injection of iodine-131-labeled lipiodol after resection of hepatocellular carcinoma. Hepatology 2003;38:1237–41.

92. Kubo S, Nishiguchi S, Hirohashi K, et al. Effects of long-term postoperative interferon-alfa therapy on intrahepatic recurrence after resection of hepatitis c virus-related hepatocellular carcinoma. Ann Intern Med 2001;134:963–7.

93. Ikeda K, Arase Y, Saitoh, S, et al. Interferon beta prevents recurrence of hepatocellular carcinoma after complete resection or ablation of the primary tumor—a prospective randomized study of hepatitis C virus related liver cancer. Hepatology 2000;32:228–32.

94. Bismuth H, Majno P, Adam R. Liver transplantation for hepatocellular carcinoma. Semin Liver Dis 1999;19:311–28.

95. Koneru B, Cassavilla A, Bowman J, et al. Liver transplantation for malignant tumors. Gastroenterol Clin North Am 1988;17:177–93.

96. Mazzaferro V, Regalia E, Doci R, et al. Liver transplantation for the treatment of small hepatocellular carcinomas in patients with cirrhosis. N Engl J Med 1996;334:693–9.

97. Lee J, Chu I, Heo J, et al. Classification and prediction of sur-

vival in hepatocellular carcinoma by gene expression profiling. Hepatology 2004;40:667–76.

98. Jonas S, Bechstein W, Steinmuller T, et al. Vascular invasion and histopathologic grading determine outcome after liver transplantation for hepatocellular carcinoma in cirrhosis. Hepatology 2001;33:1080–6.

99. Wiesner R, Freeman R, Mulligan D. Liver transplantation for hepatocellular carcinoma: the impact of the MELD allocation policy. Gastroenterology 2004;127:S261–7.

100. Yao F, Bass N, Nikolai B, et al. Liver transplantation for hepatocellular carcinoma: analysis of survival according to the intention-to-treat principle and dropout from the waiting list. Liver Transpl 2002;8:873–83.

101. Malinchoc M, Kamath P, Gordon, F, et al. A model to predict poor survival in patients undergoing transjugular intrahepatic portosystemic shunts. Hepatology 2000;31:864–71.

102. Majno PE, Adam R, Bismuth H, et al. Influence of preoperative transarterial lipiodol chemoembolization on resection and transplantation for hepatocellular carcinoma in patients with cirrhosis. Ann Surg 1997;226:688–701.

103. Mazzaferro V, Battiston C, Perrone S, et al. Radiofrequency ablation of small hepatocellular carcinoma in cirrhotic patients awaiting liver transplantation: a prospective study. Ann Surg 2004;240:900–9.

104. Roayaie S, Frischer J, Emre S, et al. Long-term results from multimodal adjuvant therapy and liver transplantation for the treatment of hepatocellular carcinomas larger than 5 centimeters. Ann Surg 2002;235:533–9.

105. Adult-to-adult living donor liver transplantation cohort study (A2ALL). Hepatology 2003;38:792.

106. Lencioni R, Cioni D, Crocetti L, et al. Percutaneous ablation of hepatocellular carcinoma: state-of-the-art. Liver Transpl 2004;10(2 Suppl 1):S91–7.

107. Shiina S, Tagawa K, Unuma T, et al. Percutaneous ethanol injection therapy for hepatocellular carcinoma: a histopathologic study. Cancer 1991;68:1524–30.

108. Giorgio A, Tarantino L, de Stefano G, et al. Ultrasound-guided percutaneous ethanol injection under general anesthesia for the treatment of hepatocellular carcinoma on cirrhosis: long-term results in 268 patients. Eur J Ultrasound 2000;12:145–54.

109. Di Stasi M, Buscarini L, Livraghi T, et al. Percutaneous ethanol injection in the treatment of hepatocellular carcinoma. A multicenter survey of evaluation practices and complication rates. Scand J Gastroenterol 1997;32:1168–73.

110. Shiina S, Tagawa K, Niwa Y, et al. Percutaneous ethanol injection therapy for hepatocellular carcinoma: results in 146 patients. AJR Am J Roentgenol 1993;160:1023–8.

111. Teratani T, Ishikawa T, Shiratori Y, et al. Hepatocellular carcinoma in elderly patients: beneficial therapeutic efficacy using percutaneous ethanol injection therapy. Cancer 2002;95:816–23.

112. Livraghi T, Bolondi L, Buscarini L, et al. No treatment, resection and ethanol injection in hepatocellular carcinoma: a retrospective analysis of survival in 391 patients with cirrhosis. Italian Cooperative HCC Study Group. J Hepatol 1995;22:522–6.

113. Shiina S, Teratani T, Obi S, et al. Nonsurgical treatment of hepatocellular carcinoma: from percutaneous ethanol injection therapy and percutaneous microwave coagula-

tion therapy to radiofrequency ablation. Oncology 2002; 62 Suppl 1:64–8.

114. Ohnishi K, Yoshioka H, Ito S, et al. Prospective randomized controlled trial comparing percutaneous acetic acid injection and percutaneous ethanol injection for small hepatocellular carcinoma. Hepatology 1998;27:67–72.

115. Huo TI, Huang YH, Wu JC, et al. Comparison of percutaneous acetic acid injection and percutaneous ethanol injection for hepatocellular carcinoma in cirrhotic patients: a prospective study. Scand J Gastroenterol 2003; 38:770–8.

116. Yoon HK, Song HY, Sung KB, et al. Percutaneous hot saline injection therapy: effectiveness in large hepatocellular carcinoma. J Vasc Interv Radiol 1999;10:477–82.

117. Goldberg SN, Gazelle GS, Mueller PR. Thermal ablation therapy for focal malignancies: a unified approach to underlying principles, techniques, and diagnostic imaging guidance. AJR Am J Roentgenol 2000;174:323–31.

118. Lencioni R, Goletti O, Armillotta N, et al. Radio-frequency thermal ablation of liver metastases with a cooled-tip electrode needle: results of a pilot clinical trial. Eur Radiol 1998;8:1205–11.

119. Rossi S, Buscarini E, Garbagnati F, et al. Percutaneous treatment of small hepatic tumors by an expandable RF electrode needle. AJR Am J Roentgenol 1998;170:1015–22.

120. Livragi T, Solbiati L, Meloni MF, et al. Treatment of focal liver tumors with percutaneous radio-frequency ablation: complications encountered in a multicenter study. Radiology 2003;226:441–51.

121. Rhim H, Dodd GD, Chintapalli KN, et al. Radiofrequency thermal ablation of abdominal tumors: lessons learned from complications. Radiographics 2004;24:41–52.

122. Lencioni R, Allgaier HP, Cioni D, et al. Small hepatocellular carcinoma in cirrhosis: randomized comparison of radiofrequency thermal ablation versus percutaneous ethanol injection. Radiology 2003;228:235–40.

123. Lencioni R, Cioni D, Crocetti L, et al. Early-stage hepatocellular carcinoma in cirrhosis: long-term results of percutaneous image-guided radiofrequency ablation. Radiology 2005;234:961–7.

124. Sato M, Watanabe Y, Ueda S, et al. Microwave coagulation therapy for hepatocellular carcinoma. Gastroenterology 1996;110:1507–14.

125. Lu MD, Chen JW, Xie XY, et al. Hepatocellular carcinoma: US-guided percutaneous microwave coagulation therapy. Radiology 2001;221:167–72.

126. Dong B, Liang P, Yu X, et al. Percutaneous sonographically guided microwave coagulation therapy for hepatocellular carcinoma: results in 234 patients. AJR Am J Roentgenol 2003;180:1547–55.

127. Seki T, Wakabayashi M, Nakagawa T, et al. Percutaneous microwave coagulation therapy for patients with small hepatocellular carcinoma: comparison with percutaneous ethanol injection therapy. Cancer 1999;85:1694–702.

128. Shibata T, Iimuro Y, Yamamoto Y, et al. Small hepatocellular carcinoma: comparison of radio-frequency ablation and percutaneous microwave coagulation therapy. Radiology 2002;223:331–7.

129. Bolondi L, Sofia S, Siringo S. et al. Surveillance programme of cirrhotic patients for early diagnosis and treatment of

hepatocellular carcinoma: a cost-effectiveness analysis. Gut 2001;48:251–9.

130. Konno T. Targeting cancer chemotherapeutic agents by use of lipiodol contrast medium. Cancer 1990;66:1897–903.

131. Bruix J, Sala M, Llovet JM. Chemoembolization for hepatocellular carcinoma. Gastroenterology 2004;127:S179–88.

132. Chan A, Yuen MF, Hui CK, et al. A prospective study regarding the complications of transcatheter intraarterial lipiodol chemoembolization in patients with hepatocellular carcinoma. Cancer 2002;94:1747–52.

133. Llovet JM, Bruix J. Systematic review of randomized trials for unresectable hepatocellular carcinoma: chemoembolization improves survival. Hepatology 2003;37:429–42.

134. Llovet JM, Real MI, Montana X, et al. Arterial embolisation or chemoembolisation versus symptomatic treatment in patients with unresectable hepatocellular carcinoma: a randomized controlled trial. Lancet 2002;359:1734–9.

135. Lo CM, Ngan H, Tso WK, et al. Randomized controlled trial of transarterial lipiodol chemoembolization for unresectable hepatocellular carcinoma. Hepatology 2002;35:1164–71.

136. Kamel IR, Bluemke DA, Ramsey D, et al. Role of diffusion-weighted imaging in estimating tumor necrosis after chemoembolization of hepatocellular carcinoma. AJR Am J Roentgenol 2003;181:708–10.

137. Morimoto M, Shirato K, Sugimori K, et al. Contrast-enhanced harmonic gray-scale sonographic-histologic correlation of the therapeutic effects of transcatheter arterial chemoembolization in patients with hepatocellular carcinoma. AJR Am J Roentgenol 2003;181:65–9.

138. Ho CL, Yu Sc, Yeung DW. ^{11}C-acetate PET imaging in hepatocellular carcinoma and other liver masses. J Nucl Med 2003;44:213–21.

139. Ng IO, Liu CL, Fan ST, et al. Expression of P-glycoprotein in hepatocellular carcinoma: a determinant of chemotherapy response. Am J Clin Pathol 2000;113:355–63.

140. Di Maio M, De Maio E, Perrone F, et al. Hepatocellular carcinoma: systemic treatments. J Clin Gastroenterol 2002;35:109–14.

141. Lai CL, Wu PC, Chan GC, et al. Doxorubicin versus no antitumor therapy in inoperable hepatocellular carcinoma. A prospective randomized trial. Cancer 1988;62:479–83.

142. Brans B, Van Lare K, Gemmel F, et al. Combining iodine-131 lipiodol therapy with low-dose cisplatin as a radiosensitiser: preliminary results in hepatocellular carcinoma. Eur J Nucl Med Mol Imaging 2002;29:928–32.

143. Lu YS, Hsu C, Li CC, et al. Phase II study of combination doxorubicin, interferon-alpha and high-dose tamoxifen treatment for advanced hepatocellular carcinoma. Hepatogastroenterology 2004;51:815–9.

144. Pignata S, Daniele B, Gallo C, et al. Endocrine treatment of hepatocellular carcinoma. Any evidence of benefit? Eur J Cancer 1998:34:25–32.

145. Simonetti RG, Liberati A, Angiolini C, et al. Treatment of hepatocellular carcinoma: a systematic review of randomized controlled trials. Ann Oncol 1997; 8:117–36.

146. Chao Y, Chan WK, Wang SS, et al. Phase II study of megestrol acetate in the treatment of hepatocellular carcinoma. J Gastroenterol Hepatol 1997;12:277–81.

147. Villa E, Ferretti I, Grottola A, et al. Hormonal therapy with megestrol in inoperable hepatocellular carcinoma characterized by variant oestrogen receptors. Br J Cancer 2001; 84:881–5.

148. Manesis EK, Giannoulis G, Zoumboulis P, et al. Treatment of hepatocellular carcinoma with combined suppression and inhibition of sex hormones: a randomized controlled trial. Hepatology 1995;21:1535–42.

149. Kouroumalis E, Skordilis P, Thermos K, et al. Treatment of hepatocellular carcinoma with octreotide: a randomised controlled study. Gut 1998;42:442–7.

150. Yuen MF, Poon RT, Lai CL, et al. A randomized placebo-controlled study of long-acting octreotide for the treatment of advanced hepatocellular carcinoma. Hepatology 2002;36:687–91.

17

Simian Virus 40 and Human Malignancy

ERIC A. ENGELS

The potential for animal viruses to cross over into humans and cause severe disease is an important public health topic. The development of modern medicine has led to opportunities for animal-to-human transmission of infectious agents through the use of animal tissues in the production of medical products, including vaccines. Simian virus 40 (SV40), a macaque polyomavirus, was present as a contaminant in poliovirus vaccines used widely throughout the world during the 1950s and early 1960s.

There is presently substantial research and public health interest regarding whether human exposures to SV40 through contaminated vaccines or other routes have led to an increase in cancer. Multiple lines of evidence bear on this question, and the data are complex and at times inconsistent. Laboratory data show that SV40 is capable of transforming and immortalizing cells in tissue culture and is able to induce malignancies in experimental animals. Furthermore, multiple reports in recent years have described the molecular detection of SV40 DNA in human tumor tissues of various types, most notably mesothelioma, brain tumors, bone sarcomas, and non-Hodgkin's lymphoma (NHL). These studies directly raise the possibility that SV40 is a cause of cancer in humans. However, other studies have not found SV40 DNA in human tumors, and interpreting results from these various studies is challenging. Another major line of evidence, pointing away from SV40 as a cause of cancer, derives from epidemiologic studies. Epidemiologic studies have not found an increased risk of cancer in recipients of SV40-contaminated vaccines, nor have they found an increased prevalence of exposure to or infection with SV40 among individuals with cancer.

A critical review of available data can serve to frame the issues in this unsettled research area. The following sections review the laboratory and epidemiologic data in detail and discuss their strengths and weaknesses. In the concluding sections, a framework is presented for considering these data in the context of causality: do the data together indicate that SV40 is a cause of cancer in humans? Avenues for future research are also discussed.

EXPERIMENTAL EVIDENCE FOR SV40 AS A CANCER-CAUSING VIRUS

The replication of SV40 and steps leading to transformation and immortalization of infected cells have been reviewed in detail elsewhere.[1] The DNA genome of SV40, like other polyomaviruses, is relatively short (5,000 base pairs) and encodes few genes, which can be classified as "early" or "late" based on the timing of their expression during infection. The early portion of the SV40 genome encodes two proteins, large T antigen and small t antigen, so named because sera from animals with SV40-induced *tumors* react with these proteins. The T antigen and t antigen proteins act to increase the production of cellular enzymes necessary for DNA replication and stimulate the cell, if resting, to reenter the cell cycle. These steps facilitate the replication of viral DNA. The late genes of SV40 encode for the viral capsid proteins VP1, VP2, and VP3. These genes are expressed efficiently only after the start of viral DNA replication. The coordinated expression of early and late viral gene proteins, leading to efficient DNA replication, virion assembly, cell lysis, and release of virus progeny, is termed "productive" viral infection (Figure 17–1). Cells supporting productive infection are said to be "permissive." Macaque cells are permissive for SV40 replication.

In contrast, nonproductive infection occurs when viral replication does not proceed to completion, such as in rodent cells.[1] Nonproductive infection arises when the T antigen cannot interact effectively with cellular replication factors. Although virions are not produced under such conditions, T antigen still stimulates cell cycling and proliferation. Importantly, T antigen binds to and inactivates the protein products of two cellular tumor suppressor genes, *TP53* and *pRb*. These actions facilitate cell division and prevent apoptosis. If episomal SV40 DNA does not also replicate in conjunction with the dividing cells, then the viral genome and the SV40 T antigen will eventually be lost from the cells, causing proliferation to cease. However, at a low frequency, SV40 DNA can become integrated into the host genome and be passed constitutionally with the cellular DNA into daughter cells with continuing cell division (see Figure 17–1).

The continued expression of T antigen in cells with integrated SV40 DNA is responsible for development of a "transformed" phenotype; that is, the proliferation of cells under normally adverse conditions. Transformed cells will grow to an abnormally great density, piling close upon one another. Additionally, cells with this phenotype may become "immortalized"; that is, they continue replication for an indefinite number of doublings, when normally they would stop dividing after a limited number of cycles. The transformation and immortalization of nonpermissive cells by SV40 provide a model for how SV40 can cause malignancy in animals. Indeed, SV40 is not known to cause malignancy in macaque species, since cells from these animals support productive infection. In contrast, SV40 can cause malignancies of various types in experimental rodents whose cells are nonpermissive.

Experimental data regarding the effects of SV40 on human cell lines support the possibility that SV40 could cause cancer in humans. Although many human cell types are readily infected and lysed by SV40, and are thus permissive for infection, other cell types (eg, fibroblasts) can be transformed by SV40.[2] However, the efficiency of transformation is somewhat lower for human cells than for rodent cells, a type of infection sometimes termed "semipermissive."[3] Recently, Bocchetta and colleagues described the efficient transformation of human mesothelial cells by SV40, which would be consistent with the hypothesis that SV40 may cause mesothelioma.[4] On the other hand, Shaikh and col-

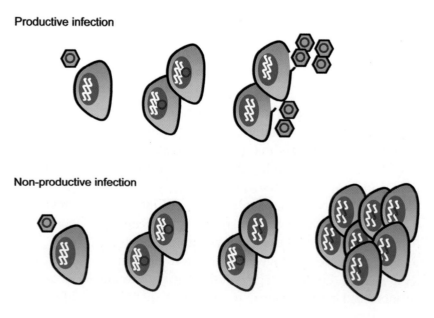

Figure 17–1. Productive and nonproductive infection by simian virus 40 (SV40). Cells are depicted as *pink ovals* with *blue* nuclei. Under productive infection, SV40 virions (shown as *green hexagons*) infect cells permissive for the entire replication cycle of the virus. SV40 T antigen, expressed early in replication, activates the cell cycle and causes replication of the SV40 genome (shown as a *red circle*) and production of viral structural proteins. This eventually leads to lysis of the infected cells and release of progeny virions. During nonproductive infection, early SV40 infection still leads to activation of the cell cycle and cell division. However, the complete replication cycle of SV40 is not supported, and virions are not produced. Rather, the incorporation of SV40 DNA into cellular genomic DNA (in the figure, human DNA is depicted as irregular *white lines* in the nucleus of the cell, whereas SV40 DNA is depicted as a *short red segment*) leads to the continued expression of T antigen, continued cell division, and the phenotypic characteristics of transformation and immortalization.

Productive infection

Non-productive infection

leagues were unable to demonstrate that SV40 can infect human lymphocytes, arguing against a direct role for this virus in human lymphomas.[5]

The inoculation of SV40 into laboratory rodents induces several malignancies. In 1961, Eddy and colleagues described the induction of soft tissue sarcomas in newborn hamsters injected subcutaneously with extracts of monkey kidney cells.[6] Sweet and Hilleman reported the isolation of SV40 in the same year, and Eddy and her colleagues subsequently demonstrated that the tumor-causing agent in their extracts was indeed SV40.[7,8] Other studies later showed that SV40 infection of hamsters can lead to ependymoma, lymphoma and leukemia, and mesothelioma.[9–11] Implantation into hamsters of SV40-tranformed cells also induces the development of large tumors.[12]

As will be discussed in more detail below, several aspects of these experimental studies in animals are relevant in considering the potential for SV40 to act as a human carcinogen. First, in some experimental models of SV40-induced carcinogenesis, SV40 was injected in extremely high inocula and by unique routes, directly into the tissue of interest. For example, ependymomas in newborn hamsters followed direct inoculation of 10 million median tissue culture infective dose ($TCID_{50}$) units of SV40 directly into the brain ($TCID_{50}$ corresponds to the dose at which 50% of monkey kidney cells would be infected in tissue culture).[9] Similarly, mesothelioma in hamsters arose in the lining of the heart, lung, or abdominal organs following direct inoculation of 200 million or more plaque-forming units of SV40 into these sites.[11] The dose was clearly important. In one experiment, 96% of newborn hamsters developed tumors when inoculated with 320,000 $TCID_{50}$ units of SV40, 18% when inoculated with 3,200 $TCID_{50}$ units, and 0% when inoculated with only 32 $TCID_{50}$ units.[13] Humans who were exposed to SV40 via contaminated vaccines received only low levels of SV40, which might have been insufficient to induce cancer (see "Epidemiology of SV40 Infection in Humans," below).

A second relevant observation from animal experiments is that the occurrence of cancer was related to the age at SV40 infection. In one experiment, cancer developed in 96% of hamsters infected with SV40 in the neonatal period, in 60% of those

infected at 7 days of age, in 23% of those infected at 1 month of age, and in 0% of those infected at 3 months of age.[13] A third observation is that SV40 T antigen expression was detected within each tumor cell, consistent with the presence of viral DNA in each tumor cell; that is, chromosomal integration of SV40.[10,12,14] Finally, animals with SV40-induced tumors produced measurable antibody responses to SV40 viral capsids and T antigen.[10,15,16]

In 1964, Jensen and colleagues reported on an experiment in humans that might not be considered ethical today but also bears on the question of whether SV40 could cause cancer in humans.[17] With the purpose of evaluating "the neoplastic character of the SV40-transformed human cultures," 79 patients with "terminal cancer" received subcutaneous implantation or inoculation of several types of transformed cells (including human cells transformed by SV40), SV40-infected but untransformed cells, or normal cells. Most notably, 8 patients received SV40-infected cells derived from cultures of their own skin or buccal mucosa. Of the 6 individuals inoculated with SV40-infected cells that had not yet manifested transformation in culture, none developed a nodule or an inflammatory response at the site of implantation. However, the two other patients who received implants of their own cells transformed by SV40 developed subcutaneous nodules, characterized histologically as sarcomas. Both of these nodules resolved spontaneously, in one case accompanied by a vigorous local inflammatory response. Although this study by Jensen and colleagues highlights the potential oncogenic role for SV40 in humans, it is noteworthy that tumors did not arise in the patients who were injected with untransformed cells, and that SV40-induced tumors resolved in the two others, at least one of whom developed an effective host response. Thus, the study results could be interpreted to indicate that if humans were to be infected with SV40, the host response could prevent the development of SV40-induced malignancies.

In summary, the available experimental data indicate that SV40 is a transforming virus in nonpermissive cells or, less effectively, in semipermissive cells. Furthermore, SV40 can cause malignancies in experimental rodents, although sometimes under conditions in which high viral inocula are injected directly into the tissue in question. Based on the study by Jensen and colleagues, it is not clear that SV40 infection in humans could readily cause cancer.[17] Nonetheless, the experimental studies in animals have led to several predictions for studies in humans. First, infection early in life, such as through childhood exposure to SV40-contaminated vaccines, might be expected to be associated with an especially high cancer risk. Second, the integration of SV40 DNA into host chromosomes in malignant cells would lead to the expectation that SV40 would be present in each cell in human tumors. Finally, one would predict that individuals with SV40-induced malignancies would make readily detectable antibodies to SV40-expressed proteins.

LABORATORY STUDIES OF DETECTION OF SV40 DNA IN HUMAN TUMORS

Reports on the detection of SV40 DNA in human cancers date back at least to 1981.[18] However, a 1992 study by Bergsagel and colleagues represents the first investigation to use the polymerase chain reaction (PCR), a technique that uses specific pairs of primers to amplify target DNA fragments from biologic samples.[19] PCR methods form a cornerstone of modern experimental methods for detecting viral signatures in human specimens. PCR is highly sensitive, typically detecting as few as 10 copies of the target sequence. Additionally, PCR has relatively low cost, and the techniques are widely available in clinical and basic science laboratories. For these reasons, PCR techniques have been applied extensively to the study of SV40 in human cancer following the Bergsagel report, as reviewed below.

Based on experimental data in animals showing that polyomaviruses can induce brain tumors, Bergsagel and colleagues tested archived ependymomas and choroid plexus tumors obtained from US children.[19] The investigators initially used a set of PCR primers capable of amplifying T antigen sequences from SV40 and from the related human polyomaviruses BK and JC. They noted that several brain tumor specimens had amplifiable T antigen DNA that hybridized most strongly with an SV40 DNA probe, and direct sequencing of two samples

confirmed that the PCR product corresponded to the SV40 T antigen gene. Some of these specimens may have had SV40 at very low levels, because results were intermittently positive in repeated experiments and with varying PCR primers. Nonetheless, using a PCR primer set designated as SV.for3/SV.rev (where "for" and "rev" stand for forward and reverse, respectively), Bergsagel and colleagues reported amplification of SV40 T antigen sequences in 10 of 11 (91%) ependymomas, 10 of 20 (50%) choroid plexus tumors, and only 1 of 19 (5%) control tissues (consisting of neuroblastoma tumors and non-neoplastic brain tissue).

Since the study by Bergsagel and colleagues, other investigators have attempted to replicate the detection of SV40 in human ependymomas and choroid plexus tumors.[19-27] Detection rates have varied widely (0 to 91% for ependymoma, 0 to 83% for choroid plexus tumors; Table 17–1). Reconciling these diverse results has proven difficult and requires a careful consideration of the studies' laboratory methods and findings (see Table 17–1). Four studies from Austria and Germany (where SV40-contaminated poliovirus vaccines would have been the likely route of SV40 exposure) and India (where SV40 infections might have occurred through contacts with macaques) produced negative results.[20-23] A Finnish study was also negative, but this could have been due to a lack of poliovirus vaccine contamination in Finland.[24] In two negative studies, all of the specimens were fixed in formalin, which might have degraded the DNA and hindered PCR amplification.[21,23] However, two other studies used fresh frozen tissues and yielded negative results, and other studies using only formalin-fixed tissues produced positive results.[20,22,26,27]

It is also possible that the positive results in some studies were due to laboratory artifact.[19,25-27] SV40 DNA sequences are present in hundreds of cloning vectors used by laboratories worldwide, which could lead to low-level PCR contamination of specimens or reagents.[28] In this regard, one positive study did not include negative control tissues, and none described masked extraction and testing of specimens.[26] In one study, SV40 DNA was found in a wide range of tumor types and normal cells, and almost all specimens also had detectable BK virus

DNA, calling into question the specificity of testing.[25] Finally, none of the positive studies quantified the amount of SV40 DNA present in tumor specimens. Indeed, one study repeated the PCR cycling to increase sensitivity, which would have increased the likelihood of amplification and detection of low-level contaminants.[25]

Aside from ependymoma and choroid plexus tumors, SV40 DNA has been detected in other malignancies (Table 17–2). Mesothelioma, brain tumors, and NHL have been the most studied, but a diverse set of other types is represented. Notably, although this spectrum of cancers resembles those induced by SV40 in rodents, it also includes others (such as lung cancer and breast cancer) for which there is no corresponding animal model. This lack of specificity of association raises questions about an etiologic relationship between SV40 and cancer.[29] It seems implausible that SV40 causes all of the malignancies noted in Table 17–2, yet it is unclear how to distinguish etiologic from non-etiologic findings. Similarly, other studies reported detection of SV40 DNA across a range of normal tissues.[25,30,31] Without clearly negative findings for normal tissues, assigning an interpretation to the amplification of SV40 DNA from other specimens is problematic.

The extensive literature reporting on the PCR-based detection of SV40 in mesothelioma is especially challenging to synthesize. The principal cause of mesothelioma is asbestos, to which males were heavily exposed in occupational settings in the 1940s to 1970s. In 1994, Carbone and colleagues described the PCR-based detection of SV40 DNA in 29 of 48 (60%) mesothelioma specimens from the United States.[32] This report was followed by dozens of studies conducted in multiple laboratories, using specimens predominantly obtained in North America and Europe.[33] PCR detection rates in these studies have ranged extremely widely, from 0 to 86%.[34,35]

It is unlikely that geographic differences in the source of the mesothelioma specimens explain all of the variability manifested in the results reported for mesothelioma.[33] Rather, as for studies of brain tumors (see Table 17–1), some of the differences probably arise from differences in laboratory methods or quality control of PCR procedures. For example, many studies did not include appropriate normal

Table 17–1. STUDIES REPORTING ON PCR DETECTION OF SV40 IN HUMAN EPENDYMOMAS AND CHOROID PLEXUS TUMORS

Study (Reference)	Country	No. Positive/ No. Tested (%)*	PCR Primers‡	PCR Cycles	Tissue Type†	Negative Controls/ Masking§	Quantification of SV40 DNA
Bergsagel et al, 1992[19]	United States	E: 10/11 (91), C: 10/20 (50)	SV.for3 / SV.rev	45–60	Fresh, formalin	Yes / No	No
Krainer et al, 1995[21]	Austria	E: 0/10 (0)	SVO.for /SVO.rev (SV.for3 / SV.rev nested)	45–60	Formalin	No / No	No
Martini et al, 1996[25]	Italy	E: 8/11 (73), C: 5/6 (83)	PYV.for / PYV.rev	35–105	Fresh, formalin	Yes / No	No
Suzuki et al, 1997[27]	Japan	E: 4/13 (31)	SV.for2/SV.rev	45	Formalin	Yes / No	No
Huang et al, 1999[26]	Switzerland	E: 9/16 (56), C: 6/16 (38)	SVTAGP1 / P2, SVTAGP1 / P3	45	Formalin	No / No	No
Ohgaki et al, 2000[24]	Finland	E: 0/10 (0), C: 0/7 (0)	SVTAGP1 / P2, SVTAGP1 / P3	45	ND	No / No	No
Weggen et al, 2000[20]	Germany	E: 2/27 (7)	SV.for3 /SV.rev, LA1 / LA2	40	Fresh	Yes / No	No
Reuther et al, 2001[22]	Germany	E: 3/62 (5)	SV.for3 /SV.rev, RA1 / RA2	36	Fresh, formalin	No / No	No
Engels et al, 2002[23]	India	E: 0/33 (0), C: 0/14 (0)	SV.for3 / SV.rev	50	Formalin	Yes / Yes	Yes

DNA = deoxyribonucleic acid; PCR = polymerase chain reaction; SV40 = simian virus 40.
*Entries are for ependymoma (E) and choroid plexus tumors (C).
†See Bergsagel DJ et al[19] and Reuther FJ et al[22] for descriptions of PCR primer pairs.
‡Tissue type: fresh = fresh frozen; formalin = formalin-fixed paraffin-embedded; ND = not described.
§Negative controls = inclusion of biologic tissues as negative control; masking = documentation that both extraction of DNA and PCR were done under masked conditions.
Adapted from Engels EA et al.[23]

Table 17–2. MOLECULAR DETECTION OF SV40 DNA IN HUMAN NEOPLASMS

Neoplasm	Representative Studies Reporting Detection of SV40 DNA	Detection Rate in Representative Studies (%)
Brain tumors/neural tumors		
Ependymoma	Bergsagel et al, 1992[19]	91
Choroid plexus tumor	Bergsagel et al, 1992[19]	50
Astrocytoma/glioma	Huang et al, 1999[26]; Martini et al, 1996[25]	11–59
Medulloblastoma	Huang et al, 1999[26]; Krynska et al,1999[101]	22–29
Meningioma	Martini et al, 1996[25]; Arrington et al, 2004[102]	14
Mesothelioma	Carbone et al,1994[32]	60
Non-Hodgkin's lymphomas		
Diffuse large B-cell lymphoma	Vilchez et al, 2002[38]; Shivapurkar et al, 2002[103]	45–48
Burkitt's lymphoma	Vilchez et al, 2002[38]; Shivapurkar et al, 2002[103]	35–100
Follicular lymphoma	Vilchez et al, 2002[38]; Shivapurkar et al, 2002[103]	31–46
Mantle cell lymphoma	Shivapurkar et al, 2002[103]	50
Small lymphocytic lymphoma	Martini et al, 1998[44]	17
T-cell lymphoma	Shivapurkar et al, 2002[103]	27
AIDS-related lymphoma	Vilchez et al, 2002; Shivapurkar et al, 2002[103]	33–46
Posttransplant lymphoproliferative disorder	Rizzo et al, 1999[104]	24
Hodgkin's lymphoma	Shivapurkar et al, 2002[103]; Martini et al, 1998[44]	9–16
Sarcomas		
Osteosarcoma	Carbone et al, 1996[51]	32
Chondrosarcoma	Carbone et al, 1996[51]	27
Ewing's sarcoma	Martini et al, 2002[31]	21
Giant cell tumor	Carbone et al, 1996[51]; Martini et al, 2002[31]	67–80
Nonsmall cell lung cancer	Galateau-Salle et al, 1998[36]	29
Breast cancer	Shivapurkar et al, 2002[103]	10
Papillary thyroid cancer	Vivaldi et al, 2003[105]	66
Medullary thyroid cancer	Vivaldi et al, 2003[105]	90
Hepatoblastoma	Shivapurkar et al, 2002[103]	7
Wilm's tumor	Martini et al, 2002[31]	25

AIDS = acquired immune deficiency syndrome; SV40 = simian virus 40.
The table includes malignant and benign neoplasms for which SV40 DNA has been detected by molecular methods from two or more cases.

tissues as negative controls.[33] The need for such negative controls was highlighted by results of one study, which found SV40 DNA sequences in 48% of mesothelioma specimens, 29% of lung cancer specimens (various histologic types), and 13% of normal lung tissues.[36] The high frequency of SV40 DNA detection in normal lung tissues calls into question the specificity of the PCR testing.

Only one study of mesothelioma used quantitative PCR methods to estimate the amount of SV40 in tumor tissues.[37] In that study, based in the United States, SV40 DNA was detected in only two mesothelioma specimens (6%), at a level below one SV40 genome copy per 134 cells.[37] Because animal models suggest that SV40 DNA is integrated into host chromosomes and thus present in each tumor cell, such low-level detection raises problems for an etiologic interpretation of the detection of SV40 DNA in human tumors.

Some laboratories have sequenced PCR products to confirm the detection of SV40 in the tumor tissues. Sequencing of the T antigen region can distinguish between SV40, BK, and JC.[19,38] Furthermore, whereas commonly used laboratory strains of SV40 contain a duplicated 72–base pair enhancer in the regulatory region of the genome, some sequences amplified from human tissues contain only a single copy of the enhancer.[39,40] Additionally, variability in sequences amplified from the carboxy-terminal domain of the T antigen gene has been described.[38–40] Interestingly, Vilchez and colleagues reported the amplification of DNA from the carboxy-terminal of the SV40 T antigen gene from NHL tumors that was similar to a sequence found in a vial of poliovirus vaccine preserved from 1955.[38] In contrast, others have reported that amplified SV40 sequences were identical to the sequences found in laboratory strains.[31,41] Although reported differences among SV40 sequences amplified from human tumors and other tissues argue against PCR contamination as a ready explanation for detection of SV40 DNA, the lack of standardized methods for SV40 DNA detection and inconsistent results across laboratories have precluded a definitive conclusion.

The difficulties in study interpretation arising from the lack of standardized molecular methods and poor assay reproducibility were highlighted in a multi-institutional study of mesothelioma.[42] Nine laboratories jointly participated in a masked evaluation of DNA extracts, which were all prepared in a single central laboratory. Eight of the testing laboratories used a common set of PCR primers (SV5/SV6) previously reported to detect SV40 DNA in mesothelioma, and several also used their own PCR assays; the remaining laboratory performed Southern blot analyses without PCR amplification. Under blinded conditions, the laboratories each evaluated DNA from the same 25 mesothelioma specimens (each of which was provided in duplicate) and 25 normal lung tissues, along with positive and negative controls. One testing laboratory detected SV40 DNA in 40% of mesothelioma specimens. However, this laboratory also found SV40 DNA in 28% of normal lung specimens, and almost all of the SV40-positive mesothelioma specimens in that laboratory were positive in only 1 of the 2 duplicates. These anomalous results were attributed to SV40 DNA contamination of PCR primers in this laboratory. In other laboratories, SV40 DNA detection was more sporadic: < 10% of mesothelioma specimens were positive in all but one laboratory, which had a detection rate of 24%. Importantly, PCR detection results were inconsistent, both across duplicates within the same testing laboratory and across laboratories. The low prevalence of SV40 DNA detection was not likely due to inadequate assay sensitivity, since most laboratories could detect as few as 5 to 50 copies of SV40 DNA when present in control specimens. Notably, one entire batch of negative-control specimens was contaminated with SV40 in the central processing laboratory, leading to widespread positive results for this batch in the testing laboratories.

As demonstrated in this multicenter study, PCR contamination, introduced in either the processing or testing stages, can occur readily and lead to artifactual results.[42] Without the masking of laboratory investigators and inclusion of multiple types of negative and positive controls, it is possible that such artifacts could be interpreted as indicating actual detection of SV40 DNA in tumor specimens. Unfortunately, as noted above, many molecular studies have not incorporated such careful designs.

Recently, Lopez-Rios and colleagues provided additional data regarding the possibility of PCR contamination as an explanation for the many reported detections of SV40 DNA.[43-45] Using two sets of PCR primers located in the T-antigen region of SV40 (SV5–SV6 and SV5–SV6b), these investigators amplified SV40 DNA sequences from 56 to 62% of mesothelioma specimens. However, they observed that their results were inconsistent across experiments, and that the negative-control specimens were occasionally positive as well. Lopez-Rios and colleagues then realized that their PCR primers would also be expected to amplify SV40 sequences that had previously been incorporated into multiple cloning vectors.[43] In response, they selected alternative PCR primers from a region of SV40 not present in these plasmids (SVINT.for and SVINT.rev, from an intron region of T antigen). Using these primers, only 6% of mesotheliomas were positive for SV40 DNA, and the amount of SV40 appeared very low. In a last experiment, they also used primers that spanned two discontinuous regions of SV40 DNA that had been artificially joined together in the construction of plasmids. This set of PCR primers amplified SV40 sequences in 36% of mesothelioma specimens. Remarkably, however, in each case of amplification, SV40 DNA was of the length predicted by the joining together of the two distant regions in the plasmids, rather than corresponding to the much longer sequence, including the intervening region, that would have been amplified from SV40 itself. Finally, the investigators reviewed prior published studies on SV40 DNA detection in mesothelioma and noted that reported detection rates for SV40 DNA were consistently higher using "high-risk" primers (those that would be predicted also to amplify cloning vector DNA) than using "low-risk" primers (those targeting DNA not included in vectors). The authors concluded that the inconsistent low-level detection of SV40 DNA in mesothelioma specimens in their laboratory, and perhaps in other laboratories, was likely the result of contamination of PCR reagents or tissue specimens by cloning vectors. The study by Lopez-Rios and colleagues represents the first rigorous attempt to account for the perplexing phenomenon of widespread but inconsistent detection of SV40 DNA across laboratories.[43]

In principle, immunohistochemistry methods could provide supportive evidence for the presence of SV40 in human malignancies by visually demonstrating the presence and physical location of SV40 proteins within tumor cells. Immunohistochemical staining for SV40 T antigen has been performed in studies covering a range of tumors, such as choroid plexus tumors and ependymomas, mesothelioma, NHL, and bone sarcomas.[19,32,41,46,47] Although these experiments have been interpreted as supporting the presence of SV40 in these types of human cancers, there are several caveats. First, immunohistochemistry photomicrographs have not always reproduced well in journal publications, complicating the formation of independent assessments. Second, although T antigen staining in animal tumors is present in all tumor cells and exclusively displays a nuclear pattern, staining in human tumor specimens appears to be more variable in terms of the proportion of cells staining positive (< 1 to 50%) and the location (nucleus or cytoplasm) of the staining.[10–12,14] Third, there has not been complete concordance of PCR and immunohistochemistry results, with some tumors appearing positive by one method but not by another.[19,32] Finally, questions about the specificity of antibodies used in some immunohistochemistry experiments were raised by Pilatte and colleagues, who found a previously unidentified protein contaminating two different commercially available monoclonal antibodies against SV40 T antigen (Ab-1 and pAb-101).[48] As these investigators demonstrated, this contaminating protein can generate false-positive cytoplasmic staining of SV40-negative cells. These antibodies had been used previously in some of the studies that reported T antigen staining of human tumor specimens.[32,41,44] Lopez-Rios and colleagues also noted nonspecific cytoplasmic staining of mesothelioma tissues using a commercially available antibody.[43]

Together, these considerations raise questions about the validity of published immunohistochemical staining results on human tumors.

Interesting data suggesting a role for SV40 in human cancer were provided in a study of individuals with Li-Fraumeni syndrome.[49] Li-Fraumeni syndrome is characterized by the early onset and familial clustering of characteristic malignancies (sarcomas, breast cancer, adrenocortical carcinoma, brain tumors, and leukemia). The syndrome is due to inheritance of a defective *TP53* tumor suppressor gene. Individuals develop cancer when a somatic cell loses the remaining normal *TP53* allele because of a mutation (termed "loss of *TP53* heterozygosity"). In some instances, however, tumors do not exhibit loss of the second *TP53* allele, indicating that other mechanisms are involved. Malkin and colleagues studied two children with Li-Fraumeni syndrome.[49] The first child developed a rhabdomyosarcoma and a choroid plexus tumor, but only the rhabdomyosarcoma exhibited loss of *TP53* heterozygosity. The second child developed a choroid plexus tumor and renal cell carcinoma, neither of which showed loss of *TP53* heterozygosity, as well as an osteosarcoma (not evaluable for loss of *TP53* heterozygosity). Interestingly, SV40 DNA sequences were detected by PCR in both the choroid plexus tumors and the renal cell carcinoma, whereas SV40 sequences were not detected in the rhabdomyosarcoma. Immunohistochemistry studies using an antibody against T antigen revealed punctate nuclear and cytoplasmic staining of a minority of tumor cells in the PCR-positive tumors. These data suggest that SV40 can contribute to development of cancer in Li-Fraumeni patients, via T antigen inactivation of TP53 protein (which is presumably expressed at relatively low levels because of the constitutional presence of only a single normal copy of the *TP53* gene). Although provocative, these conclusions are based on a small number of tumors and limited by some of the same considerations raised above.

A final perplexing aspect of some PCR-based studies has been the reported detection of SV40 DNA in individuals too young to have received poliovirus vaccines contaminated with SV40 (last present in vaccines in 1962).[19,38,49–51] Taken at face value, these reports suggest that there are additional routes of SV40 infection, perhaps including direct person-to-person transmission. However, given the difficulties with interpretation of PCR-based studies, it has not been possible to conclude from these studies that such transmission has occurred or is ongoing. Evidence regarding the prevalence of SV40 infection in humans and routes of transmission is reviewed in the next section.

EPIDEMIOLOGY OF SV40 INFECTION IN HUMANS

Vaccine-Related Exposures to SV40

The conquest of poliomyelitis in developed countries represents one of the great public health accomplishments of the twentieth century. A cornerstone of the program of eradication of poliomyelitis in these nations was the development of poliovirus vaccines and their deployment in large-scale vaccination campaigns beginning in the 1950s. These poliovirus vaccines, produced in kidney tissue cells harvested from macaques, also represented the most widespread, generally recognized route of exposure of humans to SV40.

In the United States, the majority of poliovirus vaccine used during the 1950s and early 1960s was a parenterally administered formalin-inactivated poliovirus vaccine (IPV) developed by Jonas Salk and colleagues. IPV was field-tested in 1954 in an enormous field trial involving over 400,000 US schoolchildren. Following its reported success in preventing poliomyelitis, IPV was licensed in early 1955. By July 1955, IPV had been administered to 6 million US schoolchildren. Over time, as more vaccine became available, vaccination campaigns with IPV were implemented much more widely, involving additional age groups. By 1957, 60 million people under the age of 50 years had received one or more doses of IPV. As of September 1961, 98 million people under the age of 60 years (62% of the population in that age range) had received at least one dose, and many had received multiple doses (Table 17–3).[52] For children under the age of 20 years, who were especially targeted by public health officials, 88% had received at least one dose and nearly 50% had received at least four doses of IPV.

Oral poliovirus vaccine (OPV) was a live vaccine developed by several research groups led by Albert Sabin, Herald Cox, and Hilary Koprowski. OPV was not used widely in the United States until 1963, when the Sabin vaccine was first licensed. Nonetheless, OPV was used in the United States in several field trials before 1963 (eg, in Florida, Louisiana, Minnesota, and Ohio).[53] For example, Flipse and colleagues described the vaccination of over 400,000 children and young adults with OPV in 1960 in Dade County, Florida.[54] From 1960 to 1962, OPV was also

		Percentage Vaccinated, by No. of Doses*					Population Prevalence of SV40 Exposure, by Frequency of SV40 Contamination in IPV Doses†		
Age (Years)	Population (Millions)	1	2	3	4+	Any Doses	10% Doses	20% Doses	30% Doses
0	4.3	13.1	18.8	19.7	3.4	55.0	11%	21%	29%
1–4	16.8	3.7	9.2	32.3	42.0	87.2	25%	45%	59%
5–9	19.7	2.0	4.8	24.9	61.6	93.3	29%	51%	66%
10–14	18.0	1.6	4.5	29.3	58.1	93.5	29%	51%	66%
15–19	13.6	1.9	5.9	32.5	43.9	84.2	25%	44%	58%
Total, children	72.4	2.9	6.7	28.8	49.7	88.1	26%	46%	61%
20–29	21.1	3.0	8.2	24.4	28.0	63.6	18%	32%	42%
30–39	23.5	3.1	6.8	20.9	24.1	54.9	16%	27%	36%
40–49	22.5	2.3	4.1	11.7	10.6	28.7	8%	14%	19%
50–59	18.4	1.1	1.7	4.5	2.9	10.2	3%	5%	6%
Total	157.9	2.6	5.9	21.8	31.9	62.2	18%	32%	42%

Table 17–3. EXPOSURE OF US POPULATION TO PRE-1963 INACTIVATED POLIOVIRUS VACCINE AND SV40

IPV = inactivated poliovirus vaccine; SV40 = simian virus 40.
*Data are the cumulative percentage of the US population vaccinated with inactivated poliovirus vaccine, as of September 1961. Data are from Communicable Disease Center.[50]
†Table entries are the prevalence of SV40 exposure resulting from receipt of one or more doses of SV40-contaminated inactivated poliovirus vaccine, calculated from the number of doses of vaccine received and various hypothesized contamination rates of the vaccine.

given to neonates in much smaller vaccine immunogenicity trials.[55] During this early period of poliovirus vaccination, OPV was used extensively in the Soviet Union, Eastern Europe, and Africa.

Poliovirus grown for both IPV and OPV was produced in cultures of monkey kidney cells. SV40 commonly infects rhesus macaques in the wild, and SV40 is readily transmitted among rhesus and from rhesus to other Old World monkeys, including cynomolgus macaques, in captivity.[56] Additionally, SV40 establishes lifelong latency in kidney cells in infected macaques. Thus, SV40 was frequently present in kidneys harvested for poliovirus vaccine production. Two methods were used to grow pools of vaccine virus.[54] In the first ("Maitland") method, poliovirus was grown in a cell culture prepared from the minced kidney of a single animal. In the second ("monolayer") method, vaccine virus was produced in a kidney cell monolayer derived from the kidneys of dozens of monkeys. In both methods, any contaminating SV40 was carried along with poliovirus in the final steps of vaccine production. Notably, the monolayer method would be expected to produce vaccine virus pools almost universally contaminated with SV40, because the vaccine product was derived from the kidneys of many animals. In the United States, the major vaccine manufacturer used Maitland cultures.[56]

The final step in IPV production involved treatment with formalin to inactivate the poliovirus. However, SV40 is relatively resistant to formalin inactivation.[57] Therefore, low levels of live SV40 frequently remained in lots of finished IPV. Because most lots in the United States were produced using the Maitland culture method and because formalin inactivated much, although not all, of the live SV40 in the finished product, it has remained uncertain how frequently IPV was contaminated with SV40 and how much live SV40 was present. In 1961, Gerber and colleagues reported the presence of live SV40 in 50% of 8 IPV lots prepared by US manufacturers.[57] Larger-scale testing of lots released for the first year of public vaccination campaigns (1955) in the United States indicated that 71% of used lots of IPV that contained live SV40, and that these states together included 80% of US children in the 6- to 8-year-old age range.[58]

Because formalin partially inactivates SV40, the amount of live SV40 present in IPV doses was substantially lower than in the cultures from which it was derived, although the exact levels are not known with certainty. Gerber and colleagues estimated that some IPV doses contained up to 2,000 viral particles/mL of vaccine.[55] The amount of live SV40 that neonates received by injection in an IPV immunogenicity trial was < 50 $TCID_{50}$, lower than the amount typically required to induce tumors in experimental animals.[13,53]

Another measure of SV40 present in IPV is provided by data on the development of SV40 antibody (ie, seroconversion) following vaccination. Seroconversion rates provide an upper bound on the proportion of people becoming infected with SV40, since individuals could also seroconvert owing to the presence of formalin-inactivated virus proteins or rapid clearance of live SV40. Estimates for the proportion of individuals who seroconverted to SV40 following one or more doses of pre-1963 IPV have varied widely (4 to 92%) in studies based in the United States and United Kingdom.[7,59–62] This wide variability may reflect the uneven contamination of IPV produced using the Maitland method, the variable amounts of live SV40 in vaccines, or differences in assay methods.

It has been difficult to synthesize these limited data regarding the prevalence of SV40 in IPV and seroconversion following vaccination, to estimate the overall frequency of SV40 contamination of IPV in the United States, and on a related note, how many individuals would have been exposed to live SV40 through vaccinations. Shah and Nathanson estimated that 10 to 30% of the 98 million people who had received IPV by 1961 were exposed to live SV40 through vaccination.[56]

The estimates by Shah and Nathanson are supported by analyses presented in Table 17–3. The table shows published data on the cumulative receipt of IPV by the US population as of September 1961, and highlights that many people who received IPV actually received multiple doses, which would have increased their likelihood of exposure to live SV40 on at least one occasion.[52] Based on these data, one can calculate the prevalence of SV40 exposure (receipt of at least one dose of SV40-contaminated vaccine), given various rates of SV40 contamination in IPV (see Table 17–3). For example, if 30% of vaccine doses contained live SV40, then 42% of the population under age 60 years (including 61% of children) would have received at least one dose of SV40-contaminated vaccine. If only 10% of vaccine doses contained live SV40, then 18% of the population under age 60 years (26% of children) would have received at least one dose of SV40-contaminated vaccine. Regardless of the frequency of SV40 contamination of US IPV, a substantial proportion of the US population was exposed to live SV40 through vaccination. Higher proportions of US children than adults were exposed to live SV40 on at least one occasion.

As mentioned above, OPV was not licensed in the United States until 1963, and so was not administered as widely as IPV. Because OPV was not formalin-inactivated, live SV40 was present in much higher titers than in IPV. For example, Mortimer and colleagues reported titers of live SV40 of $10^{4.5}$ to 10^7 $TCID_{50}$ units per 1 mL dose of OPV.[53] Some studies reported that SV40 was shed in stool for several weeks following OPV ingestion, suggesting that SV40 can transiently infect cells at enteric sites.[56] However, SV40 seroconversion following receipt of OPV was not observed, indicating that even though OPV contained large amounts of live SV40, systemic infection probably did not occur after oral exposure.[7,59]

Another type of vaccine that was widely contaminated with live SV40 was the adenovirus vaccine used by the US military. Several versions of this vaccine were developed by various manufacturers and evaluated in field trials in the US Army and Navy.[63–65] In adenovirus vaccine production, adenovirus was propagated in kidney tissue from macaques. Importantly, adenoviruses grow poorly in monkey kidney tissue unless SV40 is also present as a "helper virus."[66] Therefore, as a result of this strong positive selection, nearly all adenovirus seeds and vaccine pools grown from them became contaminated with SV40.[7,67] This situation is unlike poliovirus vaccine contamination, which was not uniform, because SV40 is not a necessary cofactor for poliovirus replication in vitro. In the final step of vaccine manufacture, vaccine pools were treated with formalin to inactivate live adenovirus. How-

ever, as for poliovirus vaccines, formalin would not have inactivated all of the live SV40 present. In 1961, Gerber and colleagues tested three samples of formalin-inactivated adenovirus vaccine, and all had live SV40.[57] Additionally, in a 1956 adenovirus vaccine trial conducted at Fort Dix, New Jersey, 100% of 9 evaluated subjects seroconverted to SV40.[7] Available evidence thus points to frequent SV40 contamination of this vaccine. Because this vaccine was used routinely only in the US Army over a limited time period (1960 to 1961), it has not been considered a major source for SV40 exposure in the US population.

The only other vaccine with demonstrated contamination by SV40 was an experimental respiratory syncytial virus vaccine.[66] This vaccine, administered to fewer than 50 individuals, is of interest because of the route of administration. The inoculum of vaccine was administered as a nebulized mist into the nose and mouth, and an additional 0.5 mL of vaccine (containing 5,000 $TCID_{50}$ of SV40 per mL) was dropped into each nostril. Vaccination was not associated with any symptoms attributable to SV40 infection. SV40 neutralizing antibodies were detectable in some subjects at 3 weeks after vaccination, generally at low titers. Although antibody titers declined further over the ensuing months, these data suggest that SV40 might be able infect humans when transmitted by a respiratory route. Still, the relevance of these data is uncertain, because it is unclear how frequently, if ever, other humans have been exposed by this route.

The 1961 report of the discovery of SV40 led to changes in the manufacture and testing of vaccines, which eliminated SV40 from US vaccine products.[56] A July 1961 memorandum from the director of the National Institutes of Health's Division of Biologics Standards stated that no lots of IPV could subsequently be released without negative results from a tissue culture test for SV40. However, previously released vaccine lots were not withdrawn. Because IPV could be stored for a year and had a shelf life of 6 months, SV40-contaminated IPV would likely have been in use in the United States through the end of 1962; but, beginning in 1963, IPV in use in the United States was free of SV40. The Army's adenovirus vaccine was withdrawn in mid-1961 because of manufacturing difficulties and concerns about SV40 contamination. An SV40-free oral adenovirus vaccine was later reintroduced into US military use.

OPV was required to be SV40-free upon licensure in 1963. The absence of SV40 contamination was supported by steps in vaccine production and testing specified in US regulations and incorporated by manufacturers. SV40 was eliminated from poliovirus vaccine seeds using SV40-specific antisera. One major US manufacturer has described detailed production methods for OPV, involving multiple steps to safeguard vaccine from SV40 contamination.[69] Using PCR techniques, Sierra-Honigmann and Krause did not find SV40 DNA sequences in any of 30 OPV lots produced by various manufacturers and released in the United States from 1972 to 1996.[70] Similarly, Sangar and colleagues did not find SV40 sequences in OPV lots used in the United Kingdom from 1966 through the 1990s.[71]

Other Potential Routes of Exposure to SV40

An important question is whether SV40 can be transmitted to humans by routes other than administration of SV40-contaminated vaccines. The principal route of infection with polyomaviruses is generally thought to be via exposures to virus-contaminated urine (eg, through inhalation of aerosols or contact with fomites). In macaques, SV40 is shed in urine.[72] Similarly, the related human polyomaviruses, BK and JC, are shed in urine.[73] It is therefore telling that PCR-based testing suggests that SV40 is not commonly present in human urine. In the largest published study, Shah and colleagues did not find SV40 DNA sequences in urine from any of 166 individuals, including 88 persons who were immunocompromised owing to HIV infection (in contrast, BK and JC viruses were detected in 14% and 34% of urines, respectively).[71] In a much smaller study, Li and colleagues reported detection of SV40 DNA in 1 of 22 (5%) urine specimens from healthy volunteers.[74]

Additionally, Bofil-Mas and colleagues reported results of PCR testing of sewage samples for polyomavirus DNA.[75] Evaluation of sewage samples provides an opportunity to examine the cumulative community-wide shedding of viruses in stool or urine. Similar methods have been used to measure shedding of poliovirus, adenovirus, and hepatitis viruses. Importantly, in samples obtained from France, Spain, Sweden, and South Africa, SV40 DNA was not detected.[75] In contrast, adenovirus, BK virus, and JC virus were frequently detected. The investigators estimated that 10^2 to 10^4 copies of JC virus and 10^1 to 10^3 copies of BK virus were detected per 4 mL of sewage sample analyzed. The sensitivity of the PCR methods for SV40 was estimated to be five copies per sewage sample, so the negative results for SV40 detection rule out its presence at levels substantially lower than observed for the two human polyomaviruses. Overall, these data indicate that SV40 is shed in human urine infrequently (if ever), or is shed at much lower levels than BK or JC viruses, and point away from person-to-person transmission of this virus.

Additionally, several serology-based studies have indicated that SV40 is an uncommon infection in humans.[76–81] Antibodies that react to SV40 capsid protein are detectable in 3 to 10% of individuals in the United States and Europe. Importantly, however, several lines of evidence indicate that these results largely reflect nonspecific antibody cross-reactivity against other viruses, most likely BK or JC. First, SV40 antibody is generally present at a low level; that is, at a much lower titer than observed in SV40-infected macaques and at lower levels than seen for antibodies to BK and JC viruses in humans.[77–82] Second, SV40 antibody levels in humans are correlated with BK and JC virus antibody levels, and SV40 antibodies are frequently absorbed by the addition of BK or JC particles.[75,80–82] Finally, although one study has found suggestive evidence for an increased SV40 seroprevalence in people born before 1963 (ie, individuals exposed to SV40-contaminated vaccines), other studies have not found a clear relationship between SV40 seroprevalence and birth year or age.[78–81] A demonstrable relationship with birth year or age would be expected if SV40 seroprevalence reflects past exposure to SV40-contaminated vaccines or continued acquisition of SV40 infection throughout life. Because much of the measured SV40 antibody reactivity is likely nonspecific, SV40 seroprevalence estimates are most useful in providing an upper bound for the prevalence of SV40 exposure or infection in the general population. Albeit limited, these data indicate that SV40 is not a common infection of humans.

An additional possible route by which some humans might become infected with SV40 is through contact with nonhuman primates. SV40 infection is endemic among rhesus macaques living in northern India, Nepal, and Pakistan.[83] Humans live in close contact with rhesus in this region, and with the continuing destruction of woodlands for human agriculture, macaques have become increasingly common in towns and cities.[84] Given this ecology, human contacts with monkeys occur frequently during everyday life, and it is conceivable that SV40 might be transmitted from monkeys to humans. For example, since SV40 is shed in macaque urine, transmission to humans might occur through ingestion of contaminated food or water.[72] Providing limited support to the presence of macaque-to-human transmission in India, low-titer SV40 neutralizing antibodies were detected in 6 to 11% of the general population in Uttar Pradesh.[85]

Evidence from studies of individuals who have occupational contacts with nonhuman primates further supports the possibility of direct animal-to-human transmission of SV40.[85,86] In a 1966 study of workers at two monkey export firms in northern India, Shah observed that 10 of 37 (27%) workers exhibited SV40 neutralizing antibodies, generally at low titer (median titer, 1:8).[85] The prevalence of SV40 neutralizing antibody increased with duration of service, from 6% in those with < 6 years employment, to 31% with 6 to 10 years employment, to 71% with 11 to 13 years employment. More recently, Engels and colleagues evaluated 254 workers at North American zoos for SV40, BK, and JC antibodies using virus-like particle enzyme immunoassays.[86] SV40-specific seroreactivity was more common among workers with primate contacts than among other workers (10% versus 3%; $p = .04$). Although these two studies suggest that SV40 can be acquired from nonhuman primates, they do not provide data regarding which primate species can transmit SV40 to humans, specific risk factors and routes for transmission, or the likelihood of transmission per contact.

Discussion of SV40 Epidemiology in Humans

Available data provide strong evidence that humans in many countries were exposed to SV40 through contaminated vaccines in the period 1954 to 1962. In the United States, SV40 was present in IPV, which was very widely administered, and two other vaccines (OPV and adenovirus vaccine) that were given to hundreds of thousands of persons. Although the frequency of contamination with live SV40 in IPV is not known with certainty, under even conservative assumptions, it is possible to conclude that 28 million people (ie, 18% of 157.9 million persons; see Table 17–3) were given at least one dose of IPV that contained live SV40. Through IPV campaigns, many individuals would have been parenterally exposed to live SV40 as children and on multiple occasions.

Epidemiologic evidence does not suggest that ongoing transmission of SV40 represents an important source of infection in humans. It is likely that much of the infrequent and low-level SV40 antibody reactivity observed in seroprevalence surveys reflects cross-reactivity with the common human polyomaviruses BK and JC.[76] Based on limited testing, the absence of SV40 in human urine and sewage argues against human shedding of SV40. Nonetheless, the available data cannot definitively rule out infrequent transmission of SV40 or transmission through as yet undefined routes. Although it is possible that SV40 can be transmitted directly from primates to humans, this route is not of major importance for geographic areas outside the natural range of rhesus macaques.

Finally, of great relevance is the overarching question of whether humans can actually be infected with SV40. There are at least three possible outcomes to consider for individuals with meaningful exposures to live SV40, such as via vaccination or contact with primates: (1) transient SV40 infection (abortive infection or clearance of infection by the immune system); (2) persisting SV40 infection of cells in one or more tissues, without completion of the viral life cycle ("nonproductive infection")[1]; and (3) persistent SV40 infection with viral replication ("productive infection"). In their natural hosts, polyomaviruses (such as BK and JC viruses in humans,

SV40 in macaques) manifest the last of these possibilities: the viruses establish lifelong infections in the kidney, and viral DNA can be detected in urine and peripheral blood mononuclear cells even from immunocompetent individuals.[87] Productive infection would seem to be necessary for sustained transmission of SV40 among humans. By contrast, it is nonproductive infection (eg, in experimental rodents) that leads to malignancy.

Available studies do not provide a clear answer as to which of these possible outcomes is most relevant for humans. For example, serologic data for recipients of SV40-contaminated IPV and workers exposed to nonhuman primates indicate only that immunologically significant exposure to SV40 occurred, but they do not demonstrate the establishment of ongoing SV40 infection in these individuals. Indeed, the low levels of SV40 antibody that are detected, and the absence of SV40 in human urine and sewage, actually point away from the possibility for productive SV40 infection in humans. On the other hand, studies reporting on the molecular detection of SV40 DNA in human tumors and other tissues would suggest that nonpermissive SV40 infections occur and are biologically relevant. However, data from these studies are controversial and have proven difficult to interpret, as reviewed above and discussed elsewhere.[33]

RETROSPECTIVE COHORT STUDIES OF VACCINE RECIPIENTS

A major line of epidemiologic evidence concerning the potential relationship between SV40 and cancer derives from retrospective cohort studies of recipients of SV40-contaminated poliovirus vaccines. The premise of these studies is that if SV40 causes cancer, then cancer incidence or mortality will be higher in groups exposed to SV40 through vaccination than in groups not exposed in this manner. The studies thus rely on documentation that SV40 contamination was present in the vaccine under consideration and that it can be determined whether individuals actually received the vaccine. Retrospective cohort studies have ascertained cancer outcomes in vaccine-exposed and unexposed cohorts through active follow-up of these individuals or through the use of

population-based cancer registries. These studies are summarized in Table 17–4, and several of these studies are reviewed in detail in the following paragraphs.

Mortimer and Colleagues (1981) and Carroll-Pankhurst and Colleagues (2001)

From 1960 to 1962, 1,073 neonates (1 to 3 days old) in Cleveland, Ohio, participated in a study of the immunogenicity of poliovirus vaccine given in the first few days of life.[55] Eighty-six percent of these infants received OPV, and 14% received IPV. Notably, testing subsequently revealed that all of the lots of vaccines used in this trial contained live SV40 at varying titer.[55] Given the documented exposure of these children to live SV40 at a very young age, this cohort provides valuable information on the effects of early-life exposure to SV40. However, a limitation of the data from follow-up studies of this cohort (most of whom received OPV) is that it is unclear whether oral exposures to SV40 can lead to systemic infection.

Two long-term follow-up studies of this cohort have been published.[55,88] In the first study, Mortimer and colleagues contacted parents about the health status of the vaccinated children in 1976 to 1979, when the children were 13 to 19 years old.[55] They also matched a list of the vaccinated children against hospital, cancer registry, and death certificate information. Fifteen children had died, but none of the deaths was from cancer. One child had developed a "mixed tumor" of the salivary gland reported to have a "low degree of malignancy." No other cancers were noted.

In the second study, Carroll-Pankhurst and colleagues matched identifying information on these individuals against the US national death certificate registry to ascertain additional deaths through 1996.[88] A total of 44 deaths were found, of which four were due to cancer (relative risk [RR], 1.3 compared to the general population; 95% CI, 0.3–3.2). Two deaths were due to leukemia, but these were of different types and did not represent a significant excess (RR, 4.2; 95% CI, 0.5–16). Two deaths were attributed to testicular cancer (RR, 37; 95% CI, 4.5–133). The increased mortality from testicular cancer was unexpected, since no data from animal experiments support an etiologic link with SV40. The authors specu-

Table 17–4. MAJOR COHORT STUDIES OF RECIPIENTS OF SV40-CONTAMINATED POLIOVIRUS VACCINES

Study	Population	Exposure/Measure	Major Outcomes*	Follow-Up Duration/Method	Association of Cancer Outcome with Vaccine Exposure
Fraumeni et al, 1963[58]	7.6 million US children, 6–8 years old, vaccinated in 1955	IPV with varying levels of documented SV40; birth cohort	Leukemia; mortality	4 years, registry	No increase
Mortimer et al, 1981[55]; Carroll-Pankhurst et al, 2001[88]	1,073 US children, neonates, vaccinated in 960–1962 as part of trial	IPV or OPV with documented SV40	All cancer types; incidence and mortality	36 years, direct follow-up and registry	No increased incidence; only 4 cancer deaths (RR, 1.3 versus general population)
Strickler et al, 1998[90]	US SEER areas, children vaccinated in 1956–1962	IPV with presumed SV40; birth cohort	Ependymoma, osteosarcoma, mesothelioma; incidence	38 years, registry	No increase
Engels et al, 2003[106]	39,468 US persons with AIDS, vaccinated as children in 1955–1962	IPV with presumed SV40; birth cohort	AIDS-associated NHL; incidence	41 years, registry	No increase compared with persons with AIDS who did not receive vaccine
Engels et al, 2003[89]	Denmark, children vaccinated 1955–1962	IPV with documented SV40; almost all children received multiple doses	Ependymoma, osteosarcoma, mesothelioma, NHL; incidence	42 years, registry	No increase
Strickler et al, 2003[91]	US SEER areas, children and adults vaccinated in 1955–1962	IPV with presumed SV40; birth cohort	Mesothelioma; incidence	42 years, registry	No increase
Engels et al, 2004[62]	54,796 US children whose mothers received vaccine during pregnancy	IPV or OPV with presumed SV40; maternal interview and records	Hematologic malignancies, neural tumors; incidence	8 years, direct follow-up	Increase in hematologic malignancies, largely leukemia (RR, 2.5), and neural tumors, largely neuroblastoma (RR, 2.5). See text for further details

AIDS = acquired immunodeficiency syndrome; IPV = inactivated poliovirus vaccine; OPV = oral poliovirus vaccine; NHL = non-Hodgkin's lymphoma; RR = relative risk; SEER = Surveillance, Epidemiology, and End Results; SV40 = simian virus 40.

*Major outcomes: types of cancer evaluated and measure of risk (incidence or mortality).

lated that this increase arose because of late diagnosis or poor treatment of testicular cancer, since the cohort was composed largely of persons from inner-city Cleveland, a medically underserved population.[88] A subsequent cohort study in Denmark did not identify an increased incidence of testicular carcinoma among SV40-exposed individuals.[89]

Strickler and Colleagues (1998)

Strickler and colleagues conducted a registry-based study in the United States using data collected by the Surveillance, Epidemiology, and End Results (SEER) program.[90] The SEER data covered nine areas with approximately 10% of the US population for the period 1973 to 1993. The investigators divided individuals in these areas into three birth cohorts: persons born in 1947 to 1952 (who would have been young children at the initiation of IPV vaccination campaigns in the United States in 1955 and thus first exposed to SV40 after infancy), persons born in 1956 to 1962 (ages 0 to 1 years at the start of vaccination campaigns, or born during the campaigns, and so first exposed to SV40 as infants), and those born in 1964 to 1969 (born after vaccines were cleared of SV40, and so unexposed to SV40-contaminated poliovirus vaccine). Given the scope of the vaccination campaigns and level of SV40 contamination of vaccines, it was considered probable that individuals in the first two birth cohorts would have received SV40-contaminated vaccine on at least one occasion, and those exposed as infants might have the highest cancer risk.[13,56]

For a range of malignancies, the data relating birth cohort (the proxy measure for SV40 exposure) with cancer incidence did not suggest an etiologic link with SV40. For example, for all brain tumors combined, the incidence in the birth cohort exposed as infants was similar to that in the unexposed cohort (age-adjusted RR, 0.90; 95% CI, 0.82–0.99), while the incidence in the birth cohort exposed as children was actually less than that in the unexposed cohort (RR, 0.82; 95% CI, 0.73–0.92). Similar results were found for ependymoma, osteosarcoma, and mesothelioma (although data were limited for this last outcome, due to the young attained ages of these birth cohorts).

Strickler and Colleagues (2003)

This group of investigators subsequently extended their results for mesothelioma in the United States using SEER data for additional birth cohorts, specifically including individuals who would have been adults in the period 1955 to 1962.[91] This approach allowed an evaluation of data for persons who had attained an age during follow-up (in their 50s, 60s, and 70s), when mesothelioma incidence becomes appreciable. For both males and females, they noted generally increasing incidence over time during 1975 to 1997, but mesothelioma remained extraordinarily rare among females (0.21 per 100,000 person-years versus 1.29 per 100,000 person-years in males; Figure 17–2). The authors noted that this pattern was inconsistent with an effect of SV40-contaminated poliovirus vaccine on mesothelioma risk, since males and females were vaccinated equally. Instead, the pattern supports the well-established relationship between occupational exposures to asbestos in men and subsequent development of mesothelioma.[92]

In additional analyses, Strickler and colleagues examined mesothelioma incidence by birth cohort as a function of the proportion of individuals in each cohort who had received one or more doses of SV40-contaminated vaccine.[91] In Figure 17–3, results of one such analysis are shown. Among men, adjacent birth cohorts were compared both with respect to mesothelioma incidence and prevalence of exposure to contaminated vaccine. Across a range of differences in exposure prevalence, there was little difference in mesothelioma incidence. These results again provide little support for a relationship between SV40 and mesothelioma.

Engels and Colleagues (2003)

Highly informative data on cancer risk associated with SV40 exposure come from Denmark.[89] IPV was first administered there in April 1955, shortly after vaccination campaigns began in the United States. Danish public health officials mounted a concerted campaign to administer IPV to a large proportion of the Danish population, especially children and young adults, and these efforts were maintained throughout the late 1950s and early 1960s. As

Engels and colleagues examined cancer incidence in Denmark for three birth cohorts with varying exposures to SV40-contaminated IPV: the 1946 to 1952 birth cohort, who were vaccinated in 1955 when vaccine first became available (exposed as children); the 1955 to 1961 birth cohort, who were vaccinated at approximately 9 months of age or soon thereafter (exposed as infants); and the 1964 to 1970 birth cohort, who were unexposed, since they were born after vaccines were cleared of SV40 contamination. Cancer incidence data were obtained from the Danish cancer registry for the period 1943 to 1997.

Figure 17–4 illustrates the age-specific incidence of all cancers combined and several specific cancer types of interest. For each cancer outcome, the two cohorts exposed to SV40-contaminated IPV as infants or children had similar incidence

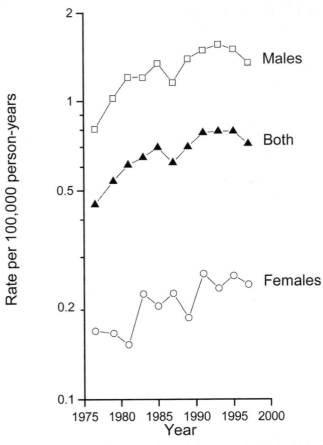

Figure 17–2. Pleural mesothelioma incidence rates in the United States based on data from the Surveillance, Epidemiology, and End Results Program. Shown are age-standardized pleural mesothelioma incidence rates in males, females, and both combined, for the 3-year periods 1975 to 1977 through 1993 to 1995, and 1996 to 1997. Reproduced with permission from Strickler HD et al.[91]

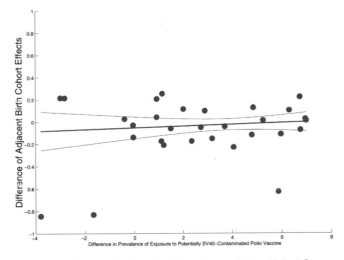

Figure 17–3. Mesothelioma incidence in men in the United States, as a function of birth cohort. Depicted are the differences between adjacent 2-year birth-cohort effects in relation to the differences in prevalence of exposure to potentially SV40-contaminated poliovirus vaccine. Individual data points are plotted as *solid circles*. Ordinates equal the differences between adjacent 2-year birth-cohort effects (eg, 1902 to 1903 versus 1900 to 1901, and 1903 to 1904 versus 1902 to 1903), and abscissas equal the corresponding differences in the prevalence of exposure to potentially SV40-contaminated vaccine. The *dark horizontal line* is the weighted regression line between the changes in cohort effects and changes in prevalence of exposure, and the *upper and lower curved lines* indicate the 95% confidence intervals for the regression line. A positive association between SV40 exposure and incidence of mesothelioma would be indicated by increasing positive differences in adjacent birth-cohort effects with increasing differences in the prevalence of exposure to SV40-contaminated vaccine (ie, a line with a positive slope). The slope of the weighted regression line did not differ statistically significantly from zero (slope = 0.0076; p = .49). Thus, short-term changes in birth-cohort effects were not related to differences in exposure to contaminated vaccine. Reproduced with permission from Strickler HD et al.[91]

of April 1962, approximately 90% of children aged 9 months or older had received at least one dose of IPV, and most had received 3 to 4 doses. Importantly, the Danish vaccine, unlike that used in the United States, was grown using a monolayer method that pooled together kidney cells from dozens of monkeys, which greatly increased the likelihood of SV40 contamination of the final product. Indeed, testing in late 1961 revealed that 9 of 9 evaluated lots of IPV, released previously for use in vaccination campaigns, contained live SV40. Vaccine production was halted, and beginning in 1963, all Danish IPV was free of SV40.

Hence, almost all Danish children alive in 1955 to 1962 were exposed to live SV40 on multiple occasions through injection. In an analysis paralleling that conducted by Strickler and colleagues (1998), compared with the unexposed cohort. Indeed, the cohort exposed to SV40-contaminated vaccine as infants had slightly lower risk than the unexposed cohort for most of these outcomes, even though neonatal exposure to SV40 carries the greatest cancer risk in experimental animal models.[13] Data for mesothelioma were again limited by small numbers, but the small number of cases itself would indicate a lack of effect of SV40 exposure on risk for this malignancy.

In another analysis, Engels and colleagues examined cancer incidence by calendar year for Danish children 0 to 4 years of age.[89] This analysis provided information on cancer outcomes in children that might be associated with a short latency after exposure. Interestingly, ependymoma incidence increased in the period when SV40-contami-

nated IPV was in use (RR, 2.59; 95% CI, 1.36–4.92), compared with earlier years (Figure 17–5). Nonetheless, incidence remained elevated in subsequent years, after vaccine no longer contained SV40. Overall, there were few ependymoma cases, and incidence actually appeared to peak in 1969, 7 years after vaccine last contained SV40 (none of the children aged 0 to 4 years in 1969 would have received contaminated vaccine). Overall, the temporal patterns of cancer incidence in Denmark did not suggest an effect of exposure to SV40-contaminated IPV on later risk of cancer.

Engels and Colleagues (2004)

A recent study evaluated the relationship between maternal receipt of SV40-contaminated poliovirus

Figure 17–4. Age-specific cancer incidence for three Danish birth cohorts with varying exposure to SV40-contaminated poliovirus vaccine. Incidence data are shown for all cancers combined *A*, mesothelioma *B*, all brain and nervous system tumors combined *C*, all bone tumors combined *D*, osteosarcoma *E*, and non-Hodgkin's lymphoma *F*. The three birth cohorts are 1946 to 1952 (exposed to SV40-contaminated poliovirus vaccine as children, *orange line*), 1955 to 1961 (exposed to SV40-contaminated poliovirus vaccine as infants, *black line*), and 1964 to 1970 (unexposed, *blue line*). Both the observed incidence (*thin lines*) and fitted estimates derived from a Poisson model (*thick lines*) are shown. Incidence is per 100,000 person-years (vertical scales vary). Reproduced with permission from Engels EA et al.[89]

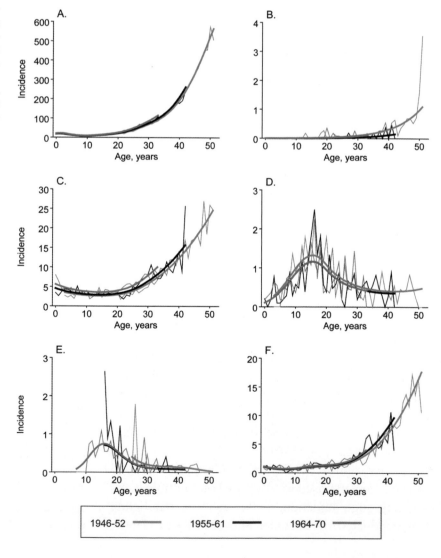

vaccines during pregnancy and risk of cancer in the subsequently born children.[62] This approach considered the possible effects of SV40 infection acquired by children in utero or immediately following birth, which might conceivably occur if primary infection of mothers during pregnancy was associated with high levels of viremia or virus shedding in urine. Engels and colleagues used data collected in the Collaborative Perinatal Project (CPP), a cohort study in 12 US cities that enrolled women in 1959 to 1966. The cohort comprised 54,796 children born to 44,621 mothers. Enrolled mothers had study visits scheduled as an integral part of prenatal medical care, and data on vaccinations during pregnancy were collected. Overall, 21,649 children (39.5%) had mothers who received poliovirus vaccine (IPV or OPV) during pregnancy: 12,334 children (22.5%) had mothers who received pre-1963 poliovirus vaccine (mostly IPV) and 9,315 (17.0%) had mothers who received only 1963+ poliovirus vaccine.

During follow-up through their eighth birthday, 52 children developed cancer, comprising 22 hematologic malignancies, 18 neural tumors, and 12 miscellaneous tumors. Notably, compared with children whose mothers received no poliovirus vaccine or only 1963+ poliovirus vaccine, those whose mothers had received pre-1963 poliovirus vaccine had an increased risk for hematologic malignancies (RR, 2.5; 95% CI, 1.1–5.6) and neural tumors (RR, 2.5; 95% CI, 1.0–6.3). However, 17 of the hematologic malig-

nancies were leukemias, whereas the most common type of neural tumor was neuroblastoma (7 cases). Laboratory studies have not identified SV40 in childhood leukemia or neuroblastoma specimens.[19,93] Conversely, considering childhood tumors with a proposed relationship to SV40, there was only one ependymoma arising among the CPP children, and no cases of choroid plexus tumor or osteosarcoma.

Thus, the distribution of cancer types does not suggest an effect of SV40. Rather, it appears likely that the relationship between maternal receipt of poliovirus vaccine and risk of cancer in children was related to risk factors other than SV40, as yet unidentified. The possible relationship between SV40 and cancer in the CPP children was explored further in a related case-control study, as described below (see "Case-Control Studies," below).[62]

Discussion of Retrospective Cohort Studies

Overall, these retrospective cohort studies indicate that individuals exposed to SV40-contaminated poliovirus vaccines do not have an increased risk for cancer compared with individuals who did not receive these vaccines. Because receipt of SV40-contaminated vaccines represents the principal route of SV40 exposure in the United States and Europe, these studies provide evidence against SV40 as a cause of cancer in humans. Furthermore, the studies

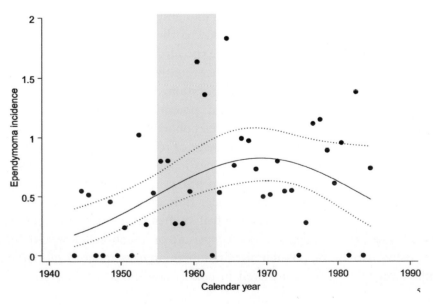

Figure 17–5. Ependymoma incidence among 0- to 4-year-old children as a function of calendar year. The shaded period corresponds to the years 1955 through 1962, when Danish poliovirus vaccine was contaminated with SV40. Also shown is a smooth curve fitted to the data using Poisson regression (*solid line* = fitted values; *dotted lines* = two-sided 95% confidence interval). On the x-axis, *tick marks* indicate the start of each year (ie, January 1), and data points are centered over the middle of each year. Incidence is per 100,000 person-years. Reproduced with permission from Engels EA et al.[89]

indicate that there has not been an "epidemic" of cancer following exposure to SV40 via contaminated vaccines, which provides some reassurance regarding any potential public health impact of SV40 exposures arising through vaccines.

Retrospective cohort studies of vaccine recipients have several strengths that should be considered in evaluating their findings in a scientific context. One strength is that they allow the evaluation of SV40-exposed children, especially SV40-exposed neonates and older infants, who can be posited to be at greatest risk for SV40-induced malignancy.[13,55,62,88] Furthermore, as noted above, most children received multiple doses of poliovirus vaccine and so might have been exposed to SV40 on multiple occasions. A second strength of some studies is that the use of cancer registries allows follow-up of millions of vaccine-exposed individuals over long periods of time, which is of value for studying rare cancer outcomes that might arise many years after SV40 exposure.[89–91]

The retrospective cohort studies relied on several assumptions that, nonetheless, point to some limitations of these studies. The studies depended on historic records to document the presence of SV40 in poliovirus vaccines and the extent of individuals' exposure to these vaccines. Given the importance attributed to the poliomyelitis epidemic by public health officials in the 1950s and 1960s, there are good extant data describing the widespread use of these vaccines, particularly for children. The quality of the data documenting the presence of SV40 in the poliovirus vaccines varies from fair (for registry-based studies in the United States) to excellent (for studies of the Cleveland cohort and Denmark), although there is little information on the actual titer of live SV40 in contaminated vaccines. In the United States, not every dose of IPV contained live SV40. Still, the multiple doses of vaccine received by US children would have increased the likelihood of SV40 exposure (see Table 17–3). The interpretation of follow-up data on OPV recipients is more limited, because it is unclear whether SV40 infection can occur via an oral exposure.

Because the cohort studies compared vaccine recipients with those who did not receive the vaccines, a further assumption of these studies was that SV40 infection is rarely acquired by other routes and that transmission effectively ceased by 1963, following clean-up of the poliovirus vaccines. Indeed, as noted above (see "Epidemiology of SV40 in Humans," above), recent serologic data indicate that SV40 infrequently, if ever, infects humans. Regardless of whether SV40 can be acquired by routes other than vaccination, it is clear that the circumstances for children in 1955 to 1962 were unique, because exposure to SV40 was ubiquitous and occurred early in life, when SV40 might be more likely to induce cancer. If SV40 infections occurred after vaccines were cleared of SV40, then they would likely have occurred at older ages, been less frequent, and been due to smaller inocula. Therefore, even without definitive evidence on whether SV40 currently infects humans, follow-up of vaccine-exposed children offers valuable information.

An additional limitation of retrospective cohort studies is the rarity of some cancer outcomes (such as choroid plexus tumor or mesothelioma). However, the rarity of these cancers itself is reassuring with respect to the possible cancer-inducing effects of SV40. Future follow-up of vaccine-exposed cohorts will provide data on cancer risk after longer latencies from exposure.

CASE-CONTROL STUDIES

Case-control studies offer a complementary approach to the cohort studies discussed above for the epidemiologic investigation of the possible association between SV40 infection and cancer. Case-control studies allow a direct comparison of measures of SV40 exposure or infection between representative cancer cases and controls sampled from the same population.

There are two potential advantages of case-control studies over cohort studies. First, by focusing on the recruitment of relatively large numbers of individuals with a particular cancer of interest, case-control studies can allow an evaluation of associations for rare cancer outcomes (eg, mesothelioma). Second, case-control studies facilitate the collection of data on SV40 exposure or infection that would not be possible for the much larger number of individuals considered in cohort studies. Most case-control studies have measured SV40 antibodies in cases and controls, which provide a direct assessment of SV40 exposure status. If SV40 causes cancer in humans, one would expect a high prevalence of SV40 antibodies in cases, and that this prevalence would be significantly higher than in controls.

Serology-based case-control studies, in which SV40 antibodies were measured in cases and controls, are summarized in Table 17–5. Several findings of these studies are notable. First, SV40 seroprevalence was low (approximately 5 to 10%) in cases, substantially lower than the rates of DNA detection often reported in PCR-based studies of tumors. Second, SV40 seroprevalence was similar in cases and controls. Third, SV40 antibodies, when present, were detected at lower levels than seen in SV40-infected macaques.[77,80,81] Fourth, several studies demonstrated that most SV40 antibody reactivity was likely due to cross-reactivity with BK or JC viruses.[77,80,81]

Engels and colleagues used the case-control design to explore further the intriguing positive association noted in the CPP cohort study between maternal poliovirus vaccination during pregnancy and risk of neural tumors and hematologic malignancies in childhood.[62] The investigators obtained paired sera from CPP mothers during pregnancy for 50 of the children with cancer and 200 control children. Two assays were used to identify SV40 antibodies. SV40 seroconversion during pregnancy (ie, the transition from seronegative to seropositive status) was used as a marker for newly acquired SV40 infection, which was postulated to carry an especially high risk of transmission from mothers to children. Remarkably, only six children with cancer had mothers who seroconverted according to either assay during pregnancy, and the malignancies that developed in these six children have not otherwise been linked with SV40 (two neuroblastomas, one astrocytoma, two leukemias, one fibrosarcoma). These observations therefore indicate that the association between maternal poliovirus vaccination and subsequent childhood cancer observed in the CPP was not likely due to SV40.

Whereas most case-control studies have used serologic methods, several have used history of receipt of SV40-contaminated vaccine to assess SV40 exposure.[94–96] A limitation of this approach is

Table 17–5. MAJOR SEROLOGY-BASED CASE-CONTROL STUDIES OF SV40 AND HUMAN CANCER

Study	Malignancy	Antibody Measurement*	SV40+ Cases/Total (%)	SV40+ Controls/Total (%)	Comments
Strickler et al, 1996[34]	Mesothelioma; osteosarcoma	Plaque neutralization assay	3/34 (9); 1/33 (3)	1/35 (3)	Low-titer antibody
Rollison et al, 2003[107]	Brain tumors (mostly astrocytic tumors)	Plaque neutralization assay, prediagnostic specimens	5/44 (11)	10/88 (11)	
de Sanjose et al, 2003[80]	Lymphoma	VLP EIA	31/520 (6)	56/587 (10)	Low-level antibody, cross-reactive with BK virus
Carter et al, 2003[77]	Osteosarcoma	VLP EIA	3/122 (2)	32/415 (8)	Low-level antibody, cross-reactive with BK and JC viruses
Engels et al, 2004[62]	Childhood malignancies	Plaque neutralization assay, VLP EIA; Seroconversions measured in mothers	3/46 (7); 4/50 (8)	8/187 (4); 6/200 (3)	Low-level antibody, no relationship between seroconversion and specific malignancies
Engels et al, 2004[81]	Non-Hodgkin's lymphoma	VLP EIA, measured in two laboratories	52/724 (7); 70/718 (10)	65/622 (11); 59/615 (10)	Low-level antibody cross-reactive with BK and JC viruses

*Antibody measurement: type of assay and comments on sera or testing methods.
EIA = enzyme immunoassay; SV40 = simian virus 40, VLP = virus-like particle.

that it relies either on subjects' potentially inaccurate recall of vaccination events, perhaps occurring in the distant past of their childhood, or the existence of medical records documenting vaccination, which can be difficult to obtain.

A case-control design was employed in the only follow-up study of individuals who received the US Army's adenovirus vaccine.[95] As described above (see "Epidemiology of SV40 in Humans," above), there is substantial evidence that this vaccine was widely contaminated with SV40. The US Army began routine use of this parenteral adenovirus vaccine in 1960. According to a 1961 article by the chief of the US Army's Communicable Disease Branch, adenovirus vaccine was given to all recruits entering Army service in February through April 1960, but production difficulties then interrupted vaccination until August 1960, when vaccination resumed.[63] Recruits were again routinely vaccinated from August 1960 through May 1961, when vaccination ceased because "supplies once more became limited." Other evidence indicates that adenovirus vaccine was withdrawn in 1961 because of concern regarding contamination with SV40.[97]

To examine the possible relationship between receipt of SV40-contaminated adenovirus vaccine and risk of cancer, Rollison and colleagues used Veterans Administration records to identify patients with mesothelioma, brain tumors, NHL, colon cancer, or lung cancer.[95] The first three diagnoses were considered as types of cases, whereas colon and lung cancer patients were treated as controls, since these malignancies are not generally thought to be related to SV40. A linkage of Veterans Administration and military databases allowed assignment of exposure status (entry into the Army during a period of use or non-use of SV40-contaminated adenovirus vaccine) to these subjects. Results are shown in Table 17–6. The odds ratios were all close to 1.00 and not significantly different from this null value, indicating no association between exposure to this SV40-contaminated vaccine and risk for mesothelioma, brain tumors, or NHL.

Overall, these case-control studies do not identify an association between SV40 exposure or infection and cancer risk. The low SV40 seroprevalence measured consistently in serology-based studies (see Table 17–5) contrasts strikingly with the high rates of PCR-based detection of SV40 reported in some tumor studies. Indeed, the low level of SV40 reactivity and the cross-reactivity of measured SV40 antibodies with BK and JC viruses in humans suggest that very few cases or controls actually have infection with SV40.[77] While such low levels of detection of SV40 antibodies have raised questions about the sensitivity of these assays, they have also highlighted other investigators' concerns about the specificity of PCR-based detection of SV40 in tumors.[98,99]

A strength of the case-control studies is that they provide a measure of association (the odds ratio) that corresponds to an estimate of the cancer risk related to SV40 exposure or infection. In contrast, studies that rely exclusively on the laboratory evaluation of human tumor tissues (eg, PCR testing of brain tumors) cannot yield a similar measure of association, since the concomitant evaluation of control tissues (eg, PCR testing of normal brain tissue) does not provide a measure of infection prevalence in controls.

SV40 AND HUMAN CANCER: SUMMARIZING THE EVIDENCE

As reviewed in this chapter, the data regarding the possible relationship between SV40 and human cancer are complex and not easily synthesized. Data bearing on the question come from multiple lines of evidence, including in vitro laboratory studies, animal experiments, laboratory evaluations of human tumors, and a range of epidemiologic studies. In broad terms, although animal studies suggest that SV40 can cause cancer and some laboratory studies have found evidence for SV40 in human tumors, epidemiologic studies (cohort studies of vaccine recipients, case-control studies) have not found evidence for an association between SV40 exposure or infection and human cancer. On balance, what do these conflicting data then suggest?

In 1965, Hill proposed nine criteria for evaluating associations between putative disease-causing agents and human disease.[29] The Hill criteria provide a useful framework for evaluating the evidence regarding SV40 and human cancer (Table 17–7). As applied to the question of SV40 and cancer, these criteria and the evidence bearing on them are as follows:

1. *Biological plausibility.* It is biologically plausible that SV40 could be a cause of human cancer, because (i) SV40 transforms and immortalizes cells (including human cells) in culture systems through well-described pathways, and (ii) SV40 causes cancer in experimental animals, albeit sometimes under conditions (eg, direct inoculation of high titers of virus into brain or body cavities) not experienced by humans.

2. *Analogy.* SV40 might be a cause of cancer in humans because of the analogy with experimental animal models—SV40 causes cancer when injected into laboratory rodents. However, the analogy is imperfect, because in some instances, animal tumors were induced only following inoculation of extremely large amounts of virus directly into the tissues of interest, which does not happen in humans.

3. *Biological coherence.* According to Hill, "The cause-and-effect interpretation of our data should not seriously conflict with the generally known facts of the natural history and biology of the disease."[29] There are two aspects of the hypothesis that SV40 causes cancer in humans that do not cohere with accepted biologic tenets. First, the amount of SV40 DNA reported in human tumors is very low, whereas SV40 is chromosomally integrated and present within each tumor cell in animals. Second, specific antibody responses against SV40 proteins are not found in cancer patients, even though systemic viral infections (including SV40 infection in animals) generally lead to antibody responses.

4. *Specificity.* This criterion requires that a single cause lead to a single effect. Although this criterion is not absolutely required (eg, smoking causes many different types of cancer and other diseases), the wide range of human tumors in which SV40 DNA has reportedly been detected is striking (see Table 17–2). Many studies did not include appropriate negative controls or reported SV40 DNA in normal tissues, further heightening concerns regarding specificity.

5. *Consistency.* The evidence for a causal association is strengthened if multiple studies of different types all point to a relationship between exposure and outcome. The laboratory data on the detection of SV40 in human tumors are inconsistent. In

Table 17–6. CASE-CONTROL STUDY OF CANCER AND HISTORY OF VACCINATION WITH ADENOVIRUS VACCINE AMONG U.S. ARMY VETERANS

Date of Entry into Army Service	Exposure to Adenovirus Vaccine	Cases			Controls	
		Brain Tumors, n (%)	Mesothelioma, n (%)	NHL, n (%)	Colon Cancer, n (%)	Lung Cancer, n (%)
Jan 1959–Jan 1960	Unexposed	58 (32.0)	3 (30.0)	59 (26.8)	45 (42.1)	39 (34.2)
Feb 1960–Apr 1960	Exposed	15 (8.3)	2 (20.0)	12 (5.5)	10 (9.3)	5 (4.4)
May 1960–Jul 1960	Unexposed	11 (6.1)	0 (0.0)	18 (8.2)	3 (2.8)	7 (6.1)
Aug 1960–May 1961	Exposed	35 (19.3)	2 (20.0)	57 (25.9)	28 (26.2)	28 (24.6)
Jun 1961–Dec 1961	Unexposed	62 (34.3)	3 (30.0)	74 (33.6)	21 (19.6)	35 (30.7)
Combined exposed		50 (27.6)	4 (40.0)	69 (31.4)	38 (35.5)	33 (29.1)
Combined unexposed		131 (72.4)	6 (60.0)	151 (68.6)	69 (64.5)	81 (70.9)
Adjusted odds ratio*		0.76	1.49	0.98	1.00 (reference)	
(95% Confidence interval)		(0.48–1.20)	(0.38–5.88)	(0.65–1.47)		

NHL = non-Hodgkin's lymphoma.

*The ratio of the odds of entering the Army during a period of adenovirus vaccination in the cases of the site hypothesized to be associated with SV40 (brain tumors, mesothelioma, NHL) to the odds of adenovirus vaccination in lung and colon cancer cases combined. Odds ratios are adjusted for age at diagnosis and race.

Adapted from Rollison DEM.[95]

	Table 17–7. HILL CRITERIA FOR SV40 AS A CAUSE OF CANCER IN HUMANS	
Hill Criterion	**Strength of Evidence in Favor of SV40 as a Cause of Cancer***	**Comment**
Biological plausibility	+++	SV40 T antigen blocks TP53 and transforms cells. SV40 causes cancer in animals.
Analogy	+++	SV40 causes cancer in animals.
Biological coherence	–	In animals, SV40 is chromosomally integrated in tumor cells, but DNA detection in humans is low-level. SV40-specific antibodies are not detected in humans.
Specificity	– –	SV40 DNA has reportedly been detected in a wide range of tumors and normal tissues.
Consistency	– – –	Laboratory studies reporting detection of SV40 in human tumors are inconsistent. Epidemiologic studies are consistently negative.
Strength of association	– – –	Epidemiologic studies consistently find a null association between SV40 exposure/ infection and cancer.
Biological gradient	–	SV40-exposed infants are not at highest cancer risk.
Temporality	– –	Recipients of SV40-contaminated vaccines are not at increased cancer risk.
Experimental evidence	–	Humans implanted with SV40-transformed cells do not develop persistent tumors.

SV40 = simian virus 40.

*Strength of evidence is presented on a scale from +++ (strong evidence in favor of a causal relationship) to — (strong evidence against a causal relationship). Adapted from Hill AB.[29]

contrast, epidemiologic data (cohort and case-control studies) are consistently negative.

6. *Strength of association.* Association is measured in terms of a relative risk or odds ratio. A strong association (ie, large relative risk or odds ratio) between SV40 exposure or infection and cancer would exist if cancer risk were much higher in SV40-exposed individuals than in SV40-unexposed individuals, or if cancer patients were much more likely to be SV40-infected than controls. As Hill argued, strong associations are most likely to be causal, since they are less likely than weak associations to arise from unknown biases in study design.[29] Cohort studies of vaccine recipients and case-control studies using serologic markers for SV40 infection have consistently yielded null associations, providing no support for a causative relationship between SV40 and cancer. Studies reporting on the PCR-based detection of SV40 DNA in tumor tissues do not provide an estimate of the strength of association between SV40 infection and cancer, because they lack appropriate controls that yield information on the prevalence of SV40 infection among individuals without cancer.

7. *Biological gradient.* This criterion refers to a dose-response relationship. One way in which this criterion can be assessed for SV40 is to evaluate can-

cer risk in SV40-exposed infants, SV40-exposed older children, and SV40-unexposed individuals. SV40-exposed infants would be expected to have the highest risk and SV40-exposed children intermediate risk, based on data from animals showing a similar gradient of decreasing risk with increasing age of infection.[13] Cohort studies of vaccine recipients that have undertaken such analyses have not identified an increased cancer risk in SV40-exposed neonates or infants.[88–90]

8. *Temporality.* It is necessary that a causal exposure precede the cancer. The most important evidence regarding temporality comes from retrospective cohort studies of recipients of SV40-contaminated vaccines. In those studies, the exposure of these individuals to SV40 was not followed by an increase in cancer incidence during extended follow-up.

9. *Experimental evidence.* By "experimental evidence," Hill does not refer to laboratory data (eg, experiments on cell cultures or animals), since these bear on the effects of SV40 in humans only indirectly, through plausibility or analogy. Rather, Hill's reference is to experiments performed on humans.[29] Since most studies that would expose humans to a potentially harmful agent are unethical, Hill pointed to data deriving from experiments in which the potentially harm-

ful agent is removed, such as the evaluation of the biologic effects of an infection through observations made in a randomized trial of a vaccine. There are no data from vaccine trials in humans showing that prevention of SV40 infection would decrease cancer risk. Remarkably, however, the human experimental data provided by Jensen and colleagues provide some limited insight.[17] In their experiments, the implantation of SV40-infected but untransformed cells did not lead to formation of a tumor. The implantation of SV40-transformed cells led transiently to the development of a tumor, but the tumors subsequently regressed in the presence of a host immune response. Although somewhat inconclusive, these data might suggest that SV40 infection would not lead readily to cancer in humans, perhaps because immune system surveillance could eliminate SV40-infected or -transformed cells.

Overall, consideration of these criteria suggests that the body of evidence supporting SV40 as a cause of cancer is not convincing. Indeed, the collected data deriving from epidemiologic studies suggest that SV40 does not cause cancer in humans. There are at least three possible models to account for the conflicting data:

Model 1. *SV40 is not present in human tumors, and SV40 is not a cause of human cancer.* As reviewed above, the laboratory data on the detection of SV40 in human tumors are inconsistent. It is possible that reports of SV40 detection, primarily by PCR but also by other means, derive from flawed experiments, and that the positive results in multiple laboratories are due to artifacts such as PCR contamination. The extremely low-level detection of SV40 DNA in tumors and the low prevalence of SV40 antibodies in cancer patients both support this conclusion. Furthermore, the absence of an increased risk of cancer in persons with exposures to SV40-contaminated vaccines supports the conclusion that SV40 is not a cause of human cancer.

Model 2. *SV40 is present in human tumors, and SV40 is a cause of human cancer.* If this model is correct, studies that have not detected SV40 DNA in human tumors must have been flawed due to methodologic problems (eg, poor specimen handling or low assay sensitivity). Additionally, this model implies that SV40 infection does not lead to the production of SV40 antibodies, since SV40-specific antibody responses have only rarely been detected in cancer patients and persons in the general population. Additionally, the negative data from cohort studies of vaccine recipients would need to be explained by an absence of frequent SV40 infection by this route and/or extremely common infection by other routes. The detection of SV40 DNA in tumors from people born after 1962 would also require transmission routes other than vaccination. However, there are no data to indicate that SV40 has been widely spread through other routes.

Model 3. *SV40 is present in human tumors, but SV40 does not cause cancer.* This potential "compromise" model raises the possibility that SV40 is present in human tumors as an "innocent bystander." Conceivably, this model could reconcile the reported detection of virus in tumors with an absence of increased cancer risk in vaccine-exposed individuals. However, this model has several major problems. First, given the in vitro and animal data supporting SV40 as a possible carcinogen, it seems unlikely that SV40, if it were in a tumor, would be playing no role in actually causing the tumor. Second, this model does not resolve the difficulty created by finding SV40 in people born after vaccines were cleared of the virus. Under this model, routes of transmission of SV40 other than vaccination would still need to be identified. Finally, this model does not explain why cancer patients would not make antibodies against SV40 proteins.

The review of available laboratory and epidemiologic data, as presented in this chapter, suggest that SV40 is not a cause of cancer in humans (Model 1). However, other scientists have reviewed the same data and concluded that SV40 is a cause of human malignancy (Model 2).[100] The question of whether SV40 is a cause of human cancer continues to be highly controversial and depends, to a large extent, on how the available data are evaluated and considered.

FUTURE RESEARCH DIRECTIONS

Several approaches seem most likely to lead to insights that could resolve existing uncertainty on whether SV40 is a cause of cancer in humans[33]:

1. *Improvements in study design and laboratory methods for detection of SV40 in human tumors and other tissues.* Because of persisting concerns regarding the specificity and reproducibility of reported detections of SV40 DNA in tumors, improved laboratory methods are required. To avoid false-positive PCR results due to contamination by plasmids, careful attention should be paid to the choice of primers, including targeting regions of the SV40 genome not included in cloning vectors.[28,43] Additionally, the use of quantitative PCR methods to provide information on the amount of SV40 DNA detected in tissues will help distinguish between the actual presence of virus and low-level contamination. The quantification of human genomic DNA in specimens should also be performed, to ensure that an adequate amount of tissue is present and that the DNA extraction was sufficiently efficient. Better standardized immunohistochemical methods for the detection of SV40 proteins in tissues would be valuable as well. Finally, methods that detect SV40 messenger RNA in tissues could also provide confirmatory information regarding the presence of SV40 in tissues and data on the expression patterns of viral genes, although this approach has not been widely used.[43] Importantly, laboratory studies must include appropriate negative-control tissues and incorporate identical treatment of tumor and control tissues, ideally using masking of specimens. Multilaboratory studies validating the detection or nondetection of SV40 DNA in tumor tissues, conducted with the utmost rigor, may ultimately be required.[42]

2. *Improvements in serologic assays for SV40 infection.* Recently developed enzyme immunoassays incorporating SV40 virus-like particles have shown promise for evaluating the potential association between SV40 and human cancer.[76] These assays appear highly sensitive and specific, and allow the identification of cross-reacting antibodies to BK or JC virus.[77,82] Additionally, assays that identify antibodies to the SV40 T antigen will be useful for studying the possible presence of SV40 in cancer patients.

3. *Additional studies of SV40 epidemiology in humans.* With improved laboratory assays, it will be possible to conduct further studies to better determine the prevalence of SV40 infection in humans and identify potential routes of SV40 transmission. If these studies identify individuals with chronic SV40 infection, it will be valuable to follow these individuals over time to characterize the virologic and clinical manifestations of infection.

4. *Studies of cancer incidence in SV40-exposed populations.* Longer-term follow-up of vaccine-exposed cohorts will provide valuable data on rare cancer outcomes as well as outcomes that increase in incidence with older age (eg, mesothelioma and NHL). Studies of cancer incidence in countries that used predominantly OPV (eg, the former Soviet Union) might be valuable. Finally, it would be of interest to compare cancer incidence in geographic regions (eg, northern India) where individuals are exposed to SV40-infected rhesus macaques with cancer incidence elsewhere. If SV40 causes cancer, one would expect a heightened incidence of SV40-related cancers in regions where rhesus macaques are common.

REFERENCES

1. Cole CN, Conzen SD. Polyomaviridae: the viruses and their replication. In: Knipe DM, Howley PM, editors. Fields virology. 4th ed. Philadelphia: Lippincott, Williams, and Wilkins; 2001. p. 2141–74.

2. O'Neill FJ, Carroll D. Amplification of papovirus defectives during serial low multiplicity infections. Virology 1981;112:800–3.

3. Huschtscha LI, Holliday R. Limited and unlimited growth of SV40-transformed cells from human diploid MRC-5 fibroblasts. J Cell Sci 1983;63:77–99.

4. Bocchetta M, Di Resta I, Powers A, et al. Human mesothelial cells are unusually susceptible to simian virus 40-mediated transformation and asbestos cocarinogenicity. Proc Natl Acad Sci U S A 2000;97:10214–9.

5. Shaikh S, Skoczylas C, Longnecker R, Rundell K. Inability of simian virus 40 to establish productive infection of lymphoblastic cell lines. J Virol 2004;78:4917–20.

6. Eddy BE, Borman GS, Berkeley WH, Young RD. Tumors induced in hamsters by injection of rhesus monkey kidney cell extracts. Proc Soc Exp Biol Med 1961;107:191–7.

7. Sweet BH, Hilleman MR. The vacuolating virus, SV40. Proc Soc Exp Biol Med 1960;105:420–7.

8. Eddy BE, Borman GS, Grubbs GE, Young RD. Identification of the oncogenic substance of rhesus monkey kidney cell culture as simian virus 40. Virology 1962;17:65–75.

9. Kirschstein RL, Gerber P. Ependymomas produced after intracerebral inoculation of SV40 into new-born hamsters. Nature 1962;195:299–300.

10. Diamandopoulos GT. Leukemia, lymphoma, and osteosarcoma induced in the Syrian golden hamster by simian virus 40. Science 1972;176:173–5.

11. Cicala C, Pompetti F, Carbone M. SV40 induces mesotheliomas in hamsters. Am J Pathol 1993;142:1524–33.

12. Rapp F, Butel JS, Melnick JL. Virus-induced intranuclear antigen in cells transformed by papovavirus SV40. Proc Soc Exp Biol Med 1964;116:1131–5.

13. Girardi AJ, Sweet BH, Hilleman MR. Factors influencing tumor induction in hamsters by vacuolating virus, SV40. Proc Soc Exp Biol Med 1963;112:662–7.

14. Pope JH, Rowe WP. Detection of specific antigen in SV40-transformed cells by immunofluorescence. J Exp Med 1964;120:121–8.

15. Black PH, Rowe WP, Turner HC, Huebner RJ. A specific complement-fixing antigen present in SV40 tumor and transformed cells. Proc Nat Acad Sci U S A 1963;50:1148–56.

16. Black PH, Rowe WP. Viral studies of SV40 tumorigenesis in hamsters. J Natl Cancer Inst 1964;32:253–65.

17. Jensen F, Koprowski H, Pagano JS, et al. Autologous and homologous implantation of human cells transformed in vitro by simian virus 40. J Natl Cancer Inst 1964;32: 917–37.

18. Shah KV. Does SV40 infection contribute to the development of human cancers? Rev Med Virol 2000;10:31–43.

19. Bergsagel DJ, Finegold MJ, Butel JS, et al. DNA sequences similar to those of simian virus 40 in ependymomas and choroid plexus tumors of childhood. N Engl J Med 1992; 326:988–93.

20. Weggen S, Bayer TA, von Deimling A, et al. Low frequency of SV40, JC and BK polyomavirus sequences in human medulloblastomas, meningiomas and ependymomas. Brain Pathol 2000;10:85–92.

21. Krainer M, Schenk T, Zielinski CC, Müller C. Failure to confirm presence of SV40 sequences in human tumours. Eur J Cancer 1995;31A:1893.

22. Reuther FJ, Löhler J, Herms J, et al. Low incidence of SV40-like sequences in ependymal tumours. J Pathol 2001;195: 580–5.

23. Engels EA, Sarkar C, Daniel RW, et al. Absence of simian virus 40 in human brain tumors from northern India. Int J Cancer 2002;101:348–52.

24. Ohgaki H, Huang H, Haltia M, et al. More about cell and molecular biology of simian virus 40: implications for human infections and disease. J Natl Cancer Inst 2000; 92:495–7.

25. Martini F, Iaccheri L, Lazzarin L, et al. SV40 early region and large T antigen in human brain tumors, peripheral blood cells, and sperm fluids from healthy individuals. Cancer Res 1996;56:4820–5.

26. Huang H, Reis R, Yonekawa Y, et al. Identification in human brain tumors of DNA sequences specific for SV40 large T antigen. Brain Pathol 1999;9:33–42.

27. Suzuki SO, Mizoguchi M, Iwaki T. Detection of SV40 T antigen genome in human gliomas. Brain Tumor Pathol 1997; 14:125–9.

28. Völter C, zur Hausen H, Alber D, de Villiers EM. A broad spectrum PCR method for the detection of polyomaviruses and avoidance of contamination by cloning vectors. Dev Biol Stand 1998;94:137–42.

29. Hill AB. The environment and disease: association or causation? Proc R Soc Med 1965;295–300.

30. David H, Mendoza S, Konishi T, Miller CW. Simian virus 40 is present in human lymphomas and normal blood. Cancer Lett 2001;162:57–64.

31. Martini F, Lazzarin L, Iaccheri L, et al. Different simian virus 40 genomic regions and sequences homologous with SV40 T antigen in DNA of human brain and bone tumors and of leukocytes from blood donors. Cancer 2002;94:1037–48.

32. Carbone M, Pass HI, Rizzo P, et al. Simian virus 40-like DNA sequences in human pleural mesothelioma. Oncogene 1994;9:1781–90.

33. Anonymous. Immunization safety review. SV40 contamination of polio vaccine and cancer. Washington (DC): National Academy Press; 2003.

34. Strickler HD, Goedert JJ, Fleming M, et al. Simian virus 40 and pleural mesothelioma in humans. Cancer Epidiol Biomarkers Prev 1996;5:473–5.

35. de Luca A, Baldi A, Esposito V, et al. The retinoblastoma gene family pRb/p105, p107, pRb2/p130 and simian virus-40 large T-antigen in human mesotheliomas. Nature Med 1997;3:913–6.

36. Galateau-Salle F, Bidet P, Iwatsubo Y, et al. SV40-like DNA sequences in pleural mesothelioma, bronchopulmonary carcinoma, and non-malignant pulmonary diseases. J Pathol 1998;184:252–7.

37. Gordon GJ, Chen C-J, Jaklitsch MT, et al. Detection and quantification of SV40 large T-antigen DNA in mesothelioma tissues and cell lines. Oncol Rep 2002;9:631–4.

38. Vilchez RA, Madden CR, Kozinetz CA, et al. Association between simian virus 40 and non-Hodgkin lymphoma. Lancet 2002;359:817–23.

39. Lednicky JA, Garcea RL, Bergsagel DJ, Butel JS. Natural simian virus 40 strains are present in human choroid plexus and ependymoma tumors. Virology 1995;212:710–7.

40. Lednicky JA, Stewart AR, Jenkins JJ, et al. SV40 DNA in human osteosarcomas shows sequence variation among T-antigen genes. Int J Cancer 1997;72:791–800.

41. Testa JR, Carbone M, Hirvonen A, et al. A multi-institutional study confirms the presence and expression of simian virus 40 in human malignant mesotheliomas. Cancer Res 1998;58:4505–9.

42. Strickler HD, International SV40 Working Group. A multi-center evaluation of assays for detection of SV40 DNA and results in masked mesothelioma specimens. Cancer Epidemiol Biomarkers Prev 2001;10:523–32.

43. Lopez-Rios F, Illei PB, Rusch V, Ladanyi M. Evidence against a role for SV40 infection in human mesotheliomas and high risk of false-positive PCR results owing to presence of SV40 sequences in common laboratory plasmids. Lancet 2004;364:1157–66.

44. Engels EA, Switzer WM, Heneine H, Viscidi RP. Serologic evidence for exposure to simian virus 40 in North American zoo workers. Journal of Infectious Diseases. 2004; 190;2065–9.

45. Engels EA, Viscidi RP, Galloway DA, et al. Case-control study of simian virus 40 and non-Hodgkin lymphoma in the United States. J Natl Cancer Inst 2004;96:1368–74.

46. Martini F, Dolcetti R, Gloghini A, et al. Simian-virus-40 footprints in human lymphoproliferative disorders of HIV- and HIV+ patients. Int J Cancer 1998;78:669–74.

47. Gamberi G, Benassi MS, Pompetti F, et al. Presence and expression of the simian virus-40 genome in human giant cell tumors of bone. Genes Chromosomes Cancer 2000;28:23–30.

48. Pilatte Y, Vivo C, Renier A, et al. Absence of SV40 large T-antigen expression in human mesothelioma cell lines. Am J Respir Cell Mol Biol 2000;23:788–93.

49. Malkin D, Chilton-MacNeil S, Meister LA, et al. Tissue-specific expression of SV40 in tumors associated with the Li-Fraumeni syndrome. Oncogene 2001;20:4441–9.

50. Nakatsuka S, Liu A, Dong Z, et al. and the Osaka Lymphoma Study Group. Simian virus 40 sequences in malignant lymphomas in Japan. Cancer Res 2003;63:7606–8.

51. Carbone M, Rizzo P, Procopio A, et al. SV40-like sequences in human bone tumors. Oncogene 1996;13:527–35.

52. Communicable Disease Center. Poliomyelitis surveillance. Atlanta. 1961. Report No.: 248.

53. Second international conference on live poliovirus vaccines. 1960. Washington (DC). Pan American Health Organization and World Health Organization.

54. Flipse ME, Erickson GM, Hoffert WR, et al. Preliminary report on a large-scale field trial with the oral Cox-Lederle attenuated poliomyelitis vaccine in Dade County (Miami), Florida. In: Proceedings of the Second International Conference on Live Poliovirus Vaccines. 1960. p. 456.

55. Mortimer EA Jr, Lepow ML, Gold E, et al. Long-term follow-up of persons inadvertently inoculated with SV40 as neonates. N Engl J Med 1981;305:1517–8.

56. Shah K, Nathanson N. Human exposure to SV40: review and comment. Am J Epidemiol 1976;103:1–12.

57. Gerber P, Hottle GA, Grubbs RE. Inactivation of vacuolating virus (SV40) by formaldehyde. Proc Soc Exp Biol Med 1961;108:205–9.

58. Fraumeni JF Jr, Ederer F, Miller RW. An evaluation of the carcinogenicity of simian virus 40 in man. JAMA 1963;185:713–8.

59. Magrath DI, Russell K, Tobin JO. Vacuolating agent. BMJ 1961;2:287–8.

60. Shah KV, McCrumb FR Jr, Daniel RW, Ozer HL. Serologic evidence for a simian-virus-40-like infection of man. J Natl Cancer Inst 1972;48:557–61.

61. Rosa FW, Sever JL, Madden DL. Absence of antibody response to simian virus 40 after inoculation with killed-poliovirus vaccine of mothers of offspring with neurologic tumors. N Engl J Med 1988;318:1469.

62. Engels EA, Chen J, Viscidi RP, et al. Poliovirus vaccination during pregnancy, maternal seroconversion to simian virus 40, and risk of childhood cancer. Am J Epidemiol 2004;160:306–16.

63. Gundelfinger BF, Hantover MJ, Bell JA, et al. Evaluation of a trivalent adenovirus vaccine for prevention of acute respiratory disease in naval recruits. Am J Hyg 1958;68:156–68.

64. Hilleman MR, Greenberg JH, Warfield MS, et al. Second field evaluation of bivalent types 4 and 7 adenovirus vaccine. Arch Intern Med 1958;102:428–36.

65. Sherwood RW, Buescher EL, Nitz RE, Cooch JW. Effects of adenovirus vaccine on acute respiratory disease in U.S. Army recruits. JAMA 1961;178:1125–7.

66. Rabson AS, O'Conor GT, Berezesky IK, Paul FJ. Enhancement of adenovirus growth in African green monkey kidney cell cultures by SV40. Proc Soc Exp Biol Med 1964;116:187–90.

67. Lewis AM Jr. SV40 in adenovirus vaccines and adenovirus-SV40 recombinants. Dev Biol Stand 1998;94:207–16.

68. Morris JA, Johnson KM, Aulisio CG, et al. Clinical and serologic responses in volunteers given vacuolating virus (SV40) by respiratory route. Proc Soc Exp Biol Med 1961;108:56–9.

69. Brock B, Kelleher L, Zlotnick B. Product quality control testing for the oral polio vaccine. Dev Biol Stand 1998;94:217–9.

70. Sierra-Honigmann A, Krause PR. Live oral poliovirus vaccines do not contain detectable simian virus 40 (SV40) DNA. Biologicals 2000;28:1–4.

71. Sangar D, Pipkin PA, Wood DJ, Minor PD. Examination of poliovirus vaccine preparations for SV40 sequences. Biologicals 1999;27:1–10.

72. Shah KV, Willard S, Meyers RE, et al. Experimental infection of rhesus with simian virus 40 (SV40). Proc Soc Exp Biol Med 1969;130:196–203.

73. Shah KV, Daniel RW, Strickler HD, Goedert JJ. Investigation of human urine for genomic sequences of the primate polyomaviruses simian virus 40, BK virus, and JC virus. J Infect Dis 1997;176:1618–21.

74. Li R-M, Branton MH, Tanawattanacharoen S, et al. Molecular identification of SV40 infection in human subjects and possible association with kidney disease. J Am Soc Nephrol 2002;13:2320–30.

75. Bofill-Mas S, Pina S, Girones R. Documenting the epidemiologic patterns of polyomaviruses in human populations by studying their presence in urban sewage. Appl Environ Microbiol 2000;66:238–45.

76. Shah KV, Galloway DA, Knowles WA, Viscidi RP. Simian virus 40 (SV40) and human cancer: a review of the serological data. Rev Med Virol 2004;14:231–9.

77. Carter JJ, Madeleine MM, Wipf GC, et al. Lack of serologic evidence for prevalent simian virus 40 infection in humans. J Natl Cancer Inst 2003;95:1522–30.

78. Knowles WA, Pipkin P, Andrews A, et al. Population-based study of antibody to the human polyomaviruses BKV and JCV and the simian polyomavirus SV40. J Med Virol 2003;71:115–23.

79. Minor P, Pipkin P, Jarzebek Z, Knowles W. Studies of neutralizing antibodies to SV40 in human sera. J Med Virol 2003;70:490–5.

80. de Sanjose S, Shah KV, Domingo-Domenech E, et al. Lack of serological evidence for an association between simian virus 40 and lymphoma. Int J Cancer 2003;104:522–4.

81. Engels EA, Viscidi RP, Galloway DA, et al. Case-control study of simian virus 40 and non-Hodgkin lymphoma in the United States. Journal of the National Cancer Institute. 2004;96:1368–74.

82. Viscidi RP, Rollison DEM, Viscidi E, et al. Serological cross-reactivities between antibodies to simian virus 40, BK virus, and JC virus assessed by virus-like-particle-based enzyme immunoassays. Clin Diagn Lab Immunol 2003;10:278–85.

83. Shah KV, Southwick CH. Prevalence of antibodies to certain viruses in sera of free-living rhesus and of captive monkeys. Ind J Med Res 1965;53:488–500.

84. Southwick CH, Siddiqi MF. Primate commensalism: the rhesus monkey in India. Rev Ecol 1994;49:223–31.

85. Shah KV. Neutralizing antibodies to simian virus 40 (SV40) in human sera from India. Proc Soc Exp Biol Med 1966; 121:303–7.

86. Engels EA, Switzer WM, Heneine W, Viscidi RP. Serologic evidence for exposure to simian virus 40 in North American zoo workers. Journal of Infectious Diseases. 2004; 190;2065–9.

87. Major EO. Human polyomavirus. In: Knipe DM, Howley PM, editors. Fields virology. 4th ed. Philadelphia: Lippincott, Williams, and Wilkins; 2001. p. 2175–96.

88. Carroll-Pankhurst C, Engels EA, Strickler HD, et al. Thirty-five year mortality following receipt of SV40-contaminated polio vaccine during the neonatal period. Br J Cancer 2001;85:1295–7.

89. Engels EA, Katki HA, Nielsen NM, et al. Cancer incidence in Denmark following exposure to poliovirus vaccine contaminated with simian virus 40. J Natl Cancer Inst 2003;95:532–9.

90. Strickler HD, Rosenberg PS, Devesa SS, et al. Contamination of poliovirus vaccines with simian virus 40 (1955–1963) and subsequent cancer rates. JAMA 1998;279:292–5.

91. Strickler HD, Goedert JJ, Devesa SS, et al. Trends in U.S. pleural mesothelioma incidence rates following simian virus 40 contamination of early poliovirus vaccines. J Natl Cancer Inst 2003;95:38–45.

92. Price B, Ware A. Mesothelioma trends in the United States: an update based on Surveillance, Epidemiology, and End Results Program data for 1973 through 2003. Am J Epidemiol 2004;159:107–12.

93. Smith MA, Strickler HD, Granovsky M, et al. Investigation of leukemia cells from children with common acute lymphoblastic leukemia for genomic sequences of the primate polyomaviruses JC virus, BK virus, and simian virus 40. Med Pediatr Oncol 1999;33:441–3.

94. Farwell JR, Dohrmann GJ, Marrett LD, Meigs JW. Effect of SV40 virus-contaminated polio vaccine on the incidence and type of CNS neoplasms in children: a population-based study. Trans Am Neurol Assoc 1979;104:261–4.

95. Rollison DEM, Page WF, Crawford H, et al. Case-control study of cancer among U.S. Army veterans exposed to simian virus 40-contaminated adenovirus vaccine. Am J Epidemiol 2004;160:317–24.

96. Brenner AV, LInet MS, Selker RG, et al. Polio vaccination and risk of brain tumors in adults: no apparent association. Cancer Epidemiol Biomarkers Prev 2003;12:177–8.

97. Jordan WS. History of the commission of the acute respiratory diseases. In: Woodward TE, editor. The Armed Forces Epidemiological Board, histories of the commissions. Washington (DC): Office of the Surgeon General; 1994. p. 38.

98. Vilchez RA, Butel JS. Re: Lack of serologic evidence for prevalent simian virus 40 infection in humans [letter]. J Natl Cancer Inst 2004;96:633.

99. Galloway DA, Carter JJ. Response [letter]. J Natl Cancer Inst 2004;96:633–4.

100. Gazdar AF, Butel JS, Carbone M. SV40 and human tumours: myth, association or causality. Nat Rev Cancer 2002;2: 957–64.

101. Krynska B, del Valle L, Croul S, et al. Detection of human neurotropic JC virus DNA sequence and expression of the viral oncogenic protein in pediatric medulloblastomas. Proc Nat Acad Sci U S A 1999;96:11519–24.

102. Arrington AS, Moore MS, Butel JS. SV40-positive brain tumor in scientist with risk of laboratory exposure to the virus. Oncogene 2004;23:2231–5.

103. Shivapurkar N, Harada K, Reddy J, et al. Presence of simian virus 40 DNA sequences in human lymphomas. Lancet 2002;359:851–2.

104. Rizzo P, Carbone M, Fisher SG, et al. Simian virus 40 is present in most United States human mesotheliomas, but it is rarely present in non-Hodgkin's lymphoma. Chest 1999;116:470S–3S.

105. Vivaldi A, Pacini F, Martini F, et al. Simian virus 40-like sequences from early and late regions in human thyroid tumors of different histotypes. J Clin Endocrinol Metab 2003;88:892–9.

106. Engels EA, Rodman LH, Frisch M, et al. Childhood exposure to simian virus 40-contaminated poliovirus vaccine and risk of AIDS-associated non-Hodgkin's lymphoma. Int J Cancer 2003;106:283–7.

107. Rollison DEM, Helzlsouer KJ, Alberg AJ, et al. Serum antibodies to JC virus, BK virus, and simian virus 40, and the risk of incident adult astrocytic brain tumors. Cancer Epidemiol Biomarkers Prev 2003;12:460–3.

18

The Human T-Lymphotropic Leukemia Viruses 1 and 2

MARK A. BEILKE

EDWARD L. MURPHY

HISTORY AND DISCOVERY OF HUMAN T-LYMPHOTROPIC VIRUSES 1 AND 2

The devastating impact of human immunodeficiency virus serotype 1 (HIV-1) has overshadowed the biologic and clinical significance of the first two described human retroviruses, human T-lymphotropic viruses 1 and 2 (HTLV-1, HTLV-2). Confusion exists among physicians and health care workers about the clinical significance of these viruses, and both professionals and lay people may incorrectly think that HTLVs cause acquired immune deficiency syndrome (AIDS). Early in the AIDS epidemic, HTLV-1 was thought to be etiologically associated with this disease.[1] Later, this hypothesis was disproved.[2] Nonetheless, antibodies reacting against HTLV-1 and -2 proteins could be detected in the sera of some patients with AIDS or AIDS-related complex.[3] Furthermore, the similar modes of transmission of the human T-lymphotropic and human immunodeficiency viruses made the possibility of simultaneous coinfection with multiple viruses more likely.[4]

HTLV-1 is the causative agent of adult T-cell leukemia/lymphoma (ATLL), tropical spastic paraparesis/HTLV-1–associated myelopathy (TSP/HAM), uveitis, polymyositis, synovitis, thyroiditis, and bronchoalveolar pneumonitis.[5–20] HTLV-2, a virus epidemic among intravenous drug users, also has the potential to cause TSP/HAM, as well as other neurologic disorders, bronchopneumonia, and immunologic conditions.[21–26]

HTLV-1 was the first human retrovirus to be described as being associated with disease.[6–9] Interest in the possible association of human retroviruses and cancer resulted in vigorous effort to detect the retroviral reverse transcriptase enzyme in the blood and tissues of patients with hematologic malignancies.[27,28] These efforts were fruitful when in 1980, American investigators at the National Cancer Institute detected and isolated type C retrovirus particles from a West Indian patient with cutaneous T-cell lymphoma (CTCL).[6] Integrated HTLV-1 proviral sequences were present in the malignant cells, but not in normal cells of the affected individual. Concurrently, Japanese investigators identified HTLV-1 as the cause of ATLL.[7,8] Yoshida and colleagues used cocultivation of leukemia cells from an ATLL patient with cord blood lymphocytes to characterize HTLV-1, which resulted in an HTLV-1-producing cell line known as MT-2.[9] Virus particles present in the MT-2 culture supernatant fluids were purified by density in a sucrose gradient, and were shown to have magnesium-dependent reverse transcriptase activity. The investigators then demonstrated that a radiolabeled cDNA probe prepared by reverse transcription was homologous with chromosomally integrated DNA present in ATLL cells.

T-cell malignancies were recognized to be among the most common lymphoproliferative disorders in certain regions of Japan. This observation followed the initial description of ATLL by Takatsuki and colleagues in 1977.[5,29] The epidemiologic clustering of ATLL within certain age groups, in distinct prefectures within southern Japan, led the Japanese investigators to suspect that the malignancy was virally induced. Following the discovery of HTLV-1 and the development of reagents to perform reliable serologic testing, it was shown that both HTLV-1 infection and ATLL are endemic in areas of high HTLV-1 seroprevalence.[30,31] Antibodies against HTLV-1 have been found in over one million individuals, and more than 700 cases of ATLL have been diagnosed each year in Japan alone.[30]

An interesting sequence of events led to reports of an unusual neurodegenerative syndrome in which HTLV-1 was implicated in the pathogenesis. Seroprevalence studies performed in Jamaica, Colombia, and Japan indicated that HTLV-1 antibodies were present in patients afflicted with a debilitating process, characterized by a slow-onset spastic paraparesis that was associated with sphincter disturbance and variable degrees of proprioceptive and sensory dysfunction.[11–14] The disorder, designated TSP/HAM, is characterized as a progressive inflammatory process with parenchymal infiltration of mononuclear cells into the gray and white matter of central nervous system tissues, resulting in severe white matter degeneration of the thoracic spinal cord.[32] Following initial studies confirming HTLV-1 as the cause of ATLL and TSP/HAM, a spectrum of HTLV-1–associated rheumatologic conditions have been described in which viral genome and/or viral proteins were detected in target tissues. These include endemic polymyositis, bronchoalveolar pneumonitis, autoimmune thyroiditis, uveitis, and arthritis.[15,16,18–20]

The second human retrovirus, HTLV-2, has previously been regarded as a bloodborne retroviral pathogen with limited disease potential.[33,34] This contention has been challenged by recent studies, especially when HTLV-2 and HIV infect the same individual.[35,36] HTLV-2 causes TSP/HAM and neurodegenerative disease but, unlike HTLV-1, is rarely found in cases of lymphoproliferative disease. Following the initial isolation and identification of HTLV-2 from a patient with T-cell variant hairy cell leukemia, a second case report described the isolation of a HTLV-2 patient with CD8$^+$ T-lymphotropic.[37,38] Case reports of other hematologic malignancies have been made, including a description of CTCL in an HIV/HTLV-2–co-infected patient, in which clonally HTLV-2–infected CD8$^+$ cells were present in the skin biopsy samples.[39]

Beyond the previously mentioned case reports, dispute remains regarding a broader role for HTLV-2 in the pathogenesis of leukemia or lymphoma. Careful investigations have essentially excluded a role for HTLV-2 in the pathogenesis of classic B-cell hairy cell leukemia and large-cell granulocytic leukemia.[38,40,41] Similarly, the possibility that retroviruses are involved in the development of HTLV-1–seronegative cases of CTCL is based on disputable evidence.[42,43] Small studies examining fresh peripheral blood mononuclear cells and cultured cell lines obtained from patients with either Sézary syndrome or mycosis fungoides suggested the possibility that the HTLV-1 regulatory gene, *tax*, could be detected in some samples, using the polymerase chain reaction (PCR).[44,45] Other laboratories have not confirmed these findings.[46–49] Furthermore, patients presenting with CTCL in the absence of ATLL had rates of seroreactivity to HTLV-1 or -2 comparable to the general population.[46]

EPIDEMIOLOGY AND MODES OF TRANSMISSION OF HTLV-1 AND HTLV-2

HTLV-1 Distribution Worldwide

Since its initial description in 1980, HTLV-1 has been described in many countries throughout the world. Its worldwide epidemiology has been the subject of several reviews.[50–53] Genetic sequence data support the hypothesis that HTLV-1 in humans is derived from simian T-lymphotropic virus in primates, with the several independent interspecies transmissions thought to have occurred in Africa, Melanesia, and perhaps other worldwide locations.[51,54]

In sub-Saharan Africa, the overall prevalence of HTLV-1 is < 5% (Figure 18–1).[55] Other areas of endemic infections include southwestern Japan, several countries in the Caribbean Basin, Brazil, Colombia, Peru, some areas in Iran, and the Pacific islands including Hawaii, Melanesia, and Papua New Guinea. Very low levels of HTLV-1 infection are also present in the United States, United Kingdom, Europe, and Australia, probably due to immigration from endemic areas. The genetic variability of HTLV-1 is very low, with only 1 to 2% nucleotide variation in worldwide isolates. Nevertheless, molecular epidemiologic studies have demonstrated several unique HTLV-1 strains that are localized to specific geographic regions such as Africa and Melanesia. In addition, the so-called cosmopolitan strain is identified in most HTLV-1–infected persons in Japan, the Caribbean, and South America.

Caution must be exercised in the interpretation and comparison of international seroprevalence studies because of differences in the age, gender, and risk profile composition of the populations studied. Furthermore, serologic screening assays such as enzyme immunoassays (EIAs) were subject to nonspecificity, especially during the 1980s. There is also a phenomenon of biologic false-positivity, particularly in Africa, which causes reactive EIAs and indeterminate Western blot patterns that may be falsely interpreted as positive.[55] This phenomenon has been attributed to possible cross-reactivity with malaria antigens.[56]

HTLV-1 Epidemiology Endemic Populations

In endemic areas, there is a general pattern of increasing HTLV-1 seroprevalence with older age, and in most countries, females have a higher sero-prevalence than males, particularly in the elderly age groups (Figure 18–2).[57,58] It is possible to interpret this age- and sex-specific seroprevalence relationship as being indicative of a pattern of ongoing mother-to-child transmission (low childhood prevalence) and sexual transmission in adulthood (cumulative increase in seroprevalence with age). The female excess of prevalence has been interpreted as indicating preferential sexual transmission from male to female compared with the opposite direction.[59] In addition, a portion of the high HTLV-1 prevalence in elderly age groups may represent an age-cohort effect; namely, higher levels of HTLV prevalence in the past compared with future generations, due to changes in breast-feeding practices or in the use of condoms for birth control.[60] Finally, HTLV-1 seroprevalence often varies on a microgeographic level, with clusters of high infection in particular socioeconomic groups, isolated villages, or in particular ecologic regions.[61,62] These are likely due to sociologic rather than biologic phenomena.

Specific examples of high HTLV-1 prevalence populations include the island of Jamaica where a large seroprevalence survey in the 1980s demonstrated prevalence increasing from < 2% (both sexes, age 10 to 19 years) to 17% (women aged 70 years and older) (see Figure 18–2A).[57] Data from the same

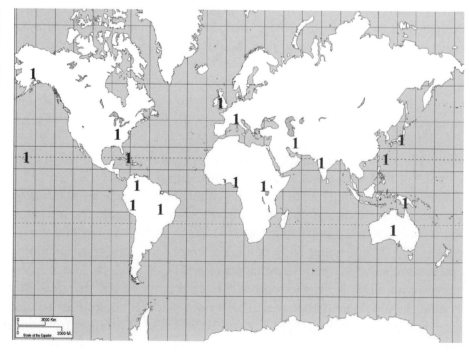

Figure 18–1. Geographic distribution of human T-lymphotropic virus 1 (HTLV-1) infection. HTLV-1–endemic populations are shown in *red* typeface, and areas with sporadic cases of HTLV-1 often due to immigration from endemic areas, are shown in *blue* typeface.

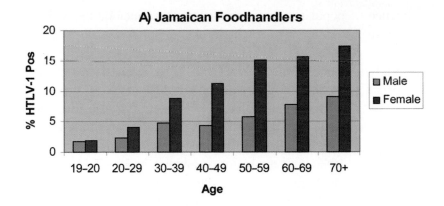

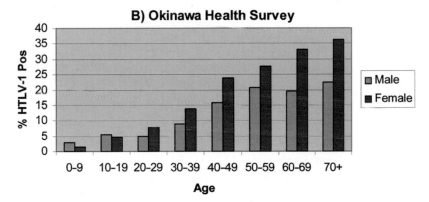

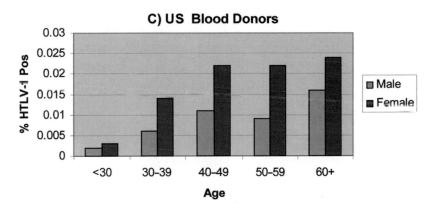

Figure 18–2. Age- and sex-specific seroprevalence of human T-lymphotropic virus 1 (HTLV-1) in several population groups. *A*, Jamaicans employed in food handling occupations.[57] *B*, Participants in a community health survey in Okinawa, Japan.[63] *C*, US blood donors with very low HTLV-1 seroprevalence.[64] All three graphs show the characteristic higher female prevalence, and rising prevalence with age.

decade in Okinawa in southwestern Japan showed a higher but similar pattern of age- and sex-specific seroprevalence, with the exception that the difference between males and females was not pronounced until the older age groups (see Figure 18–2B).[63] The reasons for this difference are unclear, but may be related to differences in sexual behavior or to the post-war promotion of condoms for birth control in Japan. Finally, data from United States blood donors in 1991 to 1995 reveal an HTLV-1 seroprevalence that is 1,000-fold lower than in Jamaica or Okinawa, but a strikingly similar pattern of age- and sex-spe-

cific seroprevalence to that of endemic areas may be seen (see Figure 18–2C).[64] In the latter study, HTLV-I seroprevalence was significantly higher in Blacks, Hispanics, and Asians, compared with Whites and in those born outside of the United States.

HTLV-2 in Indigenous People

HTLV-2 infection is endemic and widespread among many Native American populations in South, Central, and North America and among African pygmies (Figure 18–3). Tribes in the Amazon region of Brazil have some of the highest HTLV-2 seroprevalence rates in the world. Until recently, many of these indigenous populations have remained relatively isolated, both geographically as well as culturally from other tribes and urban areas, suggesting that HTLV-2 may be an ancient human pathogen in this region. HTLV-2 molecular subtypes a, b, c, and d have been useful in delineating the epidemiology and origins of this retrovirus.[51]

In South America, HTLV-2 seroprevalence in native populations ranges widely, from 1 to 58%. HTLV-2 is found more often in ethnic tribes living in the lowland regions, whereas HTLV-1 tends to be found at a lower prevalence (1 to 7%) and shows geographic clustering within groups living in the Andes highlands and among persons of African descent living in coastal regions.[65] In South America, HTLV-2b is the predominant molecular subtype within indigenous tribes, with the exception of Brazil, where HTLV-2c is the exclusive subtype. By region, these tribes include the Wayu, Guahibo, Orinoco, and Tunebo in Colombia[66-68]; the Yaruro and Guahibo in Venezuela[69]; the Toba, Mataco, and Mapuche in Argentina[70,71]; the Gran Chaco in Paraguay; and the Alacaluf and Yahgan in Chile.[65] In Brazil, HTLV-2 is highly prevalent within several Native American communities, with a particularly strong focus in the Amazon region. By

population and prevalence, these include the Kayapo (32 to 58%), Munduruku (8%), Arara do Laranjal (11%), Tyrio (15%), and Kraho (12%) tribes.[65,72,73]

In Central America, HTLV-2 has been reported among the Guaymi Indians of Panama, a tribe that inhabits isolated areas of Western Panama and Costa Rica. Several population-based studies in the region have found seroprevalence rates ranging from 8 to 10%, with the primary subtype being HTLV-2b.[74-76] One large study of 3,686 Guaymi Indians reported a marked increase of infection by age, with the most notable spike occurring at young adulthood. This, combined with a similar distribution of infection in both males and females, suggests that sexual transmission plays a strong role in the spread of infection within these communities.[74]

In North America, HTLV-2 infection is endemic among several large Native American tribes. By tribe and subtype, these include the Navajo (HTLV-1a/-2b) and Pueblo (HTLV-1a/-2b) of New Mexico and the Seminole (HTLV-2b) of Florida in the United States[77,78]; the Nuu-chah-nulth (HTLV-2a) in Canada[79]; and the Maya (HTLV-2b) in Mexico.[80] Seroprevalence rates of 2 to 3% and 13.2% have been reported among the Pueblo and Seminole tribes, respectively. Serologic screening of blood donors in the Albuquerque, New Mexico area has

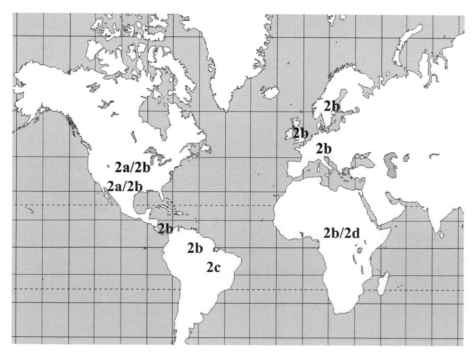

Figure 18–3. Geographic distribution of human T-lymphotropic virus 2 (HTLV-2) molecular subtypes. 2a, 2b, 2c, and 2d refer to HTLV-2 subtypes a, b, c, and d, respectively. Endemic Native American and African populations are shown in *red* typeface, and injection drug users and their sexual partners are shown in *blue* typeface.

revealed unusually high rates of HTLV-1 and -2 (0.72 per 1,000), most of which was attributed to HTLV-2.[81] Moreover, HTLV-2 seroprevalence was found to be much higher among Native American blood donors (1.0 to 1.6%) compared with non-Hispanic white donors (0.009 to 0.06%) in New Mexico.[82] Studies on Native Canadians in Canada have been limited, but one study of the Nuu-chah-nulth tribe in coastal British Columbia found a prevalence of 1.6%.[79] Similarly, HTLV-2 prevalence among indigenous Mayans in the Yucatan Peninsula of Mexico has been found to be quite low (< 1%).[80]

In Africa, few seroprevalence studies have been carried out, but HTLV-2 has been uncovered in two different pygmy tribes living in remote areas of Cameroon and the Democratic Republic of Congo (formerly Zaire), suggesting that HTLV-2 is endemic in Central Africa and has been sustained in isolated communities for a long time.[83–85] HTLV-2 has also been detected sporadically in some semi-urban populations in these same regions, including several members of a family in Gabon, where the infection appears to have spanned three generations.[86–88]

HTLV-2 Epidemic Among Injection Drug Users and HTLV/HIV Coinfection

HTLV-2 is epidemic among injection drug users (IDUs) in the United States and Europe, but has also been detected in IDUs from Southeast Asia and Brazil (see Figure 18–3). Prevalence rates as high as 20% have been observed in IDUs living in metropolitan areas of the United States, thus making them the largest high-risk population.[23] Within the United States, HTLV-2 is most prevalent among black IDUs, particularly in New Orleans, where this group showed a seroprevalence of 19%, roughly three times that of Hispanic or white IDUs.[89] Similarly, seroprevalence studies of blood donors have shown significantly higher rates of HTLV-2 infection in blacks compared with other racial groups.[64] It is unclear whether the high prevalence of HTLV-2 observed among Blacks is attributed to ancestry from endemically infected areas of Africa or whether it is the result of other sociodemographic factors.

HTLV-2 is also common among IDUs in Europe, particularly in Italy and Spain, with prevalence ranging from 1.6 to 8% and 0.4 to 11.5%, respectively, and is frequently coupled with HIV-1 infection.[90–92] In Northern Europe, HTLV-2 is found at a comparatively lower frequency among IDUs in Sweden and France.[93,94] One study in Ireland found a high seroprevalence (15%) of HTLV-2 among IDUs.[95] Extraordinarily high rates of HTLV-2 (> 60%) have also been reported among IDUs living in South Vietnam, where the infection was most likely introduced by US military personnel during the Vietnam war.[96] Furthermore, given the high seroprevalence of HTLV-2 observed in Native American populations living in the Amazon, it is not surprising that the virus has also been detected in neighboring urban populations of Brazil, such as among IDUs and blood donors.[97,98]

How HTLV-2 infection became epidemic among IDUs is unclear, but it is likely to have occurred in the United States. Intravenous drug use has infiltrated many Native American tribes living in North America, and there is evidence that sexual transmission may be a strong source of infection among non–drug-using sexual partners of IDUs.[99–102] Both of these factors probably contributed to a US epidemic of HTLV-2 among IDUs in the 1960s and 1970s, followed by dissemination to IDUs in Europe, and into the broader US population and blood donors by secondary sexual transmission (Figure 18–4).[64,103]

In 1988, routine serologic screening for HTLV-1 in all blood donations was implemented in the United States. Cross-reacting antibodies to HTLV-2 were also detected through this screening method, although at a slightly lower sensitivity. Owing to self-selection and deferral, HTLV-2 seroprevalence among US blood donors remains low, albeit higher than that of HTLV-1. A screening of more than 1.7 million blood donors from five major US cities between 1991 and 1995 detected a seroprevalence of 0.02% for HTLV-2 and 0.01% for HTLV-1 (see Figure 18–4). HTLV-2 infection was found to be significantly higher in female donors, black and Hispanic donors, and in those with a high school or lower education.[64] Major risk factors reported among US donors included a history of IDU, sex with an IDU, or a history of blood transfusion.[102] Similar rates of HTLV-2 seroprevalence have been reported among blood donors in Brazil, whereas significantly lower rates of HTLV-2

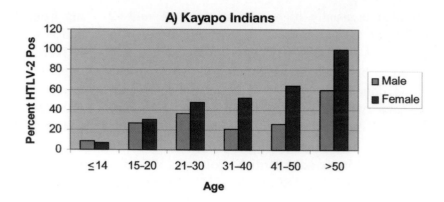

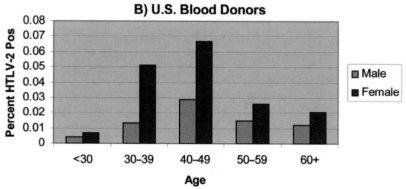

Figure 18–4. Age- and sex-specific seroprevalence of human T-lymphotropic virus 2 (HTLV-2) among the highly-endemic Kayapo Indians *A*, and in US blood donors with very low HTLV-2 seroprevalence *B*.[64,73] The Kayapo data are consistent with ongoing mother-to-child and sexual transmission within a closed population, whereas the US data suggest an age-cohort effect due to injection drug use and secondary sexual transmission in the 1960s and 1970s.

have been found among European blood donors, where HTLV-1 is more common.[104–107]

In HTLV-1–endemic countries such as Brazil, which have also experienced major epidemics of HIV, HTLV-1/HIV coinfection has been observed.[108] Risk factors include sexual promiscuity and IDU, and rates of coinfection correspond to the background prevalence of each retrovirus. Since HTLV-2 is prevalent among IDUs in the United States and Europe, coinfection with HTLV-2/HIV-1 is relatively more common, and research on coinfection is particularly relevant.[109,110] In the United States, only New York and Miami have significant levels of HTLV-1/HIV coinfection among IDUs, presumably due to immigrants from the HTLV-1–endemic Caribbean region.[111]

Modes of Transmission

HTLV-1 and -2 have several well-established modes of transmission: mother-to-child, primarily through breast-feeding; sexual transmission, predominantly heterosexual; and parenteral exposure by transfusion of infected cellular blood products or intravenous

drug use. The predominant routes of transmission vary by population, wherein mother-to-child and sexual transmissions play an important role in Native American populations and parenteral transmission is clearly a significant source of infection among IDUs.

Mother-to-Child Transmission

Vertical transmission (from mother to child), and mostly through breast-feeding, contributes to the high seroprevalence rates observed in HTLV-1– and -2–endemic populations.[112] The duration of breast-feeding appears to be important, suggesting a possible dose effect.[113] High maternal HTLV-1 antibody titer and HTLV-1 proviral load have also been associated with transmission.[113,114] Few studies have focused on mother-to-child transmission of HTLV-2, but the virus has been isolated from breast milk of infected mothers, and children born to infected mothers have a higher seropositivity compared with those born to seronegative mothers.[74,115] Moreover, high seroprevalence rates have been reported among children younger than 15 years of age in the Guaymi

(16.5%), Gran Chaco (14%), and Kayapo (12%) tribes.[71,74,116] In the absence of breast-feeding, several studies have indicated that the risk of perinatal transmission of HTLV-2 is quite low, suggesting that the predominant source of infection occurs via breast-feeding.[117–120]

Sexual Transmission

Sexual transmission of HTLV-1 has been well documented by cross-sectional studies showing sexual behaviors to be a risk factor, studies of HTLV-1 discordant couples, and prospective observation of seroconversion in sexual partners of known HTLV-1 seropositives.[58,59,121,122] In contrast to HTLV-1, sexual transmission of HTLV-2 has been less well studied, but cross-sectional studies have identified sexual transmission of HTLV-2 as an important route of infection in several populations, including Native Americans, blood donors, patients attending sexually transmitted disease clinics, and prostitutes. Endemic Native American tribes offer some of the most compelling evidence of sexual transmission, as prevalence rates are high among both men and women and show a gradual increase with age (see Figure 18–4), suggesting that sexual transmission is one of the predominant sources of infection in these communities.[72,74] A recent US prospective study of HTLV-2–infected blood donors and their seronegative sexual partners found an HTLV-2 incidence rate of 0.5 per 100 person-years, statistically no different from the rate for HTLV-1.[121]

Bloodborne Transmission

Parenteral transmission occurs for both HTLV-1 and -2. In endemic areas, blood transfusion can clearly transmit HTLV-1 when blood products are not tested for HTLV antibody. Okochi and colleagues first described transfusion-transmitted HTLV-1 in Japanese endemic regions, and recommended antibody testing of all blood donors.[123] Among Jamaican patients transfused with an HTLV-seropositive blood unit prior to the initiation of screening in that country, 44% seroconverted after a mean interval of 51 days, and antibody status correlated well with detection of human T-lymphotropic provirus.[124]

Among blood donors found to be infected with HTLV-1 or -2 soon after the initiation of blood screening in the United States in 1988, previous receipt of a blood transfusion was significantly more common than in HTLV-seronegative controls.[102,125] The risk of transfusion-transmitted HTLV-1 or -2 was estimated to be 1 in 641,000 after the introduction of antibody screening.[126] On the other hand, nucleic acid testing (NAT) of all US blood donors further reduced the risk of transfusion-transmitted HIV and hepatitis C, but NAT has not been introduced for HTLV-1 or -2, probably because current NAT systems test plasma and not white cells, and because the disease risk of HTLV-1 and -2 is underappreciated.

Injection Drug Use

Both HTLV-1 and -2 are clearly transmitted by drug injection, presumably via blood contamination of shared needles and syringes. However, in the United States, HTLV-1 has remained localized mainly in the Northeastern and Southeastern states, whereas HTLV-2 is found among IDUs throughout the country but at highest prevalence on the West coast and in Louisiana. An early study that differentiated HTLV-1 from HTLV-2, using a competitive HTLV-1 and -2 enzyme-linked immunoassay technique, reported a high seroprevalence of both HTLV-1 and -2 among IDUs in the New Jersey area.[127] In New Orleans, approximately 25% of IDUs tested were HTLV-2–positive by the PCR, and another 2% were infected with HTLV-1.[21] Sixteen percent of San Francisco IDUs were infected with HTLV-2 and risk factors included black race and the duration of heroin injection.[110] A study of primarily white IDUs from the Staten Island, New York area found PCR-determined prevalences of 11% for HTLV-2 and an additional 9% for HTLV-1.[111] Finally, measurement of HTLV-1 and -2 antibodies in sera, from the Centers for Disease Control and Prevention–sponsored HIV sentinel counties survey, yielded undifferentiated HTLV-1 and -2 prevalences among IDUs in methadone treatment centers, ranging from 0.4 (Atlanta) to 17.6% (Los Angeles).[22] Interestingly, there was little concordance in the ranking of cities by HIV prevalence compared with HTLV-1 and -2 prevalence.

BIOLOGY OF HTLV-1 AND HTLV-2 INFECTIONS

Viral Genome and Gene Products and Comparison with HIV-1

Despite the structural similarity of the HTLV viruses to HIV-1, they lead to immunologically and clinically distinct responses that appear opposite from one another. The primary defect seen in HIV-1 infection is the profound selective depletion of CD4 lymphocytes over time.[128] In contrast, HTLV-1 infection is associated with T-cell activation, proliferation, and leukemogenesis (Tables 18–1 and 18–2).[129] HTLV-1 and -2 can be differentiated from HIV-1 morphologically.[130,131] In contrast to the bullet-shaped nucleocapsid of HIV-1, the HTLV viruses contain a central round nucleocapsid structure, characteristic of delta retroviruses (Figure 18–5). Also, in contradistinction to biopsy samples from HIV/AIDS patients, HTLV-1 and -2 virions are never visualized in biopsy samples of ATLL or TSP/HAM patients and can only be observed when cells and/or tissues are cultured in vitro (Figure 18–6).

Table 18–3 summarizes the differences between HIV and HTLV-1 and -2 with respect to their morphology and genomic structure. The overall genetic structure of the three viruses is similar, in that they contain the structural (*gag, env*) and enzymatic (*pol, pro, in*[tegrase]) genes.[132] The principal differences reside in the characteristics and functions of the nonstructural genes. HIV-1 possesses a number of accessory genes that facilitate viral replication within host cells at very high levels.[133] These genes are lacking in the HTLVs.

In contrast, HTLV-1 and -2 contain a unique region at the 3′ end of their genomes, referred to as the pX region.[134–137] The pX region codes for five open reading frames, two of which encode for the regulatory proteins known as Tax and Rex. Other accessory proteins have also been identified, although their function is not entirely known.[138] Tax and Rex are vital for viral replication and viral persistence, and Tax is thought to hold a central role in cellular transformation events resulting in leukemogenesis.[139–147] Tax-1 and -2 interact in concert with a number of host transcriptional activating proteins to initiate transcription in the 5′ long terminal repeat (LTR) region of the proviral genome. Rex-1 and -2 function to produce incompletely spliced viral messenger (m)RNAs that encode for viral proteins, and may also function to downregulate Tax-mediated *trans*-activation of viral transcription.[148,149]

Although in vitro evidence suggests that Tax-1 and -2 may bind directly to the transcription start site of the human T-lymphotropic provirus, it appears that Tax-mediated activation of transcription is mediated through a complex interaction with multiple cellular proteins that bind to promoters at several adjacent regions within the U3 region of the LTR.[140]

Table 18–1. HIV-1 VS. HTLV-1/2	
HIV-1	**HTLV-1, HTLV-2**
• Rapid lytic events result in release of virus into plasma/extracellular compartments • CD8 CTL responses ultimately fail in controlling infection • Can measure HIV viral load in plasma, CSF, genital secretions, and breast milk	• Rare lytic events with no detectable virus in plasma, extracellular compartments • Persistent robust CD8 CTL responses result in life-long infection and long latency period with little disease expression • Cannot detect HTLV in cell-free fluids as virus is highly cell-associated

Table 18–2. HIV-1 VS. HTLV-1/2	
HIV-1	**HTLV-1, HTLV-2**
• Preferentially infects CD4 cells, dendritic cells, macrophages • Extracellular virions use CD4 receptor and chemokine co-receptor in addition to direct cell-cell spread of virus • Integration of genome into host DNA • Cytopathic for CD4 cells • Neurotropic	• Preferentially infects CD4 cells and CD8 cells, ? others • Cell-to-cell spread of virus is primary mode of viral entry into T lymphocytes • Integration of genome into host DNA • Not highly cytopathic • Neurotropic

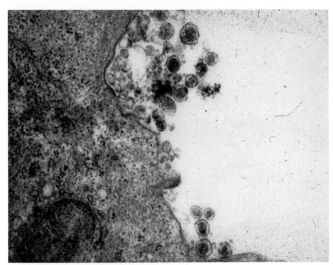

Figure 18–5. Electron micrograph of human T-lymphotropic virus 1 (HTLV-1) virions budding from cultured lymphocytes obtained from an HTLV-1–infected patient. HTLV-1 virions contain a central round nucleocapsid, characteristic of type C retroviruses. HTLV-1 virions are never identified in uncultured cells or tissues of HTLV-1–infected individuals. Reproduced with permission from Peter Didier, PhD, Tulane National Primate Research Center, Louisiana, USA.

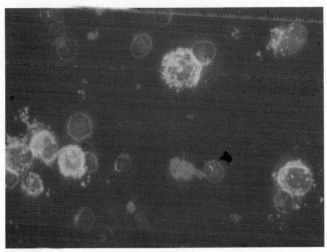

Figure 18–6. Indirect immunofluorescence micrograph of an human T-lymphotropic virus 1 (HTLV-1)-producing cell line established from an HTLV-1–infected patient. Note the abundant expression of the HTLV-1 p19 viral antigen. Cells are counterstained with Evans Blue.

Probably the most important interaction of Tax is with the cyclic adenosine monophosphate (cAMP) response-element–binding protein/activating transcription factor (CREB/ATF) DNA-binding proteins, leading to the expression of viral proteins (Figure 18–7). Several publications carefully elaborate upon these complex interactions.[135,140,141,146]

In addition to the vital function of transcriptional activation, Tax-1 and -2 function to *trans*-activate a number of important cellular genes (primarily through interaction with host cell transcriptional activating proteins), resulting in cellular activation, transformation, and intracellular and extracellular expression of cytokines (Table 18–4).[150–163] Of these interactions, the most notable is the activation of both the interleukin-2 (IL-2) and interleukin-2 receptor (IL-2R) genes in T cells,

TABLE 18–3. MORPHOLOGIC AND STRUCTURAL CHARACTERISTICS OF HIV-1 VERSUS HTLV-I AND -2[130-137]		
	HIV-1	**HTLV-1/HTLV-2**
Taxonomy/Morphology	Lentivirus "Bullet shaped" nucelocapsid 100-120 nm	Oncornaviruses Round Nucleocapsid 100 nm
Detection of virions in biopsy samples by electron microscopy	yes	no
Structural Genes	gag (p17, p24, p2, p7, p1, p6) pol (Reverse transcriptase, integrase, protease) env (gp120, gp41)	gag (p19, p24,p15) pro (protease) pol (reverse transcriptase, ?integrase) env (gp46, p21)
Accessory Genes	Six: 1. vif (virion infectivity protein) 2. vpr (viral protein R, enhances viral replication) 3. tat (viral transactivator) 4. rev (regulator of expression of viral protein) 5. vpu (Viral protein U, enhances virion release from cell) 6. nef (negative regulatory factor)	At least two: 1. tax (transcriptional activator) 2. rex (posttranscriptional modification) (there may be other accessory genes but their function is unknown)

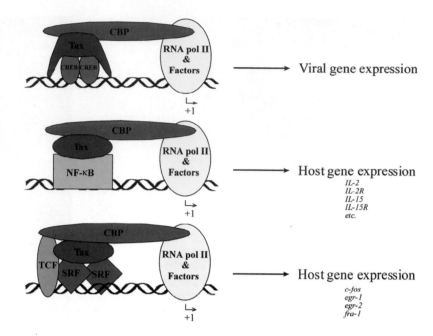

Figure 18–7. A simple model of Tax transcriptional activation. *Top panel*: Tax activates viral gene expression by interacting with the GC-rich region of the viral CRE (vCRE), CREB, and CBP. *Middle panel*: Tax activates host gene expression by interacting with NF-κB and CBP. *Bottom panel*: Tax activates host immediate-early gene expression by interacting with SRF, TCF, and CBP. (CRE = cyclic AMP responsive element, CREB = cyclic AMP responsive-element–binding protein, CBP = CREB-binding protein, NF-κB = nuclear factor-kappa B, SRF = serum response factor, TCF = ternary complex factor. 1+ designates the transcription start site (AUG). Reproduced with permission from Maureen Shuh, PhD, Loyola University, Louisiana, USA.

which appears central to the polyclonal expansion of HTLV-1 infected cells in early infection.[164–168] HTLV-1 *trans*-activation of the IL-2R promoter region is due to the interaction between Tax-1 and the nuclear factor-κ B transcription factors and CREB-binding protein (CBP)/p300.[139]

Cellular Tropism and Viral Entry

Both HTLV-1 and -2 preferentially infect T cells, with the CD4+ T cell as primary host for HTLV-1 and the CD8+ T cell as primary host for HTLV-2.[169,170] However, as will be discussed below, HTLV-1 and -2 viral entry into CD4+ and CD8+ T cells does not appear to require the CD4 or CD8 receptor. Both HTLV-1 and -2 share tropism for a variety of nonlymphoid cells, suggesting the possibility that the viruses use a more ubiquitous cellular receptor for viral binding and entry.[171,172] At least one laboratory has presented evidence suggesting that nearly all vertebrate cell lines express a functional HTLV envelope receptor.[173] Interestingly, the receptor may be underexpressed (or perhaps absent) on human resting T cells and is expressed only upon T-cell activation. However, recent evidence suggests that receptor-mediated viral entry is probably unnecessary for infection of T lymphocytes. It is now clear that HTLV-1 may spread between lymphocytes without actual budding from the donor cell.[174,175] In fact, it has been suggested that

persistent HTLV-1 infection may occur without any requirement to make extracellular virions. Instead, cell–cell contact may initiate polarization of the cellular cytoskeleton of the infected cell to the cell–cell junction. In the context of these polarization events, it appears that HTLV-1 gag proteins and genome accumulate in concert with cellular cytoskeletal proteins, with resultant transfer of viral protein and nucleic acid into the recipient cell.

Viral Replication and Persistence

The epidemiologic evidence provided above strongly supports the conclusion that the two primary modes of HTLV-1 transmission include mother-to-child (via breast milk) and sexual transmissions.[176] HTLV-2 transmission may also occur through these common modes, although the epidemic among IDUs implies a much greater role for bloodborne transmission of HTLV-2 via shared needles. Therefore, with the exception of blood-borne transmission, the initial targets of HTLV-1 and -2 infections are mucosal surfaces, just as for HIV-1. HTLV-1–infected CD4+ T cells are present in abundant quantities in both breast milk and seminal fluid. In fact, evidence suggests that seminal fluid enhances replication of HTLV-1, perhaps through cytokine-mediated up-regulation of viral transcription.[177] In the scenario of mother-to-child transmission, ingestion of breast

Table 18–4. PRINCIPAL CELLULAR GENES WHICH ARE TRANS-ACTIVATED BY HTLV-1 TAX PROTEIN[150-167]; (NOT AN EXHAUSTIVE LIST)

Cytokines and Receptors IL-1 IL-2 and IL-2Rα GM-CSF IL-6 IL-8 IL-10 IL-13 IL-15 TNF-β MIP-1α, MIP-1β	Activity upregulated	Polyclonal expansion of HTLV-1 and HTLV-2 infected cells.
Host transcription factors (c-fos, c-sis, c-rel, c-myc, erg-1, erg-2, fra-1)	Activity upregulated	Cellular transformation
Adhesion molecules (ICAM-1, vimentin, CD54)	Activity upregulated	Lymphocyte tracking into involved tissues
Pro-apoptotic factors (bax, p53)	Activity down-regulated	Cellular transformation and leukemogenesis
DNA repair enzymes	Activity down-regulated	Cellular transformation and leukemogenesis

milk by the infant and subsequent infection most likely involves cell–cell contact between maternal HTLV-1–infected T cells and the infant's mucosal lymphoid and/or dendritic cells. Sexual transmission similarly results from cell–cell contact on vaginal or penile mucosal surfaces. As with HIV-1, genital ulcerations may enhance rates of male-to-female and female-to-male transmission events. Blood-borne transmission of HTLV-1 and -2 through transfusions or via injection drug use enables virally infected lymphoid cells to rapidly disseminate and infect host target cells, possibly resulting in higher levels of viral burden during early infection.[178,179]

Beyond initial sites of viral replication, it is presumed that initial infection occurs locally within the regional lymphatics. Trafficking of HTLV-1-infected cells via the lymphatics and the blood stream may result in dissemination of infection to various reservoirs of infection, including the skin, thymus, liver and spleen, mucosally associated lymphoid tissues, and perivascular locations within the central nervous system. The risk of developing ATLL appears to be greatest in individuals who acquire HTLV-1 via mother-to-child transmission.[180] One suggestion is that infection of thymocytes early in life may correlate with the later development of ATLL.[181] This hypothesis is substantiated by experiments demonstrating that in vitro infection of both mature (CD2$^+$, CD3$^+$) or immature (CD2$^+$, CD3$^-$) thymocytes resulted in the IL-2-dependent proliferation of HTLV-1 positive thymocytes expressing CD2$^+$, CD3$^-$, CD4$^+$ phenotypes.[182] Efficient replication of HTLV-1 and -2 within their respective target cells follows the paradigm of mammalian retroviruses.[183] Following entry of the target cell via cell–cell fusion or endocytosis of virions, the single-stranded viral RNA is copied into an RNA–DNA hybrid by the HTLV-1 and -2 reverse transcriptase enzyme. The RNA template is then degraded and the reverse transcriptase copies the single-stranded DNA into a double-stranded DNA–DNA hybrid during multiple steps. The full-length double-stranded DNA undergoes one of two fates: (1) the hybrid may circularized and exist in a nonintegrated episomal form, or (2) the DNA–DNA hybrid may be transported into the cell nucleus where it becomes integrated within the host genome at random sites.[184] Viral latency may then ensue, or in activated T cells, activation of viral transcription may be initiated. The initiation of transcription, or the maintenance of viral latency, is under strong control by the HTLV-1 and -2 regulatory proteins Tax and Rex.

Transformation and Leukemogenesis

Development of ATLL follows a remarkably extended period of time—years to decades of chronic and latent infection with HTLV-1. The cumulative risk of development of ATLL among HTLV-1–infected individuals is approximately 4%.[185] The low probability of developing ATLL in the setting of prolonged clinical latency would seem to imply that cellular transformation and leukemogenesis must involve several complex events within host cells over an extended period.

Abundant evidence supports the contention that the HTLV-1 Tax protein is the principal viral oncoprotein mediating leukemogenesis. First, it is known that Tax is able to transform primary CD4+ T lymphocytes in vitro, resulting in clonal cell lines of genetically identical lineage.[186] Second, Tax-transgenic mouse models of lymphoma and mesenchymal tumors have been developed.[187,188] In the latter model, the transgene was expressed in many organs, including the brain, salivary gland, spleen, thymus, skin, muscle, and mammary gland. The investigators found that the expression of the c-*fos* and c-*jun* genes was augmented 2- to 20-fold in histologically normal skin and muscle of the mice. Additionally, a large group of cellular genes involved in T-cell growth are activated by Tax (see Table 18–4). Tax induces genetic instability and represses expression of DNA repair through multiple mechanisms, and induces cell-cycle dysregulation.[141,189–192] For example, Tax has been shown to alter the ability of cells to undergo G_1-phase cycle arrest, facilitating genomic stability of infected host cells.[191] Finally, Tax mediates repression of the tumor suppressor $p53$ function, thereby suppressing growth arrest and apoptosis of transformed cells.[162,193]

Ultimately, HTLV-1 Tax–mediated transformation of T cells results in emergence of multiple clones of CD4+ T cells containing the integrated human T-lymphotropic provirus. During the extended period of clinical latency prior to development of leukemia, there is the eventual emergence of a predominant clone of transformed T cells that undergoes uncontrolled cell cycling and expansion, with resultant clinical manifestation of ATLL.[194] Mature ATLL cells may contain the entire human T-lymphotropic proviral genome or defective genomes, and may have little or no potential to generate mature human T-lymphotropic viral progeny.[195–197] However, the HTLV Tax mRNA may be detected in ATLL cells by in situ hybridization.[198]

Immune Responses to Infection

The establishment of lifelong HTLV-1 and -2 infection with persistent clinical latency occurs in the setting of a robust host humoral and cellular immune response to infection.[199] Characteristic of vertebrate retroviral infections, the virus is able to evade destruction through its ability to integrate into the host genome and propagate itself during the normal physiologic process of cellular division. In addition, viral spread from cell to cell may occur without production of extracellular virions.[174,175]

Infection with HTLV-1 results in development of antibodies within 1 to 2 months, after which levels of antibody persist at a stable level for life.[200] Proviral nucleic acid sequences can be detected during the window phase prior to seroconversion. Additional studies have shown a fairly good correlation with levels of antibody, proviral load, and clinical disease manifestations.[178] Patients developing TSP/HAM appear to mount the most robust humoral immune responses, followed by pre-ATLL patients, with asymptomatic carriers generally exhibiting lower antibody titers and lower levels of human T-lymphotropic proviral burden.[201,202] Viral neutralizing antibodies directed at epitopes within the envelope region can be detected in asymptomatic carriers of HTLV-1, but do not appear to be correlates of protective immunity in vivo.[201,202] Nonetheless, the potential for protection against infection, via induction of viral neutralizing antibodies, by HTLV-1 vaccines is under investigation.[203,204]

Both HTLV-1 and -2 infections are associated with spontaneous proliferative responses in vitro, which can be observed early in the course of infection.[170,205] HTLV-1–infected CD4+ T-cell lines, established from ATLL patients and normal donors by infecting their CD4+ T cells with the virus, express CD80, CD86, and human leukocyte antigen-DR, and induce proliferation of autologous and allogenic CD4+ T cells.[205] The induction of proliferation of noninfected CD4+ cells has been suggested as a mechanism to generate additional targets for spread of HTLV-1 infection to uninfected lymphocytes.[170]

HTLV-1–specific CD4[+] T cells respond in vitro to HTLV-1–infected targets, and these responses appear more robust in patients with TSP/HAM.[170] Cellular cytotoxic immune responses appear to be strong and persistent among HTLV-1–infected individuals.[206] HTLV-1–specific cytotoxic T lymphocytes (CTL) control human T-lymphotropic viral burden by eliminating HTLV-1–infected CD4[+] T lymphocytes. Despite the documented high frequency of HTLV-1–specific CTL cells, CTL is ineffective in eradicating the entire viral reservoir. In fact, CTL activity appears to contribute directly to development of disease, especially TSP/HAM.[207,208] Expansion of HTLV-1 Tax–specific CTL clones is pathognomonic of TSP/HAM, and is strongly HLA-restricted.[209,210]

In contrast to TSP/HAM, patients with ATLL or smoldering ATLL appear to have a decline in HTLV-1–specific CTL responses.[211] This may be in part explained by down-regulation of HTLV-1 Tax expression in ATLL cells, or by mutation of the *tax* gene.[212,213] A proof-in-concept of this hypothesis was demonstrated in a rat model of ATLL, where adoptively transferred T cells from donors who were immunized with a DNA *tax* vaccine replenished HTLV-1 Tax–specific CTL responses and prevented the development of ATLL.[214]

CLINICAL SPECTRUM OF HTLV-1-ASSOCIATED DISEASES

The largest case series describing the clinical spectrum of ATLL come from Japan.[30,215] Smaller case series include those from the West Indies, Africa, and South America.[216–219] The malignancy is very rare in Europe and the United States, and therefore, descriptions of ATLL in these areas exist principally as case reports.[220] An earlier, yet very comprehensive review of the clinical and laboratory features of ATLL and so-called smoldering ATLL is provided in a publication by Catovsky and Foa.[221] This section will focus on the typical clinical presentation of ATLL, chronic ATLL, cutaneous manifestations of ATLL (CTCL), and nonhematologic and infectious complications associated with HTLV-1 infections (Table 18–5).

ATLL and Smoldering ATLL

ATLL is a spectrum of diseases that is generally categorized in four forms: acute, chronic, smoldering, and lymphoma-type.[222] The acute form of ATLL comprises 55 to 75% of all ATLLs, with the chronic forms and cutaneous forms comprising the remaining 25%.[222,223] These variant forms appear to be described more frequently in Japan, and the authors speculate that earlier recognition and diagnosis could account for these differences. ATLL is reported to present typically among individuals in their fifth decade of life. In the Jamaican series, patients presented at a younger age.

Classic ATLL is almost invariably associated with lymphadenopathy, both in the periphery as well as within body cavities. Hepatosplenomegaly is the next most common manifestation, described in approximately 50% of patients. These findings may be preceded by, or occur co-incidentally with, cutaneous manifestations. Skin lesions are generally described as indolent, nodular, and sometimes indurated (Figure 18–8). Occasionally patients are reported to present with a more diffuse rash with exfoliation and erythroderma (Figure 18–9). Pulmonary, central nervous system, and intestinal involvement are variably reported, as well as more unusual extranodal sites.[215,224]

The leukemic phase of ATLL tends to spare the bone marrow. Therefore, significant anemia and thrombocytopenia is not predominant early in disease. White blood cell (WBC) counts, while occasionally normal, are nearly always elevated and may range into the hundred-thousands. Higher WBC counts, and the degree of lactate dehydrogenase and calcium elevations are markers of a poorer prognosis. Peripheral blood smears will reveal the pleomorphic, multilobulated, atypical lymphoid cells with significant nuclear abnormality (Figure 18–10). Hematopathologists will make a distinction between ATLL cells and Sézary cells, in that the nuclear convolutions appear more evident in ATLL cells. The surface phenotype of ATLL cells is usually CD3[+], CD4[+], CD7[-], CD8[-], CD25[+], CD30[+] and terminal deoxynucleotidyl transferase negative. The acid phosphatase reaction is reported to be moderately positive in most cases and shows a granular pattern.[221] Integrated HTLV-1 provirus and clonally rearranged T-cell

Table 18–5. CLINICAL MANIFESTATIONS OF HTLV-1 AND HTLV-2 INFECTIONS

	HTLV-I		HTLV-2	
	Disease	Evidence	Disease	Evidence
Malignancies	Acute ATLL Chronic ATLL Smoldering ATLL T-cell non-Hodgkin's lymphoma	1. Isolation of HTLV-1 from ATLL cells 2. Detection of integrated HTLV-I provirus 3. Clonal T-cell receptor V-β and V-γ gene rearrangements 4. Preferential tropism for CD4+ T cells 5. Transgenic HTLV-1 tax mouse models 6. In vitro studies on HTLV-1-tax trans-activation of cellular genes 7. Epidemiologic evidence	Rare CD8+ cutaneous lymphomas	1. Detection of integrated HTLV-2 provirus 2. Clonal T-cell receptor gene rearrangements 3. Preferential tropism for CD8+ T cells
Neurologic manifestations	TSP/HAM	1. Isolation of HTLV-1 in CSF of TSP/HAM patients 2. Intrathecal synthesis of HTLV-1 IgG 3. Infiltration of HTLV-1 tax–specific CTL cells in CNS tissues 4. detection of proviral genome in involvement tissues 5. Epidemiologic evidence	TSP/HAM ? Peripheral neuropathy	1. Isolation of HTLV-2 from CSF of a TSP/HAM patient 2. Detection of HTLV-2 proviral gene sequences in biopsy specimens
Autoimmune disorders	Polymyositis Arthritis Uveitis Thyroiditis Pneumonitis Sjogren's syndrome	1. Detection of HTLV-1 proviral sequences in involved tissues 2. Detection of high levels of HTLV-1–infected CD4+ T cells in vitrious fluids and inflammatory tissues 3. HTLV-1 tax–specific CD8 cells mediate tissue damage	Arthritis, ? Pneumonitis	Epidemiologic evidence
Infectious Diseases	Opportunistic infections in ATLL patients CMV pneumonitis, *P. carinii* pneumonia, disseminated herpes zoster, Asperillosis, Cryptococcosis, Disseminated *M. avium* infection Miliary tuberculosis	Case reports	Bacterial pneumonia	1. Epidemiologic evidence 2. Host immune defects in HTLV-2 infected may increase susceptibility to infectious diseases
	Infective dermatitis in children	1. Case reports; 2. Detection of HTLV-1 proviral genome in skin biopsies	Tuberculosis	
	Stongyloides stercoralis infections	Individuals infected with HTLV and *S. stercoralis* have a reduction in the production of IL-4, IL-5, IL-13 and parasitic IgE response, all of which are factors participating in the defense mechanism against *S. stercoralis*	Urinary tract infections	

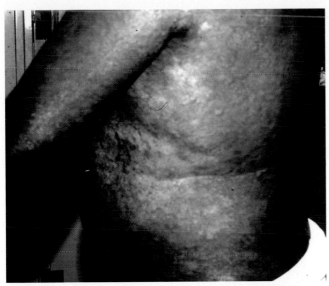

Figure 18–8. Cutaneous involvement in adult T-lymphotropic/lymphoma. Lesions are generalized, nodular, and indurated. Reproduced with permission from Erin Boh, MD, Tulane University Health Sciences Center, Louisiana, USA.

receptors V-β and V-γ can be detected by Southern hybridization analysis.[221]

Hypercalcemia is described in approximately 30 to 60% of patients with ATLL, and is frequently associated with lytic bone lesions.[222,223] The pathogenesis of the hypercalcemia may involve Tax-mediated overexpression of parathyroid hormone-related peptide in HTLV-1-infected T cells.[225] More recent evidence suggests that ATLL cells overexpress the

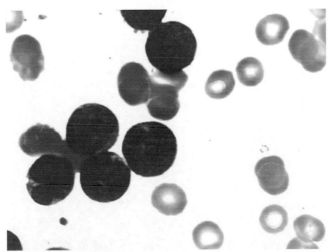

Figure 18–10. Peripheral blood smear in adult T-lymphotropic/lymphoma (ATLL). ATLL cells (sometimes described as "flower cells") appear pleomorphic, multilobulated, and have a significant nuclear convolutions. Reproduced with permission by John Krause, MD, Tulane University Health Sciences Center, Louisiana, USA.

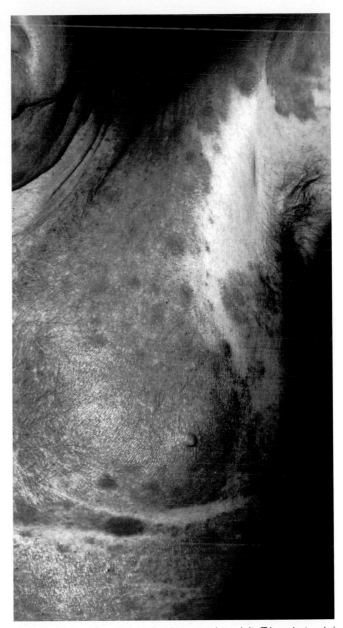

Figure 18–9. Cutaneous involvement in adult T-lymphotropic/lymphoma. Occasionally, patients present with a more diffuse rash with exfoliation and erythroderma. Reproduced with permission from Erin Boh, MD, Tulane University Health Sciences Center, Louisiana, USA.

receptor activator of nuclear factor-κ B (*RANK*) ligand gene.[226] Expression of this gene was shown to induce differentiation of human hematopoietic precursor cells into osteoclasts in vitro, in the presence of macrophage colony-stimulating factor.

Without treatment, ATLL is invariably rapidly fatal, with pulmonary complications, opportunistic infections, and sepsis emerging as the principal causes of death. Uncontrolled hypercalcemia also contributes to fatality.

The chronic and smoldering forms of ATLL comprise more infrequent presentations. Monoclonal HTLV-1 integration appears to present in both forms, and thus many of these individuals will eventually transform to acute forms of ATLL after many years. Chronic ATLL presents with minor cutaneous involvement and persistent lymphocytosis, with fewer cells exhibiting the typical flower cell morphology. Differentiation of chronic from smoldering forms of ATLL seems to be mainly the extent of lymphocytosis and lymphoid cell morphology.[5] In the smoldering form, abnormal lymphocytes comprise < 3% of the cells seen on peripheral smear.

Lymphoma and Cutaneous T-Cell Lymphoma

HTLV-1-associated T-cell lymphoma may present in the absence of blood or bone marrow involvement in approximately 10 to 15% of cases of ATLL. T-cell lymphomas typically present with large and firm peripheral lymphadenopathy, but may also present as primary central nervous system or body cavity lymphomas. Lymph node biopsies show leukemic-type infiltration with medium-sized lobulated lymphoid cells, and may closely resemble non-Hodgkin's lymphomas, and apparent Reed-Sternberg cells are sometimes present. However, the presence of T-cell markers and detection of HTLV-1 proviral sequences, along with HTLV-1 seropositivity, differentiates these tumors. Hypercalcemia is absent, and eosinophilia has been reported.

The hallmark of ATLL is the presence of cutaneous involvement in over one-third of cases. It is important to differentiate HTLV-1–associated cutaneous lymphoma from primary CTCL in HTLV-1–seronegative patients.[227] In the latter forms, nodal or leukemic involvement is initially absent. The clinical and histopathologic appearances of the cutaneous tumors in HTLV-seropositive versus HTLV-seronegative cases are essentially identical (Figure 18–11). Integrated HTLV-1 provirus is detected only in biopsies from HTLV-1-seropositive patients. Some investigators have reported the detection of HTLV *tax/rex* sequences in fresh biopsy specimens of HTLV-1-seronegative CTCL biopsy samples, but these findings have not been reproduced in other laboratories.[46–49]

Primary CTCL represents a spectrum of T-cell neoplasms that originate in the skin, and include mycosis fungoides and Sézary syndrome. Occasionally, these HTLV-seronegative CTCLs will eventually progress to involve the lymph nodes, blood, and peripheral organs. Tumors may range (using the TNM classification) from clinically and/or histopathologically suspicious lesions (T0) to generalized plaques, papules, or erythematous patches involving > 10% of the skin surface (T2), tumors of more than one (T3), and generalized erythroderma (T4).[227] The beneficial clinical response to psoralen plus ultraviolet A (PUVA) therapy has been well described (Figure 18–12).[228]

Neurologic Complications

Shortly after it was established that HTLV-1 was the causative agent of ATLL, investigators in the Caribbean established an epidemiologic link between HTLV-1 and TSP/HAM, followed by similar reports from Japan.[12–14] The occasional presentation of ATLL in TSP/HAM patients (and vice versa) has also been reported.[229–232] The most prominent feature of TSP/HAM includes chronic inflammatory changes in the spinal cord, most notably a meningomyelitis of the lower thoracic cord. Inflammatory changes emerge primarily circumferentially around venules and capillaries in early disease. In cases of longer disease duration, these inflammatory

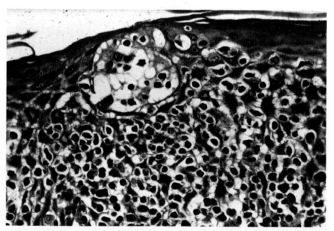

Figure 18–11. Histopathology of a skin biopsy from an human T-lymphotropic virus 1 seronegative patient with cutaneous T-cell lymphoma. The biopsy is histologically identical to those obtained from adult T-lymphotropic/lymphoma patients with cutaneous involvement.

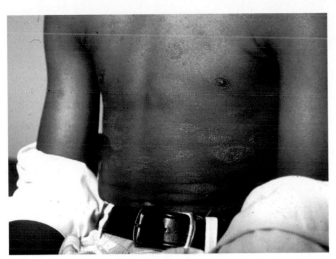

Figure 18–12. Beneficial response to psoralen plus ultraviolet A (PUVA) therapy in cutaneous T-cell lymphoma. This patient's lesions have involuted significantly with PUVA therapy. Reproduced with permission from Erin Boh, MD, Tulane University Health Sciences Center, Louisiana, USA.

changes persist in a perivascular localization and are accompanied by hyalinosis of blood vessels, meningeal fibrosis, and glial scars.[32]

HTLV-1 has been implicated as the cause of TSP/HAM through several lines of evidence: (1) HTLV-1 has been isolated from the cerebrospinal fluid (CSF) of TSP/HAM patients[233]; (2) intrathecal synthesis of HTLV-1 antibodies within the CSF can be detected in some patients[234]; (3) viral genome can be detected within involved tissues by PCR and by in situ hybridization[235,236]; and (4) TSP/HAM has been shown to develop following blood transfusion to an HTLV-1–seronegative recipient from an HTLV-1–infected donor.[237]

TSP/HAM typically develops after years of infection with HTLV-1. Although some of the youngest patients reported were still in their first decade of life, the majority of individuals present in their fourth or fifth decade.[238] Epidemiologic evidence suggests that sexual transmission of HTLV-1 is the predominant mode of transmission leading to the later development of TSP/HAM. This contention is supported by the observed female predominance of TSP/HAM and by sexual activity at an earlier age and higher frequency.[239,240] Additionally, a study examining fresh uncultured peripheral blood mononuclear cells in male TSP/HAM patients and in their spouses, for the presence of HTLV-1 *tax/rex* mRNA by in situ hybridization in TSP/HAM,

revealed higher numbers of HTLV-1 mRNA–positive cells in the female spouses.[241]

TSP/HAM (or HAM/TSP as designated in the Japanese literature) is gradual in onset.[242,243] Lower back pain was evident in two-thirds of patients on presentation. Complaints of burning, pins and needles, cramps, numbness, and tingling exist in approximately 50% of cases. Many patients eventually seek medical treatment because of loss of bladder control or erectile dysfunction. The principle disability is spasticity of the lower legs, and patients will frequently require a walker or a wheelchair. TSP/HAM appears to occur frequently in patients co-infected with HIV-1 and HTLV-1, although HIV vacuolar myelopathy needs to be excluded in cases of coinfection.[244]

Autoimmune Diseases

An entire spectrum of rheumatologic syndromes have been linked epidemiologically to HTLV-1 (and possibly HTLV-2) infection, as alluded to in the beginning of this chapter.[15–20,245] However, with the exception of HTLV-I uveitis, epidemiologic proof of association between HTLV-1 and autoimmune diseases is weak. In the example of HTLV-associated uveitis, human T-lymphotropic viral sequences can be detected in vitreous fluid in conjunction with higher numbers of HTLV-1–infected T lymphocytes compared with the peripheral blood compartment.[15,246] Concurrent autoimmune-mediated disorders, including polymyositis (Figure 18–13), Grave's disease, arthritis, and TSP/HAM, have been described in several case series. In most of these reports, HTLV-1 proviral sequences can be readily detection, whereas viral antigen expression is low or absent in areas with extensive lymphocytic infiltration. Existing evidence suggests that restricted viral gene expression by antigen-presenting cells in the affected tissues triggers a vigorous CD4$^+$ and CD8$^+$ immune response directed toward HTLV Tax or some other gene product.[247,248]

Infectious Diseases

Infectious diseases and fatal opportunistic infections occur most frequently in the context of acute ATLL.

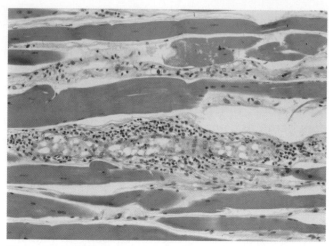

Figure 18–13. Human T-lymphotropic virus 1 (HTLV-1) polymyositis. This patient, co-infected with human immunodeficiency virus serotype 1 and HTLV-1, had severe steroid-responsive polymyositis. Note the extensive lymphoid infiltration of muscle. HTLV-1 *tax/rex* mRNA gene products were detected in the biopsy sample. Reproduced with permission from Faruk Ayden, MD, Tulane University Health Sciences Center, Louisiana, USA.

These include *Pneumocystis carinii* infection, pulmonary aspergillosis, cytomegalovirus (CMV) pneumonitis, disseminated herpes zoster, *Cryptococcus neoformans*, *Mycobacterium avium-intracellulare*, and hyperinfection syndrome with *Strongyloides stercoralis*.[249–251] Trimethoprim/sulfamethoxazole prophylaxis against *P. carinii* infection should be administered to patients with acute forms of ATLL, and possibly to patients with chronic ATLL, as well. Monitoring of peripheral blood for the development of CMV antigenemia may be advised so that pre-emptive ganciclovir can be administered prior to development of overt CMV pneumonitis. Patients with prior tuberculin reactivity, or residency in countries with high rates of tuberculosis, should be considered for isoniazid prophylaxis, although hepatic involvement with ATLL may preclude the use of hepatotoxic drugs.

Some HTLV-1– and -2–infected carriers without ATLL also appear to have immune deficiency associated with an increased risk for certain infectious disease complications, including strongyloidiasis.[251,252] HTLV-1–infected individuals in areas of high endemicity for *S. stercoralis* should probably undergo examination for stool ova and parasites, although there is no formal recommendation in this regard. Other infections associated with HTLV-1 and -2 infections (single case reports) include Nor-wegian scabies, disseminated molluscum contagiosum, and extrapulmonary histoplasmosis. Finally, staphylococcal and streptococcal skin infections are common in the infectious dermatitis syndrome described in Jamaica.[253]

CLINICAL SPECTRUM OF HTLV-2–ASSOCIATED DISEASES

Neurologic Complications

HTLV-2 has been most strongly associated with the neurologic syndrome TSP/HAM. As in HTLV-1, TSP/HAM is characterized by weakness of the legs, spasticity, hyperreflexia, loss of vibration sense, and bladder symptoms and signs consistent with spinal cord damage. Neurologic dysfunction predominates in the lower extremities. The upper extremities, except for occasional hyperreflexia, and cognitive function are spared. Symptoms of TSP/HAM are similar for both HTLV-1 and -2, but HTLV-2 TSP/HAM generally presents with milder and more slowly progressive signs and symptoms.

As summarized in a recent critical review, there are currently about a dozen known cases of HTLV-2–associated myelopathy.[254] This includes four cases from a well-defined prospective cohort of 405 HTLV-2–infected blood donors (cumulative prevalence, 1.0%; 95% CI, 0.3–2.5) followed over more than 10 years.[255] In this same study, six cases of HTLV-1–associated myelopathy were detected among 160 donors (cumulative prevalence, 3.7%; 95% CI, 1.4–8.0), suggesting that the risk of acquiring HAM may be lower in HTLV-2 carriers. Lehky and colleagues reported another four cases of TSP/HAM in patients with HTLV-2, including four African American patients, of whom which three were also of Native American decent.[256] Magnetic resonance imaging from three of these patients showed white matter disease and HTLV-2 antibodies in the cerebrospinal fluid and serum. HTLV-2 RNA was also detected from a spinal cord biopsy in one patient.[256] These clinical findings along with other case reports of TSP/HAM support a neuropathogenic role for HTLV-2.[24,257,258]

In addition to TSP/HAM, HTLV-2 may be associated with several other neurologic disorders, including an ataxic variant of HAM, peripheral neuropathy, and spinocerebellar syndrome. Ataxic HAM shares many of the same signs and symptoms of classic HAM, namely paraparesis and spasticity, but is distinguished by prominent ataxia, neuropathy, and mental changes. Several cases of ataxic HAM have been reported.[25,78,259] In addition, studies on IDUs have found an increased incidence of sensory neuropathy in persons infected with HTLV-2.[260] The exact role of HTLV-2 in the pathogenesis of peripheral neuropathy is unknown, however. In one case report, HTLV-2 nucleic acid sequences were detected in and around peripheral nerves in a biopsy sample.[35] Peripheral neuropathy in the absence of myelopathy has also been described in association with HTLV-2 infection, particular in the setting of HIV-1 coinfection.[35,261] The risk of developing peripheral neuropathy was shown to be three times higher in HTLV-2/HIV co–infected patients than in patients infected with HIV-1 alone.[262]

Pneumonia, Bronchitis, and Other Infections

HTLV-2 has been associated with an increased incidence of pneumonia, bronchitis, tuberculosis, bladder or kidney infection, and abscess. Although several studies have found that respiratory disorders were significantly higher among persons infected with HTLV-2, particularly pneumonia and bronchitis, the pathologic mechanism has yet to be determined.[26,34,263,264] HTLV-2 has also been associated with increased incidence of tuberculosis (TB) in studies involving IDUs and blood donors.[26,265] Moreover, a serologic survey in Nigeria, found a high seroprevalence (3%) of HTLV-2 among TB patients compared with 0.9% in blood donors, although rates were not adjusted for age, a frequent confounding variable with TB infection.[266]

A recent study found no significant difference in pulmonary function and diffusing capacity in asymptomatic HTLV-1 and -2 carriers as compared with uninfected controls.[267] However, clinical or subclinical pulmonary inflammation and progressive loss of pulmonary function over time would not have been detected during this cross-sectional pulmonary function study. Another recent study found

normal production and function of antipneumococcal antibody in response to pneumococcal vaccination in HTLV-2 seropositives.[268] However, baseline levels of antipneumococcal antibody were increased in the HTLV-2–seropositive compared with the seronegative subjects. Murphy and colleagues hypothesized that increased incidence of pneumonia and acute bronchitis in HTLV-2 may be the result of transient inflammatory or autoimmune reaction within the bronchoalveolar regions of the lungs, with or without concomitant respiratory infections.[263] A similar effect has been demonstrated in HTLV-1 patients, in which bronchoalveolar lavage fluid has been found to contain cytokines and other inflammatory markers.[269–273]

Skin and soft-tissue infections are common among IDUs, a population in which HTLV-2 is prevalent. The incidence of abscess and the risk factors associated with its occurrence among IDUs has received limited investigation. A cross-sectional study found that HTLV-2–seropositive IDUs were more vulnerable to skin and soft-tissue abscess than were seronegative IDUs.[264] However, the findings of this study may have been confounded by factors related to both abscess and HTLV-2 seropositivity, such as sex, race, and frequency of drug injection. Subsequent case-control studies with better control for possible confounding variables did not find a significant association between abscess and HTLV-2 infection.[274,275]

Autoimmune Diseases

The notion that HTLV-2 may induce an autoimmune response within the host is further supported by a recent report finding an increased incidence of arthritis and asthma in a prospective cohort of HTLV-2. Compared with seronegative controls, individuals with HTLV-2 were more than twice as likely to have arthritis (odds ratio [OR], 2.66; 95% CI, 1.58–4.45) and more than three times as likely to have asthma (OR, 3.28; 95% CI, 1.57–6.84).[263]

HIV-1/HTLV-2 Coinfection

Since HTLV-2 is prevalent among IDUs in the United States and Europe, coinfection with HIV-1 is common, and therefore research on HIV-1/HTLV-2 coinfection is particularly relevant. Recently, investigation has focused on HTLV-2 as a potential modifier of HIV disease progression.[261] Earlier studies on HIV-1/HTLV coinfection did not differentiate between HTLV-1 and -2. More recent findings have been contradictory, with some studies suggesting that HTLV-2 coinfection accelerates HIV disease progression, whereas other studies have shown no significant effect. [108,109,262,276–279] Many of the studies had limitations, however, including a cross-sectional design and small numbers of co-infected patients. Thus controlling for potential confounding variables such as age, gender, and duration of HIV infection (seroconversion date) may have been difficult.

Addressing many of the limitations of prior studies, the best analysis on HIV-1/HTLV-2 coinfection included pooled longitudinal data on 370 HIV-infected IDUs from four cohort studies.[109] The investigators took into account possible confounding variables, such as age and sex. More importantly, the dates of HIV seroconversion for each subject were clearly defined, thereby allowing for the prospective monitoring of clinical AIDS development or AIDS-related mortality in IDUs with and without HTLV-2 coinfection. The rates of decline in CD4 cell percent were similar in singly infected HIV-1 and co-infected HIV-1/HTLV-2 IDUs, and the study concluded that HTLV-2 coinfection did not independently affect HIV disease progression overall. In contrast to these findings, Beilke and colleagues observed a delayed rate of progression to AIDS and a survival benefit among HIV/HTLV-2 co-infected clinic patients, even after matching for baseline CD4, age, race, injection drug use, and exposure to antiretroviral therapy.[261]

Data concerning the effect of HIV-1 coinfection on HTLV-2 viral load have been limited. One study found no significant difference in viral load between HTLV-2–infected and HIV-1/HTLV-2-co–infected individuals, and similarly, no correlation was seen between HTLV-2 viral load and $CD4^+$ or $CD8^+$ counts in HIV-1–co-infected individuals.[280] Another study, examining HIV-1/HTLV-2 coinfection and sensory neuropathy, found that patients affected by neuropathy had higher mean HTLV-2 proviral loads than patients without the disorder. Interestingly, the patients with neuropathy and the highest proviral loads also exhibited the broadest tropism of HTLV-2

for different cell subpopulations, including peripheral blood mononuclear cells, $CD3^+$, $CD8^+$, $CD14^+$, and $CD19^+$ cells.[281]

Another focus of current research has been on the effects of highly active antiretroviral therapy (HAART) on HIV-1/HTLV-2 coinfection. Preliminary data suggest that HAART may have a paradoxic affect of raising HTLV-2 proviral load. Two separate case series found a similar and marked increase in HTLV-2 proviral load after initiating treatment, which was then followed by a decrease in viral load over time; however, the degree of decline in HTLV-2 proviral load differed between the two studies. A study of one HIV-1/HTLV-2–co-infected patient demonstrated a 1-log peak in viral load after initiating HAART, followed by a 1-log decrease.[282] In contrast, another study of two co-infected patients observed a greater (2-log) increase, followed by a gradual decline in HTLV-2 viral expansion, although viral load remained well above baseline after 15 months of treatment.[283] The $CD4^+$ lymphocyte count of these two patients also increased in concert with HTLV-2 proviral load, suggesting that integrated HTLV-2 provirus was amplified in expanding T-cell clones during HAART.

An increased HTLV-2 proviral load following HAART may predispose HIV–co-infected patients to HTLV-2–related pathology. This may include conditions such as HTLV-myelopathy, cutaneous lymphoma, or peripheral neuropathy.[35,39,255,260,262] It would be premature to draw conclusions about HAART, based solely on these few case reports; further studies are needed to better understand the outcomes of antiretroviral therapy in patients with HIV-1/HTLV-2 coinfection.

Mortality

There have been few studies on mortality associated with HTLV-1 and -2, and two recent HTLV-2 analyses have found conflicting results. One study of 6,570 IDUs, who were tested for antibodies to HIV and HTLV-2 and then matched by age, sex, race, and year to the National Death Index, found that for HTLV-2 infection alone, all-cause mortality was reduced (relative risk [RR], 0.8; 95% CI, 0.7–0.9), with no statistically significant reduction or elevation in cause-specific mortality. They did find, however, a non-significant excess of tuberculosis deaths with HTLV-2 (RR, 4.6; 95% CI, 0.8–25.2), but no association was seen between mortality and any other HTLV-2–related disorder.[265] In contrast, a prospective survival analysis on 1,340 blood donors (138 HTLV-1, 358 HTLV-2, and 759 seronegative controls) found that HTLV-2 was associated with an overall increased risk of mortality when compared with uninfected controls (hazard ratio [HR], 2.3; 95% CI, 1.1–4.9), but no single cause of death appeared to be responsible for the increased mortality (Figure 18–14).[284] This same study found an increased HTLV-1 mortality (HR, 1.9; 95% CI, 0.8–4.6) that did not reach statistical significance; ongoing follow-up will be needed to confirm

these findings and to determine which causes of death are linked with HTLV-1 and -2.

DIAGNOSIS AND TREATMENT

Serologic and Nucleic Acid Testing for HTLV-1 and HTLV-2

In November 1988, the Food and Drug Administration issued recommendations to screen all whole blood donations in the United States for HTLV-1.[285] Initial testing of blood donors employed the use of commercially obtained EIA systems, in which HTLV-1 viral lysates were used to capture serum antibodies. Subsequent serologic detection systems have incorporated

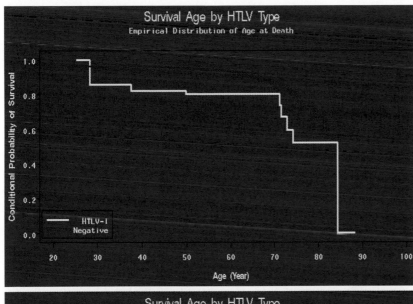

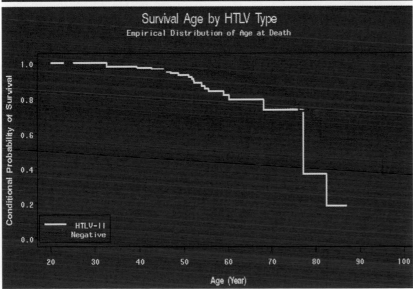

Figure 18–14. Mortality in a prospective cohort study of US blood donors followed for a median of 8.6 years since 1992. The Kaplan-Meier curves show the unadjusted probability of survival at a given age among 138 human T-lymphotropic virus 1 (HTLV-1)-infected subjects (*top*), and 358 HTLV-2-infected subjects (*bottom*), both relative to 759 uninfected controls. Reproduced with permission from Orland JR et al.[284]

the use of recombinant peptides, with improved level of detection of HTLV-2 seropositivity.[286]

A problem arising from broadly implemented testing for HTLV-1 and -2 infections in low-risk populations is the high rate of false-positive EIA tests. Frequently, blood donors are notified of their testing result and are rejected as future donors. Moreover, these individuals may suffer emotional trauma and mistakenly think they have contracted AIDS. Ultimately, these individuals will be referred to an infectious diseases specialist. Confirmation of HTLV-1 or -2 infection has been recommended using Western blot and/or PCR, which are offered through many reference laboratories.[287,288] Even so, many of these tests lack adequate specificity or sensitivity, and none are licensed for supplemental testing in the blood donor setting.[289] In low-prevalence populations such as blood or sperm donors, only 20 to 40% of EIA-positive tests are positive on confirmatory tests, with the remainder being indeterminate (some reactivity short of positive criteria) or negative. One study undertaken in Brazil demonstrates the problems associated with confirming HTLV-1–indeterminate results.[290] Out of 191 EIA reactive individuals, 118 were Western blot seroindeterminate and 73 were seropositive for HTLV-1 and -2. In the PCR analysis of 41 whole blood seroindeterminate individuals, 9 (22%) were positive and 32 (78%) were negative for HTLV-1 and -2. In contrast, a study in US blood donors found only 1.5% of indeterminate Western blot samples to be HTLV-positive by PCR, perhaps reflecting the lower pretest probability of HTLV infection in US donors.[291]

Evaluation and Treatment of HTLV-1– and HTLV-2–Infected Carriers

Patients referred to infectious diseases physicians or hematologists because of a positive HTLV-1 or -2 blood test require education and counseling about the significance of a positive serologic test. Recommendations for counseling and treatment have been published by the Centers for Disease Control.[292] A history should be obtained to determine if there may be underlying risk factors for HTLV-1 and -2 infection exposure, including (1) residence in an endemic area, (2) having parents or sexual partners from an endemic area or ethnic population (see "Epidemiology and Modes of Transmission of HTLV-1 and HTLV-2," above), (3) history of blood transfusions prior to 1988 in the United States, (4) history of injection drug use, (5) having a sexual partner with a history of injection drug use, and (6) having multiple sexual partners without condom protection. These latter risk factors should alert the clinician to the possibility that the individual may have HIV-1 coinfection. Self-reporting of any of these risk factors increases the pretest probability of HTLV-1 or -2 infection, and lowers the likelihood of a false-positive test. Confirmatory testing and discriminatory testing for HTLV-1 versus HTLV-2 with Western blot analysis, immunofluorescence assays (IFA), and/or PCR should be performed in all cases. Patients with indeterminate Western blot tests and no risk factors can be offered retesting in 6 months, but most of these patients remain indeterminate and probably do not require follow-up. Because it also carriers the risk of false-positivity, PCR testing should be reserved for cases with inconclusive Western blot or IFA and an increased pretest probability of infection, or when the consequences of a missed infection are serious (sperm and organ donors). PCR can also be useful in diagnosing HTLV-1 and -2 in infants born of HTLV-infected mothers, when maternal HTLV antibody may be present.

Patients with confirmed HTLV-1 or -2 infections should, at minimum, receive a complete history and physical examination, with focus on skin, mucous membranes, thyroid, lymph nodes, liver, spleen, and neurologic examinations. The authors recommend the following baseline laboratory studies: complete blood count (CBC) with WBC differential and platelet counts, along with serum chemistries, lactate dehydrogenase, syphilis serology, and tuberculin skin testing. A chest radiography should be considered.

If baseline testing is found to be within normal limits, then HTLV-2–infected carriers should be assured that the likelihood of developing neurologic disease is low and the risk for cancer or leukemia negligible, and emphasis should be placed on focusing on positive lifestyles (such as smoking cessation and risk-reduction behavior). Because of recent evidence suggesting that HTLV-2 may be associated with an increased risk for recurrent bacterial infections and pneumonia, immunization with pneumococcal conjugate vaccine is a consideration, along with annual influenza immunization. There are no definitive recommendations for long-term follow-up or management of persons with asymptomatic HTLV-2 infection, but they should be counseled to see their physician if they develop persistent problems with gait or bladder control.

Because HTLV-1–infected carriers are at a greater risk for development of malignancies, autoimmune disorders (including uveitis, arthritis, polymyositis, thyroiditis), and neurologic complications, the authors would recommend that these individuals receive annual follow-up evaluations, including a thorough review of systems and physical examination. At minimum, a CBC, differential, and platelet count should be ordered. Patients found to have abnormal CBCs at baseline or follow-up (lymphocytosis or abnormal lymphocytes) should be referred to a hematologist for closer monitoring.

In the scenario of HIV/HTLV coinfection, there may be a rationale for initiation of antiretroviral therapy during the asymptomatic stages of HIV infection. This contention is supported by studies suggesting that HIV/HTLV coinfection is associated with higher levels of HTLV-1 and -2 virus expression and clinical disease.[261,293] The nucleoside analogues zidovudine and lamivudine are often used as initial therapy for HIV-1 infection, and both drugs have been demonstrated to have antiviral activity against HTLV-1 in vitro.[294] However recent reports of increased HTLV-2 proviral load following antiretroviral therapy may mitigate against early treatment.[282,283]

Treatment of ATLL and TSP/HAM

The diagnosis of ATLL is confirmed in a patient with serum antibodies to HTLV-1, who has the classic features of ATLL, including (1) age of onset in the fourth or fifth decade, (2) presence of abnormal lymphoid cells expressing the T-cell phenotype, (3) peripheral and/or body cavity lymph node enlargement, (4) hypercalcemia with no other explanation, and (4) evidence of clonal T-cell receptor gene rearrangements and detection of integrated HTLV-1 DNA provirus by Southern hybridization.[295] Chronic and smoldering forms of ATLL may be more difficult to diagnose, but establishment of clonal T-cell receptor gene rearrangements in skin biopsies or blood and detection of human T-lymphotropic provirus strongly support the diagnosis.

Patients diagnosed with ATLL should always be referred to a tertiary care center with expertise in the treatment of HTLV-1–associated malignancies. Conventional chemotherapy, which is active against other lymphoid malignancies, is ineffective for treating aggressive forms of ATLL. Therefore, treatment of ATLL has become the target of several clinical studies for the purpose of improving therapeutic outcomes. Combination chemotherapy exclusively designed for ATLL has considerably elevated the treatment response rate in ATLL patients, but it has not sufficiently extended the median survival time of < 2 years with standard cytotoxic regimens (eg, cyclophosphamide, doxorubicin, vincristine, prednisone). One trial, recently initiated in the United States, employs the use of oral zidovudine in combination with high doses of interferon-α, administered daily.[296] Recent evidence suggests that arsenic trioxide may induce cell cycle arrest and apoptosis of ATLL cells in vitro, and is in consideration as an adjuvant chemotherapeutic agent in combination with interferon-α.[297] Several reports from Japan have employed the successful use of allogeneic stem cell transplantation following cytoreductive chemotherapy.[298,299] Other trials (championed by Waldmann and colleagues at the National Cancer Institute) have attempted immunotherapy using humanized monoclonal antibodies directed against the IL-2 and other receptors expressed on ATLL cells.[300,301]

Additional adjuvant treatments for extranodal complications of ATLL include the use of external-beam radiation for lytic bone tumors and tumors within the spinal cord, PUVA for CTCL lesions, and bisphosphonates for the treatment of hypercalcemia.[302]

Efforts to treat of TSP/HAM and HTLV-1–associated autoimmune diseases, using various antiretroviral compounds, has been disappointing.[303] Corticosteroids and immunosuppressive agents such as azathioprine may ameliorate disease progression, but are unsuitable for chronic use because of their adverse effects.[304] Immunotherapy with interferon-α has produced minimal to moderate results, depending on the degree of inflammation and tissue destruction within the involved tissue.[305,306]

Vaccine Development

Despite enthusiasm about developing an effective HTLV-1 vaccine, interest in advancing a candidate vaccine into clinical trials has not been realized. This may be partially due to the fact that most economically prosperous nations have a very low seroprevalence of HTLV-1 infection. An HTLV-2 vaccine could be beneficial in high-risk groups such as IDUs. The greatest interest in developing a vaccine may not be for protection of infection, but rather as an immunomodulatory agent in the treatment of smoldering or chronic ATLL.[307]

Prototype peptide vaccines developed from HTLV-1-Tax and other regions of the genome have been shown to induce viral neutralizing antibodies and robust CTL responses.[203,308] Naked DNA vaccines have been shown to induce protective immunity in monkey models.[309]

REFERENCES

1. Schupbach J, Popovic M, Gilden RV, et al. Serological analysis of a subgroup of human T-lymphotropic retroviruses (HTLV-III) associated with AIDS. Science 1984;224:503–5.

2. Gonda MA, Wong-Staal F, Gallo RC, et al. Sequence homology and morphologic similarity of HTLV-III and visna virus, a pathogenic lentivirus. Science 1985;227:173–7.

3. Essex M, McLane MF, Lee TH, et al. Antibodies to cell membrane antigens associated with human T-cell leukemia virus in patients with AIDS. Science 1983;220:859–62.

4. Chang KS, Wang LC, Gao CL, et al. Concomitant infection of HTLV-I and HIV-1: prevalence of IgG and IgM antibodies in Washington, D.C. area. Eur J Epidemiol 1988;4:426–34.

5. Takatsuki K, Yamaguchi K, Kawano F, et al. Clinical diversity in adult T-cell leukemia-lymphoma. Cancer Res 1985;45:4644s–5s.

6. Poiesz BJ, Ruscelli FW, Gazfar AF, et al. Detection and isolation of type C retrovirus particles from fresh and cultured lymphocytes of a patient with cutaneous T-cell lymphoma. Proc Natl Acad Sci USA 1980;77:7415–9.

7. Hinuma Y, Nagata K, Hanaoka M, et al. Adult T-cell leukemia: antigen in an ATL cell line and detection of antibodies to the antigen in human sera. Proc Natl Acad Sci USA 1981;78:6476–80.

8. Miyoshi I, Kubonishi I, Yoshimoto S, et al. Type C virus particles in a cord T-cell line derived by co-cultivating normal human cord leukocytes and human leukaemic T cells. Nature 1981;294:770–1.

9. Yoshida M, Seiki M, Yamaguchi K, Takatsuki K. Monoclonal integration of human T-cell leukemia provirus in all primary tumors of adult T-cell leukemia suggests causative role of human T-cell leukemia virus in the disease. Proc Natl Acad Sci USA 1984;81:2534–7.

10. Cruikshank EK. A neuropathic syndrome of uncertain origin. West Indian Med J 1956;5:147–58.

11. Rodgers PE. The clinical features and aetiology of the neuropathic syndrome in Jamaica. West Indian Med J 1965;14:36–47.

12. Gessain A, Barin F, Vernant JC, et al. Antibodies to human T-lymphotropic virus type-I in patients with tropical spastic paraparesis. Lancet 1985;2:407–10.

13. Rodgers-Johnson P, Gajdusek DC, Morgan OS, et al. HTLV-I and HTLV-III antibodies and tropical spastic paraparesis. Lancet 1985;2:1247–8.

14. Osame M, Usuki I, Izumo S, et al. HTLV-I associated myelopathy, a new clinical entity [letter]. Lancet 1986;1:1031–2.

15. Mochizuki M, Watanabe T, Yamaguchi K, et al. Uveitis associated with human T lymphotropic virus type I: seroepidemiologic, clinical, and virologic studies. J Infect Dis 1992;166:943–44.

16. Inose M, Higuchi I, Yoshimine K, et al. Pathological changes in skeletal muscle in HTLV-I-associated myelopathy. J Neurol Sci 1992;110:73–8.

17. Beilke MA, Traina-Dorge V, England JD, Blanchard JL. Polymyositis, arthritis, and uveitis in a macaque experimentally infected with human T lymphotropic virus type I. Arthritis Rheum 1996;39:610–5.

18. Sowa JM. Human T lymphotropic virus I, myelopathy, polymyositis and synovitis: an expanding rheumatic spectrum. J Rheumatol 1992;19:316–8.

19. Kawai H, Inui T, Kashiwagi S, et al. HTLV-I infection in patients with autoimmune thyroiditis (Hashimoto's thyroiditis). J Med Virol 1992;38:138–41.

20. Kimura I. [HABA (HTLV-I associated bronchiolo-alveolar disorder)]. Nihon Kyobu Shikkan Gakkai Zasshi 1992;30:787–95.

21. Lee H, Swanson P, Shorty VS, et al. High rate of HTLV-II infection in seropositive IV drug abusers in New Orleans. Science 1989;244:471–5.

22. Khabbaz RF, Onorato IM, Cannon RO, et al. Seroprevalence of HTLV-1 and HTLV-2 among intravenous drug users and persons in clinics for sexually transmitted diseases. N Engl J Med 1992;326:375–80.

23. Briggs NC, Battjes RJ, Cantor KP, et al. Seroprevalence of human T cell lymphotropic virus type II infection, with or without human immunodeficiency virus type 1 coinfection, among US intravenous drug users. J Infect Dis 1995;172:51–8.

24. Biglione MM, Pizarro M, Salomon HE, Berria MI. A possible case of myelopathy/tropical spastic paraparesis in an Argentinian woman with human T lymphocyte virus type II. Clin Infect Dis 2003;37:456–8.

25. Hjelle B, Appenzeller O, Mills R, et al. Chronic neurodegenerative disease associated with HTLV-II infection. Lancet 1992;339:645–6.

26. Murphy EL, et al. Increased prevalence of infectious diseases and other adverse outcomes in human T lymphotropic virus types I- and II-infected blood donors. Retrovirus Epidemiology Donor Study (REDS) Study Group. J Infect Dis 1997;176:1468–75.

27. Gallo RC. On the etiology of human acute leukemia. Med Clin North Am 1973;57:343–54.

28. Gallo RC. Summary of recent observations on the molecular biology of RNA tumor viruses and attempts at application to human leukemia. Am J Clin Pathol 1973;60:80–7.

29. Takatsuki K. Kenneth MacGredie Memorial Lectureship. Adult T-cell leukemia/lymphoma. Leukemia 1997;11 Suppl 3:54–6.

30. Yamaguchi K, Watanabe T. Human T lymphotropic virus type-I and adult T-cell leukemia in Japan. Int J Hematol 2002;76 Suppl 2:240–5.

31. Mueller N, Okayama A, Stuver S, Tachibana N. Findings from the Miyazaki Cohort Study. J Acquir Immune Defic Syndr Hum Retrovirol 1996;13 Suppl 1:S2–7.

32. Iwasaki Y. Pathology of chronic myclopathy associated with HTLV-I infection (HAM/TSP). J Neurol Sci 1990;96:103–23.

33. Manns A, Blattner WA. The epidemiology of the human T-cell lymphotrophic virus type I and type II: etiologic role in human disease. Transfusion 1991;31:67–75.

34. Murphy EL, Glynn SA, Fridey J, et al. Increased incidence of infectious diseases during prospective follow-up of human T-lymphotropic virus type II- and I-infected blood donors. Retrovirus Epidemiology Donor Study. Arch Intern Med 1999;159:1485–91.

35. Zehender G, De Maddalena C, Osio M, et al. High prevalence of human T cell lymphotropic virus type II infection in patients affected by human immunodeficiency virus type 1-associated predominantly sensory polyneuropathy. J Infect Dis 1995;172:1595–8.

36. Berger JR, Svenningsson A, Raffanti S, Resnick L. Tropical spastic paraparesis-like illness occurring in a patient dually infected with HIV-1 and HTLV-II. Neurology 1991;41:85–7.

37. Kalyanaraman VS, Sarngadharan MG, Robert-Guroff M, et al. A new subtype of human T-cell leukemia virus (HTLV-II) associated with a T-cell variant of hairy cell leukemia. Science 1982;218:571–3.

38. Loughran TP Jr, Coyle T, Sherman MP, et al. Detection of human T-cell leukemia/lymphoma virus, type II, in a patient with large granular lymphocyte leukemia. Blood 1992;80:1116–9.

39. Poiesz B, Dube D, Dube S, et al. HTLV-II-associated cutaneous T-cell lymphoma in a patient with HIV-1 infection. N Engl J Med 2000;342:930–6.

40. Rosenblatt JD, Giorgi JV, Golder DW, et al. Integrated human T-cell leukemia virus II genome in CD8+ T cells from a patient with "atypical" hairy cell leukemia: evidence for distinct T and B cell lymphoproliferative disorders. Blood 1988;71:363–9.

41. Loughran TP Jr, Sherman MP, Ruscetti FW, et al. Prototypical HTLV-I/II infection is rare in LGL leukemia. Leuk Res 1994;18:423–9.

42. Pancake BA, Zucker-Franklin D. The difficulty of detecting HTLV-1 proviral sequences in patients with mycosis fungoides. J Acquir Immune Defic Syndr Hum Retrovirol 1996;13:314–9.

43. Ghosh SK, Abrams JT, Terunuma H, Vonderheid EC, DeFreitas E. Human T-cell leukemia virus type I tax/rex DNA and RNA in cutaneous T-cell lymphoma. Blood 1994;84:2663–71.

44. Hall WW, Liu CR, Schneewind O, et al. Deleted HTLV-I provirus in blood and cutaneous lesions of patients with mycosis fungoides. Science 1991;253:317–20.

45. Zucker-Franklin D, Pancake BA, Najfeld V. Localization of HTLV-I tax proviral DNA in mononuclear cells. Blood Cells Mol Dis 2003;31:1–6.

46. Bazarbachi A, Soriano V, Pawson R, et al. Mycosis fungoides and Sezary syndrome are not associated with HTLV-I infection: an international study. Br J Haematol 1997;98:927–33.

47. Kikuchi A, Nishikawa T, Ikeda Y, Yamaguchi K. Absence of human T-lymphotropic virus type I in Japanese patients with cutaneous T-cell lymphoma. Blood 1997;89:1529–32.

48. Wood GS, Schaffer JM, Boni R, et al. No evidence of HTLV-I proviral integration in lymphoproliferative disorders associated with cutaneous T-cell lymphoma. Am J Pathol 1997;150:667–73.

49. Fouchard N, Flageul B, Bagot M, et al. Lack of evidence of HTLV-I/II infection in T CD8 malignant or reactive lymphoproliferative disorders in France: a serological and/or molecular study of 169 cases. Leukemia 1995;9:2087–92.

50. Manns A, Hisada M, La Grenade L. Human T-lymphotropic virus type I infection. Lancet 1999;353:1951–8.

51. Slattery JP, Franchini G, Gessain A. Genomic evolution, patterns of global dissemination, and interspecies transmission of human and simian T-cell leukemia/lymphotropic viruses. Genome Res 1999;9:525–40.

52. Ferreira OC Jr, Planelles V, Rosenblatt JD. Human T-cell leukemia viruses: epidemiology, biology, and pathogenesis. Blood Rev 1997;11:91–104.

53. Taylor GP, Tosswill JH, Matutes E, et al. Prospective study of HTLV-I infection in an initially asymptomatic cohort. J Acquir Immune Defic Syndr 1999;22:92–100.

54. Mahieux R, Pecon-Slattery J, Gessain A. Molecular characterization and phylogenetic analyses of a new, highly divergent simian T-cell lymphotropic virus type 1 (STLV-1marc1) in Macaca arctoides. J Virol 1997;71:6253–8.

55. Mauclere P, Le Hesran JY, Mahieux R, et al. Demographic, ethnic, and geographic differences between human T cell lymphotropic virus (HTLV) type I-seropositive carriers and persons with HTLV-I Gag-indeterminate Western blots in Central Africa. J Infect Dis 1997;176:505–9.

56. Mahieux R, Horal P, Mauclere P, et al. Human T-cell lymphotropic virus type 1 gag indeterminate western blot patterns in Central Africa: relationship to *Plasmodium falciparum* infection. J Clin Microbiol 2000;38:4049–57.

57. Murphy EL, Figueroa JP, Gibbs WN, et al. Human T-lymphotropic virus type I (HTLV-I) seroprevalence in Jamaica: I. Demographic determinants. Am J Epidemiol 1991;133:1114–24.

58. Kajiyama W, Kashiwagi S, Hayashi J, et al. Intrafamilial clustering of anti-atla-positive persons. Am J Epidemiol 1986;124:800–6.

59. Murphy EL, Figueroa JP, Gibbs Wn, et al. Sexual transmission of human T-lymphotropic virus type I (HTLV-I). Ann Intern Med 1989;111:555–60.

60. Morofuji-Hirata M, Kajiyama W, Nakashima, et al. Prevalence of antibody to human T-cell lymphotropic virus type I in Okinawa, Japan, after an interval of 9 years. Am J Epidemiol 1993;137:43–8.

61. Maloney EM, Murphy EL, Figueroa, et al. Human T-lymphotropic virus type I (HTLV-I) seroprevalence in Jamaica: II. Geographic and ecologic determinants. Am J Epidemiol 1991;1331125–34.

62. Stuver SO, Tachibana N, Okayama A, et al. Determinants of HTLV-I seroprevalence in Miyazaki Prefecture, Japan: a cross-sectional study. J Acquir Immune Defic Syndr 1992;5:12–8.

63. Kajiyama W, Kashiwagi S, Nomura H, et al. Seroepidemiologic study of antibody to adult T-cell leukemia virus in Okinawa, Japan. Am J Epidemiol 1986;123:41–7.

64. Murphy EL, Watanabe K, Nass CC, et al. Evidence among blood donors for a 30-year-old epidemic of human T lymphotropic virus type II infection in the United States. J Infect Dis 1999;180:1777–83.

65. Fujiyoshi T, Li HC, Lou H, et al. Characteristic distribution of HTLV type I and HTLV type II carriers among native ethnic groups in South America. AIDS Res Hum Retroviruses 1999;15:1235–9.

66. Zaninovic V, Sanzon F, Lopez F, et al. Geographic independence of HTLV-I and HTLV-II foci in the Andes highland, the Atlantic

coast, and the Orinoco of Colombia. AIDS Res Hum Retroviruses 1994;10:97–101.

67. Fujiyoshi T, Yashiki S, Fujiyama C, et al. Ethnic segregation of HTLV-I and HTLV-II carriers among South American native Indians. Int J Cancer 1995;63:510–5.

68. Duenas-Barajas E, Bernal JE, Vaught DR, et al. Human retroviruses in Amerindians of Colombia: high prevalence of human T cell lymphotropic virus type II infection among the Tunebo Indians. Am J Trop Med Hyg 1993;49:657–63.

69. Leon-Ponte M, Echevarria de Perez G, Bianco N, et al. Endemic infection with HTLV-IIB in Venezuelan Indians: molecular characterization. J Acquir Immune Defic Syndr Hum Retrovirol 1998;17:458–64.

70. Ferrer JF, Del Pino N, Esteban E, et al. High rate of infection with the human T-cell leukemia retrovirus type II in four Indian populations of Argentina. Virology 1993;197:576–84.

71. Ferrer JF, Esteban E, Dube S, et al. Endemic infection with human T cell leukemia/lymphoma virus type IIB in Argentinean and Paraguayan Indians: epidemiology and molecular characterization. J Infect Dis 1996;174:944–53.

72. Ishak R, Harrington WJ Jr, Azevedo VN, et al. Identification of human T cell lymphotropic virus type IIa infection in the Kayapo, an indigenous population of Brazil. AIDS Res Hum Retroviruses 1995;11:813–21.

73. Maloney EM, Biggar RJ, Neel JV, et al. Endemic human T cell lymphotropic virus type II infection among isolated Brazilain Amerindians. J Infect Dis 1992;166:100–7.

74. Vitek CR, Gracia FI, Giusti R, et al. Evidence for sexual and mother-to-child transmission of human T lymphotropic virus type II among Guaymi Indians, Panama. J Infect Dis 1995; 171:1022–6.

75. Reeves WC, Cutler JR, Gracia F, et al. Human T cell lymphotropic virus infection in Guaymi Indians from Panama. Am J Trop Med Hyg 1990;43:410–8.

76. Pardi D, Hjelle B, Folks TM, Lal RB. Genotypic characteristics of HTLV-II isolates from Amerindian and non-Indian populations. Virus Genes 1995;10:27–35.

77. Hjelle B, Zhu SW, Takahashi H, Ijichi S, Hall WW. Endemic human T cell leukemia virus type II infection in southwestern US Indians involves two prototype variants of virus. J Infect Dis 1993;168:737–40.

78. Lowis GW, Sheremata WA, Wickman PR. HTLV-II risk factors in Native Americans in Florida. Neuroepidemiology 1999;18: 37–47.

79. Peters AA, Coulthart MB, Oger JJ, et al. HTLV type I/II in British Columbia Amerindians: a seroprevalence study and sequence characterization of an HTLV type IIa isolate. AIDS Res Hum Retroviruses 2000;16:883–92.

80. Gongora-Biachi RA, Lal RB, Rudolph DL, et al. Low prevalence of HTLV-II in Mayan Indians in the Yucatan Peninsula, Mexico. Arch Med Res 1997;28:555–8.

81. Hjelle B, Scalf R, Swenson S. High frequency of human T-cell leukemia-lymphoma virus type II infection in New Mexico blood donors: determination by sequence-specific oligonucleotide hybridization. Blood 1990;76:450–4.

82. Hjelle B, Mills R, Swenson S, et al. Incidence of hairy cell leukemia, mycosis fungoides, and chronic lymphocytic leukemia in first known HTLV-II-endemic population. J Infect Dis 1991;163:435–40.

83. Gessain A, Mauclere P, Froment A, et al. Isolation and molecular characterization of a human T-cell lymphotropic virus type II (HTLV-II), subtype B, from a healthy Pygmy living in a remote area of Cameroon: an ancient origin for HTLV-II in Africa. Proc Natl Acad Sci U S A 1995;92:4041–5.

84. Vandamme AM, Salemi M, Van Brussel M, et al. African origin of human T-lymphotropic virus type 2 (HTLV-2) supported by a potential new HTLV-2d subtype in Congolese Bambuti Efe Pygmies. J Virol 1998;72:4327–40.

85. Goubau P, Liu HF, De Lange GG, Vandamme Am, Desmyter J. HTLV-II seroprevalence in Pygmies across Africa since 1970. AIDS Res Hum Retroviruses 1993;9:709–13.

86. Goubau P, Desmyter J, Swanson P, et al. Detection of HTLV-I and HTLV-II infection in Africans using type-specific envelope peptides. J Med Virol 1993;39:28–32.

87. Nyambi PN, Ville Y, Louwagie J, et al. Mother-to-child transmission of human T-cell lymphotropic virus types I and II (HTLV-I/II) in Gabon: a prospective follow-up of 4 years. J Acquir Immune Defic Syndr Hum Retrovirol 1996;12:187–92.

88. Tuppin P, Gessain A, Kazanji M, et al. Evidence in Gabon for an intrafamilial clustering with mother-to-child and sexual transmission of a new molecular variant of human T-lymphotropic virus type-II subtype B. J Med Virol 1996;48:22–32.

89. Lee HH, Weiss SH, Brown LS, et al. Patterns of HIV-1 and HTLV-I/II in intravenous drug abusers from the middle Atlantic and central regions of the USA. J Infect Dis 1990;162:347–52.

90. Giuliani M, Rezza G, Lepri AC, et al. Risk factors for HTLV-I and II in individuals attending a clinic for sexually transmitted diseases. Sex Transm Dis 2000;27:87–92.

91. Giacomo M, Franco EG, Claudio C, et al. Human T-cell leukemia virus type II infection among high risk groups and its influence on HIV-1 disease progression. Eur J Epidemiol 1995;11: 527–33.

92. Henrard DR, Soriano V, Robertson E, et al. Prevalence of human T-cell lymphotropic virus type 1 (HTLV-1) and HTLV-2 infection among Spanish drug users measured by HTLV-1 assay and HTLV-1 and -2 assay. HTLV-1 and HTLV-2 Spanish Study Group. J Clin Microbiol 1995;33:1735–8.

93. Krook A, Albert J, Andersson S, et al. Prevalence and risk factors for HTLV-II infection in 913 injecting drug users in Stockholm, 1994. J Acquir Immune Defic Syndr Hum Retrovirol 1997;15:381–6.

94. Vignoli C, Zandotti C, De Lamballerie X, et al. Prevalence of HTLV-II in HIV-1-infected drug addicts in Marseille. Eur J Epidemiol 1993;9:351–2.

95. Egan JF, O'Leary B, Lewis MJ, et al. High rate of human T lymphotropic virus type IIa infection in HIV type 1-infected intravenous drug abusers in Ireland. AIDS Res Hum Retroviruses 1999;15:699–705.

96. Fukushima Y, Takahashi H, Hall WW, et al. Extraordinary high rate of HTLV type II seropositivity in intravenous drug abusers in south Vietnam. AIDS Res Hum Retroviruses 1995;11:637–45.

97. Dourado I, Andrade T, Galvao-Castro B. HTLV-I in Northeast Brazil: differences for male and female injecting drug users. J Acquir Immune Defic Syndr Hum Retrovirol 1998;19:426–9.

98. Segurado AA, Malaque CM, Sumita LM, Pannuti CS, Lal RB. Laboratory characterization of human T cell lymphotropic virus types 1 (HTLV-1) and 2 (HTLV-2) infections in blood donors from Sao Paulo, Brazil. Am J Trop Med Hyg 1997;57:142–8.

99. Hepatitis B and injecting-drug use among American Indians— Montana, 1989–1990. MMWR Morb Mortal Wkly Rep 1992; 41:13–4.

100. Strathdee SA, Patrick DM, Currie SL, et al. Needle exchange is not enough: lessons from the Vancouver injecting drug use study. AIDS 1997;11:F59–65.

101. Diamond C, Davidson A, Sorvillo F, Buskin S. HIV-infected American Indians/Alaska natives in the Western United States. Ethn Dis 2001;11:633–44.

102. Schreiber GB, Murphy EL. Horton JA,et al. Risk factors for human T-cell lymphotropic virus types I and II (HTLV-I and -II) in blood donors: the Retrovirus Epidemiology Donor Study. NHLBI Retrovirus Epidemiology Donor Study. J Acquir Immune Defic Syndr Hum Retrovirol 1997;14:263–71.

103. Liu H, Leung P, Glynn S, Murphy EL. Human T-lymphotropic virus type II RFLP subtypes a0 and b4/b5 are associated with different demographic and geographic characteristics in the United States. Virology 2001;279:90–6.

104. Colin DD, Alcantara Junior LC, Santos FL, Uchoa R, Tavares-Neto J. [Seroprevalence of human T cell lymphotropic virus infection and associated factors of risk in blood donors of Rio Branco city, AC, Brazil (1998–2001)]. Rev Soc Bras Med Trop 2003;36:677–83.

105. Dickmeiss E, Christiansen AH, Smith E. [Screening of donor blood for viral markers. Anti-HIV, HBsAg and anti-HTLV-I/II in Denmark 1990–1999]. Ugeskr Laeger 2001;163:2623–8.

106. Boni J, Bisset LR, Burckhardt JJ, et al. Prevalence of human T-cell leukemia virus types I and II in Switzerland. J Med Virol 2004;72:328–37.

107. Pillonel J, David D, Pinget R, Laperche S. [Prevalence of HBV, HCV, HIV and HTLV in autologous blood donors in France between 1993 and 2000]. Transfus Clin Biol 2002;9:289–96.

108. Brites C, Harrington W Jr, Pedroso C, Martins Netto E, Badaro R. Epidemiological characteristics of HTLV-I and II coinfection in Brazilian subjects infected by HIV-1. Braz J Infect Dis 1997;1:42–7.

109. Hershow RC, Galai N, Fukuda K, et al. An international collaborative study of the effects of coinfection with human T-lymphotropic virus type II on human immunodeficiency virus type 1 disease progression in injection drug users. J Infect Dis 1996;174:309–17.

110. Feigal E, Murphy E, Vranizan K, et al. Human T cell lymphotropic virus type I and II in intravenous drug users in San Francisco: risk factors associated with seropositivity. J Infect Dis 1991;164:36–42.

111. Ehrlich GD, Glaser JB, LaVigne K, et al. Prevalence of human T-cell leukemia/lymphoma virus (HTLV) type II infection among high-risk individuals: type-specific identification of HTLVs by polymerase chain reaction. Blood 1989;74:1658–64.

112. Hino S, Yamaguchi K, Katamine S, et al. Mother-to-child transmission of human T-cell leukemia virus type-I. Jpn J Cancer Res 1985;76:474–80.

113. Wiktor SZ, Pate EJ, Rosenberg PS, et al. Mother-to-child transmission of human T-cell lymphotropic virus type I associated with prolonged breast-feeding. J Hum Virol 1997;1:37–44.

114. Ureta-Vidal A, Angelin-Duclos C, Tortevoye P, et al. Mother-to-child transmission of human T-cell-leukemia/lymphoma virus type I: implication of high antiviral antibody titer and high proviral load in carrier mothers. Int J Cancer 1999;82:832–6.

115. Heneine W, Woods T, Green D, et al. Detection of HTLV-II in breastmilk of HTLV-II infected mothers. Lancet 1992;340:1157–8.

116. Black FL, Biggar RJ, Neel JV, Maloney EM, Waters DJ. Endemic transmission of HTLV type II among Kayapo Indians of Brazil. AIDS Res Hum Retroviruses 1994;10:1165–71.

117. Kaplan JE, Abrams E, Shaffer N, et al. Low risk of mother-to-child transmission of human T lymphotropic virus type II in non-breast-fed infants. J Infect Dis 1992;166:892–5.

118. Gallo D, Petru A, Yeh ET, Hanson CV. No evidence of perinatal transmission of HTLV-II. J Acquir Immune Defic Syndr 1993;6:1168–70.

119. Chironna M, Quarto M, Barbuti S. Lack of HTLV-II infection in newborns born from HIV-1 infected mothers in southern Italy. Eur J Epidemiol 1997;13:121–2.

120. Caterino-de-Araujo A, de los Santos-Fortuna E. No evidence of vertical transmission of HTLV-I and HTLV-II in children at high risk for HIV-1 infection from Sao Paulo, Brazil. J Trop Pediatr 1999;45:42–7.

121. Roucoux DH, et al. Prospective study on sexual transmission of HTLV-I and HTLV-II [abstract O62]. AIDS Res Hum Retroviruses 2003;19 Suppl:S25.

122. Iga M, Okayama A, Stuver S, et al. Genetic evidence of transmission of human T cell lymphotropic virus type 1 between spouses. J Infect Dis 2002;185:691–5.

123. Okochi K, Sato H, Hinuma Y. A retrospective study on transmission of adult T cell leukemia virus by blood transfusion: seroconversion in recipients. Vox Sang 1984;46:245–53.

124. Manns A, Wilks RJ, Murphy EL, et al. A prospective study of transmission by transfusion of HTLV-I and risk factors associated with seroconversion. Int J Cancer 1992;51:886–91.

125. Eble BE, Busch MP, Guiltinan AM, Khayam-Bashi H, Murphy EL. Determination of human T lymphotropic virus type by polymerase chain reaction and correlation with risk factors in northern California blood donors. J Infect Dis 1993;167:954–7.

126. Schreiber GB, Busch MP, Kleinman SH, Korelitz JJ. The risk of transfusion-transmitted viral infections. The Retrovirus Epidemiology Donor Study. N Engl J Med 1996;334:1685–90.

127. Robert-Guroff M, Weiss SH, Giron JA, et al. Prevalence of antibodies to HTLV-I, -II, and -III in intravenous drug abusers from an AIDS endemic region. JAMA 1986;255:3133–7.

128. Schnittman SM, Psallidopoulos MC, Lane HC, et al. The reservoir for HIV-1 in human peripheral blood is a T cell that maintains expression of CD4. Science 1989;245:305–8.

129. Gallo RC. The first human retrovirus. Sci Am 1986;255:88–98.

130. Levy JA, Hoffman AD, Kramer SM, et al. Isolation of lymphocytopathic retroviruses from San Francisco patients with AIDS. Science 1984;225:840–2.

131. Orenstein JM. Ultrastructural pathology of human immunodeficiency virus infection. Ultrastruct Pathol 1992;16:179–210.

132. Matsuoka M. Human T-cell leukemia virus type I and adult T-cell leukemia. Oncogene 2003;22:5131–40.

133. Haseltine WA. Molecular biology of the human immunodeficiency virus type 1. FASEB J 1991;5:2349–60.

134. Pavlakis GN, Felber BK, Ciminale V, et al. Structure, regulation and oncogenic mechanisms of HTLV-I and HTLV-II. Leukemia 1992;6 Suppl 3:176S–80S.

135. Poiesz B, Poiesz M, Choi D. Human T-cell lymphoma/leukemia virus-associated T-cell lymphoma and leukemia. In: Wiernik P, et al, editors. Neoplastic diseases of the blood. New York: Cambridge Univ. Press; 2003. p. 141–63.

136. Seiki M, Hattori S, Hirayama Y, Yoshida M. Human adult T-cell leukemia virus: complete nucleotide sequence of the provirus genome integrated in leukemia cell DNA. Proc Natl Acad Sci U S A 1983;80:3618–22.

137. Shimotohno K, Takahashi Y, Shimizu N, et al. Complete nucleotide sequence of an infectious clone of human T-cell leukemia virus type II: an open reading frame for the protease gene. Proc Natl Acad Sci U S A 1985;82:3101–5.

138. Albrecht B, Lairmore MD. Critical role of human T-lymphotropic virus type 1 accessory proteins in viral replication and patho-

genesis. Microbiol Mol Biol Rev 2002;66:396–406; table of contents.

139. Jeang KT. Functional activities of the human T-cell leukemia virus type I Tax oncoprotein: cellular signaling through NF-kappa B. Cytokine Growth Factor Rev 2001;12:207–17.

140. Yoshida M. Molecular biology of HTLV-I: recent progress. J Acquir Immune Defic Syndr Hum Retrovirol 1996;13 Suppl 1: S63–8.

141. Gatza ML, Watt JC, Marriott SJ. Cellular transformation by the HTLV-I Tax protein, a jack-of-all-trades. Oncogene 2003;22: 5141–9.

142. Green PL, Chen IS. Regulation of human T cell leukemia virus expression. FASEB J 1990;4:169–75.

143. Hauber J. Nuclear export mediated by the Rev/Rex class of retroviral trans-activator proteins. Curr Top Microbiol Immunol 2001;259:55–76.

144. Johnson JM, Harrod R, Franchini G. Molecular biology and pathogenesis of the human T-cell leukaemia/lymphotropic virus type-1 (HTLV-1). Int J Exp Pathol 2001;82:135–47.

145. Ye J, Silverman L, Lairmore MD, Green PL. HTLV-1 Rex is required for viral spread and persistence in vivo but is dispensable for cellular immortalization in vitro. Blood 2003; 102:3963–9.

146. Hollsberg P. Mechanisms of T-cell activation by human T-cell lymphotropic virus type I. Microbiol Mol Biol Rev 1999;63: 308–33.

147. Franchini G, Nicot C, Johnson JM. Seizing of T cells by human T-cell leukemia/lymphoma virus type 1. Adv Cancer Res 2003;89:69–132.

148. Hidaka M, Inoue J, Yoshida M, Seiki M. Post-transcriptional regulator (rex) of HTLV-1 initiates expression of viral structural proteins but suppresses expression of regulatory proteins. EMBO J 1988;7:519–23.

149. Rimsky L, Dodon MD, Dixon EP, Greene WC. Trans-dominant inactivation of HTLV-I and HIV-1 gene expression by mutation of the HTLV-I Rex transactivator. Nature 1989;341:453–6.

150. Rosenblatt JD, Miles S, Gasson JC, Prager D. Transactivation of cellular genes by human retroviruses. Curr Top Microbiol Immunol 1995;193:25–49.

151. Nimer SD, Gasson JC, Hu K, et al. Activation of the GM-CSF promoter by HTLV-I and -II tax proteins. Oncogene 1989;4:671–6.

152. Ejima E, Rosenblatt JD, Massari M, et al. Cell-type-specific transactivation of the parathyroid hormone-related protein gene promoter by the human T-cell leukemia virus type I (HTLV-I) tax and HTLV-II tax proteins. Blood 1993;81:1017–24.

153. Nakajima T, Katamura K, Yamashita N, et al. Constitutive expression and production of tumor necrosis factor-beta in T-cell lines infected with HTLV-I and HTLV-II. Biochem Biophys Res Commun 1993;191:371–7.

154. Uchijima M, Sato H, Fujii M, Seiki M, et al. Tax proteins of human T-cell leukemia virus type 1 and 2 induce expression of the gene encoding erythroid-potentiating activity (tissue inhibitor of metalloproteinases-1, TIMP-1). J Biol Chem 1994;269:14946–50.

155. Mori N, Prager D. Transactivation of the interleukin-1alpha promoter by human T-cell leukemia virus type I and type II Tax proteins. Blood 1996;87:3410–7.

156. Owen SM, Rudolph DL, Dezzutti CS, et al. Transcriptional activation of the intercellular adhesion molecule 1 (CD54) gene by human T lymphotropic virus types I and II Tax is mediated through a palindromic response element. AIDS Res Hum Retroviruses 1997;13:1429–37.

157. Tanaka Y, Hayashi M, Takagi S, Yoshie O. Differential transactivation of the intercellular adhesion molecule 1 gene promoter by Tax1 and Tax2 of human T-cell leukemia viruses. J Virol 1996;70:8508–17.

158. Nakamura N, Fujii M, Tsukahara T, et al. Human T-cell leukemia virus type 1 Tax protein induces the expression of STAT1 and STAT5 genes in T-cells. Oncogene 1999;18:2667–75.

159. Mariner JM, Lantz V, Waldmann TA, Azimi N. Human T cell lymphotropic virus type I Tax activates IL-15R alpha gene expression through an NF-kappa B site. J Immunol 2001;166:2602–9.

160. Sharma V, Lorey SL. Autocrine role of macrophage inflammatory protein-1 beta in human T-cell lymphotropic virus type-I tax-transfected Jurkat T-cells. Biochem Biophys Res Commun 2001;287:910–3.

161. Miyazaki T, Liu ZJ, Taniguchi T. Selective cooperation of HTLV-1-encoded p40tax-1 with cellular oncoproteins in the induction of hematopoietic cell proliferation. Oncogene 1996;12:2403–8.

162. Uittenbogaard MN, Giebler HA, Reisman D, Nyborg JK. Transcriptional repression of p53 by human T-cell leukemia virus type I Tax protein. J Biol Chem 1995;270:28503–6.

163. Waldele K, Schneider G, Ruckes T, Grassmann R. Interleukin-13 overexpression by tax transactivation: a potential autocrine stimulus in human T-cell leukemia virus-infected lymphocytes. J Virol 2004;78:6081–90.

164. Marriott SJ, Trinh D, Brady JN. Activation of interleukin-2 receptor alpha expression by extracellular HTLV-I Tax1 protein: a potential role in HTLV-I pathogenesis. Oncogene 1992;7:1749–55.

165. McGuire KL, Curtiss VE, Larson EL, Haseltine WA. Influence of human T-cell leukemia virus type I tax and rex on interleukin-2 gene expression. J Virol 1993;67:1590–9.

166. Waldmann TA. IL-2 receptor expression in the haematologic malignancies: a target for immunotherapy. Cancer Surv 1989; 8:891–903.

167. Tendler CL, Greenberg SJ, Blattner WA, et al. Transactivation of interleukin 2 and its receptor induces immune activation in human T-cell lymphotropic virus type I-associated myelopathy: pathogenic implications and a rationale for immunotherapy. Proc Natl Acad Sci U S A 1990;87:5218–22.

168. Wano Y, Feinberg M, Hosking JB, Bogerd H, Greene WC, et al. Stable expression of the tax gene of type I human T-cell leukemia virus in human T cells activates specific cellular genes involved in growth. Proc Natl Acad Sci U S A 1988;85:9733–7.

169. Cereseto A, Mulloy JC, Franchini G. Insights on the pathogenicity of human T-lymphotropic/leukemia virus types I and II. J Acquir Immune Defic Syndr Hum Retrovirol 1996;13 Suppl 1: S69–75.

170. Goon PK, Igakura T, Hanon E, et al. Human T cell lymphotropic virus type I (HTLV-I)-specific CD4+ T cells: immunodominance hierarchy and preferential infection with HTLV-I. J Immunol 2004;172:1735–43.

171. Trejo SR, Ratner L. The HTLV receptor is a widely expressed protein. Virology 2000;268:41–8.

172. Jassal SR, Pohler RG, Brighty DW. Human T-cell leukemia virus type 1 receptor expression among syncytium-resistant cell lines revealed by a novel surface glycoprotein-immunoadhesin. J Virol 2001;75:8317–28.

173. Manel N, Kim FJ, Kinet S, et al. The ubiquitous glucose transporter GLUT-1 is a receptor for HTLV. Cell 2003;115:449–59.

174. Bangham CR. The immune control and cell-to-cell spread of human T-lymphotropic virus type 1. J Gen Virol 2003; 84(Pt 12):3177–89.

175. Igakura T, Stinchcombe JC, Goon PK, et al. Spread of HTLV-I

between lymphocytes by virus-induced polarization of the cytoskeleton. Science 2003;299:1713–6.

176. Kashiwagi K, Furusyo N, Nakashima H, et al. A decrease in mother-to-child transmission of human T lymphotropic virus type I (HTLV-I) in Okinawa, Japan. Am J Trop Med Hyg 2004; 70:158–63.

177. Moriuchi M, Moriuchi H. Transforming growth factor-beta enhances human T-cell leukemia virus type I infection. J Med Virol 2002;67:427–30.

178. Manns A, Miley WJ, Wilks RJ, et al. Quantitative proviral DNA and antibody levels in the natural history of HTLV-I infection. J Infect Dis 1999;180:1487–93.

179. Saxton EH, Lee H, Swanson P, et al. Detection of human T-cell leukemia/lymphoma virus type I in a transfusion recipient with chronic myelopathy. Neurology 1989;39:841–4.

180. Wilks RJ, LaGrenade L, Hanchard B, et al. Sibling adult T-cell leukemia/lymphoma and clustering of human T-cell lymphotropic virus type I infection in a Jamaican family. Cancer 1993;72:2700–4.

181. Maguer V, Casse-Ripoll H, Gazzolo L, Dodon MD. Human T-cell leukemia virus type I-induced proliferation of human immature CD2+CD3- thymocytes. J Virol 1993;67:5529–37.

182. Maguer-Satta V, Gazzolo L, Dodon MD. Human immature thymocytes as target cells of the leukemogenic activity of human T-cell leukemia virus type I. Blood 1995;86:1444–52.

183. Green P, Chen ISY. Human T-cell leukemia virus types 1 and 2. In: Knipes D, Howley P, editors. Fields virology. Philadelphia: Lippincott, Williams and Wilkins; 2001. p. 1941–69.

184. Ohshima K, Ohgami A, Matsuoka M, et al. Random integration of HTLV-1 provirus: increasing chromosomal instability. Cancer Lett 1998;132:203–12.

185. Murphy EL, Hanchard B, Figueroa JP, et al. Modelling the risk of adult T-cell leukemia/lymphoma in persons infected with human T-lymphotropic virus type I. Int J Cancer 1989;43:250–3.

186. Grassmann R, Berchtold S, Radant I, et al. Role of human T-cell leukemia virus type 1 X region proteins in immortalization of primary human lymphocytes in culture. J Virol 1992;66:4570–5.

187. Grossman WJ, Ratner L. Cytokine expression and tumorigenicity of large granular lymphocytic leukemia cells from mice transgenic for the tax gene of human T-cell leukemia virus type I. Blood 1997;90:783–94.

188. Iwakura Y, Tosu M, Yoshida E, et al. Augmentation of c-fos and c-jun expression in transgenic mice carrying the human T-cell leukemia virus type-I tax gene. Virus Genes 1995;9:161–70.

189. Jeang KT, Widen SG, Semmes OJ 4th, Wilson SH. HTLV-I trans-activator protein, tax, is a trans-repressor of the human beta-polymerase gene. Science 1990;247:1082–4.

190. Miyake H, Suzuki T, Hirai H, Yoshida M. Trans-activator Tax of human T-cell leukemia virus type 1 enhances mutation frequency of the cellular genome. Virology 1999;253:155–61.

191. Saggioro D, Majone F, Forino M, Turchetto L, Chieco-Bianchi L. Studies on the mechanisms of HTLV-I leukemogenesis. Leukemia 1992;6 Suppl 3:64S–6S.

192. Lemoine FJ, Marriott SJ. Genomic instability driven by the human T-cell leukemia virus type I (HTLV-I) oncoprotein, Tax. Oncogene 2002;21:7230–4.

193. Reid RL, Lindholm PF, Mireskandari A, Dittmer J, Brady JN. Stabilization of wild-type p53 in human T-lymphocytes transformed by HTLV-I. Oncogene 1993;8:3029–36.

194. Fujimoto T, Hata T, Itoyama T. et al. High rate of chromosomal abnormalities in HTLV-I-infected T-cell colonies derived from prodromal phase of adult T-cell leukemia: a study of IL-2-stim-ulated colony formation in methylcellulose. Cancer Genet Cytogenet 1999;109:1–13.

195. Kamihira S, Dateki N, Sugahara K, et al. Real time polymerase chain reaction for quantification of HTLV-1 proviral load: application for analyzing aberrant integration of the proviral DNA in adult T-cell leukemia. Int J Hematol 2000;72:79–84.

196. Takeda S, Maeda M, Morikawa S, et al. Genetic and epigenetic inactivation of tax gene in adult T-cell leukemia cells. Int J Cancer 2004;109:559–67.

197. Hanai S, Nitta T, Shoda M, et al. Integration of human T-cell leukemia virus type 1 in genes of leukemia cells of patients with adult T-cell leukemia. Cancer Sci 2004;95:306–10.

198. Ohshima K, Hashimoto K, Izumo S, Suzumiya J, Kikuchi M. Detection of human T lymphotrophic virus type I (HTLV-I) DNA and mRNA in individual cells by polymerase chain reaction (PCR) in situ hybridization (ISH) and reverse transcription (RT)-PCR ISH. Hematol Oncol 1996;14:91–100.

199. Bangham CR. Human T-lymphotropic virus type 1 (HTLV-1): persistence and immune control. Int J Hematol 2003;78:297–303.

200. Okayama A, Chen YM, Tachibana N, et al. High incidence of antibodies to HTLV-I tax in blood relatives of adult T-cell leukemia patients. J Infect Dis 1991;163:47–52.

201. Blanchard S, Astier-Gin T, Moynet D, Edouard E, Guillemain B. Different HTLV-I neutralization patterns among sera of patients infected with cosmopolitan HTLV-I. Virology 1998; 245:90–8.

202. Astier-Gin T, Portail JP, Londos-Gagliardi D, Moynet D, et al. Neutralizing activity and antibody reactivity toward immunogenic regions of the human T cell leukemia virus type I surface glycoprotein in sera of infected patients with different clinical states. J Infect Dis 1997;175:716–9.

203. Sundaram R, Lynch MP, Rawale SV, et al. De novo design of peptide immunogens that mimic the coiled coil region of human T-cell leukemia virus type-1 glycoprotein 21 transmembrane subunit for induction of native protein reactive neutralizing antibodies. J Biol Chem 2004;279:24141–51.

204. de The G, Kazanji M. An HTLV-I/II vaccine: from animal models to clinical trials? J Acquir Immune Defic Syndr Hum Retrovirol 1996;13 Suppl 1:S191–8.

205. Takamoto T, Makino M, Azuma M, et al. HTLV-I-infected T cells activate autologous CD4+ T cells susceptible to HTLV-I infection in a costimulatory molecule-dependent fashion. Eur J Immunol 1997;27:1427–32.

206. Hanon E, Hall S, Taylor GP, et al. Abundant tax protein expression in CD4+ T cells infected with human T-cell lymphotropic virus type I (HTLV-I) is prevented by cytotoxic T lymphocytes. Blood 2000;95:1386–92.

207. Kubota R, Kawanishi T, Matsubara H, Manns A, Jacobson S. Demonstration of human T lymphotropic virus type I (HTLV-I) tax-specific CD8+ lymphocytes directly in peripheral blood of HTLV-I-associated myelopathy/tropical spastic paraparesis patients by intracellular cytokine detection. J Immunol 1998;161:482–8.

208. Ureta-Vidal A, Pique C, Garcia Z, et al. Human T cell leukemia virus type I (HTLV-I) infection induces greater expansions of CD8 T lymphocytes in persons with HTLV-I-associated myelopathy/tropical spastic paraparesis than in asymptomatic carriers. J Infect Dis 2001;183:857–64.

209. Bieganowska K, Hollsberg P, Buckle GJ, et al. Direct analysis of viral-specific CD8+ T cells with soluble HLA-A2/Tax11-19 tetramer complexes in patients with human T cell lymphotropic virus-associated myelopathy. J Immunol 1999;162:1765–71.

210. Yashiki S, Fujiyoshi T, Arima N, et al. HLA-A*26, HLA-B*4002, HLA-B*4006, and HLA-B*4801 alleles predispose to adult T cell leukemia: the limited recognition of HTLV type 1 tax peptide anchor motifs and epitopes to generate anti-HTLV type 1 tax CD8(+) cytotoxic T lymphocytes. AIDS Res Hum Retroviruses 2001;17:1047–61.

211. Arnulf B, Thorel M, Poirot Y, et al. Loss of the ex vivo but not the reinducible CD8+ T-cell response to Tax in human T-cell leukemia virus type 1-infected patients with adult T-cell leukemia/lymphoma. Leukemia 2004;18:126–32.

212. Nomura M, Ohashi T, Nishikawa K, et al. Repression of tax expression is associated both with resistance of human T-cell leukemia virus type 1-infected T cells to killing by tax-specific cytotoxic T lymphocytes and with impaired tumorigenicity in a rat model. J Virol 2004;78:3827–36.

213. Furukawa Y, Kubota R, Tara M, et al. Existence of escape mutant in HTLV-I tax during the development of adult T-cell leukemia. Blood 2001;97:987–93.

214. Ohashi T, Hanabuchi S, Kato H, et al. Prevention of adult T-cell leukemia-like lymphoproliferative disease in rats by adoptively transferred T cells from a donor immunized with human T-cell leukemia virus type 1 Tax-coding DNA vaccine. J Virol 2000;74:9610–6.

215. Shimamoto Y, Yamaguchi M. HTLV-I induced extranodal lymphomas. Leuk Lymphoma 1992;7:37–45.

216. Gibbs WN, Lofters WS, Campbell M, et al. Non-Hodgkin lymphoma in Jamaica and its relation to adult T-cell leukemia-lymphoma. Ann Intern Med 1987;106:361–8.

217. Fouchard N, Mahe A, Huerre M, et al. Cutaneous T cell lymphomas: mycosis fungoides, Sezary syndrome and HTLV-I-associated adult T cell leukemia (ATL) in Mali, West Africa: a clinical, pathological and immunovirological study of 14 cases and a review of the African ATL cases. Leukemia 1998;12:578–85.

218. Gotuzzo E, Arrango C, de Queiroz-Campos A, et al. Human T-cell lymphotropic virus-I in Latin America. Infect Dis Clin North Am 2000;14:211–39, x–xi.

219. de Oliveira Mdo S, et al. HTLV-I infection and adult T-cell leukemia in Brazil: an overview. Rev Paul Med 1996;114:1177–85.

220. Ratner L, Poiesz BJ. Leukemias associated with human T-cell lymphotropic virus type I in a non-endemic region. Medicine 1988;67:401–22.

221. Catovsky D, Foa R. The lymphoid leukaemias. London: Butterworth & Co.; 1990. p. 218–67.

222. Yamaguchi K, et al. Pathogenesis of adult T-cell leukemia from clinical pathologic features. In: Blattner WA, editor. Human retrovirology: HTLV. New York: Raven Press; 1990. p. 163–71.

223. Hanchard B, et al. Adult T-cell leukemia/lymphoma (ATL) in Jamaica. In: Blattner WA, editor. Human retrovirology: HTLV. New York: Raven Press; 1990. p. 173–83.

224. Isomoto H, Ohnita K, Mizuta Y, et al. Clinical and endoscopic features of adult T-cell leukemia/lymphoma with duodenal involvement. J Clin Gastroenterol 2001;33:241–6.

225. Nosaka K, Miyamoto T, Sakai T, et al. Mechanism of hypercalcemia in adult T-cell leukemia: overexpression of receptor activator of nuclear factor kappaB ligand on adult T-cell leukemia cells. Blood 2002;99:634–40.

226. Ikeda K, Inove D, Okazaki R, et al. Parathyroid hormone-related peptide in hypercalcemia associated with adult T cell leukemia/lymphoma: molecular and cellular mechanism of parathyroid hormone-related peptide overexpression in HTLV-I-infected T cells. Miner Electrolyte Metab 1995;21:166–70.

227. Boh EE. Cutaneous lymphomas and leukemias. In: Lim HW, editor. The clinic atlas of office procedures. Pennsylvania: WB Saunders; 2000. p. 443–55.

228. McBurney E, Marrogi A, Boh E. Cutaneous T-cell lymphoma. In: Miller SJ, Maloney ME, editors. Cutaneous oncology-pathophysiology, diagnosis, and management. Malden (MA): Blackwell Science, Inc.; 1998. p. 921–53.

229. Kasahata N, Kawaamura M, Shiota J, et al. [A case of acute type adult T cell leukemia and human T-lymphotropic virus type I associated myelopathy who presented with meningitis and polyradiculoneuropathy and improved with steroid treatment]. No To Shinkei 2000;52:1003–6.

230. Freitas V, Gomes I, Bettencourt A, Fernandes D, Melo A. Adult T-cell leukemia-lymphoma in a patient with HTLV-I/II associated myelopathy. Arq Neuropsiquiatr 1997;55:325–8.

231. Kawai H, Nishida Y, Takagi M, Nakamura S, Saito S. [HTLV-I associated myelopathy (HAM) with adult T-cell leukemia (ATL)]. Rinsho Shinkeigaku 1989;29:588–92.

232. Case records of the Massachusetts General Hospital. Weekly clinicopathological exercises. Case 36-1989. A 34-year-old Jamaican man with fever, hepatic failure, diarrhea, and a progressive gait disorder. N Engl J Med 1989;321:663–75.

233. Bhagavati S, Ehrlich G, Kula RW, et al. Detection of human T-cell lymphoma/leukemia virus type I DNA and antigen in spinal fluid and blood of patients with chronic progressive myelopathy. N Engl J Med 1988;318:1141–7.

234. Gessain A, Caudie C, Gout O, et al. Intrathecal synthesis of antibodies to HTLV-I and presence of IgG oligoclonal bands in the cerebro-spinal fluid of patients with endemic tropical spastic paraparesis. J Infect Dis 1988;157:1226–34.

235. Iannone R, Sherman MP, Rodgers-Johnson PE, et al. HTLV-I DNA sequences in CNS tissue of a patient with tropical spastic paraparesis and HTLV-I-associated myelopathy. J Acquir Immune Defic Syndr 1992;5:810–6.

236. Lehky TJ, Fox CH, Koenig S, et al. Detection of human T-lymphotropic virus type I (HTLV-I) tax RNA in the central nervous system of HTLV-I-associated myelopathy/tropical spastic paraparesis patients by in situ hybridization. Ann Neurol 1995;37:167–75.

237. Gout O, Baulac M, Gessain A, et al. Rapid development of myelopathy after HTLV-I infection acquired by transfusion during cardiac transplantation. N Engl J Med 1990;322:383–8.

238. McKhann G II, Gibbs CJ Jr, Mora CA, et al. Isolation and characterization of HTLV-I from symptomatic family members with tropical spastic paraparesis (HTLV-I encephalomyeloneuropathy). J Infect Dis 1989;160:371–9.

239. Maloney EM, Cleghorn FR, Morgan OS, et al. Incidence of HTLV-I-associated myelopathy/tropical spastic paraparesis (HAM/TSP) in Jamaica and Trinidad. J Acquir Immune Defic Syndr Hum Retrovirol 1998;17:167–70.

240. Kramer A, Maloney EM, Morgan OS, et al. Risk factors and cofactors for human T-cell lymphotropic virus type I (HTLV-I)-associated myelopathy/tropical spastic paraparesis (HAM/TSP) in Jamaica. Am J Epidemiol 1995;142:1212–20.

241. Beilke MA, Riding In D, Hamilton R, et al. In situ hybridization detection of HTLV-I RNA in peripheral blood mononuclear cells of TSP/HAM patients and their spouses. J Med Virol 1991;33:64–71.

242. Nakagawa M, Izumo S, Ivichi S, et al. HTLV-I-associated myelopathy: analysis of 213 patients based on clinical features and laboratory findings. J Neurovirol 1995;1:50–61.

243. Rodgers-Johnson PE, Ono SG, Asher DM, Gibbs CJ Jr. Tropical

spastic paraparesis and HTLV-I myelopathy: clinical features and pathogenesis. Res Publ Assoc Res Nerv Ment Dis 1990; 68:117–30.

244. Harrison LH, Vaz B, Taveira DM, et al. Myelopathy among Brazilians coinfected with human T-cell lymphotropic virus type I and HIV. Neurology 1997;48:13–8.

245. Yokoi K, Kawai H, Akaike M, Mine H, Saito S. Presence of human T-lymphotropic virus type II-related genes in DNA of peripheral leukocytes from patients with autoimmune thyroid diseases. J Med Virol 1995;45:392–8.

246. Ono A, Mochizuki M, Yamaguchi K, Miyata N, Watanabe T. Immunologic and virologic characterization of the primary infiltrating cells in the aqueous humor of human T-cell leukemia virus type-1 uveitis. Accumulation of the human T-cell leukemia virus type-1-infected cells and constitutive expression of viral and interleukin-6 messenger ribonucleic acids. Invest Ophthalmol Vis Sci 1997;38:676–89.

247. Sugaya T, Ishizu A, Ikeda H, et al. Clonotypic analysis of T cells accumulating at arthritic lesions in HTLV-I env-pX transgenic rats. Exp Mol Pathol 2002;72:56–61.

248. McCallum RM, Patel DD, Moore JO, Haynes BF. Arthritis syndromes associated with human T cell lymphotropic virus type I infection. Med Clin North Am 1997;81:261–76.

249. Suzumiya J, Marutsuka K, Nabeshima K, et al. Autopsy findings in 47 cases of adult T-cell leukemia/lymphoma in Miyazaki prefecture, Japan. Leuk Lymphoma 1993;11:281–6.

250. Tashiro T. [Pulmonary complications in patients with adult T-cell leukemia]. Nihon Kyobu Shikkan Gakkai Zasshi 1992;30:756–62.

251. Satoh M, Toma H, Sugahara K, et al. Involvement of IL-2/IL-2R system activation by parasite antigen in polyclonal expansion of CD4(+)25(+) HTLV-1-infected T-cells in human carriers of both HTLV-1 and S. stercoralis. Oncogene 2002;21:2466–75.

252. Marsh BJ. Infectious complications of human T cell leukemia/lymphoma virus type I infection. Clin Infect Dis 1996;23:138–45.

253. La Grenade L, Schwartz RA, Janniger CK. Childhood dermatitis in the tropics: with special emphasis on infective dermatitis, a marker for infection with human T-cell leukemia virus I. Cutis 1996;58:115–8.

254. Araujo A, Hall WW. Human T-lymphotropic virus type II and neurological disease. Ann Neurol 2004;56:10–9.

255. Orland JR, Engstorm J, Fridey J, et al. Prevalence and clinical features of HTLV neurologic disease in the HTLV Outcomes Study. Neurology 2003;61:1588–94.

256. Lehky TJ, Flerlage N, Katz D, et al. Human T-cell lymphotropic virus type II-associated myelopathy: clinical and immunologic profiles. Ann Neurol 1996;40:714–23.

257. Silva EA, et al. HTLV-II infection associated with a chronic neurodegenerative disease: clinical and molecular analysis. J Med Virol 2002;66:253–7.

258. Macedo O, Ribeiro-Lima TV, Linhares Ade O, et al. Human T-cell lymphotropic virus types I and II infections in a cohort of patients with neurological disorders in Belem, Para, Brazil. Rev Inst Med Trop Sao Paulo 2004;46:13–7.

259. Castillo LC, Gracia F, Roman GC, et al. Spinocerebellar syndrome in patients infected with human T-lymphotropic virus types I and II (HTLV-I/HTLV-II): report of 3 cases from Panama. Acta Neurol Scand 2000;101:405–12.

260. Dooneief G, Marlink R, Bell K, et al. Neurologic consequences of HTLV-II infection in injection-drug users. Neurology 1996;46:1556–60.

261. Beilke MA, Theall KP, O'Brien M, et al. Clinical outcomes and disease progression among patients coinfected with HIV and human T lymphotropic virus types 1 and 2. Clin Infect Dis 2004;39:256–63.

262. Zehender G, Colasante C, Santambrogio S, et al. Increased risk of developing peripheral neuropathy in patients coinfected with HIV-1 and HTLV-2. J Acquir Immune Defic Syndr 2002;31:440–7.

263. Murphy EL, Wang B, Sacher RA, et al. Respiratory and urinary tract infections, arthritis, and asthma associated with HTLV-I and HTLV-II infection. Emerg Infect Dis 2004;10:109–16.

264. Modahl LE, Young KC, Varney KF, et al. Are HTLV-II-seropositive injection drug users at increased risk of bacterial pneumonia, abscess, and lymphadenopathy? J Acquir Immune Defic Syndr Hum Retrovirol 1997;16:169–75.

265. Goedert JJ, Fung MW, Felton S, et al. Cause-specific mortality associated with HIV and HTLV-II infections among injecting drug users in the USA. AIDS 2001;15:1295–302.

266. Olaleye DO, Bernstein L, Sheng Z, et al. Type-specific immune response to human T cell lymphotropic virus (HTLV) type I and type II infections in Nigeria. Am J Trop Med Hyg 1994;50:479–86.

267. Murphy EL, Ownby HE, Smith JW, et al. Pulmonary function testing in HTLV-I and HTLV-II infected humans: a cohort study. BMC Pulm Med 2003;3:1.

268. Jarvis GA, Janoff EN, Cheng H, et al. Assessment of antibody responses to pneumococcal polysaccharide and tetanus toxoid vaccines in HTLV-II-infected adults [abstract P44]. AIDS Res Hum Retroviruses 2003;19 Suppl):S41.

269. Mukae H, Kohno S, Morikawa N, et al. Increase in T-cells bearing CD25 in bronchoalveolar lavage fluid from HAM/TSP patients and HTLV-I carriers. Microbiol Immunol 1994;38:55–62.

270. Mita S, Sugimoto M, Nakamura M, et al. Increased human T lymphotropic virus type-1 (HTLV-1) proviral DNA in peripheral blood mononuclear cells and bronchoalveolar lavage cells from Japanese patients with HTLV-1-associated myelopathy. Am J Trop Med Hyg 1993;48:170–7.

271. Seki M, Higashiyama Y, Mizokami A, et al. Up-regulation of human T lymphotropic virus type 1 (HTLV-1) tax/rex mRNA in infected lung tissues. Clin Exp Immunol 2000;120:488–98.

272. Seki M, Higashiyama Y, Kadota J, et al. Elevated levels of soluble adhesion molecules in sera and BAL fluid of individuals infected with human T-cell lymphotropic virus type 1. Chest 2000;118:1754–61.

273. Yamazato Y, Miyazato A, Kawakami K, et al. High expression of p40(tax) and pro-inflammatory cytokines and chemokines in the lungs of human T-lymphotropic virus type 1-related bronchopulmonary disorders. Chest 2003;124:2283–92.

274. Murphy EL, DeVita D, Liu H, et al. Risk factors for skin and soft-tissue abscesses among injection drug users: a case-control study. Clin Infect Dis 2001;33:35–40.

275. Safaeian M, Wilson LE, Taylor E, Thomas DL, Vlahov D. HTLV-II and bacterial infections among injection drug users. J Acquir Immune Defic Syndr 2000;24:483–7.

276. Eskild A, Samdal HH, Heger B. Co-infection with HIV-1/HTLV-II and the risk of progression to AIDS and death. The Oslo HIV Cohort Study Group. APMIS 1996;104:666–72.

277. Bessinger R, Beilke M, Kissinger P, et al. Retroviral coinfections at a New Orleans HIV outpatient clinic. J Acquir Immune Defic Syndr Hum Retrovirol 1997;14:67–71.

278. Rezza G. Determinants of progression to AIDS in HIV-infected

individuals: an update from the Italian Seroconversion Study. J Acquir Immune Defic Syndr Hum Retrovirol 1998;17 Suppl 1: S13–6.

279. Visconti A, Visconti L, Bellocco R, et al. HTLV-II/HIV-1 coinfection and risk for progression to AIDS among intravenous drug users. J Acquir Immune Defic Syndr 1993;6:1228–37.

280. Woods TC, et al. Investigation of proviral load in individuals infected with human T-lymphotropic virus type II. AIDS Res Hum Retroviruses 1995;11:1235–9.

281. Zehender G, Meroni L, Varchetta S, et al. Human T-lymphotropic virus type 2 (HTLV-2) provirus in circulating cells of the monocyte/macrophage lineage in patients dually infected with human immunodeficiency virus type 1 and HTLV-2 and having predominantly sensory polyneuropathy. J Virol 1998;72:7664–8.

282. Machuca A, Soriano V. In vivo fluctuation of HTLV-I and HTLV-II proviral load in patients receiving antiretroviral drugs. J Acquir Immune Defic Syndr 2000;24:189–93.

283. Murphy EL, Grant RM, Kropp J, et al. Increased human T-lymphotropic virus type II proviral load following highly active retroviral therapy in HIV-coinfected patients. J Acquir Immune Defic Syndr 2003;33:655–6.

284. Orland JR, Wang B, Wright DJ, et al. Increased mortality associated with HTLV-II infection in blood donors: a prospective cohort study. Retrovirology 2004;1:4.

285. Anonymous. Human T-lymphotropic virus type I screening in volunteer blood donors—United States, 1989. MMWR Morb Mortal Wkly Rep 1990;39:915, 921–4.

286. Caterino-de-Araujo A, de los Santos-Fortuna E, Meleiro MC, et al. Sensitivity of two enzyme-linked immunosorbent assay tests in relation to Western blot in detecting human T-cell lymphotropic virus types I and II infection among HIV-1 infected patients from Sao Paulo, Brazil. Diagn Microbiol Infect Dis 1998;30:173–82.

287. Centers for Disease Control Model Evaluation Program (2001). Analysis of the May 5, 1997 Performance evaluation testing results for HTLV Type I and II antibody reported to the Centers for Disease Control and Prevention (CDC) by participant laboratories in the model performance evaluation program. Available at: http://www.phppo.cdc.gov/mpep/pdf/htlv/9705anal.pdf.

288. Estes MC, Sevall JS. Multiplex PCR using real time DNA amplification for the rapid detection and quantitation of HTLV I or II. Mol Cell Probes 2003;17:59–68.

289. Thorstensson R, Albert J, Andersson S. Strategies for diagnosis of HTLV-I and -II. Transfusion 2002;42:780–91.

290. Santos Tde J, Costa CM, Goubau P, et al. Western blot seroindeterminate individuals for human T-lymphotropic virus I/II (HTLV-I/II) in Fortaleza (Brazil): a serological and molecular diagnostic and epidemiological approach. Braz J Infect Dis 2003;7:202–9.

291. Busch MP, et al. Accuracy of supplementary serologic testing for human T-lymphotropic virus types I and II in US blood donors. Retrovirus Epidemiology Donor Study. Blood 1994;83:1143–8.

292. Anonymous. Recommendations for counseling persons infected with human T-lymphotropic virus, types I and II. MMWR Morb Mortal Wkly Rep 1993;42:RR9.

293. Beilke MA, Japa S, Vinson DG. HTLV-I and HTLV-II virus expression increase with HIV-1 coinfection. J Acquir Immune Defic Syndr Hum Retrovirol 1998;17:391–7.

294. Hill SA, Lloyd PA, McDonald S, et al. Susceptibility of human T cell leukemia virus type I to nucleoside reverse transcriptase inhibitors. J Infect Dis 2003;188:424–7.

295. Sugahara K, Yamada Y. [Southern blot hybridization analysis for lymphoid neoplasms]. Rinsho Byori 2000;48:702–7.

296. Ramos JC, et al. Successful treatment with AZT and IFNa in adult T-cell leukemia-lymphoma is characterized by in vivo induction of TRAIL and AP-1 activity [abstract O68]. AIDS Res Hum Retroviruses 2003;19 Suppl:S26.

297. Nasr R, Rosenwald A, El-Sabban ME, et al. Arsenic/interferon specifically reverses 2 distinct gene networks critical for the survival of HTLV-1-infected leukemic cells. Blood 2003;101: 4576–82.

298. Ishikawa T. Current status of therapeutic approaches to adult T-cell leukemia. Int J Hematol 2003;78:304–11.

299. Abe Y, Yashiki S, Choi I, et al. Eradication of virus-infected T-cells in a case of adult T-cell leukemia/lymphoma by nonmyeloablative peripheral blood stem cell transplantation with conditioning consisting of low-dose total body irradiation and pentostatin. Int J Hematol 2002;76:91–3.

300. Waldmann TA. Anti-IL-2 receptor monoclonal antibody (anti-Tac) treatment of T-cell lymphoma. Important Adv Oncol 1994: 131–41.

301. Zhang Z, Zhang M, Goldman CK, Ravetch JV, Waldmann TA. Effective therapy for a murine model of adult T-cell leukemia with the humanized anti-CD52 monoclonal antibody, Campath-1H. Cancer Res 2003;63:6453–7.

302. Kaplan MH, Hall W, Susin M, et al. Syndrome of severe skin disease, eosinophilia, and dermatopathic lymphadenopathy in patients with HTLV-II complicating human immunodeficiency virus infection. Am J Med 1991;91:300–9.

303. Taylor GP, et al. The Bridge Study: a double-blind placebo controlled trial of zidovudine plus lamivudine for treatment of patients with HTLV-I associated myelopathy [abstract O23]. AIDS Res Hum Retroviruses 2003;19 Suppl:S13.

304. Nakagawa M, Nakahara K, Maruyama Y, et al. Therapeutic trials in 200 patients with HTLV-I-associated myelopathy/tropical spastic paraparesis. J Neurovirol 1996;2:345–55.

305. Saito M, Nakagawa M, Kaseda S, et al. Decreased human T lymphotropic virus type I (HTLV-I) provirus load and alteration in T cell phenotype after interferon-alpha therapy for HTLV-I-associated myelopathy/tropical spastic paraparesis. J Infect Dis 2004;189:29–40.

306. Feng J, Misu T, Fujihara K, et al. Interferon-alpha significantly reduces cerebrospinal fluid CD4 cell subsets in HAM/TSP. J Neuroimmunol 2003;141:170–3.

307. Kannagi M, Harashima N, Kurihara K, et al. Adult T-cell leukemia: future prophylaxis and immunotherapy. Expert Rev Anticancer Ther 2004;4:369–76.

308. Sundaram R, Sun Y, Walker CM, et al. A novel multivalent human CTL peptide construct elicits robust cellular immune responses in HLA-A*0201 transgenic mice: implications for HTLV-1 vaccine design. Vaccine 2003;21:2767–81.

309. Kazanji M, Tartaglia J, Franchini G, et al. Immunogenicity and protective efficacy of recombinant human T-cell leukemia/lymphoma virus type 1 NYVAC and naked DNA vaccine candidates in squirrel monkeys (Saimiri sciureus). J Virol 2001; 75:5939–48.

19

Non–AIDS-Defining Cancers in HIV-Infected Individuals

ELIZABETH Y. CHIAO
SUSAN E. KROWN

Human immunodeficiency virus (HIV) infection increases the risk for a number of malignant neoplasms.[1,2] Kaposi's sarcoma, non-Hodgkin's lymphoma, and cervical cancer have been included in the CDC case definition of acquired immune deficiency syndrome (AIDS).[3] In addition to the three AIDS-defining malignancies, HIV-infected people are also at significantly higher risk for anal cancer and Hodgkin's disease, malignancies not included in the AIDS definition. Recent cohort studies and linked AIDS/cancer registry studies have also documented an increased incidence of other non–AIDS-defining cancers including testicular cancer, basal cell cancer of the skin, squamous cell cancer of the skin, melanoma, lung cancer, and head and neck cancer.[2–8]

The non–AIDS-defining malignancies in HIV-infected patients present an evolving clinical picture. As the life expectancy of people with HIV disease continues to increase because of highly active antiretroviral therapy (HAART),[9,10] the proportion of deaths attributable to non–AIDS-defining malignancies has increased among AIDS patients.[11] It is likely that non–AIDS-defining malignancies will become more prevalent as the HIV-positive cohort ages. However, there are many unresolved questions regarding the epidemiology, natural history, and outcomes for non–AIDS-defining malignancies. For example, it is unclear if the predisposition to these cancers in HIV-infected patients is associated with factors specific to HIV and chronic immunosuppression, or whether the predisposition is attributable to other factors, such as smoking. In addition, it is unclear if non–AIDS-related neoplastic processes, such as lung cancer, present at later stages and have a more aggressive course in HIV-infected patients compared to the general non–HIV-infected population.[12–14] Finally, the data regarding optimal therapy for HIV-infected people with non–AIDS-defining malignancies continue to evolve. This chapter focuses on non–AIDS-defining malignancies, excluding Hodgkin's disease and anal cancer. Specific emphasis will be placed on the following non–AIDS-defining malignancies: lung cancer, skin cancer, head and neck cancer, conjunctival cancer, testicular cancer, leiomyosarcoma, hepatocellular carcinoma, breast cancer, multiple myeloma, leukemia, colon cancer, and prostate cancer.

EPIDEMIOLOGY

The epidemiology of HIV disease in the United States, Europe, Australia, and other countries with widespread HAART access has changed significantly. Causes of mortality have changed since the advent of HAART, including a higher proportion of deaths caused by non-AIDS malignancies.[11] Louie and colleagues[11] analyzed deaths among persons with AIDS reported from 1994 to 1998 in San Francisco and found that non–AIDS-defining malignancies as a cause of death increased from 6.4% in 1994 to 10.9% in 1998 ($p < .01$).[11]

In the pre-HAART era, two cohort studies failed to convincingly show an increased risk of non–AIDS-related malignancy in HIV-infected people.[15,16] However, more recent linkage analyses of data from AIDS and cancer registries have shown statistically significant increases in the age-standardized incidence ratio (SIR) or relative risk (RR) of non–AIDS-defining malignancies for HIV-infected cohorts compared to a standardized population (Table 19–1),[1,2,4,5,17–21] In addition, two prospective studies have been performed that included data on the development of non–AIDS-defining malignancies after the introduction of HAART.[8,20] Patel and colleagues[8] evaluated 7,893 patients from two Chicago clinics and 4,053 patients enrolled in the HIV Outpatient Study (HOPS) in the HAART era (from 1996–2000). In an analysis of the HOPS data adjusted for age, race, smoking, and gender, the RRs for developing lung cancer, Hodgkin's disease, anorectal cancer, and melanoma were found to be significantly elevated compared to the general US population. They also analyzed data from the two Chicago clinics and found that the RRs for developing lung cancer, Hodgkin's disease, anorectal cancer, melanoma, and head and neck cancer were also significantly elevated compared to the general population of Chicago (Table 19–2).

Table 19–1. COMPARISON OF PUBLISHED HIV/AIDS CANCER MATCH REGISTRY STUDIES

Reference	Years of Study	Cohort	Number of Patients	SIR/RR of all non-AIDS Malignancies	Specific Malignancies	SIR/RR*
Serraino et al[5] 2000	1988–1992	Italy and France HIV and AIDS Cohort Men 20–49	5,281	1.9 (1.2–2.8)	Hodgkin's disease Salivary gland	8.7 (3.4,18.0) 33.6 (3.2–123.5)
Gallagher et al[18] 2001	1981–1994	New York State AIDS Cohort Men 15–69	122,993	2.6 (2.41–2.7)	Hodgkin's disease Anal cancer Lung cancer Testicular cancer Liver cancer Multiple myeloma Brain cancer Skin (non-KS) Soft/Connective tissue	8.0 (5.05–9.33) 3.3 (2.6–3.75) 3.0 (2.37–3.69) 1.5 (1.05–2.03) 5.1(3.57–7.07) 2.7 (1.57–4.19) 3.1 (2.26–4.24) 19.8 (15.0–23.5) 5.6 (4.13–7.34)
Frisch et al[4] 2001	1978–1996	US AIDS Cohort Men and Women	302,834	2.7 (2.7–2.8)*	Hodgkin's disease Anal cancer Lung cancer Testicular cancer Lip cancer Melanoma Liver cancer Multiple myeloma Brain cancer Leukemia Soft/Connective tissue	11.5 (10.6–12.5)* 33.8 (29.5–38.6)* 4.5 (4.2–4.8)* 2.0 (1.7–2.4)* 3.1 (1.9–4.8)* 1.3 (1.1–1.6)* 7.7 (6.1–9.4)* 2.6 (1.9–3.4)* 3.5 (3.0–4.1)* 2.1 (1.5–2.9)* 3.3 (2.6–4.1)*
Allardice et al[19] 2003	1980–1996	Scotland HIV and AIDS Cohort Men and Women	2,574	1.8 (1.1–2.6)	Skin Lung Liver	2.8 (1.04–6.2) 4.1 (1.3–9.5) 22 (2.7–80.2)
Grulich et al[2] 1999	1980–1999	Australia AIDS Cohort Men and Women	13,067	3.0 (2.3–3.84)	Hodgkin's disease Anal cancer Lip cancer Multiple myeloma Leukemia Soft /Connective tissue	7.85 (4.4–13) 37.1 (17.8–68.3) 2.26 (1.08–4.16) 4.15 (1.34–9.67) 3.38 (1.80–5.78) 9.71 (5.93–15.0)
Dal Maso et al[21] 2003	1982–2000	Italy AIDS Cohort Men and Women	12,104	2.3 (2.0–2.7)	Hodgkin's disease Anal cancer Lung Brain Leukemia	16.2 (11.8–21.7) 33.6 (12.1–73.6) 2.4 (1.5–3.7) 4.4 (2.2–8.0) 5.3 (2.8–9.2)

*RR = relative risk; SIR = age-standardized incidence ratio.

However, the RRs of breast, colon, and prostate cancer were not increased.

Herida and colleagues[20] evaluated 77,025 HIV-infected patients in France followed from 1992 to 1999. The median follow-up was 32 months. The period of study enrollment was divided into two periods: 1992 to 1995 (P1) and 1996 to 1999 (P2). They reported an overall increase of non–AIDS-defining malignancies among HIV-infected men, but not among women, during both study periods. Among men, they found that the incidence of Hodgkin's disease was elevated in both P1 and P2. However, oral cancer; colon, rectal, and anal cancer; stomach cancer; and CNS cancer were all statistically significantly elevated in P1, but none of these cancers was elevated in P2. Instead, only lung cancer and kidney cancer were elevated in P2. Among women, the overall risk of non–AIDS-defining malignancies was not higher than the general population, but the incidence of Hodgkin's disease was higher during both P1 and P2, and, as in men, the incidence of lung cancer was higher during P2. Of note, the incidence of breast cancer was significantly lower in HIV-infected women than in the general French population during both P1 and P2. They concluded that HAART did not have a measurable impact on the incidence of non–AIDS-defining cancers.[20]

The AIDS/cancer-linked registry studies have retrospectively linked national AIDS registries and cancer registries. These studies were able to investigate the cancer pattern in the years surrounding the time of AIDS diagnosis (see Table 19–1). All of the studies found an increased risk of Hodgkin's disease in the cohorts.[2,4,5,18,19,21] Four of the five studies showed an increased risk of anal cancer[2,4,18,19,21] and lung cancer.[4,18,19,21] In addition, three of the six studies found an increased risk of liver cancer,[4,18,19] mul-

tiple myeloma,[2,4,18] brain (non-lymphoma) cancer,[4,18,21] and leukemia.[2,4,21] Two studies found an increased risk of soft/connective tissue cancers,[2,18] lip cancer,[2,4] testicular cancer,[4,18] and skin cancer.[18,19] (Of note, the majority of cancer registries do not reliably include non-melanoma skin cancer cases.) Only one out of the six studies found an increased risk of melanoma[4] or salivary gland cancer.[5] None of the studies found an increased risk of breast cancer, colon cancer, or prostate cancer.[2,4,5,18,19,21] Frisch and colleagues[4] and Gallagher and colleagues[18] both found a statistically significant decrease in the risk of prostate and bladder cancer, and Gallagher and colleagues[18] found a statistically significant decreased risk of esophagus and colon cancer.

Several studies also attempted to evaluate the risk of cancer based on the level of immunosuppression. Frisch and colleagues[4] and Gallagher and colleagues[18] used the timing of cancer diagnosis with respect to development of AIDS. Frisch and colleagues[4] defined three criteria suggesting that non–AIDS-defining cancers were associated with immunosuppression: (1) the overall RR for the period from 60 months before to 27 months after AIDS was significantly elevated, (2) the RR in the early post-AIDS period was significantly elevated, and (3) there was a statistically significant increasing trend in the RRs from before to after AIDS onset. Using a test for trend, they found that Hodgkin's disease, lung cancer, penile cancer, soft tissue malignancies, lip cancer, and testicular seminoma met the three criteria associated with immunosuppression.[4] Mbulaiteye and colleagues[6] used a subset of the AIDS/cancer-linked registry to evaluate the effect of decreasing CD4 count on various AIDS- and non–AIDS-related malignancies. They found that the RR for oropharynx cancer decreased with worsening immunity. Otherwise, none

Table 19–2. INCIDENCE OF NON–AIDS-DEFINING MALIGNANCIES IN THE HIV OUTPATIENT STUDY (HOPS)[8]

Non–AIDS-Defining Malignancy	Adjusted Relative Risk	
	HOPS *N* = 4,053	Chicago Outpatient Clinics *N* = 7,893
Hodgkin's disease	4.58 (3.10, 6.77)	77.43 (19.37, 309.55)
Anorectal cancer	10.13 (7.48, 13.72)	5.03 (4.76, 5.33)
Lung cancer	2.13 (1.06, 4.27)	3.63 (2.18, 6.05)
Melanoma	2.99 (1.71, 5.22)	4.10 (1.71, 5.22)
Head and neck cancer	Not reported	9.96 (2.49, 39.79)

of the non–AIDS-defining malignancies were affected by level of immunity.[6]

Gallagher and colleagues[18] used similar criteria for defining immunosuppression-related cancers. They divided the time intervals for developing cancer into four time periods: 5 to 2 years prior to AIDS, 2 years to 6 months prior to AIDS, within 6 months before to 3 months after an AIDS diagnosis, and 3 months to 5 years after an AIDS diagnosis. Using similar criteria to those used by Frisch and colleagues,[4] they found that cancers of the rectum, rectosigmoid and anus; trachea, bronchus and lung; skin; and connective tissues among males were associated with increasing immunosuppression.[18]

PATHOGENESIS

Substantial progress has been made in understanding AIDS-related neoplasms, but the exact pathogenesis of these malignancies is still not fully elucidated. Many of the HIV-associated cancers are also associated with infection with other viruses.[22] For example, Epstein-Barr virus (EBV) has been implicated as an important agent in the development of non-Hodgkin's lymphoma,[23] human herpesvirus 8 (HHV-8) is essential for the development of Kaposi's sarcoma (KS),[24] and oncogenic types of human papillomavirus (HPV) have been associated with cervical and anogenital neoplasia.[22] There are, however, fewer specific associations with non–AIDS-related malignancies and viruses, nor have other etiologic factors been clearly identified.

There have been several hypotheses and in vitro findings that suggest molecular mechanisms of pathogenesis in non–AIDS-related malignancies, but there are few definitive findings.[25] HIV-1 Tat is a nonstructural viral protein essential for replication. It is a potent transactivator of the HIV LTR.[26] It has also been shown to transactivate several endogenous cellular genes, including cytokines, extracellular matrix proteins, and proto-oncogenes.[27] Exogenous Tat has also been found in the extracellular environment of HIV-infected cells.[28] De Falco and colleagues[29] showed that levels of pRB2/p130 mRNA increased in the presence of Tat. They also found that Tat can inhibit the growth control activity exerted by pRB2/p130 in the T98G cell line, and that the interaction between Tat and pRB2/p130 results

in the deregulation of the control exerted by pRB2/p130 on the cell cycle. They hypothesized that the inhibition of pRB2/p130 by HIV Tat may implicate HIV itself as an oncogenic virus.[29] Altavilla and colleagues[30] showed that in a population of Tat-transgenic mice exposed to urethane, there was a statistically significant increase of preneoplastic lesions of the liver but not of lymphomas or lung tumors.[30] Chipitsyna and colleagues[31] described that Tat production causes an increase in the survival of Tat-transfected cells after treatment with genotoxic agents. They exposed cells to cisplatin and found reduced DNA breakage in Tat-transfected cells as compared to control cells. They also found that cells expressing Tat had elevated levels of Rad51 (a key regulator of homologous recombination) and a slight decrease of Ku70 (one of the components on the non-homologous end-joining repair pathway). In addition, they found that repair of DNA double-strand breaks by homologous recombination was increased in Tat-producing cells, and protein extracts from Tat-producing cells had reduced ability in end-rejoining linearized DNA as compared to protein extract from control cells. They concluded that Tat may affect the expression of genes involved in DNA repair and thus influence host genomic integrity.[31]

Microsatellite alterations (MA) are another molecular phenomenon demonstrated in non–AIDS-defining malignancies. MAs probably represent evidence of some form of genomic instability.[32–34] Wistuba and colleagues[25] evaluated MA and loss of heterozygosit (LOH) in lung tumors from 11 HIV-positive people and 35 people of indeterminate HIV status. The overall frequency of LOH was similar in the HIV-positive and HIV negative tumors. However, the number of MA present in the HIV-associated tumors was six-fold higher ($p < .03$) than in the tumors from HIV-indeterminate people. The molecular changes were independent of tumor stage and gender. They did not find any HIV or HPV sequences in the tumor cells.[35]

INDIVIDUAL TUMORS

Lung Cancer

The incidence of lung cancer in the United States in 2000 was greater than 70 per 100,000, and approximately 160,000 new cases were diagnosed in 2000. Lung cancer is the leading cause of cancer deaths in the United States among both men and women.[36] The HIV-infected population, in particular, may be at increased risk of lung cancer.[1,4,8,18,20,37] As shown in Table 19–1, Serraino and colleagues[5] and Grulich and colleagues[2] did not find an increased risk of lung cancer in 2 cohorts of HIV-infected patients from Italy and Australia. Similarly, Cooksley and colleagues[38] did not find an increased risk of lung cancer in an AIDS/cancer-linked registry study from Harris County, Texas. However, Frisch and colleagues[4] and Gallagher and colleagues[18] found an increased SIR/RR when AIDS/cancer-linked registry data were analyzed. Engels and colleagues[39] conducted an age-stratified analysis of the AIDS/cancer-linked registry match and found that patients under age 50, particularly those in the 30 to 49 age group, had a significantly increased incidence of lung cancer. Goedert and colleagues[1] used the AIDS/cancer-linked registry data to evaluate risk of cancer based on the level of immunosuppression estimated by time of cancer diagnosis in relation to the onset of AIDS. They found that although lung cancer incidence did not increase with increasing immunosuppression, the risk of lung adenocarcinoma was 2.5 (1.0–5.1) in the time period 4 to 27 months after the diagnosis of AIDS. Parker and colleagues,[37] in a retrospective analysis of the Texas Department of Health cancer and HIV registries, showed a 6.5-fold increase in the incidence of lung cancer in HIV-infected people compared to the general US population.

Other smaller cohort studies have also reported an increased risk of lung cancer. Ricaurte and colleagues[40] reported an incidence rate of 191 per 100,000 for lung cancer in a cohort of 2,616 HIV patients followed at an urban clinic. They reported that this rate is 7.4 times the rate in US males between ages 35 and 54.[40] Cailhol and colleagues[41] reported 5 lung cancer cases in a cohort of 247 HIV-infected men in France aged 40 to 74 years. The SIR was 4.6 (1.5–10.7) compared to the general population of French men aged 40 to 74.[41] Finally, as shown in Table 19–2, Patel and colleagues[8] found an increased risk of lung cancer in 2 cohorts of HIV-positive individuals, despite controlling for age, gender, race, and smoking.

The majority of studies in the post-HAART era show an increased risk of lung cancer, but there is no consensus on whether the risk of lung cancer has changed since the introduction of HAART. Some studies have found that the risk of lung cancer has increased since the introduction of HAART, whereas other studies have found lung cancer risk to be unchanged. In their analysis of a prospective HIV hospital cohort, Herida and colleagues[20] found an increased SIR for lung cancer in the HAART period (1996–1999), but not in the pre-HAART period (1992–1995). Bower and colleagues[42] analyzed a prospectively acquired data base of 8,400 HIV-infected patients between 1986 and 2001. They found 11 lung cancer cases. The incidence of lung cancer increased from 0.8 per 100,000 (0.2–3.2) in the pre-HAART era to 6.7 per 100,000 (3.1–13.9) in the post-HAART era. In the post-HAART era, the RR of lung cancer in the HIV-infected population was comparable to that of the general population in southeast England, which was 8.93 (4.92–19.98).[42] However, Dal Maso and colleagues,[43] using data from the Italian Cancer and AIDS Registries Study, found that HIV-infected individuals were at higher risk for lung cancer, but the risk did not change in the post-HAART era. The overall SIR was 7.4 (4.6–11.3) in the pre-HAART period, and 7.9 (2.1–20.4) in the post-HAART period. A total of 21 lung cancers were identified from 1985 to 1998.[43]

Contribution of Smoking Tobacco to Risk of HIV-Related Lung Cancer

The increased risk of lung cancer seen in large epidemiologic studies has frequently been attributed to increased smoking rates in HIV-positive individuals. Serraino and colleagues[5] found that the risk of lung cancer was not significantly increased in a mixed population of male HIV-positive intravenous drug users and non-intravenous drug users, but it was significantly elevated in a cohort of HIV-negative male intravenous drug users. Additionally, Dal Maso and colleagues[43] reported that the risk of lung cancer was significantly higher in intravenous drug users with HIV compared to HIV-positive patients from other HIV exposure categories. They found that the SIR of lung cancer was 23.9 (11.9–43.0) among intravenous drug users with HIV, and 4.2 (2.0–7.7) for other HIV-exposure categories.[43] Both Serraino and Dal Maso suggested that intravenous drug users, regardless of HIV status, were at higher risk of lung cancer because of increased tobacco use.[5,43] Although smoking information was not specifically collected, Gallagher and colleagues[18] reported that men whose HIV risk factors were either homosexual contact or intravenous drug use were all at higher risk for lung cancer. In addition, they found that women in all HIV exposure groups were at higher risk for lung cancer.[18] Furthermore, Patel and colleagues[8] found an increased risk of lung cancer in a prospective cohort of HIV-infected individuals despite controlling for smoking behavior.

Diminished tumor immune surveillance as a result of chronic HIV-related immunosuppression has been postulated as another variable accounting for the increased risk of lung cancer in this population.[39,44] Wistuba and colleagues[35] found microsatellite instability in a significantly higher proportion of lung tumor specimens from HIV-infected patients compared to non–HIV-infected controls, and hypothesized that immunosuppressive states may result in microsatellite instability, which, in turn, may play a role in tumor development. Other factors that have been linked to increased lung cancer risk in HIV-infected patients include opportunistic lung infections,[45] intravenous drug use, and the increasing age of HIV patients in the HAART era.[20,39]

Clinical Characteristics of HIV-Positive Patients with Lung Cancer

Several case series reporting on HIV-associated lung cancers have been published in the last several years (Table 19–3). Although the mean age of lung cancer patients in the general population is 68 years,[46] the mean age at diagnosis in the HIV population ranged from 38 to 49 years. In the majority of published series, the most common histology was adenocarcinoma, and many patients presented with advanced stage, non-resectable disease. Adenocarcinoma accounted for between 25 and 60% of cases, whereas 0 to 20% showed small cell histology. The authors of these series reported between a 30- to 60-pack per year median tobacco history. Between 13 and 57% of HIV-positive patients had a history of tuberculosis (TB) or *Pneumocystis carinii* pneumonia (PCP). A large proportion of cases presented with late stage disease (67–100%), and 0 to 26% were treated with surgery. The median survival was 1.8 to 14 months.[12,13,37,41,42,45,47,48]

Symptoms at the time of lung cancer presentation in the HIV-positive population have been

Table 19–3. COMPARISON OF PUBLISHED HIV AND LUNG CANCER SERIES

	Author/Reference Number							
	Bazot[47]	Parker[37]	Sridar[12]	Vyzula[13]	Tirelli[45]	Bower[42]	Cailhol[41]	Burke[48]
Dates of Study	1988–1994	1990–1995	1986–1991	1988–1995	1986–1998	1996–2001	1999–2001	1999–2002
Number of cases	15	36	19	16	36	9	5	4
Homosexual (%)	40	47	31	31	17	89	80	100
Receiving HAART (%)	0	0	0	0	8	66	100	100
Mean age at lung cancer diagnosis	48	49	47	45.3	38	44	50	42.3
Small cell histology (%)	13	8	5	12	13	11	20	0
Adenocarcinoma histology (%)	47	NA	42	50	36	44	60	25
Median CD4 count (cells/mm³)	136	NA	121	184	150	180	449	373.5
Pack years (tobacco smoked [median range])	40 (15–100)	NA	60 (0–100)	30 (15–90)	40 cigarettes /day (median)	40 (25–60)	40 (7–50)	40 (20–40)
% with history of PCP or TB	13	NA	57	NA	22	33	NA	NA
Stage IIIB/IV (%)	67	89	79	81	71	100	100	100
Median survival (months)	14	NA	3	1.8	5	2	6	3

HAART = highly active anti-retroviral therapy; PCP = Pneumocystis carinii pneumonia; TB = tuberculosis.

reported to be similar to those in the HIV-negative population. Case reports note that patients present with cough, chest pain, shortness of breath, hemoptysis, wasting, fatigue, Horner's syndrome, bone pain, clubbing or hypercalcemia.[12,13,37,42,45,47,48] Patients may also present with only abnormal chest x-ray findings. Although it has been suggested that HIV-positive patients present more frequently with advanced stage disease, recent studies have shown that the distribution of stages at presentation in HIV-positive patients is similar to that of HIV-negative patients.[12,45] However, performance status at time of diagnosis, which has been shown to be an adverse prognostic factor in lung cancer survival,[49] was shown to be decreased in HIV-positive patients compared to age-matched controls.[42,45]

Patients in the pre-HAART and HAART eras appear to have similar presentations of disease. Bower and colleagues[42] found that the only major difference was the median length of time from HIV diagnosis to lung cancer diagnosis, which was 2 months in the pre-HAART era and 10 months in the HAART era. Another recent HAART era study by Powles and colleagues[50] compared the presentation and outcomes of 9 HIV-positive non–small-cell lung cancer patients with 27 HIV-negative age- and stage-matched controls. Seven of the 9 HIV-positive patients were on HAART at the start of treatment. The median age was similar in the HIV-positive patients and the HIV-negative controls (45 and 48 years, respectively). Sixty-six percent of HIV-positive patients had adenocarcinoma histology compared to 70% of HIV-negative patients, and 66% of HIV-positive patients and 70% of HIV-negative controls presented with stage IV disease. The HIV-negative patients had a better performance status than the HIV-positive patients; 52% of HIV-negative patients and 22% of the HIV-positive patients presented with ECOG performance status less than two.

Treatment and Outcomes

Powles and colleagues[50] found that a smaller percentage of the HIV-negative controls received chemotherapy (66% of HIV-negative patients versus 88% of the HIV-positive patients). In addition, chemotherapy was stopped early in 3 HIV-positive patients, 2 because of progression of disease and 1 because of toxicity. Overall survival was the same for HIV-positive and HIV-negative patients at 4 months ($p = .55$). Cancer-related death rates were similar in the HIV-negative and HIV-positive patients (74 versus 77%).[50] The findings of Powles and colleagues[50] contrast with previous reports that show inferior survival for HIV-positive patients compared to HIV-negative patients.[12,13,45] The earlier studies hypothesized either that lung cancer was a more aggressive disease in HIV-positive patients, or that fewer HIV-positive than HIV-negative patients were candidates for curative surgical resection because of poor lung function as a result of multiple previous opportunistic infections. Poor performance status may have also contributed to decreased rates of surgical resection or chemotherapy treatment. The study by Powles and colleagues[14] was not able to address the issue of surgical resection because all of the patients in the study presented with advanced stage disease. However, they hypothesized that the poor outcomes in both the HIV-positive cases and HIV-negative controls may reflect advanced and aggressive disease behavior in young people who present with lung cancer as a whole, and that lung cancer does not appear to be more aggressive in HIV-positive individuals. They report that advanced non–small-cell lung cancer in HIV-infected individuals treated with HAART is still associated with a poor outcome, but the outcomes are similar to HIV-negative controls matched for age and stage.[14]

HAART may improve outcomes in HIV-infected patients with lung cancer. Although there are no data that directly compare the survival between the pre-HAART era and the HAART era, pooled data from the pre-HAART era indicate that the median survival was approximately 2 months.[12,13,51,52] Powles and colleagues[14] reported that the survival in the HAART era was 4 months. They hypothesized that HAART may decrease HIV-related mortality and increase the ability to tolerate treatment.[14]

Based on the data published to date, HIV infection per se should not be a contraindication for surgical intervention or palliative therapy. The available data suggest that HIV-positive patients with lung cancer should be treated in a similar fashion to HIV-negative patients based on stage and performance status.[50] When investigating the diagnosis and stage of lung cancer in HIV-infected individuals, it is important to note that there is a higher likelihood of non-malignant causes of abnormal mediastinal lymph node enlargement in the HIV-infected. Therefore, in HIV-positive individuals, mediastinoscopy may be recommended if there is any doubt regarding the etiology of mediastinal lymphadenopathy. In addition, palliative chemotherapy and radiotherapy should be considered for possible improvement in quality of life. Hematopoietic growth factors may be necessary to support HIV-positive patients during treatment. Prophylaxis against opportunistic infection during chemotherapy and radiation therapy, and avoidance of anemia-inducing anti-retroviral medications, such as zidovudine, should be standard adjunctive treatment measures.

HIV-positive patients appear to be at a higher risk for lung cancer, particularly since the introduction of HAART. Although survival appears to have improved slightly, patients presenting with advanced disease continue to demonstrate overall poor survival. Because surgical resection of early stage disease is the only therapy that has been associated with long-term survival, active screening to increase early diagnosis of lung cancer in patients can be recommended. Finally, smoking is also a significant risk factor for other chronic diseases besides lung cancer for which HIV-positive patients are at risk, including coronary artery disease,[53] emphysema,[54] and head and neck cancers.[55] A systematic approach to smoking cessation programs for HIV-positive individuals may be of great benefit in this population.

Head and Neck Cancer

Head and neck cancers comprise a wide array of anatomic and histologic entities. It is unclear from large cohort studies if patients with HIV disease are at higher risk for head and neck cancer.[2,4,5,18,19,43] Frisch and colleagues[4] and Grulich and colleagues[2] both found an elevated risk of lip cancer in the HIV-positive populations they studied. In addition, when the data were adjusted for differential survival in the HIV-positive population, Gallagher and colleagues[18] found an elevated risk of tongue, gum, pharynx, and larynx cancers in the New York State AIDS/cancer-

linked registry. More recently, Powles and colleagues,[55] in an analysis of the Chelsea and Westminster Hospital database of HIV seropositive people between 1986 and 2001, found that head and neck cancer occurred more frequently in the HIV-positive population than in age-matched HIV-negative controls. They also found that the incidence of head and neck cancer in HIV-positive patients was not significantly altered in the post-HAART period.

The oncogenic viruses, HPV and EBV, have both been implicated in the development of certain head and neck cancers in immunocompetent patients.[56,57] Whereas EBV infection has been associated with the development of nasopharyngeal cancers, recent epidemiological and laboratory studies have shown a strong and consistent association between high-risk HPV (overwhelmingly HPV-16) and head and neck squamous cell cancer (HNSCC) arising in the lingual and palatine tonsils.[58] HNSCC arising in other sites was not associated with HPV infection. The association of HPV with HNSCC is not, however, confined to tumors of tonsillar origin. In patients with Fanconi anemia, who show a marked increase in the incidence of anogenital squamous cell cancers (SCCs) and non-tonsillar HNSCCs,[59,60] a recent case-control study [61] detected high-risk HPV DNA in 21 (84%) of 25 such tumors, but in only 18 (36%) of 50 site-matched tumors from control subjects without Fanconi anemia ($p < .001$). Whereas none of the 18 Fanconi anemia-associated HNSCCs contained *p53* mutations, 12 (39%) of 31 control HNSCCs contained such a mutation. The risk of SCC in Fanconi anemia patients was associated with a specific genetic polymorphism of the *p53* tumor suppressor gene, homozygosity for arginine at codon 72, suggesting that this *p53* polymorphic variant is associated with a higher susceptibility to degradation by the HPV E6 oncoprotein.[61,62] Another molecular profile which is distinct for HPV-positive HNSCC is up-regulation of the p16 tumor suppressor protein. The HPV E7 oncogene product inhibits the activity of the pRb protein, leading to p16 up-regulation via loss of negative feedback control of pRb expression. In HPV-negative HNSCC, the *p16* gene is usually silenced by genetic or epigenetic mechanisms. However, in HPV-positive HNSCC, diffuse nuclear and cytoplasmic *p16* staining by immunohistochemistry correlates strongly with the presence of HPV by both in situ hybridization and quantitative PCR.[63–65]

Thus far, the role of HPV and the potential contribution of *p53* genetic polymorphisms to HNSCC susceptibility have not been studied systematically in HIV-positive individuals, but there are suggestions that HPV may be a contributing factor in some cases. Frisch and colleagues[66] used data from the Surveillance, Epidemiology and End Results (SEER) program and found that the incidence of tonsillar cancer increased significantly from 1973 to 1995 in unmarried men, whereas the incidence at all other oral sites remained constant. They hypothesized that unmarried status is a proxy for male homosexuality and that HIV/AIDS-related immunosuppression may be a contributing factor to the recent increase among young men. In addition, Kreimer and colleagues,[67] in a cross-sectional study of HPV prevalence in the oral cavity in a cohort of HIV-seropositive and HIV-seronegative adults, found that the prevalence of high-risk HPV infection was greater in the HIV-seropositive cohort than in the seronegative cohort (13.7 versus 4.5%; *p* < .001). However, Roland and colleagues[68] found HPV in only 2 of 8 head and neck cancers in HIV-positive patients. Powles and colleagues[55] found EBV in all 4 head and neck cancers in a cohort of HIV-positive patients but did not evaluate for HPV. The majority of studies on head and neck cancer in HIV-infected patients identified smoking cigarettes and excess alcohol consumption as the most consistent risk factors,[55] whereas a low incidence of smoking and alcohol consumption was reported in Fanconi anemia patients with HPV-associated SCCs.[61]

In the pre-HAART era, several publications noted that HIV-infected patients were younger at presentation, presented with more aggressive disease, and had poorer survival compared to HIV-negative patients.[68–71] Powles and colleagues[55] evaluated 7 HIV-positive patients with head and neck cancer in the pre-HAART and HAART eras. Only 1 patient in that series had received prior HAART. Three of the patients had asymptomatic HIV infection, and 2 had an AIDS-defining diagnosis. The median nadir CD4 cell count prior to the diagnosis of head and neck cancer was 143 cells/mm^3 (10–340/mm^3). Four of

the 7 patients presented with stage I or II disease. After receiving standard therapy, 4 of the 7 patients showed a complete response, and 3 of 7 showed a partial response. However, 5 patients relapsed after a median of only 5 months. The median overall survival was 28 months. Six of the 7 patients had died at the time of the report, and one patient was alive at 96 months. Patients whose disease relapsed had marked toxicity from subsequent treatment and short overall survival. Chemotherapy and radiotherapy decreased the CD4 cell count in this population, and the authors advocated instituting opportunistic infection prophylaxis when starting chemotherapy or radiation therapy for head and neck cancer in HIV-positive patients.

Non-Melanoma Skin Cancer

The incidence of non-melanoma skin cancers in HIV-positive populations is difficult to determine because data on SCC and basal cell cancers (BCC) of the skin are not usually reported to cancer registries. Franceschi and colleagues[17] found an increased incidence of non-melanoma skin cancers in HIV-positive patients. Of the 8 non-melanoma skin cancers, 5 were BCCs. Lobo and colleagues[72] also found that the incidence of BCC is likely increased in HIV-infected individuals.

BCCs in HIV-positive patients are mostly superficial, multicentric, and appear more commonly on the trunk or extremities. This is in contrast to cases in the general population, in which the most common presentation is on the head or neck. Decreasing CD4 cell counts do not appear to influence the risk of SCC or BCC.[17,72] It has been reported that both BCCs and SCCs present more frequently as multiple synchronous tumors in HIV-positive than in HIV-negative patients.[72,73] HPV has been hypothesized to play a role in tumorigenesis of non-melanomatous neoplasms in HIV-positive individuals.[74] However, Maurer and colleagues[75] did not find HPV sequences in the majority of SCCs or BCCs collected from 24 HIV-positive patients. They found that 90% of SCCs and BCCs from HIV-infected cases stained for *p53*, compared to only 50% of lesions from the general population. These authors and others have suggested that ultraviolet light has an important role in SCC and BCC tumorigenesis in HIV-infected patients.[25,75]

Nguyen and colleagues[73] recently reported on a retrospective case series of 10 patients with SCCs. They found that HIV-infected patients with SCCs presented at a significantly younger age than the general population. Four of the 10 patients were receiving HAART. The median CD4 count was 244.5 cells/mm^3 (34–464). They found that 20% of tumors recurred after curettage and electrodesiccation and reported that SCC in this population behaves in a particularly aggressive fashion. These authors found significant morbidity and mortality from SCC (50% mortality within 41 months). They recommended primary prevention with sunscreen and sun avoidance, as well as aggressive management of precancerous lesions for all HIV-positive patients.[73]

Melanoma

In addition to cutaneous non-melanoma neoplasms such as BCC and SCC, the risk of melanoma also appears to be increased in patients infected with HIV.[4,17,76] Using AIDS/cancer match registries, Frisch and colleagues[4] and Franceschi and colleagues[17] both found a statistically significant increase in malignant melanoma. Melanoma appears to present at a younger age in HIV-positive patients than in the general population.[77,78] Calista and colleagues[78] summarized a total of 31 cases of melanoma in HIV-positive patients reported in the literature. The average age was 38.4 years. Sixty-seven percent presented with lesions on the trunk, 13.3% presented with a limb lesion, and 10% presented with a head and neck lesion,[78] compared to 36% of cases presenting on the trunk for men and 44% of cases presenting on the lower extremities for females in a cohort of HIV-negative melanoma cases from Spain.[79] Rodrigues and colleagues[80] conducted a retrospective cohort analysis of 17 HIV-infected patients diagnosed with melanoma and compared them to 34 randomly matched HIV-negative patients with melanoma. The HIV-negative patients were matched for melanoma subtype, tumor thickness, Clark level, sex, age, and, when possible, location of the primary tumor, but they noted that a smaller percentage of HIV-positive patients had ulcerated lesions compared to the con-

trols (12 versus 41%). HIV-positive melanoma patients had a more aggressive clinical course than HIV-negative patients. Of note, 8 of the 17 HIV-positive patients were receiving HAART at the time of diagnosis, and the median CD4 cell count at diagnosis was 422 cells/mm^3. Although there have been previous reports of melanoma thickness correlating inversely with CD4 count,[81] no such association was found in this study. However, the median disease-free survival for HIV-positive patients was significantly shorter than for matched HIV-negative controls (p = .03). Overall survival was also significantly shorter among the HIV-positive patients compared to the HIV-negative controls (2.8 versus 6.4 years, p = .045).

Ocular Surface Squamous Neoplasia

Ocular surface squamous neoplasia (OSSN) involves a spectrum of diseases ranging from mild squamous dysplasia, to moderate dysplasia, carcinoma in situ, and invasive squamous carcinoma of the cornea and conjunctiva. These are rare in most parts of the world, but the prevalence is increasing in parts of sub-Saharan Africa. Ateenyi-Agaba[82] found that the incidence of conjunctival squamous-cell carcinoma increased in Uganda from 6 per million from 1970–1988 to 35 per million in 1992. In addition, 36 of 48 (75%) patients diagnosed at the New Mulago Hospital from 1990 to 1991 were HIV positive, compared to 19% of matched controls without conjunctival squamous cancer. They concluded that the increase seen in squamous cell carcinoma in Uganda and neighboring countries was related to the HIV epidemic and proposed that other factors, including conjunctival papillomavirus infection and exposure to ultraviolet light, might also contribute to the high incidence of these tumors in Africa.[82] Poole[83] also found a sharp increase in incidence rates of squamous conjunctival cancers in Tanzania between 1995 and 1997 and reported that the disease course of these cancers was relatively aggressive.

Multiple other studies have also noted that the odds ratio (OR) for HIV infection among patients presenting with SCC or carcinoma in situ of the conjunctiva was significantly higher than in patients without SCC or carcinoma in situ of the conjunctiva.[84–86] Newton and colleagues[85] reported an OR of

10.1 (95% CI, 5.2–19.4) for HIV infection in patients with conjunctival carcinoma in Uganda compared to patients presenting with other types of cancers. Waddell and colleagues[86] reported an OR of 13.1 for HIV-infected patients with OSSN in Uganda. They also reported that the percentage of OSSN attributable to HIV infection in Malawi from 1993 to 1994 was 86% of tested patients. Mahomed and colleagues[87] reported on 41 OSSN lesions in 40 black South African patients. Twelve of 17 (70.6%) patients who agreed to HIV testing were found to be HIV positive. All 12 patients were under 50 years of age.[87]

HPV may play a role in the development of squamous cell cancer of the conjunctiva. Recent studies in both HIV-positive and HIV-status unknown specimens have reported inconsistent results. Among HIV status–unknown specimens, Scott and colleagues[88] found either HPV 16 or HPV 18 E6 sequences by PCR in 20 to 40% of tumor specimens from 10 consecutive patients with conjunctival intraepithelial neoplasia (CIN), but no HPV E6 sequence in conjunctival specimens without CIN. However, Eng and colleagues[89] did not find HPV sequences by PCR in any of 20 conjunctival tumor samples from HIV-status unknown patients in Taiwan. Similarly, Newton and colleagues[85] found that patients with SCC of the conjunctiva were no different from control subjects with respect to HPV antibody detection from the serum. However, HPV antibody screening may not be sufficiently sensitive to detect active HPV infection in tumor tissue. These authors did find a positive correlation between a "cultivating" occupation (and therefore increased exposure to direct sunlight) and SCC of the conjunctiva.[85,90]

Treatment for OSSN has traditionally been mainly surgical. Recurrence rates after surgery have been reported to range from 15 to 52%.[91–93] Therefore, adjuvant therapies, including cryotherapy, radiotherapy, and topical chemotherapies, are commonly employed.[91,94] Topical Mitomycin C and 5-FU have been shown in several studies to decrease the recurrence rate after surgical excision.[91,95,96] No studies specifically evaluating treatment in HIV-infected patients have been conducted; however, there is no evidence that HIV-infected patients should receive anything other than standard therapy.

Testicular Cancer

Testicular cancer in HIV-infected individuals remains relatively rare, and the number of cases in many studies is small. Although several large HIV-cancer match registry studies from the United States, Australia, and Europe found no association between HIV and testicular cancer,[2,8,21] several other large cohort and AIDS/cancer linkage studies have shown a significantly increased risk of germ cell tumors (GCT) in HIV-infected men. The Multicenter AIDS Cohort Study found that the SIR for GCTs was 3.9 in HIV-positive men compared to an HIV-seronegative population of men who have sex with men.[97] Frisch and colleagues,[4] using the national AIDS-cancer-linked registries, showed that the relative risk (RR) of seminoma, but not nonseminomatous GCT (NSGCT), was increased among HIV-positive men (see Table 19–1). Gallagher and colleagues,[18] using the New York State AIDS/cancer-linked registry, found the SIR of testicular cancer was 1.5 (1.05–2.03) among HIV-positive individuals compared with the general population. Finally, in a large English cohort study, Powles and colleagues[98] showed that HIV-positive men had a significantly elevated RR of GCT (RR = 4.36) and seminoma (RR = 5.45) compared to age- and sex-matched controls in the general southeast England population. However, they did not find an increased RR for NSGCT.[98] It has been previously shown that lack of tumor infiltrating lymphocytes predicts relapse in patients with stage I seminoma who are treated by orchiectomy and surveillance.[99] Therefore, Powles and colleagues[98] hypothesized that chronic immunosuppression may contribute to the increased risk of seminoma seen in HIV-positive men. In addition, using the AIDS/cancer-linked database, Frisch and colleagues[4] found that testicular seminoma met the criteria for a malignancy associated with immunosuppression based on their specific criteria.

Although many HIV-related malignancies are associated with a virus infection, no definitive viral links have been found for HIV-associated GCT. There have been several viral infections implicated in the etiology of GCT, including mumps orchitis,[100] EBV,[101–103] HPV,[104] parvovirus B19,[105] and retrovirus K10 (HERV-K10).[106] However, none of these entities have been specifically associated with GCT and HIV infection. Goedert and colleagues[107] found that the seroprevalence of HERV-K10 is low in HIV-positive patients, and the seroprevalence rates among HIV-positive and HIV-negative patients with GCT are similar.

Several recent studies have evaluated treatment outcomes of HIV-infected men with GCT. Three of the largest series reported cases in the pre-HAART era from 1983 to 1996. Between 15 and 66% of the cases had AIDS prior to the GCT diagnosis, and between 0 and 20% died from GCT, whereas 20 to 40% died of HIV. The overall 2-year survival was between 62 and 74%.[108–110] However, a more recent study reported by Powles and colleagues[98] included cases from the post-HAART era. They reported on 35 cases of HIV-related GCT and found the median age at time of GCT diagnosis was 34 years. The median CD4 count was 315 cells/mm^3. Seventy-four percent were seminoma and 26% were NSGCT. Only 11% had AIDS prior to the diagnosis of GCT, and 60% had stage I disease. Eleven percent had relapse of GCT, 8% died from GCT and the overall 2-year survival was 81%.[98] The authors also conducted a case-control study to compare the outcomes of these HIV-infected patients with HIV-negative age- and stage-matched controls.[111] The distributions of International Germ Cell Consensus Collaboration prognostic class groups were similar in the HIV-positive and HIV-negative patients. The relapse-free survival was similar between the HIV-positive cases and controls ($p = .78$). However, overall survival was significantly decreased among the HIV-positive cases ($p = .03$). They found that HIV was responsible for 70% of the mortality, and overall survival of HIV-positive patients in the pre-HAART era was significantly worse than in the controls. In addition, they reported that HIV-positive patients with stage I GCT treated with orchiectomy and surveillance were not at higher risk of relapse than HIV-negative controls. They commented that intravenous drug users or patients at risk for poor compliance with follow-up visits should be encouraged to have some form of adjuvant treatment to reduce the risk of relapse. The authors concluded that HIV-positive patients with GCT tolerated standard treatments well and that HIV-positive GCT patients should be treated in a similar fashion to HIV-negative patients.[111]

Leiomyosarcoma

Although leiomyosarcoma is an extremely rare smooth muscle tumor in children that occurs at a rate of 1 case per million, the incidence in HIV-positive children has been reported to be approximately 1 case per 5,000 children.[112–114] Pollock and colleagues[115] reported data from the Pediatric Oncology Group, showing that after lymphoid malignancies, leiomyosarcomas are the second most common malignancy in HIV-positive children. In this study, leiomyosarcoma accounted for 8% of all tumors in HIV-positive children.[115] Biggar and colleagues[116] used AIDS/cancer registry–matched data to evaluate cancer incidence in HIV-positive children 14 years of age or younger. They reported that the relative risk of leiomyosarcoma during the time period 2 to 5 years after AIDS onset was 1,915 (232–6,915).[116] Granovsky and colleagues[117] conducted a retrospective evaluation of cancer cases in HIV-positive children collected from the Children's Cancer Group and the National Cancer Institute. They found that leiomyomas or leiomyosarcomas accounted for 17% of tumors in HIV-infected children.[117]

Unlike leiomyosarcomas in immunocompetent individuals, EBV may play an etiologic role in HIV-associated cases. EBV is detected by in situ hybridization and polymerase chain reaction in virtually all leiomyosarcomas associated with HIV.[114,115,118,119] In addition, leiomyosarcomas have been reported in uncommon locations, including the spleen, pleural space, adrenal glands, lung, orbit, and iris.[120,121] Although the prevalence of EBV-related smooth muscles tumors and leiomyosarcomas is not as high in HIV-infected adults, several cases in adults have been reported in the literature,[122–124] and adults may also be at higher risk for these tumors.

Whereas leiomyomas in HIV-infected children are usually indolent in nature, most leiomyosarcoma cases in HIV-infected children behave in an aggressive fashion. Granovsky and colleagues[117] reported that the median survival after diagnosis was 12 months. In addition, smooth muscle tumors in children are generally resistant to chemotherapy.[125]

Therefore, radiation therapy and local excision should be first-line therapy in these children.

Hepatocellular Carcinoma

Coinfection with HIV and hepatitis viruses is common because of their shared routes of transmission.[126] Although hepatitis B virus (HBV) is considered to be the most common cause of hepatocellular carcinoma (HCC) worldwide, hepatitis C virus (HCV) appears to be the predominant risk factor for HCC in developed countries. The immunodeficiency associated with HIV infection seems to accelerate the course of chronic HCV infection and leads to earlier onset of cirrhosis.[127] Three of the AIDS/cancer-linked studies found a significantly higher risk of liver cancer among AIDS patients. Gallagher and colleagues[18] reported that the SIR of liver cancer among AIDS patients was 5.1 times that of the general population. Frisch and colleagues[4] reported that the relative risk of liver cancer during the period before AIDS diagnosis was 7-fold greater, and during the early post-AIDS period, there was a 3.3-fold greater risk than in the general population. However, they did not find an increase in observed risk with increased length of time since HIV infection. Finally, Allardice and colleagues[19] reported that the SIR was 22 for liver cancer among HIV-infected patients compared to the general population. Garcia-Samaniego and colleagues[128] reported on a series of 7 HIV-infected patients with HCC. They compared the HIV-infected group with a total of 31 consecutive non–HIV-infected patients with HCV-related HCC and found that the HIV-infected patients were significantly younger (median age 42.2) compared to the control group (median age 68.9), and the duration of HCV infection was significantly shorter in the HCV/HIV-co-infected group (17.8 years) compared to the control group (28.1 years). As HIV-infected people live longer, the association between HCC and HIV/HCV coinfection may continue to increase. Thus, efforts to aggressively treat HCV in HCV/HIV-coinfected patients should be pursued.

Breast Cancer

Among women, breast carcinoma is the most common neoplasm in developed countries. However, multiple cohort studies and AIDS/cancer-linked studies show no increase in the risk of breast cancer among HIV-positive women compared to the general population.[2,4,18,129] In particular, Gallagher and colleagues,[18] Frisch and colleagues,[4] and Herida and colleagues[20] found that the risk of breast cancer is significantly lower in HIV-positive women than in the general population. Although, Herida and colleagues[20] found that the risk of breast cancer in a cohort of HIV-positive women was significantly lower than the general female population in both the pre-HAART and HAART eras, they hypothesized that this may have been due to under-reporting of breast cancer cases in their registries. Yet, Frisch and colleagues[4] found that the risk of breast cancer among HIV-positive women using the AIDS/cancer registry was significantly lower in the early AIDS period (4–27 months after AIDS diagnosis), and Gallagher and colleagues[18] also found a significantly lower risk of breast cancer in their registry, despite relatively complete cancer registry data for both studies. Recent data from the Women's Interagency HIV Study (WIHS) also found a deficit in the expected number of breast cancer cases in their cohort of 2,058 women.[130] Potential explanations for the deficit of breast cancer cases in HIV-positive women in industrialized countries may be related to other variables attributed to the study cohort that may protect against breast cancer. These include early age at first childbirth, high parity, and lower social economic class.[130] In addition, certain authors have raised the possibility that immunosuppression may protect against developing breast cancer.[131] Finally, in Africa, Makwaya and colleagues[132] performed a retrospective comparison of HIV infection rates in women with breast cancer and those without. They found that women younger than 50 years of age with breast cancer were significantly less likely to be HIV positive than women in the general population (OR 0.18, $p = .01$).

Several reviews have summarized multiple case reports of breast cancer cases in HIV-positive women.[133,134] These reviews suggested that breast cancer in the setting of HIV infection tended to occur at a relatively early age and was more likely to present with bilateral disease and to show unusual histologies, such as poorly differentiated or mixed tumors. They also reported frequent early metastatic spread with a poor outcome.[133] In addition, two case series have evaluated the natural history of breast cancer in HIV-positive women. Voutsadakis and Silverman[134] reported on 4 cases of breast cancer in HIV-positive women. The women presented with breast cancer at a young age and generally had aggressive disease. However, Hurley and colleagues[135] evaluated 20 HIV-positive women with breast cancer. They found that the natural history of breast cancer in HIV-positive women is similar to that in HIV-negative women of the same age range and stage. Of the 20 patients, 18 presented with local disease, 9 of whom were still alive (5 were alive > 5 years), and 7 had died (4 from complications of AIDS). The authors noted that the seven patients who received cytotoxic chemotherapy tolerated treatment poorly.[135]

It is difficult to draw conclusions from these small case series. In general, breast cancers occurring in women younger than 40 years of age and in African American women appear to have more aggressive courses.[136,137] Regardless of the influence of HIV on the incidence or natural history of breast cancer, the survival improvement associated with wide-spread HAART is likely to be associated with an increase in the incidence of women affected by both diseases. Further information is needed to evaluate the effect of HIV-related immunosuppression on the risk of developing breast cancer and to develop optimal screening and treatment recommendations for HIV-positive women.

Multiple Myeloma

Multiple myeloma is a malignancy of post-germinal center B cells. The disease is characterized by infiltration and uncontrolled proliferation of malignant plasma cells in the bone marrow.[138] These cells produce monoclonal immunoglobulin, usually IgG or IgA, and are believed to develop from clonal, transformed lymphocytic precursors that are antigen-independent. These cells may then be stimulated to differentiate into plasma cells. Although the most common hematologic AIDS-related malignancy is high-grade non-Hodgkin's lymphoma, HIV-infected individuals also appear to be at higher risk for plasma cell malignancies.[2,4,18] Gallagher and colleagues,[18] Frisch and colleagues,[4] and Grulich and colleagues[2] each found an increased risk of multiple myeloma in their respective AIDS-cancer match registry studies (see Table 19–1). In addition, plasmablastic lymphoma has been recently recognized more frequently in HIV-infected individuals.[139]

Paraproteinemias have been commonly shown in patients with HIV infection. Several studies have reported monoclonal or oligoclonal serum protein electrophoresis spikes in 3.2%,[140] 12%,[141] 26%,[142] and up to 56%[143] of HIV-positive patients compared with 0.15% of the general population.[144] In a longitudinal study of the general population, 24% of patients with monoclonal gammopathy of unknown significance developed plasma cell malignancy within 10 years of diagnosis.[145] Malignant transformation of clonal myeloma precursors may occur when these cells are stimulated by reconstituted T-cells, c-myc over-expression, increased levels of interleukin-6 (IL-6), and chronic antigen exposure to various infectious diseases, including EBV, HHV-8, or HIV.[144]

There are few studies that have systematically evaluated the long-term outcome of AIDS patients with gammopathy, and no studies have characterized this population in the HAART era. Lefrere and colleagues[140] evaluated HIV-positive patients with mono- and oligoclonal gammopathies with up to 69 months of follow-up. They found that several patients had only transient gammopathies; however, the size of the monoclonal spike appeared to correlate with persistence of the monoclonal spike. Although the authors did not include plasma cell neoplasms in their survey, they reported that none of the HIV-positive patients followed developed other B-cell lineage malignancies during the 2 to 4 years of study follow-up.[140,146]

Information regarding the clinical course of gammopathy, plasmacytoma, and myeloma in HIV-positive patients is limited to data from case series. In general, it appears that gammopathy, plasmacytoma and myeloma occur at earlier ages in AIDS patients. The median age at diagnosis of plasma cell disorders was 31 years among HIV-positive patients versus 64 years in the general population.[147–149] In addition, HIV-positive patients with myeloma appear to present more commonly with extramedullary disease, including serous effusions and solitary osseous plasmacytomas.[148–151] Large series documenting treatment and outcome data are currently lacking.

Leukemia

Although early cohort series of HIV-infected patients showed no increase in the risk of acute myelocytic leukemia (AML), three recent AIDS/cancer registry linkage studies found a significantly increased risk of leukemia among patients with AIDS compared to the general population (see Table 19–1).[2,4,21] However, the impact of immunosuppression on leukemogenesis in patients with HIV is unclear. Frisch and colleagues[4] found a statistically significant increase in the relative risk of leukemia in HIV-infected individuals compared with the general population, but they did not find an increased risk of leukemia with progressive immunosuppression. Several authors have hypothesized that the increased risk of leukemia associated with HIV seen in these studies may be related to secondary AML in patients who have received prior chemotherapy for KS or non-Hodgkin's lymphoma.[152] Additionally, the increased incidence of myelodysplasia documented in patients with HIV disease may further increase the risk of AML in the HIV-infected population.[153]

Two case series from the pre-HAART era described the characteristics, treatments, and outcomes of HIV-infected patients with AML. Pulick and colleagues,[154] in a review of 18 cases, found that a higher-than-expected proportion of AML from HIV-infected patients with AML were derived from the monocyte/macrophage cell lineage (M4, M5). Whereas 19 to 36% of AML cases in the general population present with M4 or M5 disease, 72% of the HIV-infected cases presented with M4 or M5 disease. They also found that the HIV-infected patients showed a higher-than-expected proportion of extramedullary presentations. The mean survival in patients who were not treated with chemotherapy was 2.7 weeks. Patients who received chemotherapy tolerated it well, and the mean survival for adequately treated patients was 9.8 months.[154] Sutton and colleagues[152] also conducted a retrospective evaluation of 18 HIV-infected patients with AML. Based on their single institution experience, they calculated the SIR for AML in the HIV-positive population at 2.05 (95% CI, 1.17–3.34). Forty-four percent of their cases presented with M4 or M5 disease. The majority of patients tolerated conventional cytotoxic chemotherapy, and 73% achieved a complete remission. However, the overall survival rate at 5 years was only 19%; and on univariate analysis, they found that a CD4 cell count below 200 cells/mm^3 and duration of HIV infection greater than 48 months at the time of AML diagnosis were correlated with shortened survival.[152] Thus far, there have been no publications describing the clinical characteristics, treatment, and outcomes of patients with AML and HIV infection in the HAART era.

Colorectal Cancer

Several common cancers do not appear to have any association with HIV infection. Colorectal cancer is the third leading cause of cancer deaths in both genders in the United States.[155] Although Cooksley and colleagues,[38] using AIDS/cancer registry linkage data from Harris County, Texas, found that the SIR for colon cancer among HIV-positive women was 4.0 (95% CI, 1.1–10.2), none of the recent AIDS/cancer linkage registry studies corroborate this finding (with the exception of those studies that were unable to separate colorectal cancers from anal cancers). There are no large series describing the characteristics, treatment, and outcomes of HIV-infected patients with colon cancer. As survival improves for HIV-infected individuals because of HAART, the number of colon cancer cases seen in this population is likely to increase. Thus, as the HIV-infected population ages, practitioners should emphasize age-appropriate cancer screening.

Prostate Cancer

In the United States, prostate cancer is the most common cancer diagnosed in men.[155] Neither the large cohort studies nor the AIDS/cancer-linked registry studies have shown an increased risk of prostate cancer in HIV-infected individuals. Additionally, Frisch and colleagues[4] found a significantly decreased RR of 0.7 (95% CI 0.6–0.9) of prostate cancer compared to the general population. There have been several case reports of prostate cancer in HIV-infected individuals published in the literature. Earlier studies suggested that patients presented with aggressive disease and had a poor outcome.[156,157] Crum and colleagues[158] reported on three cases presenting within 18 months in their clinic of 155 HIV patients. All three men were over age 40 and tolerated subsequent treatment well. They hypothesized that, with prolonged survival owing to HAART, there may be an increase of prostate cancer in older HIV-infected individuals.[158] As with colon cancer, clinicians will need to discuss age-appropriate prostate cancer screening with older HIV-infected men.

CONCLUSIONS

HAART has prolonged the survival of HIV-infected individuals and significantly changed the epidemiology of HIV-associated morbidity and mortality.[11] HAART has decreased the incidence of some AIDS-defining malignancies, including KS, non-Hodgkin's lymphoma, and primary CNS lymphomas,[159] but the influence of HAART on non–AIDS-defining malignancies is less clear. Many of the epidemiologic studies documenting elevated risks of non–AIDS-defining cancers were conducted in the pre-HAART era. In addition, HAART was introduced fewer than 10 years ago, and, therefore, studies that have attempted to compare cancer risks in the pre-HAART and post-HAART eras do not include long-term post-HAART follow-up.[20,160,161] Because chronic immunosuppression may contribute to an increased risk for non–AIDS-defining malignancies in HIV-infected individuals, it will be important to closely monitor this population for emerging epidemiologic trends.

Other HAART or HIV-related adverse effects may also have an impact on cancer risk. Metabolic abnormalities associated with HAART, such as fat redistribution from the periphery to the abdomen and breast, elevated body mass indices, undesirable serum lipid levels, and elevated waist-hip ratios, have been associated with breast cancer risk and survival.[162–164] In addition, adjunctive therapies may be associated with an increased risk for tumor growth. For example, there has been one report in the litera-

ture of a growth hormone receptor-expressing carcinoid tumor discovered in an HIV-positive patient after growth hormone was administered to treat lipodystrophy.[165] In addition, testosterone, which is commonly used to treat HIV-related hypogonadism, may stimulate prostate cancer growth.

HIV-infected individuals are at higher risk for certain non–AIDS-defining malignancies compared to the general population. Currently, there are no data to support alternative screening, evaluation, or treatment strategies for HIV-infected patients with non–AIDS-defining malignancies. The majority of case series published in the literature indicate that HIV-infected patients who are not severely immunocompromised can tolerate standard treatment regimens. Many authors advocate the use of HAART to preserve immune function during administration of chemotherapy, despite the potential for adverse drug interactions. In addition, standard prophylaxis against *Pneumocystis jiroveci* (formerly *carini*) pneumonia and hematopoietic growth factor support may prevent complications from chemotherapy.[166] Further studies to evaluate the epidemiology, natural history, and optimal treatments for HIV-associated malignancies are needed. In addition, clinicians need to emphasize the role of smoking cessation, patient education, and age-appropriate cancer screening in HIV-infected people.

REFERENCES

1. Goedert JJ, Cote TR, Virgo P, et al. Spectrum of AIDS-associated malignant disorders. Lancet 1998;351(9119):1833–9.
2. Grulich A, Wan X, Law M, et al. Risk of cancer in people with AIDS. AIDS 1999;13(7):839–43.
3. Jones JL, Hanson DL, Dworkin MS, et al. Surveillance for AIDS-defining opportunistic illnesses, 1992–1997. MMWR CDC Surveill Summ 1999;48(2):1–22.
4. Frisch M, Biggar R, Engels E, Goedert J. Association of cancer with AIDS-related immunosuppression in adults. JAMA 2001;285(13):1736–45.
5. Serraino D, Boschini A, Carrieri P, et al. Cancer risk among men with, or at risk of, HIV infection in southern Europe. AIDS 2000;14(5):553–9.
6. Mbulaiteye S, Biggar R, Goedert J, Engels E. Immune deficiency and risk for malignancy among persons with AIDS. J Acquir Immune Defic Syndr 2003;32(5):527–33.
7. Petruckevitch A, Del Amo J, Phillips A, et al. Risk of cancer in patients with HIV disease. London African HIV/AIDS Study Group. Int J STD AIDS 1999;10(1):38–42.
8. Patel P, Tong T, Behari A, et al. Incidence of non–AIDS-defining malignancies in the HIV Outpatient Study (HOPS). Proceedings of the 11th Conference on Retro-

viruses and Opportunistic Infections, 2004; San Francisco, CA.

9. Palella FJ Jr, Delaney KM, Moorman AC, et al. Declining morbidity and mortality among patients with advanced human immunodeficiency virus infection. HIV Outpatient Study Investigators. N Engl J Med 1998;338:853–60.

10. Mocroft A, Brettle R, Kirk O, et al. Changes in the cause of death among HIV positive subjects across Europe: results from the EuroSIDA study. AIDS 2002;16:1663–71.

11. Louie JK, Hsu LC, Osmond DH, et al. Trends in causes of death among persons with acquired immunodeficiency syndrome in the era of highly active antiretroviral therapy, San Francisco, 1994–1998. J Infect Dis 2002;186:1023–7.

12. Sridar S, Flores MR, Raub WA Jr, et al. Lung cancer in patients with human immunodeficiency virus infection compared with historic control subjects. Chest 1992; 102:1704–8.

13. Vyzula R. Lung cancer in patients with HIV-infection. Lung Cancer 1996;15:325–39.

14. Powles T, Thirwell C, Newsom-Davis T, et al. Does HIV adversely influence the outcome in advanced non-small–cell lung cancer in the era of HAART? Br J Cancer 2003;89:457–9.

15. Hajjar M, Lacoste D, Brossard G, et al. Non-acquired immune deficiency syndrome-defining malignancies in a hospital-based cohort of human immunodeficiency virus-infected patients: Bordeaux, France, 1985–1991. Groupe d'Epidemiologie Clinique du SIDA en Aquitaine. J Natl Cancer Inst 1992;84:1593–5.

16. Biggar RJ, Curtis RE, Cote TR, et al. Risk of other cancers following Kaposi's sarcoma: relation to acquired immunodeficiency syndrome. Am J Epidemiol 1994;139:362–8.

17. Franceschi S, Dal Maso L, Arniani S, et al. Risk of cancer other than Kaposi's sarcoma and non-Hodgkin's lymphoma in persons with AIDS in Italy. Cancer and AIDS Registry Linkage Study. Br J Cancer 1998;78:966–70.

18. Gallagher B, Zhengyan W, Schymura M, et al. Cancer incidence in new york state acquired immunodeficiency sydnrome patients. Am J Epidemiol 2001;154:544–56.

19. Allardice GM, Hole DJ, Brewster DH, et al. Incidence of malignant neoplasms among HIV-infected persons in Scotland. Br J Cancer 2003;89:505–7.

20. Herida M, Mary-Krause M, Kaphan R, et al. Incidence of non–AIDS-defining cancers before and during the highly active antiretroviral therapy era in a cohort of human immunodeficiency virus-infected patients. J Clin Oncol 2003;21:3447–53.

21. Dal Maso L, Franceschi S, Polesel J, et al. Risk of cancer in persons with AIDS in Italy, 1985–1998. Br J Cancer 2003;89:94–100.

22. Kieff E. Current perspectives on the molecular pathogenesis of virus-induced cancers in human immunodeficiency virus infection and acquired immunodeficiency syndrome. J Natl Cancer Inst Monogr 1998:7–14.

23. Knowles DM. Etiology and pathogenesis of AIDS-related non-Hodgkin's lymphoma. Hematol Oncol Clin North Am 1996;10:1081–109.

24. Jenner RG, Boshoff C. The molecular pathology of Kaposi's sarcoma-associated herpesvirus. Biochim Biophys Acta 2002;1602:1–22.

25. Wistuba II, Behrens C, Gazdar AF. Pathogenesis of non–AIDS-defining cancers: a review. AIDS Patient Care STDS 1999;13:415–26.

26. Gatignol A, Jeang KT. Tat as a transcriptional activator and a potential therapeutic target for HIV-1. Adv Pharmacol 2000;48:209–27.

27. Vene R, Benelli R, Noonan DM, Albini A. HIV-Tat dependent chemotaxis and invasion, key aspects of tat mediated pathogenesis. Clin Exp Metastasis 2000;18:533–8.

28. Frankel AD, Bredt DS, Pabo CO. Tat protein from human immunodeficiency virus forms a metal-linked dimer. Science 1988;240:70–3.

29. De Falco G, Bellan C, Lazzi S, et al. Interaction between HIV-1 Tat and pRb2/p130: a possible mechanism in the pathogenesis of AIDS-related neoplasms. Oncogene 2003;22:6214–9.

30. Altavilla G, Caputo A, Trabanelli C, et al. Prevalence of liver tumours in HIV-1 tat-transgenic mice treated with urethane. Eur J Cancer 2004;40:275–83.

31. Chipitsyna G, Slonina D, Siddiqui K, et al. HIV-1 Tat increases cell survival in response to cisplatin by stimulating Rad51 gene expression. Oncogene 2004;23:2664–71.

32. Loeb LA. Microsatellite instability: marker of a mutator phenotype in cancer. Cancer Res 1994;54:5059–63.

33. Gaidano G, Pastore C, Gloghini A, et al. Microsatellite instability in KSHV/HHV-8 positive body-cavity–based lymphoma. Hum Pathol 1997;28:748–50.

34. Bedi GC, Westra WH, Farzadegan H, et al. Microsatellite instability in primary neoplasms from HIV + patients. Nat Med 1995;1:65–8.

35. Wistuba I, Behrens C, Michgrub S. Comparison of molecular changes in lung cancers in HIV-positive and HIV-indeterminate subjects. JAMA 1998;279:1154–9.

36. Cancer facts and figures. Atlanta: American Cancer Society; 2000.

37. Parker ML. AIDS-related bronchogenic carcinoma: fact or fiction. Chest 1998;113:154–61.

38. Cooksley CD, Hwang LY, Waller DK, Ford CE. HIV-related malignancies: community-based study using linkage of cancer registry and HIV registry data. Int J STD AIDS 1999;10:795–802.

39. Engels EA. Human immunodeficiency virus infection, aging, and cancer. J Clin Epidemiol 2001;54(Suppl 1): S29–34.

40. Ricaurte JC, Hoerman MF, Nord JA, Tietjen PA. Lung cancer in HIV-infected patients: a one-year experience. Int J STD AIDS 2001;12:100–2.

41. Cailhol J, Calatroni MI, Roudiere L, et al. Increased incidence of lung neoplasms among HIV-infected men and the need for improved prevention. J Acquir Immune Defic Syndr 2003;34:247–9.

42. Bower MP, Powles T, Nelson M, et al. HIV-related lung cancer in the era of highly active antiretroviral therapy. AIDS 2003;17:371–5.

43. Dal Maso L, Polesel J, Serraino D, Franceschi S. Lung cancer in persons with AIDS in Italy, 1985–1998. AIDS 2003;17:2117–9.

44. Vaccher E, Spina M, Tirelli U. Clinical aspects and management of Hodgkin's disease and other tumours in HIV-infected individuals. Eur J Cancer 2001;37:1306–15.

45. Tirelli U, Spina M, Sandri S, et al. Lung carcinoma in 36 patients with human immunodeficiency virus infection. The Italian Cooperative Group on AIDS and Tumors. Cancer 2000;88:563–9.

46. Kosary C, Reiss L, Miller B, et al. SEER Cancer statistics review, 1973–1992: tables and graphs. Bethesda, MD: NIH publication 96-2789; 1995.

47. Bazot M, Cadranel J, Khalil A, et al. Computed tomographic diagnosis of bronchogenic carcinoma in HIV-infected patients. Lung Cancer 2000;28:203–9.

48. Burke M, Furman A, Hoffman M, et al. Lung cancer in patients with HIV infection: is it AIDS-related? HIV Med 2004;5:110–4.

49. Hoffman PC, Mauer AM, Vokes EE. Lung cancer. Lancet 2000;355:479–85.

50. Powles T, Nelson M, Bower M. HIV-related lung cancer—a growing concern? Int J STD AIDS 2003;14:647–51.

51. Remick SC. Non–AIDS-defining cancers. Hematol Oncol Clin North Am 1996;10:1203–13.

52. Alshafie MT, Donaldson B, Oluwole SF. Human immunodeficiency virus and lung cancer. Br J Surg 1997;84:1068–71.

53. Friis-Moller N, Sabin CA, Weber R, et al. Combination antiretroviral therapy and the risk of myocardial infarction. N Engl J Med 2003;349:1993–2003.

54. Diaz PT, King MA, Pacht ER, et al. Increased susceptibility to pulmonary emphysema among HIV-seropositive smokers. Ann Intern Med 2000;132:369–72.

55. Powles T, Powles J, Nelson M, et al. Head and neck cancer in patients with human immunodeficiency virus-1 infection: incidence, outcome and association with Epstein-Barr virus. J Laryngol Otol 2004;118:207–12.

56. Almadori G, Galli J, Cadoni G, et al. Human papillomavirus infection and cyclin D1 gene amplification in laryngeal squamous cell carcinoma: biologic function and clinical significance. Head Neck 2002;24:597–604.

57. Gillison ML, Shah KV. Human papillomavirus-associated head and neck squamous cell carcinoma: mounting evidence for an etiologic role for human papillomavirus in a subset of head and neck cancers. Curr Opin Oncol 2001;13:183–8.

58. Gillison ML, Koch WM, Capone RB, et al. Evidence for a causal association between human papillomavirus and a subset of head and neck cancers. J Natl Cancer Inst 2000;92:709–20.

59. Rosenberg PS, Greene MH, Alter BP. Cancer incidence in persons with Fanconi anemia. Blood 2003;101:822–6.

60. Kutler DI, Auerbach AD, Satagopan J, et al. High incidence of head and neck squamous cell carcinoma in patients with Fanconi anemia. Arch Otolaryngol Head Neck Surg 2003;129:106–12.

61. Kutler DI, Wreesmann VB, Goberdhan A, et al. Human papillomavirus DNA and p53 polymorphisms in squamous cell carcinomas from Fanconi anemia patients. J Natl Cancer Inst 2003;95:1718–21.

62. Hafkamp HC, Speel EJ, Haesevoets A, et al. A subset of head and neck squamous cell carcinomas exhibits integration of HPV 16/18 DNA and overexpression of p16INK4A and p53 in the absence of mutations in p53 exons 5-8. Int J Cancer 2003;107:394–400.

63. Klussmann JP, Gultekin E, Weissenborn SJ, et al. Expression of p16 protein identifies a distinct entity of tonsillar carcinomas associated with human papillomavirus. Am J Pathol 2003;162:747–53.

64. Fregonesi PA, Teresa DB, Duarte RA, et al. p16(INK4A) immunohistochemical overexpression in premalignant and malignant oral lesions infected with human papillomavirus. J Histochem Cytochem 2003;51:1291–7.

65. Begum S, Gillison ML, Ansari-Lari MA, et al. Detection of human papillomavirus in cervical lymph nodes: a highly effective strategy for localizing site of tumor origin. Clin Cancer Res 2003;9:6469–75.

66. Frisch M, Hjalgrim H, Jaeger AB, Biggar RJ. Changing patterns of tonsillar squamous cell carcinoma in the United States. Cancer Causes Control 2000;11:489–95.

67. Kreimer AR, Alberg AJ, Daniel R, et al. Oral human papillomavirus infection in adults is associated with sexual behavior and HIV serostatus. J Infect Dis 2004;189:686–98.

68. Roland JT Jr, Rothstein SG, Mittal KR, Perksy MS. Squamous cell carcinoma in HIV-positive patients under age 45. Laryngoscope 1993;103:509–11.

69. Singh B, Balwally AN, Shaha AR, et al. Upper aerodigestive tract squamous cell carcinoma. The human immunodeficiency virus connection. Arch Otolaryngol Head Neck Surg 1996;122:639–43.

70. Singh B, Sabin S, Rofim O, Shaha A, Har-El G, Lucente FE. Alterations in head and neck cancer occurring in HIV-infected patients—results of a pilot, longitudinal, prospective study. Acta Oncol 1999;38:1047–50.

71. Kao GD, Devine P, Mirza N. Oral cavity and oropharyngeal tumors in human immunodeficiency virus-positive patients: acute response to radiation therapy. Arch Otolaryngol Head Neck Surg 1999;125:873–6.

72. Lobo DV, Chu P, Grekin RC, Berger TG. Nonmelanoma skin cancers and infection with the human immunodeficiency virus. Arch Dermatol 1992;128:623–7.

73. Nguyen P, Vin-Christian K, Ming M. Aggressive squamous cell carcinomas in persons infected with the human immunodeficiency virus. Arch Dermatol 2002;138:758–63.

74. Harwood CA, McGregor JM, Proby CM, Breuer J. Human papillomavirus and the development of non-melanoma skin cancer. J Clin Pathol 1999;52:249–53.

75. Maurer TA, Christian KV, Kerschmann RL, et al. Cutaneous squamous cell carcinoma in human immunodeficiency virus-infected patients. A study of epidemiologic risk factors, human papillomavirus, and p53 expression. Arch Dermatol 1997;133:577–83.

76. McGregor JM, Newell M, Ross J, et al. Cutaneous malignant melanoma and human immunodeficiency virus (HIV) infection: a report of three cases. Br J Dermatol 1992;126:516–9.

77. Aboulafia D. Malignant melanoma in an HIV-infected man: a case report and literature review. Cancer Invest 1998;16:217–24.

78. Calista D. Five cases of melanoma in HIV positive patients. Eur J Dermatol 2001;11:446–9.

79. Ocana-Riola R, Martinez-Garcia C, Serrano S, et al. Population-based study of cutaneous malignant melanoma in the Granada province (Spain), 1985–1992. Eur J Epidemiol 2001;17:169–74.

80. Rodrigues L, Klencke B, Vin-Christian K. Altered clinical course of malignant melanoma in HIV-positive patients. Arch Dermatol 2002;138:765–70.

81. Tindall B, Finlayson R, Mutimer K, et al. Malignant melanoma associated with human immunodeficiency virus infection in three homosexual men. J Am Acad Dermatol 1989;20:587–91.

82. Ateenyi-Agaba C. Conjunctival squamous-cell carcinoma associated with HIV infection in Kampala, Uganda. Lancet 1995;345:695–6.

83. Poole TR. Conjunctival squamous cell carcinoma in Tanzania. Br J Ophthalmol 1999;83:177–9.

84. Porges Y, Groisman GM. Prevalence of HIV with conjunctival squamous cell neoplasia in an African provincial hospital. Cornea 2003;22:1–4.

85. Newton R, Ziegler J, Ateenyi-Agaba C, et al. The epidemiology of conjunctival squamous cell carcinoma in Uganda. Br J Cancer 2002;87:301–8.

86. Waddell KM, Lewallen S, Lucas SB, et al. Carcinoma of the conjunctiva and HIV infection in Uganda and Malawi. Br J Ophthalmol 1996;80:503–8.

87. Mahomed A, Chetty R. Human immunodeficiency virus infection, Bcl-2, p53 protein, and Ki-67 analysis in ocular surface squamous neoplasia. Arch Ophthalmol 2002;120:554–8.

88. Scott IU, Karp CL, Nuovo GJ. Human papillomavirus 16 and 18 expression in conjunctival intraepithelial neoplasia. Ophthalmology 2002;109:542–7.

89. Eng HL, Lin TM, Chen SY, et al. Failure to detect human papillomavirus DNA in malignant epithelial neoplasms of conjunctiva by polymerase chain reaction. Am J Clin Pathol 2002;117:429–36.

90. Newton R, Ferlay J, Reeves G, et al. Effect of ambient solar ultraviolet radiation on incidence of squamous-cell carcinoma of the eye. Lancet 1996;347:1450–1.

91. Basti S, Macsai MS. Ocular surface squamous neoplasia: a review. Cornea 2003;22:687–704.

92. Erie JC, Campbell RJ, Liesegang TJ. Conjunctival and corneal intraepithelial and invasive neoplasia. Ophthalmology 1986;93:176–83.

93. Lee GA, Hirst LW. Ocular surface squamous neoplasia. Surv Ophthalmol 1995;39:429–50.

94. Fraunfelder FT, Wingfield D. Management of intraepithelial conjunctival tumors and squamous cell carcinomas. Am J Ophthalmol 1983;95:359–63.

95. Yeatts RP, Engelbrecht NE, Curry CD, et al. 5-Fluorouracil for the treatment of intraepithelial neoplasia of the conjunctiva and cornea. Ophthalmology 2000;107:2190–5.

96. Chen C, Louis D, Dodd T, Muecke J. Mitomycin C as an adjunct in the treatment of localised ocular surface squamous neoplasia. Br J Ophthalmol 2004;88:17–8.

97. Lyter D, Bryant J, Thackeray R, et al. Incidence of human immunodeficiency virus-related and nonrelated malignancies in a large cohort of homosexual men. J Clin Oncol 1995;13:2540–6.

98. Powles T, Bower M, Daugaard G, et al. Multicenter study of human immunodeficiency virus-related germ cell tumors. J Clin Oncol 2003;21:1922–7.

99. Parker C, Milosevic M, Panzarella T, et al. The prognostic significance of the tumour infiltrating lymphocyte count

100. Kaufman J, Bruce P. Testicular atrophy following mumps. A cause of testis tumour? BJU Int 1963;35:67–9.

101. Fend F, Hittmair A, Rogatsch H, et al. Seminomas positive for Epstein-Barr virus by the polymerase chain reaction: viral RNA transcripts (Epstein-Barr–encoded small RNAs) are present in intratumoral lymphocytes but absent from the neoplastic cells. Mod Pathol 1995;8:622–5.

102. Shimakage M, Oka T, Shinka T, et al. Involvement of Epstein-Barr virus expression in testicular tumors. J Urol 1996;156:253–7.

103. Akre O, Lipworth L, Tretli S, et al. Epstein-Barr virus and cytomegalovirus in relation to testicular-cancer risk: a nested case-control study. Int J Cancer 1999;82:1–5.

104. Rajpert-De Meyts E, Hording U, Nielsen HW, Skakkebaek NE. Human papillomavirus and Epstein-Barr virus in the etiology of testicular germ cell tumours. APMIS 1994;102:38–42.

105. Diss TC, Pan LX, Du MQ, et al. Parvovirus B19 is associated with benign testes as well as testicular germ cell tumours. Mol Pathol 1999;52:349–52.

106. Sauter M, Schommer S, Kremmer E, et al. Human endogenous retrovirus K10: expression of Gag protein and detection of antibodies in patients with seminomas. J Virol 1995;69:414–21.

107. Goedert J, Sauter M, Jacobson L. High prevalence of antibodies against HERV-K10 in patients with testicular cancer but not with AIDS. Cancer Epidemiol Biomarkders Prev 1999;8:293 6.

108. Fizazi K, Amato R, Beuzeboc P. Germ cell tumors in patients infected by the human immunodeficiency virus. Cancer 2001;92:1460–7.

109. Timmerman JM, Northfelt DW, Small EJ. Malignant germ cell tumors in men infected with the human immunodeficiency virus: natural history and results of therapy. J Clin Oncol 1995;13:1391–7.

110. Bernardi D, Salvioni R, Vaccher E, et al. Testicular germ cell tumors and human immunodeficiency virus infection: a report of 26 cases. Italian Cooperative Group on AIDS and Tumors. J Clin Oncol 1995;13:2705–11.

111. Powles T, Bower M, Shamash J, et al. Outcome of patients with HIV-related germ cell tumours: a case-control study. Br J Cancer 2004;90:1526–30.

112. Chadwick E, et al. Tumors of smooth muscle origin in HIV-infected children. JAMA 1990;263:3182–4.

113. Levin T, Adam H, van Hoeven K, et al. Hepatic spindle cell tumors in HIV positive children. Pediatr Radiol 1994;24:78–9.

114. McCain L, Leach C, Jenson H, et al. Association of Epstein-Barr virus with leiomyosarcomas in children with AIDS. N Engl J Med 1995;332:12–8.

115. Pollock BH, Jenson HB, Leach CT, et al. Risk factors for pediatric human immunodeficiency virus-related malignancy. JAMA 2003;289:2393–9.

116. Biggar RJ, Frisch M, Goedert JJ. Risk of cancer in children with AIDS. AIDS-Cancer Match Registry Study Group. JAMA 2000;284:205–9.

117. Granovsky MO, Mueller BU, Nicholson HS, et al. Cancer in human immunodeficiency virus-infected children: a case

series from the Children's Cancer Group and the National Cancer Institute. J Clin Oncol 1998;16:1729–35.

118. Jenson H, Leach C, McClain K, et al. Benign and malignant smooth muscle tumors containing Epstein-Barr virus in children with AIDS. Leuk Lympoma 1997b;27:303–14.

119. Jenson H, Montalvo E, McClain K, et al. Characterization of natural Epstein-Barr virus infection and replication in smooth muscle cells from a leiomyosarcoma. J Med Viral 1999;57:36–46.

120. Mueller B. Cancers in children infected with the human immunodeficiency virus. Oncologist 1999;4:309–17.

121. Tulvatana W, Pancharoen C, Mekmullica J, et al. Epstein-Barr virus-associated leiomyosarcoma of the iris in a child infected with human immunodeficiency virus. Arch Ophthalmol 2003;121:1478–81.

122. Zetler PJ, Filipenko JD, Bilbey JH, Schmidt N. Primary adrenal leiomyosarcoma in a man with acquired immunodeficiency syndrome (AIDS). Further evidence for an increase in smooth muscle tumors related to Epstein-Barr infection in AIDS. Arch Pathol Lab Med 1995;119:1164–7.

123. Bluhm JM, Yi ES, Diaz G, et al. Multicentric endobronchial smooth muscle tumors associated with the Epstein-Barr virus in an adult patient with the acquired immunodeficiency syndrome: a case report. Cancer 1997;80:1910–3.

124. Brown HG, Burger PC, Olivi A, et al. Intracranial leiomyosarcoma in a patient with AIDS. Neuroradiology 1999;41:35–9.

125. Miser J, Triche T, Kinsella T, et al. Other soft tissue sarcomas of childhood. In: Pizzo A, Poplack D, editors. Principles and practice of pediatric oncology. Philadelphia: Lippincott-Raven; 1997. p. 865–88.

126. Thomas DL, Vlahov D, Solomon L, et al. Correlates of hepatitis C virus infections among injection drug users. Medicine 1995;74:212–20.

127. Sanchez-Quijano A, Andreu J, Gavilan F, et al. Influence of human immunodeficiency virus type 1 infection on the natural course of chronic parenterally acquired hepatitis C. Eur J Clin Microbiol Infect Dis 1995;14:949–53.

128. Garcia-Samaniego J, Rodriguez M, Berenguer J, et al. Hepatocellular carcinoma in HIV-infected patients with chronic hepatitis C. Am J Gastroenterol 2001;96:179–83.

129. Spano JP, Atlan D, Breau JL, Farge D. AIDS and non–AIDS-related malignancies: a new vexing challenge in HIV-positive patients. Part II. Cervical and anal squamous epithelial lesions, lung cancer, testicular germ cell cancers, and skin cancers. Eur J Intern Med 2002;13:227–32.

130. Preston-Martin S, Seaberg J, Orenstein J, et al. Breast cancer among HIV-infected women: Findings from the Women's Interagency HIV Study (WIHS). Proceedings of the 7th International Conference on Malignancies in AIDS and other Immunodeficiencies, 2003 Apr 28–29; Bethesda, Maryland.

131. Pantanowitz L, Dezube BJ. Reasons for a deficit of breast cancer among HIV-infected patients. J Clin Oncol 2004;22:1347–50.

132. Makwaya A, Mbonde M, Schwartz-Albiez R. Breast cancer during the HIV epidemic in an African population. Oncol Rep 2001;8:659–61.

133. Pantanowitz L, Connolly JL. Pathology of the breast associated with HIV/AIDS. Breast J 2002;8:234–43.

134. Voutsadakis I, Silverman L. Breast cancer in HIV-positive women: a report of four cases and review of the literature. Cancer Invest 2002;20:452–7.

135. Hurley J, Franco S, Gomez-Fernandez C. Breast cancer and human immunodeficiency virus: a report of 20 cases. Clin Breast Cancer 2001;Oct:215–20.

136. Chung M, Chang J, Bland K, et al. Younger women with breast cancer have a poorer prognosis than older women. Cancer 1996;77:97–103.

137. Lannin DR, Mathews HF, Mitchell J, Swanson MS. Impacting cultural attitudes in African-American women to decrease breast cancer mortality. Am J Surg 2002;184:418–23.

138. Bataille R, Harousseau JL. Multiple myeloma. N Engl J Med 1997;336:1657–64.

139. Delecluse HJ, Anagnostopoulos I, Dallenbach F, et al. Plasmablastic lymphomas of the oral cavity: a new entity associated with the human immunodeficiency virus infection. Blood 1997;89:1413–20.

140. Lefrere J, Debbia M, Lambin P. Prospective follow-up of monoclonal gammopathies in HIV-infected individuals. Br J Haematol 1993;84:151–5.

141. Crapper R, Deam D, Mackay I. Paraproteinemias in homosexual men with HIV infection. Am J Clin Pathol 1987;88:348–51.

142. Sala P, Mazzolini S, Tonutti E, et al. Monoclonal immunoglobulins in HTLV 3 positive sera. Clin Chem 1986;32:574.

143. Heriot K, Hallquist A, Tomar R. Paraproteinemia in patients with acquired immunodeficiency syndrome (AIDS) or lymphadenopathy syndroms (LAS). Clin Chem 1985;31:1224–6.

144. Fiorino A, Atac B. Parapoteinemia, plasmacytoma, myeloma and HIV infection. Leukemia 1997;11:2150–6.

145. Kyle R. Monoclonal gammopathy of undetermined significance. Blood Rev 1994;8:135–141.

146. Lefrere JJ, Fine JM, Marneux M, et al. Follow-up of monoclonal gammopathies in asymptomatic HIV-infected subjects. Clin Chem 1989;35:338–9.

147. Fine J, Lambin P, Derycke C. Systematic survey of monoclonal gammopathies in the sera from blood donors. Transfusion 1979;19:332–5.

148. Kumar S, Kumar D, Schnadig V. Plasma cell myeloma in patients who are HIV-positive. Am J Clin Pathol 1994;102:633–9.

149. Lallemand F, Fritsch L, Cywiner-Golenzer C, et al. Multiple myeloma in an HIV-positive man presenting with primary cutaneous plasmcytomas and spinal cord compression. J Am Acad Derm 1998;39:506–7.

150. Trubowitz P, Gates A, Kaplan L. Non–AIDS-defining malignancies. Cancer Treat Res 2001;104:303–28.

151. Gold J, Schwam L, Castella A. Malignant plasma cell tumors in human immunodeficiency virus-infected patients. Cancer 1990;66:363–8.

152. Sutton L, Guenel P, Tanguy M. Acute myeloid leukaemia in human immunodeficiency virus-infected adults: epidmeiology, treatment feasibility and outcome. Br J Haem 2001;112:900–8.

153. Schneider D, Picker L. Myelodysplasia in the acquired immune deficiency syndrome. Am J Clin Pathol 1985;84:144–52.

154. Pulik M, Genet P, Jary L. Acute myeloid leukemias, multiple myelomas, and chronic leukemias in the setting of HIV infection. AIDS Patient Care STDs 1998;12:913–9.

155. Jemal A, Thomas A, Murray T, Thun M. Cancer statistics, 2002. CA Cancer J Clin 2002;52:23–47.

156. Kwan DJ, Lowe FC. Genitourinary manifestations of the acquired immunodeficiency syndrome. Urology 1995;45: 13–27.

157. Roach PJ, Fleming C, Hagen MD, Pauker SG. Prostatic cancer in a patient with asymptomatic HIV infection: are some lives more equal than others? Med Decis Making 1988;8:132–44.

158. Crum NF, Hale B, Utz G, Wallace M. Increased risk of prostate cancer in HIV infection? AIDS 2002;16:1703–4.

159. Eltom MA, Jemal A, Mbulaiteye SM, et al. Trends in Kaposi's sarcoma and non-Hodgkin's lymphoma incidence in the United States from 1973 through 1998. J Natl Cancer Inst 2002;94:1204–10.

160. Seaberg E, Kingsley, L, et al. The impact of HAART on cancer incidence in the Multicenter AIDS Cohort Study (MACS). Proceedings of the XIV International AIDS Conference, Barcelona, Spain. Jul 7–12, 2002.

161. McGinnis K, Skanderson M, Justice A. Pre and post HAART cancer incidence among HIV positive veterans. Proceedings of the XIV International AIDS Conference, Barcelona, Spain. Jul 7–12, 2002;

162. Agurs-Collins T, Kim KS, Dunston GM, Adams-Campbell LL. Plasma lipid alterations in African-American women with breast cancer. J Cancer Res Clin Oncol 1998; 124:186–90.

163. Schreier LE, Berg GA, Basilio FM, et al. Lipoprotein alterations, abdominal fat distribution and breast cancer. Biochem Mol Biol Int 1999;47:681–90.

164. Goodwin PJ, Boyd NF, Hanna W, et al. Elevated levels of plasma triglycerides are associated with histologically defined premenopausal breast cancer risk. Nutr Cancer 1997;27:284–92.

165. Pantanowitz L, Garcia-Caballero T, Dezube BJ. Growth hormone receptor (GH)-expressing carcinoid tumors after recombinant human GH therapy for human immunodeficiency virus-related lipodystrophy. Clin Infect Dis 2003; 36:370–2.

166. Berretta M, Cinelli R, Martellotta F, et al. Therapeutic approaches to AIDS-related malignancies. Oncogene 2003;22:6646–659.

20

Anemia in HIV Infection

CAROLINE BEHLER
PATRICIA CORNETT

Anemia is the most common hematologic abnormality in human immunodeficiency virus (HIV) infection and acquired immune deficiency syndrome (AIDS), and its prevalence and severity increase with progression of HIV disease. Estimates of prevalence range from 63 to 95%, depending on the definition of anemia used and HIV severity of the population studied.[1–5] Although use of combination anti-retroviral therapy has resulted in increased survival in HIV-infected individuals and is associated with lower risk of anemia,[4–6] anemia remains a common problem even for HIV-infected individuals successfully treated with antiretroviral agents. Not only is anemia associated with fatigue and decreased quality of life[7,8] but also it is also independently associated with decreased survival in HIV-infected individuals.[3,6,9–11] Some studies have demonstrated improvements in fatigue and quality of life in HIV-infected individuals treated for anemia.[12–14] Thus, anemia is an important comorbidity to address in individuals living with HIV infection.

ETIOLOGY

The differential diagnosis of anemia in HIV-infected individuals is broad and, in many cases, multifactorial. Table 20–1 outlines causes of anemia specific to HIV infection by mechanism: decreased production, increased destruction, increased loss, and sequestration of red blood cells.

DECREASED PRODUCTION

Decreased production of mature erythrocytes occurs through two major mechanisms. First, bone marrow suppression may occur owing to architectural distortion, cytokine effects, or drug-mediated inhibition of DNA synthesis. Second, erythropoiesis may be impaired by nutritional deficiencies or destruction of erythroid precursors, leading to ineffective erythropoiesis.

Anemia of Inflammation

Anemia of inflammation, also called anemia of chronic disease, is a common contributing factor to anemia in HIV-infected individuals. The pathogenesis is thought to be mediated by the release of cytokines by HIV-infected monocytes and macrophages, including tumor necrosis factor-alpha (TNF-α), transforming growth factor-beta (TGF-β) and interleukin-1 (IL-1), which have been shown to inhibit in vitro erythropoiesis.[15] Soluble TNF-α receptor (sTNF-α-R) levels increase with advanced HIV disease, and levels of sTNF-α-R and IL-6 have been shown to be inversely correlated with hemoglobin level in patients with HIV.[16] Several studies have shown that bone marrow stromal cells from HIV-infected individuals have altered cytokine production, including T cells (reduced IL-2), monocyte/macrophages (absent IL-1, IL-6, TNF-α, and reduced IL-12), and microvascular

Table 20–1. CAUSES OF ANEMIA IN HIV
Decreased Production
• Anemia of inflammation
• Viral infection of erythroid precursors (HIV, parvovirus B19)
• Bone marrow Infiltration (infectious, neoplastic)
• Drug-induced bone marrow suppression
• Nutritional deficiencies (vitamin B$_{12}$, folate, iron)
• Erythropoietin deficiency, impaired response to erythropoietin
• Androgen deficiency
Increased Destruction/Blood Loss
• Drug-induced hemolysis
• Microangiopathy (TTP/HUS)
• Autoimmune hemolysis
• Gastrointestinal bleeding (infectious, neoplastic)
• Hemophagocytic syndrome
Sequestration (Hypersplenism)
• Cirrhosis
• Lymphoma
• Infection

endothelial cells (IL-1 induced G-CSF and IL-6 production). Increased CD8$^+$ inhibitory T cells in HIV-infected patients can also have a suppressive effect on hematopoiesis.[17] Isigro and colleagues [18] have shown that levels of IL-2, IL-4, IL-10, and IFN-γ secreted by bone marrow mononuclear cell (BMMC) cultures are lower in untreated HIV-1–infected individuals than healthy controls; conversely, TNF-α levels and β-chemokines (MIP-1α and MIP-1β, RANTES) are higher. Thus, current evidence points towards altered cytokine production by bone marrow stromal cells as an important cause of impaired hematopoiesis and, specifically, erythropoiesis in HIV-infected individuals. Additionally, these cytokines may be involved either directly or indirectly in impaired bone marrow response to erythropoietin, decreased erythropoietin production, and trapping of iron in reticuloendothelial cells.

On peripheral blood smear, red blood cells appear normo- or hypochromic and normo- or microcytic. Laboratory studies show high ferritin levels, low serum iron, low total iron-binding capacity and transferrin levels, and a low reticulocyte response. Ferritin levels are increased owing to the inflammatory response in chronic HIV infection and may not accurately reflect iron stores. Soluble transferrin receptor concentration has been used to distinguish iron deficiency anemia from anemia of inflammation in non–HIV-infected individuals,[19] although its use in HIV-infected individuals has not been established.

Viral Infection of Erythroid Precursors

The presence of CD4 and CXCR4 or CCR5 on CD34$^+$ hematopoietic progenitor cells[20,21] suggests that hematopoietic stem cells are susceptible to HIV infection, although there are conflicting data as to whether this indeed is a common occurence, and there is little evidence that HIV infection results in impaired growth or differentiation.[17–25]

However, HIV infection of bone marrow stromal cells may play a role in suppression of hematopoiesis. As described above, BMMC cultures from HIV-1–infected individuals have lower levels of cytokine secretion than those of uninfected controls; however, treatment with antiretroviral therapy is associated with a statistically significant increase in IL-2 levels and a trend towards a decrease in β-chemokines. Additionally, whereas erythroid BMMC colony forming cell (CFC) assay values are lower in HIV-infected individuals compared to those of controls, anti-retroviral therapy is associated with a significant increase in CFC growth. Polymerase chain reaction analysis revealed HIV-1 DNA in bone marrow stromal cells of 3 out of 7 HIV-1–infected individuals assayed, all of which became negative after antiretroviral treatment; all CFC and long-term bone marrow culture-derived colonies were negative.[18] Wang and colleagues[26] showed that exposure of human bone marrow cells to HIV-1 in vitro resulted in HIV-1 infection of stromal colonies and, specifically, dendritic progenitor cells; mRNA levels of inflammatory cytokines (TNF-α, IL-1β, IL-6, and MIP-1β) were increased compared to non–HIV-1-exposed control stromal cultures.

Parvovirus B19 directly infects erythroid precursor cells, causing cell lysis and a block in erythropoiesis (Figure 20–1) as well as immune complex formation. In the immunocompetent host, antibody production results in viral clearance in 10 to 14 days. This disease most commonly manifests as erythema infectiosum or fifth disease in children, but adults may develop an acute viral illness, rash, arthralgias, and anemia. Those with underlying hemolytic disease may present with transient pure red cell aplasia. Patients with HIV infection may develop pancytopenia, anemia disproportionate to reductions in other cell lines, or chronic pure red cell aplasia owing to an

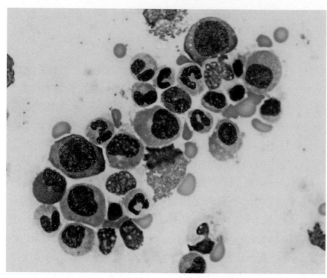

Figure 20–1. Parvovirus infection. Bone marrow aspirate smear from an AIDS patient reveals rare large/giant erythroblasts with possible intranuclear inclusions. Note absence of intermediate and late erythroid elements. Courtesy of Dr. C. Mark Lu (Wright-Giemsa).

insufficient or absent parvovirus-specific antibody response and inability to clear the virus.[27–29] Whereas parvovirus-specific IgM antibody is specific for acute parvovirus infection, an IgM response is commonly lacking in HIV-infected individuals, and dot-blot hybridization analysis is a much more sensitive assay. Therapy with intravenous immunoglobulin induces sustained remission in most cases.[29]

Bone Marrow Infiltration

Infiltration of the bone marrow by infectious or neoplastic disease should be considered in patients with AIDS and severe anemia, especially with those with pancytopenia. Infectious causes of bone marrow infiltration are typically mycobacterial (*Mycobacterium tuberculosis*, *Mycobacterium avium* complex) or fungal (*Histoplasma capsulatum*, *Cryptococcus neoformans*, coccidioidomycosis).[30,31]

Mycobacterium avium complex (MAC) infection, seen only in advanced AIDS, is particularly associated with severe anemia. Retrospective studies have demonstrated a decrease in rates of anemia and blood transfusions associated with the institution of MAC prophylaxis.[3,32] *Pneumocystis jiroveci* (formerly *carinii*) pneumonia (PCP) can also rarely infiltrate the bone marrow. Malignancies causing bone marrow infiltration are usually non-Hodgkin's lymphoma, especially Burkitt's lymphoma, other highly aggressive lymphomas, Hodgkin's lymphoma, multiple myeloma, Castleman's disease, and, rarely, Kaposi's sarcoma.[30,31]

Drugs

There are many medications used commonly in patients with HIV that can potentially cause anemia. However most of these are aimed at treating HIV infection and treatment or prevention of comorbidities that can also cause or contribute to anemia. A search for other causes of anemia should be undertaken before stopping potentially beneficial medications unless the onset of anemia can be timed specifically with the institution of a potentially offending drug and an alternative agent is readily available.

The anti-retroviral agent most commonly implicated in clinically significant anemia is AZT (3′-azido-3′-deoxythymidine, also known as zidovudine). AZT is a thymidine analog that terminates HIV reverse transcriptase activity. It can also be recognized by the human DNA polymerase, resulting in impaired erythropoiesis. Although macrocytosis occurs in most patients using AZT and mild anemia is common, pancytopenia and aplastic anemia can also rarely occur. A randomized controlled trial of AZT treatment for AIDS and AIDS-related complex in 1987 showed significantly reduced hemoglobin levels with AZT use; the AZT group also had higher rates of neutropenia and greater decline in platelet count.[33] Stavudine can also have similar hematologic effects, although less evidence is available for hematologic toxicity of the other nucleoside analogs and protease inhibitors.[2] Trimethoprim-sulfamethoxazole, commonly used in treatment and prophylaxis against PCP, acts by interfering with folic acid metabolism. Effects on human folate metabolism result in megaloblastic anemia and can result in aplastic anemia and pancytopenia as well. Other medications that can cause anemia by inhibiting hematopoiesis are listed in Table 20–2.

Nutritional Deficiencies

Patients with advanced HIV disease are at risk for poor nutrition as well as gastrointestinal pathology

Table 20–2. ANEMIA DUE TO DRUGS COMMONLY USED IN HIV

Antibacterial/Anti-protozoal
Trimethoprim-sulfamethoxazole
Pentamidine
Pyrimethamine
G6PD Deficiency: dapsone, primaquine, pyrimethamine,
trimethoprim-sulfamethoxazole[ǁ]

Antiviral
Anti-retroviral: AZT
Ganciclovir, foscarnet[*]
Interferon-α,[†,‡] Ribavirin[‡,§]

Antifungal
Flucytosine
Amphotericin

Antineoplastic

Recreational
Alcohol

[*]treatment of cytomegalovirus, herpes simplex virus; [†]treatment of hepatitis B virus; [‡]treatment of hepatitis C virus; [§]hemolytic anemia.

affecting the intake absorption of nutrients necessary for hematopoiesis, namely, iron, folate, and vitamin B_{12}.

Malignancies such as gastrointestinal lymphoma or Kaposi's sarcoma can cause not only malabsorption but also occult blood loss from the gastrointestinal tract resulting in iron deficiency. Malabsorption may also be caused by opportunistic infections such as *Mycobacterium avium–intracellulare*, cryptosporidia and microsporidia, bacterial overgrowth, HIV enteropathy (direct infection of the small bowel by HIV) and intestinal autonomic neuropathy. Vitamin B_{12} malabsorption in HIV is more commonly due to gastric pathology, with chronic inflammation and decreased secretion of intrinsic factor, not anti-intrinsic factor or parietal cell antibodies as is characteristic of pernicious anemia. Folate malabsorption is unrelated to the stage of HIV disease and is thought to be due to HIV enteropathy.[34]

Iron deficiency causes microcytosis and hypochromia and distorted red blood cell morphology. Serum ferritin, iron, and transferrin saturation are decreased; iron binding capacity and transferrin receptor levels are increased. Examination of the bone marrow shows decreased or absent iron stores. Both vitamin B_{12} and folate deficiency result in megaloblastic anemia, with macrocytic red blood cells and hypersegmented neutrophils. Diagnosis is made by measurement of serum vitamin B_{12}, methylmalonic acid, homocysteine, and red blood cell folate levels. Diagnosis can be difficult as methylmalonic acid and homocysteine levels, usually elevated in vitamin B_{12} deficiency, are often within normal limits in HIV-positive patients with clinical vitamin B_{12} deficiency. The deoxyuridine suppression test can also be used.[34]

Erythropoietin

Some studies suggest that although erythropoietin levels increase in patients with anemia of chronic disease, the erythropoietin response may be blunted. A comparison of anemic patients with AIDS and patients with uncomplicated iron deficiency anemia showed a lower degree of erythropoietin elevation for a similar severity of anemia in patients with AIDS.[35] Another study looking at anemia in patients with HIV at different stages (Centers for Disease Control [CDC] Stages I–III) and controls without chronic inflammatory or malignant disease showed lower erythropoietin response in all HIV CDC stages versus controls as well as an increasingly impaired response with more advanced HIV disease.[16] Patients with advanced HIV nephropathy or other chronic renal disease may have erythropoietin deficiency as well.

Androgen Deficiency

Hypogonadism is also common in HIV infection[36] and is associated with weight loss or AIDS-wasting syndrome.[37–39] It may also contribute to HIV-associated anemia, although this has not yet been investigated in detail. Androgens are thought to influence erythropoiesis through increased erythropoietin production in the kidney,[40] increased sensitivity to erythropoietin,[41] increased hemoglobin synthesis,[42] and by directly stimulating erythroid precursors.[41–46] Patients with hypogonadism are often anemic, and the anemia usually improves with androgen therapy; polycythemia is a known complication of supplemental androgens. One study showed a higher likelihood of anemia in HIV-infected men with higher testosterone levels and in those on supplemental androgens.[47] Randomized trials of androgen therapy in HIV-positive men for AIDS-wasting syndrome have shown increased hemoglobin and hematocrit levels in subjects treated with androgens compared to those in the placebo group.[48,49]

INCREASED DESTRUCTION/BLOOD LOSS

Individuals infected with HIV are at risk for multiple causes of reduced red blood cell longevity, including hemolytic anemia, either drug-induced or as an effect of immune dysregulation, and acute or chronic blood loss.

Drug-Mediated Hemolysis

Individuals deficient in the glucose-6-phosphate-dehydrogenase enzyme are particularly susceptible to anemia with trimethoprim-sulfamethoxazole as well as other drugs which cause oxidative stress (including dapsone, primaquine, and pyrimethamine), resulting in hemolytic anemia. A classic finding on peripheral blood smear is the presence of bite cells (Figure 20–2). The reticulocyte count may not be increased if there is concomitant bone marrow suppression, but serum lactate dehydrogenase and bilirubin concentrations are increased and haptoglobin is decreased or absent. Methemoglobinemia can also be caused by oxidant drug-induced hemolysis.[2] Ribavirin can cause a hemolytic anemia, thought to be secondary to increased susceptibility to oxidation.[50]

Microangiopathy

The combination of hemolytic anemia and thrombocytopenia should raise suspicion for microangiopathy owing to thrombotic thrombocytopenic purpura (TTP) or hemolytic uremic syndrome (HUS). Traditionally, the diagnosis of TTP has rested on five criteria: microangiopathic hemolytic anemia (schistocytes on the peripheral blood smear (Figure 20–3), markedly elevated lactate dehydrogenase), thrombocytopenia, fever, acute renal failure, and neurologic abnormalities. Although all of these features are not necessarily present, the presence of microangiopathic hemolytic anemia and thrombocytopenia in the setting of normal coagulation studies (to rule out disseminated intravascular coagulation) narrows down the diagnosis to TTP/HUS. In general, TTP is diagnosed when neurologic abnormalities predominate; HUS usually presents with renal failure but without neurologic symptoms.

The pathogenesis of TTP/HUS in HIV-infected individuals may be mediated by an acquired deficiency in the von Willebrand's factor–cleaving protease, ADAMTS-13, as indicated by case reports.[51,52] The prevalence of microangiopathy in HIV-infected individuals is thought to be higher than that of the general population; however, the prevalence may be declining with the introduction of highly active anti-

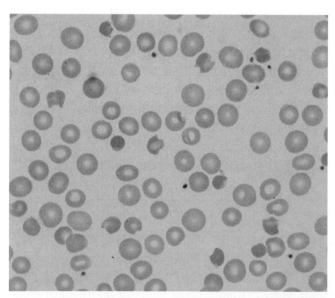

Figure 20–2. Peripheral blood smear showing several bite cells, including double-bite cells. Courtesy of Dr. C. Mark Lu) (Wright-Giemsa.

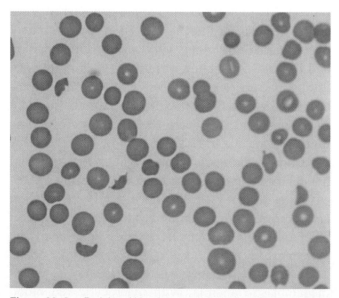

Figure 20–3. Peripheral blood smear showing marked thrombocytopenia and several fragmented erythrocytes (schistocytes, helmet cells). Courtesy of Dr. C. Mark Lu (Wright-Giemsa).

retroviral therapy (HAART). One study estimated a prevalence of 1.4% (17/1,223) in patients with AIDS prior to the introduction of highly active anti-retroviral therapy (1985–1996); no cases (0/347) were observed during 1997–2000.[53] Risk for microangiopathy may be increased in HIV-infected individuals owing to immune dysregulation as well as increased susceptibility to invasive enteric pathogens. In patients with more advanced HIV disease, HUS seems to become more common, the disease tends to be more refractory to treatment, and mortality is markedly increased (12/12 patients with AIDS died versus 1/19 with HIV only in one case series).[54] It is not clear whether anti-retroviral therapy alters the course of the disease. As in patients without HIV infection, the treatment is plasma exchange; steroids may be of benefit, and splenectomy may be indicated for refractory cases.[30]

Autoimmune Hemolytic Anemia

The prevalence of the direct antiglobulin test (DAT, or direct Coombs' test) is relatively high in patients with HIV (18–43%). Although case reports demonstrate that autoimmune hemolytic anemia occurs in HIV,[55] its incidence has not been shown definitively to be any higher in HIV-infected than non–HIV-infected individuals. Patients with a positive DAT have been shown to have lower hemoglobin levels than those with a negative DAT, although it is not clear if lower hemoglobin levels are directly caused by antiglobulin antibodies or if this is merely an association.[56,57] Autoimmune hemolytic anemia in chronic HIV infection may be due to immune activation and hypergammaglobulinemia, with nonspecific binding of excess IgG to the erythrocyte membrane.[58] Immune complex–associated IgG may be immune complex associated and bind to erythrocyte CR1 (C3b) receptors.[59] In HIV-infected individuals with autoimmune hemolytic anemia (AIHA), reticulocytopenia is uncommon, although it may occur due to other bone marrow–suppressive processes, such as a medication effect or infiltrative disease. Findings on peripheral blood smear include spherocytes, polychromatophilia and often nucleated red blood cells (Figure 20–4). Treatment is the same as for those without HIV (including prednisone, intravenous immunoglobulin, splenectomy) and appears to be similarly efficacious.

Blood Loss

Blood loss may be acute or chronic and is most commonly caused by loss through the gastrointestinal tract, but it may also be caused by internal bleeding in patients with a coagulopathy or severe thrombocytopenia. Potential causes of gastrointestinal blood loss have been described above.

Hemophagocytic Syndrome

Both ineffective erythropoiesis and sequestration from hypersplenism can be caused by hemophagocytic syndrome (also called hemophagocytic lymphohistiocytosis). Patients usually present with fever, pancytopenia, liver dysfunction, and hepatosplenomegaly. Pathologic findings include bone marrow hyperplasia with increased hemophagocytic histiocytes and infiltration of histiocytes and lymphocytes with erythrophagocytosis in the spleen, liver, and other viscera.[60] This phenomenon has been seen in mycobacterial disease (*Mycobacterium tuberculosis* and *Mycobacterium avium–intracellulare*, as well as a number of viral infections including cytomegalovirus (CMV),[2,61] Epstein-Barr virus (EBV),[2] herpes simplex virus, human herpesvirus 8 (HHV-8), and parvovirus B19.[30] T-cell non-Hodgkin's lymphoma and Kaposi's sar-

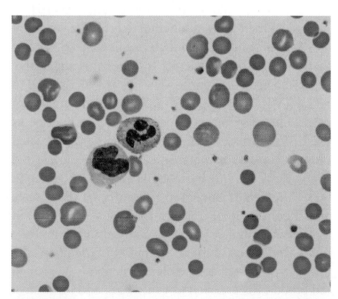

Figure 20–4. Autoimmune hemolytic anemia. Peripheral blood smear from a 66-year-old patient showing increase in polychromatic macrocytes and marked spherocytosis. Courtesy of Dr. C. Mark Lu (Wright-Giemsa).

coma have also been implicated.[30] The pathogenesis is thought to be mediated by increased cytokine production (including tumor necrosis factor-α and interferon-γ) associated with abnormal T-cell and macrophage activation and proliferation and hepatosplenomegaly.[60]

SEQUESTRATION

HIV-infected individuals may be at risk for sequestration of red blood cells from hypersplenism, based on their mode of HIV acquisition or the resulting immunodeficiency with increased risk for malignancy or infection. Individuals who acquired HIV through intravenous drug use are also at risk for chronic Hepatitis B and/or C infection, which can lead to cirrhosis, portal hypertension, and hypersplenism. Additionally, chronic hepatitis further contributes to anemia of inflammation.

HIV-infected individuals are also at increased risk of lymphoma, which can lead to anemia through both direct effects on the bone marrow as well as hypersplenism. Infections such as EBV and mycobacterial infections can lead to hypersplenism as well as hemophagocytic syndrome, as described above.

DIAGNOSTIC APPROACH

The initial laboratory evaluation of anemia in HIV-infected patients should include a reticulocyte count (< 1% or absolute reticulocyte count < 20,000/μL) in the setting of severe anemia (< 8 g/dL) is suggestive of parvovirus infection. The usual algorithm in non–HIV-infected anemic individuals using mean corpuscular volume to direct the tests may not be as useful to evaluate anemia since many HIV-infected individuals will be on medications that elevate the MCV. Review of the peripheral smear is a key step in the evaluation of anemia in HIV-infected individuals and should be done early in the course. Changes in red cell morphology often can suggest certain diagnoses and direct further testing. Microangiopathic changes with schistocytes and potentially nucleated red blood cells are seen in TTP, HUS, and infiltrative bone marrow processes, such as infections and malignancies. Spherocytes are seen in autoimmune hemolytic anemia and in drug-induced hemolysis

along with bite cells in G-6-PD deficiency. Megaloblastic changes, including macro-ovalocytes and hypersegmented granulocytes, are seen with folate and vitamin B_{12} deficiency as well as in patients treated with certain anti-retroviral drugs.

The role of performing bone marrow examinations in patients with HIV disease has been studied in multiple series. Although evaluation of a bone marrow sample often results in diagnostic results, in only about 10% of cases does bone marrow examination yield a unique diagnosis not otherwise revealed by other, often less invasive, tests.[62] A common finding on bone marrow examination of patients with AIDS is mild to moderate plasmacytosis, often with a perivascular distribution (Figure 20–5). Other nonspecific findings include normo- or hypercellularity, megaloblastic or dysplastic changes, lymphoid aggregates, and increased reticulin. Although some of these bone marrow findings may be due to concurrent drug therapy, comparisons between those who have and have not received drug treatment did not yield any significant differences.

CLINICAL CORRELATES OF ANEMIA, QUALITY OF LIFE, AND SURVIVAL

Anemia is increasingly more common with more advanced stages of HIV disease and clinical AIDS

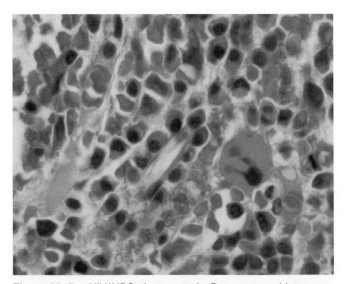

Figure 20–5.   HIV/AIDS plasmacytosis. Bone marrow biopsy section from an AIDS patient reveals focal reactive plasmacytosis. Note the perivascular distribution of the plasma cells. Courtesy of Dr. C. Mark Lu (H and E).

diagnosis.[5] It is directly associated with markers of disease progression such as lower CD4[+] T-lymphocyte counts and viral load as well as other hematologic effects, including cytpoenias (neutropenia, thrombocytopenia) and low mean corpuscular volume.[3,4,6,11,63]

Anemia is more common in women with HIV than HIV-infected men, most likely due to loss of iron stores owing to pregnancy and menstruation as in non–HIV-infected women, as well as possibly dietary intake and socioeconomic level.[64] Additionally, African-American race is associated with higher rates of anemia.[6,63] This may reflect higher rates of inherited anemias (sickle cell hemoglobin, thalassemia) and socioeconomic level as well.

Interestingly, anemia also appears to be an independent risk factor for decreased quality of life and survival. Multiple studies have shown that both clinical diagnosis of anemia or decreasing hemoglobin levels are associated with decreased survival in individuals with HIV-infection, independently of CD4+ T-lymphocyte count, clinical AIDS diagnosis, age, other cytopenias, and antiretroviral therapy (Figure 20–6).[3,9,10,11]

Although zidovudine has been associated with a higher prevalence of anemia prior to the introduction of potent combination anti-retroviral therapy,[6] in the years since anti-retroviral therapy it has been associated with a lower prevalence[63] and improvement of anemia.[4,5,6,65]

Another important aspect of anemia on HIV-infected individuals is its contribution to impaired quality of life. Fatigue is a common symptom of both chronic HIV infection as well as anemia.[7,66] Several studies have shown an improvement in both hemoglobin levels and quality of life in patients treated with erythropoietin.[12,14]

An important question is whether treatment of anemia will have any impact on survival. Retrospective studies have shown that patients with HIV who were treated for, and recovered from, anemia have improved outcomes compared to those who do not recover[3,10]; however, it is difficult to attribute improved survival directly to treatment of anemia when several other confounding factors may be contributing as well.

A growing body of data supports a strong association between anemia and survival. One possible explanation for this is a common association between anemia, other markers of HIV disease activity, such as immune activation and inflammatory cytokines, and survival. Despite this association, there is no direct evidence for a causal relationship between anemia and survival, nor is there evidence that treatment of anemia leads to improvement in survival.

TREATMENT

A rational approach to treatment of anemia in HIV-infected individuals is to identify and treat all reversible causes of anemia, including opportunistic infections and malignancies and nutritional deficiencies, then to remove potentially offending drugs if an alternative is available. Although several anti-retroviral medications can cause or contribute to anemia, multiple studies have shown that treatment of underlying HIV infection with anti-retroviral medications can protect against, and lead to, resolution or improvement of anemia. If a patient continues to have symptomatic anemia or is otherwise at high risk of morbidity from anemia (eg, coronary artery disease, heart failure), then consideration should be turned towards correction of anemia.

Blood Transfusion

In the setting of acute blood loss or severe symptomatology, transfusion may be the only option. However, several studies suggest that transfusion may be

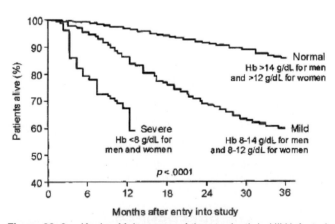

Figure 20–6. Kaplan-Meier curve of time to death in HIV-infected patients with normal hemoglobin (Hb), mild anemia, or severe anemia in the EuroSIDA study. The indicated *p* value is a log-rank statistic. Reprinted with permission from Sullivan P. J Infect Dis 2002; 185:S138–42.

associated with increased mortality in HIV and should be avoided if at all possible. Blood transfusion has been associated with increased tumor recurrence in patients with a history of malignancy, increased transplant survival in patients with a history of solid organ transplant, and suppression of inflammatory disease. Some studies suggest possible HIV and CMV activation with blood transfusion. Despite this evidence, a randomized controlled trial of blood transfusion with leukocyte-reduced versus non–leukocyte-reduced blood cells did not show a benefit with leukocyte reduction.[67] Observational data indicate that patients with anemia treated with blood transfusions have worse survival rates compared to those treated with erythropoietin.[10,68] However, the degree of potential confounding warrants that these data be interpreted with caution.

Erythropoietin

Erythropoietin has been shown to be an effective treatment for HIV-associated anemia and is likely safer than blood transfusion. Many trials have shown erythropoietin to be safe and effective for treatment of HIV-associated anemia, and it is likely safer than blood transfusion. A combined analysis of four multicenter, randomized, double-blind, controlled trials showed an increase in hemoglobin levels by > 1 g by week 2 and > 2 g by week 4 ($p \geq .05$) in patients with AIDS who were taking zidovudine, with endogenous erythropoietin levels of ≤ 500 IU/L. Also noted were significant reductions in transfusion requirements and improvements in quality of life.[12] Subsequent studies after the introduction of HAART have confirmed improvement in anemia as well as improvements in quality-of-life measures with erythropoietin therapy.[14] More recent studies also demonstrate a comparable benefit of once-weekly (40,000 IU) to three-times-weekly dosing.[69] Darbepoetin, a longer-acting recombinant erythropoietin, can be dosed even less frequently, although its use in HIV-associated anemia has not been directly studied.

REFERENCES

1. Coyle T. Hematologic complications of human immunodeficiency virus infection and the acquired immunodeficiency syndrome. Med Clin North Am 1997;81:449–70.

2. Bain BJ. Pathogenesis and pathophysiology of anemia in HIV infection. Curr Opin Hematol 1999;6:89–93.

3. Sullivan PS, Hanson DL, Chu SY, et al. Epidemiology of anemia in human immunodeficiency virus (HIV)-infected persons: results from the multistate adult and adolescent spectrum of HIV disease surveillance project. Blood 1998;91:301–8.

4. Moore RD, Forney D. Anemia in HIV-infected patients receiving highly active antiretroviral therapy. J Acquir Immune Defic Syndr 2002;19:54–7.

5. Semba RD, Shah N, Vlahov D. Improvement of anemia among HIV-infected injection drug users receiving highly active antiretroviral therapy. J Acquir Immune Defic Syndr 2001;26:315–9.

6. Semba RD, Shah N, Klein RS, et al. Prevalence and cumulative incidence of and risk factors for anemia in a multicenter cohort study of human immunodeficiency virus-infected and -uninfected women. Clin Infect Dis 2002;34:260–6.

7. Breitbart W, McDonald MV, Rosenfeld B, et al. Fatigue in ambulatory AIDS patients. J Pain Symptom Manage 1998;15:159–67.

8. Volberding P. The impact of anemia on quality of life in human immunodeficiency virus-infected patients. J Infect Dis 2002;185(Suppl 2): S110–4.

9. Saah AJ, Hoover DR, He Y, et al. Factors influencing survival after AIDS: report from the Multicenter AIDS Cohort Study (MACS). J Acquir Immune Defic Syndr 1994;7:287–95.

10. Moore RD, Keruly JC, Chaisson RE. Anemia and survival in HIV infection. J Acquir Immune Defic Syndr Hum Retrovirol 1998;19:29–33.

11. Mocroft A, Kifk O, Barton SE, et al. Anaemia is an independent predictive marker for clinical prognosis in HIV-infected patients from across Europe. AIDS 1999;13:943–50.

12. Henry DH, Gildon NB, Benson CA, et al. Recombinant human erythropoietin in the treatment of anemia associated with human immunodeficiency virus (HIV) infection and zidovudine therapy. Ann Intern Med 1992;117:739–48.

13. Abrams DI, Steinhart C, Frascino R. Epoetin alfa therapy for anaemia in HIV-infected patients: impact on quality of life. Int J STD AIDS 2000;11:659–65.

14. Revicki DA, Brown RE, Henry DH, et al. Recombinant human erythropoietin and health-related quality of life of AIDS patients with anemia. J Acquir Immune Defic Syndr 1994;7:474–84.

15. Zhang Y, Harada A, Bluethmann H, et al. TNF is a physiologic regulator of hematopoietic cells: increase of early hematopoietic progenitor cells in TNF receptor p55-deficient mice in vivo and potent inhibition of progenitor cell proliferation by TNF in vitro. Blood 1995,86(8): 2930–7.

16. Kreuzer KA, Rockstroh JK, Jelkmann W, et al. Inadequate erythropoietin response to anaemia in HIV patients: relationship to serum levels of tumour necrosis factor-alpha, interleukin-6 and their soluble receptors. Br J Haematol 1997,96:235–9.

17. Moses A, Nelson J, Bagby GC. The influence of human immunodeficiency virus-1 on hematopoiesis. Blood 1998;91:1479–95.

18. Isgro A, Aiuti A, Mezzaroma I, et al. Improvement of interleukin 2 production, clonogenic capability and restoration of stromal cell function in human immunodeficiency

virus-type-1 patients after highly active antiretroviral therapy. Br J Haematol 2002;118: 864–74.

19. Punnonen K, Irjala K, Rajamaki A. Serum transferrin receptor and its ration to serum ferritin in the diagnosis of iron deficiency. Blood 1997;89:1052–7.

20. Zauli G, Furlini G, Vitale M, et al. A subset of human CD34+ hematopoietic progenitors express low levels of CD4, the high-affinity receptor for human immunodeficiency virus-type 1. Blood 1994;80:3036–43.

21. Deichmann M, Kronenwett R, Haas R. Expression of the human immunodeficiency virus type-1 coreceptors CXCR-4 (fusin, LESTR) and CDR-5 in CD34+ hematopoietic progenitor cells. Blood 1997;89:3522–8.

22. Stanley SK, Kessler SW, Justement JS, et al. CD34+ bone marrow cells are infected with HIV in a subset of seropositive individuals. J Immunol 1992;149:689–7.

23. Neal TF, Holland HK, Baum CM, et al. CD34+ progenitor cells from asymptomatic patients are not a major reservoir for human immunodeficiency virus-1. Blood 1995;86:1749–56.

24. Sloand EM, Young NS, Sato T, et al. Secondary colony formation after long-term bone marrow culture using peripheral blood and bone marrow of HIV-infected patients. AIDS 1997;11:1547–53.

25. Weichold FF, Zella D, Barabitskaja O, et al. Neither human immunodeficiency virus-1 (HIV-1) nor HIV-2 infects most primitive human hematopoietic stem cells as assessed by long-term bone marrow cultures. Blood 1998;91:907–15.

26. Wang L, Debasis M, LarRussa VF, et al. AIDS Res Hum Retroviruses 2002;13:917–31.

27. Gyllensten K, Sönnerborg A, Jorup-Rönström et al. Parvovirus B19 infection in HIV-1 infected patients with anemia. Infection 1994;22:356–8.

28. Chernak E, Dubin G, Henry D, et al. Infection due to parvovirus B19 in patients infected with human immunodeficiency virus. Clin Infect Dis 1995;20:170–3.

29. Abkowitz JL, Brown KE, Wood RW, et al. Clinical relevance of parvovirus B19 as a cause of anemia in patients with HIV infection. J Infect Dis 1997;176:269–73.

30. Hambleton J. Hematologic complications of HIV infection. Oncology 1996;10:671–80.

31. Baker K. Human immunodeficiency virus hematology: the hematologic complications of HIV infection. Hematology 2003;1:294–313.

32. Kravcik S, Toye BW, Fyke K, et al. Impact of mycobaterium avium complex prophylaxis on the incidence of mycobacterial infections and transfusion-requiring anemia in an HIV-positive population. J Acquir Immune Defic Syndr Hum Retrovirol 1996;13:27–32.

33. Richman DD, Fischl MA, Grieco MH, et al. The toxicity of azidothymidine (AZT) in the treatment of patients with AIDS and AIDS-related complex. New Engl J Med 1987; 317:192–7.

34. Paltiel O, Falutz J, Veilleux M, et al. Clinical correlates of subnormal vitamin B12 levels in patients infected with the human immunodeficiency virus. Am J Hematol 1995; 49:318–22.

35. Spivak JL, Barnes DC, Fuchs E, Quinn TC. Serum immunoreactive erythropoietin in HIV-infected patients. JAMA 1989;261:3104–07.

36. Dobs AS, Dempsey MA, Ladenson PW, et al. Endocrine disorders in men infected with human immunodeficiency virus. Am J Med 1988;84:611–6.

37. Coodley GO, Loveless MO, Nelson HD, et al. Endocrine function in the HIV wasting syndrome. J Acquir Immune Defic Syndr 1994;7.46–51.

38. Rietschel P, Corcoran C, Stanley T, et al. Prevalence of hypogonadism among men with weight loss related to human immunodeficiency virus infection who were receiving highly active antiretroviral therapy. Clin Infect Dis 2000;31:1240–4.

39. Dobs A, Brown T. Metabolic abnormalities in HIV disease and injection drug use. J Acquir Immune Defic Syndr 2002;31(Suppl 2):S70–7.

40. Navarro JF, Mora C. Androgen therapy for anemia in elderly uremic patients. Int J Nephrol 2001;32:549–57.

41. Udupa KB, Crabtree HM, Lipschitz DA. In vitro culture of proerythroblasts: characterization of proliferative response to erythropoietin and steroids. Br J Haematol 1986;62(4):705–14.

42. Modder B, Foley JE, Fisher JW. The in vitro and in vivo effects of testosterone and steroid metabolites on erythroid colony forming cells (CFU-E). J Pharmacol Exp Ther 1978;207:1004–12.

43. Ohno Y, Fisher JW. Effects of androgens on burst forming units (BFU-E) in normal rabbit bone marrows. Life Sci 1978;22:2031–6.

44. Urabe A, Sassa S, Kappas A. The influence of steroid hormone metabolites on the in vitro development of erythroid colonies derived from human bone marrow. J Exp Med 1979;149:1314–25.

45. Claustres M, Sultan C. Androgen and erythropoiesis: evidence for an androgen receptor in erythroblasts from human bone marrow cultures. Horm Res 1988;29:17–22.

46. Gardner FH, Besa EC. Physiologic mechanisms and the hematopoietic effects of the androstanes and their derivatives. Curr Top Hematol 1983;4:123–95.

47. Behler C, Shade S, Gregory K, et al. Anemia and HIV in the antiretroviral era: potential significance of testosterone. AIDS Res and Hum Retrovir 2005;21:200–206.

48. Grinspoon S, Corcoran C, Anderson E, et al. Sustained anabolic effects of long-term androgen administration in men with AIDS wasting. Clin Infect Dis 1999;28:634–6.

49. Bhasin S, Storer TW, Asbel-Sethi N, et al. Effects of testosterone replacement with a nongenital, transdermal system, androderm, in human immunodeficiency virus-infected men with low testosterone levels. J Clin Endocrinol Metab 1998;83:3155–62.

50. De Franceschi L, Fattovich G, Turrini F, et al. Hemolytic anemia induced by ribavirin therapy in patients with chronic hepatitis C virus infection: role of membrane oxidative damage. Hepatology 2000;31:997–1004.

51. Sahud MA, Claster S, Liu L, et al. von Willebrand factor-cleaving protease inhibitor in a patient with human immunodeficiency syndrome-associated thrombotic thrombocytopenic purpura. Br J Haematol 2002;116:909–11.

52. Gruszecki AC, Wehrli G, Ragland BD, et al. Management of a patient with HIV infection-induced anemia and thrombocytopenia who presented with thrombotic thrombocytopenic purpura. Am J Hematol 2002;69:228–31.

53. Gervasoni C, Ridolfo AL, Vaccarezza M, et al. Thrombotic microangiopathy in patients with acquired immunodeficiency syndrome before and during the era of introduction of highly active antiretroviral therapy. Clin Infect Dis 2002;35:1534–40.

54. Gadallah MF, El-Shahawy MA, Campese VM, et al. Disparate prognosis of thrombotic microangiopathy in HIV-infected patients with and without AIDS. Am J Nephrol 1996;16:446–50.

55. Telen MJ, Roberts KB, Bartlett JA. HIV-associated autoimmune hemolytic anemia: report of a case and review of the literature. J Acquir Immun Defic Syndr 1990;3:933–7.

56. Toy PTCY, Reid ME, Burns M. Positive direct antiglobulin test associated with hypergammaglobulinemia in acquired immunodeficiency (AIDS). Am J Hematol 1985;19:145–50.

57. McGinniss MH, Macher AM, Rook AH, et al. Red cell autoantibodies in patients with acquired immune deficiency syndrome. Transfusion 1986;26:405–9.

58. Toy PTCY, Chin CA, Reid ME, et al. Factors associated with positive direct antiglobulin tests in pretransfusion patients: a case-control study. Vox Sang 1985;49:215–20.

59. Inada Y, Lange M, McKinley GF, et al. Hematologic correlates and the role of erythrocyte CR1 (C3b receptor) in the development of AIDS. AIDS Res 1986;2:235–47.

60. Hoffman R, Benz EJ, Shattil SJ, et al. Hematology: basic principles and practice. 3rd ed.

61. San Miguel LG, Casado JL, Canizares A, et al. High cytomegalovirus antigenemia levels and cytomegalovirus syndrome in patients with AIDS. J Acquir Immune Defic Syndr Hum Retrovirol 1997;16:307.

62. Akpek G, Lee SM, Gagnon DR, et al. Bone marrow aspiration, biopsy, and culture in the evaluation of HIV-infected patients for invasive mycobacteria and histoplasma infections. Am J Hematol 2001;67:100-6.

63. Levine AM, Berhane K, Masri-Lavine L, et al. Prevalence and correlates of anemia in a large cohort of HIV-infected women: Women's Interagency HIV Study. J Acquir Immune Defic Syndr 2001:26:28–35.

64. Semba RD. Iron-deficiency anemia and the cycle of poverty among human immunodeficiency virus-infected women in the inner city. Clin Infect Dis 2003;117:739–48.

65. Berhane K, Karim R, Cohen MH, et al. Impact of highly active antiretroviral therapy on anemia and relationship between anemia and survival in a large cohort of HIV-infected women. J Acquir Immune Defic Syndr 2004;37:1245–52.

66. Groopman JE. Fatigue in cancer and HIV/AIDS. Oncology 1998;12:335–44.

67. Collier AC, Kalish LA, Busch MP, et al. Leukocyte-reduced red blood cell transfusions in patients with anemia and human immunodeficiency virus infection. The viral activation transfusion study: a randomized controlled trial. JAMA 2001;285:1592–601.

68. Buskin SE, Sullivan PS. Anemia and its treatment and outcomes in persons infected with human immunodeficiency virus. Transfusion 2004;44:826–32.

69. Grossman HA, Goon B, Bowers P, et al. Once-weekly Epoetin alfa dosing is as effective as three times-weekly dosing in increasing hemoglobin levels and is associated with improved quality of life in anemic HIV-infected patients. J Acquir Immune Defic Syndr 2003;34:368–78.

21

Abnormalities of the Coagulation System Associated with HIV Infection

KELTY BAKER

Hematologic abnormalities are among the most commonly seen complications of infection with human immunodeficiency virus (HIV).[1] This chapter covers the various perturbations of the coagulation system found in this special patient population, focusing especially on thrombotic disorders of both the venous and arterial systems as well as thrombocytopenia and the bleeding diathesis that has been seen in some patients taking protease inhibitors.

VENOUS THROMBOEMBOLIC EVENTS

Although rarely reported in the early years of the acute immune deficiency syndrome (AIDS) epidemic, venous thromboembolic events (VTE) are now increasingly recognized as a complication of HIV infection. Both deep venous thromboses (DVT) of the lower extremities and pulmonary emboli (PE) may be found in patients at all stages of disease,[2-12] with a reported recurrence rate of 26.7% according to one retrospective study.[13] This report, which also found that hospitalized patients with HIV infection or AIDS were 10 times more likely to suffer VTE than the general population, was criticized because it used historic controls[14]; however, other studies, both retrospective and prospective, have confirmed the excess risk of VTE that HIV imparts to affected individuals relative to their age-matched peers, especially those younger than age 50.[15] For instance, a retrospective study of 42,935 patients enrolled in the Adult/Adolescent Spectrum of HIV Disease Surveillance (ASD) Project demonstrated that the overall incidence of thrombosis was 2.6 per 1,000 person-years of follow-up, with the highest risk seen in those patients with clinical AIDS as opposed to those with simple HIV infection or immunological AIDS (CD4 lymphocyte count < 200 cells/μL).[16] Similarly, a large prospective study of 37,535 HIV-infected veterans confirmed that such individuals had a 39% greater incidence of VTE relative to HIV-negative veterans in the years before 1996 (rate of VTE 11.3 per 1,000 person-years versus 7.6 per 1,000 person-years, $p < .001$), a risk that didn't change significantly once highly active anti-retroviral therapy (HAART) was introduced, declining only slightly to 33% (rate of VTE 5.7 per 1,000 person-years versus 3.3 per 1,000 person-years, $p < .001$).[14] The influence of HAART on VTE risk is somewhat controversial, however, as a much smaller study found that the incidence of thrombosis had increased with the institution of protease inhibitor (PI) therapy, rising from 0.33% before these drugs were available to 1.52% currently ($p < .001$).[12]

Accurate and timely identification of PE can be particularly problematic in HIV-infected individuals. A feature shared by many of the reported cases is that the diagnosis was rarely considered upon the patients' admission to hospital and was ultimately entertained only upon their failure to improve with initial empiric antimicrobial therapy or at the time of necropsy.[4,5,8] In fact, the incidence of previously unsuspected pulmonary emboli (PE) can be as high as 17% in decedents who undergo autopsy.[17,18] Of note, aggressive transfusion therapy should be undertaken with caution in HIV-associated autoimmune hemolytic anemia, as fatal pulmonary embolization owing to augmented hemolysis and disseminated intravascular coagulation has been reported.[19–21] Although anticoagulation therapy can be safely used in most patients who suffer PE, inferior vena cava filters are an option for those with a contraindication to such therapy.[22]

Factors associated with an increased risk of venous thromboembolic complications in HIV-positive patients include age over 45 years,[16] an advanced stage of infection,[9,16,23] the presence of cytomegalovirus (CMV) infection[16,24] or other AIDS-defining opportunistic infections,[16,23] hospitalization,[16] and therapy with indinavir sulfate[16,25] or megestrol acetate.[9,16,26] The association between thrombosis and opportunistic infections like CMV may simply reflect the prolonged immobility that results from severe illness[23]; however, CMV has been shown to alter the phenotype of endothelial cells from anticoagulant to procoagulant by promoting adhesion of neutrophils and platelets to the endothelium,[27] to induce production of antiphospholipid antibodies,[28] and to increase levels of factor VIII and von Willebrand factor.[29,30] Why indinavir predisposes to thrombosis is unclear,[16] but megestrol, like other progestational agents, can cause acquired resistance to activated protein C.[26]

In addition, individuals with HIV infection may be at increased risk for thrombosis because of decreased levels of antithrombin,[31] free protein S (see below), protein C,[32,33] or heparin cofactor II[34]); elevated levels of plasminogen activator inhibitor-1,[35] homocysteine[36,37] and factor VIII[37]; the presence of anticardiolipin antibodies (see below); coexistence of malignant, inflammatory, or autoimmune disorders; the presence of vascular damage owing to injection drug use,[38] placement of intravenous catheters,[39,40] or CMV infection[23,41,42]; and elevated markers of endothelial activation such as von Willebrand factor antigen,[32,35,43–47] soluble thrombomodulin,[45] vascular cell adhesion molecule-1 (sVCAM-1), and intercellular adhesion molecule-1 (sICAM-1).[47] Interestingly, plasma levels of von Willebrand factor antigen, sVCAM-1, and sICAM-1 all decline with institution of anti-retroviral therapy and the subsequent reduction in viral load.[46,47] Although markers of platelet activation are also increased in HIV infection, there are discrepant findings with regard to

whether these levels also decline with HAART therapy.[47,48] Finally, antithrombin deficiency can occur with HIV-associated nephropathy (HIVAN) as a result of losses in the urine. HIVAN, which predominantly affects African-American patients with full-blown AIDS, may also result in compensatory hepatic synthesis of fibrinogen and factors V and VIII induced by hypoalbuminemia and increased platelet adhesion and aggregation.[49]

Acquired Protein S Deficiency

Protein S is a vitamin K–dependent plasma protein that increases the affinity of activated protein C for phospholipid surfaces and thus serves as a nonenzymatic cofactor in the protein C–mediated proteolytic degradation of clotting factors Va and VIIIa. After its synthesis by hepatocytes, endothelial cells, or megakaryocytes, 40% of the total protein S circulates in a free, biologically active form whereas 60% is reversibly complexed to C4b-binding protein (C4b-BP), rendering it functionally inactive. Congenital dysfunction or deficiency of free or total protein S predisposes affected individuals to both arterial strokes and venous thromboembolic disease.[50] Acquired deficiency of protein S can be seen in the neonatal period, during pregnancy, with use of oral contraceptives or hormone replacement therapy, in the nephrotic syndrome, as a result of disseminated intravascular coagulation or an acute thrombotic event, and in certain inflammatory states.[51]

Acquired protein S deficiency is also found in 27 to 76% of children and adults with HIV infection, especially those with acute opportunistic infections, CD4 counts below 200 cells/μL, or full-blown AIDS,[33,35,44,50,52–55] and results in thrombotic complications in as many as 11.5%.[50] Interestingly, the low levels of free protein S seen in treatment-naïve patients increase rapidly once HAART is instituted.[56] Several possible etiologies for the observed decline in free protein S levels have been postulated: (1) the appearance in some patients of antibodies against protein S[57,58]; (2) a virally-induced disturbance in endothelial cell function that results in decreased synthesis of protein S[3]; (3) binding of protein S by antiphospholipid antibodies, which then interfere with attachment of the protein C:S complex to phospholipid surfaces[59]; and (4) elevated levels of C4b-BP, an acute phase reactant.[44] This last supposition is controversial, however, as many authors have found normal levels of C4b-BP in patients with free protein S deficiency.[3,32,52,54,60,61] Of note, the level of free protein S in HIV-infected patients can appear artificially low when assayed by the polyethylene-glycol (PEG) precipitation technique,[54,60] so that the prevalence of true protein S deficiency may actually be much lower than previously thought (about 10%). Gris and colleagues hypothesize that high titers of poorly characterized microparticles detectable by flow cytometry bind free protein S and then are removed during PEG precipitation, causing an apparent depression of free protein S levels.[54]

Antiphospholipid Antibodies and HIV Infection

Antiphospholipid antibodies (including both the lupus anticoagulant and anticardiolipin antibodies) are frequently seen in HIV-infected individuals in the absence of any thrombotic event. The former is found in 0 to 70% of patients with HIV,[33,62–65] whereas anticardiolipin antibodies can be detected in 6 to 94%,[33,35,53,55,64,66–73] depending upon the sensitivity of the assay used and the characteristics of the individuals examined. Neither is strongly associated with an increased risk of venous thromboembolic complications,[62,64–66,68,70,73,74] or with the stage of disease, CD4 cell count, or viral load.[68,72,75,76] In fact, one group found that antiphospholipid antibody levels actually decline in the late stages of HIV infection and conjecture that this is due to loss of T-helper cell type 2 functions and resultant progression of B-cell immunodeficiency.[71] Importantly, unlike autoimmune conditions such as systemic lupus erythematosus and the primary antiphospholipid syndrome, the antiphospholipid antibodies found in HIV infection are not associated with pathogenic anti–β_2-glycoprotein 1 antibodies[70,73,77–80] and are not correlated with typical markers of endothelial dysfunction.[81] It is suspected that these antibodies are clinically benign and occur when phospholipids are exteriorized by apoptotic T lymphocytes. They then cooperate with macrophages in the clearance of dead cells by an enhanced antibody-dependent cellular cytotoxicity mechanism.[82] Nonetheless, events such as DVT and PE,[5,83] transient neurological deficits[55,84] and stroke,[85] avascular necrosis of bone,[86,87] skin necrosis,[41,88–90] splenic infarction,[91] and brachial artery thrombosis[92] have occasionally been described in those with anticardiolipin antibodies. Given the high prevalence of anticardiolipin antibodies in asymptomatic HIV-infected individuals, however, these reported complications may only be coincidental.[82]

MYOCARDIAL INFARCTION AND HIV INFECTION

Beginning in 1992, several cases of coronary atheroembolic disease were reported in otherwise healthy, young HIV-infected patients without known cardiovascular risk factors.[93–95] Since then, concern has grown about an apparent increased risk of coronary artery disease (CAD) in patients with HIV infection,[96–110] with an acute myocardial infarction being the first manifestation in 94% of those patients so affected.[111] Use of HAART, especially those regimens containing PIs such as ritonavir, has been implicated since these drugs are well known to cause insulin resistance and dyslipidemia with resultant atherosclerosis[112,113] and endothelial cell dysfunction.[114,115] In fact, ritonavir has been shown to cause cytotoxicity of human endothelial cells at clinically relevant drug concentrations in vitro.[115] This topic remains controversial, however, because the published studies examining this possibility have not shown a consistent clinical association.[116,117]

For instance, a retrospective study from the University of Cincinnati did not find an association between use of protease inhibitors and ischemic cardiovascular disease; rather, the duration and severity of immunosuppression, as well as the presence of traditional risk factors for CAD, were shown to be more important.[118] Similarly, a retrospective study of 4,159 HIV-positive men receiving care at the Kaiser Permanente Medical Care Program of Northern California demonstrated that such patients were hospitalized for coronary heart disease more often than HIV-negative individuals but did not find an increase in hospitalization rates after either the beginning of the HAART era or following institution of PI therapy.[119] A large retrospective study of 36,766 HIV-positive patients receiving care at Veterans Affairs facilities also failed to discover an increase in the rate of cardiovascular or cerebrovascular events or related mortality following the introduction of PI-containing HAART.[120] Finally, a retrospective analysis of pooled, industry-sponsored, phase II and III studies comparing treatment with PI with or without nucleoside reverse transcriptase inhibitors (NRTI) to NRTI therapy alone failed to show an association between PI therapy and myocardial infarction (MI).[121]

On the other hand, several large retrospective cohort studies have reported a four- to fivefold increase in the rate of myocardial infarction in HIV-infected patients taking PI compared with those taking other forms of HAART.[122,123] Perhaps some of these discrepant results can be attributed to differences in the length of PIs therapy and overall follow-up in the various studies. For instance, in a large French cohort of 19,795 patients, Mary-Krause and colleagues found a positive association between the rate of MI and duration of PI therapy, and also a higher rate of MI in HIV-positive patients taking PI therapy compared with the general French population. Unfortunately, the authors did not include comparative data for HIV-positive patients not exposed to PI therapy.[124] Similarly, recent results from the Data Collection on Adverse Events of Anti-HIV Drugs study showed that both MI[125] and a combined end point of MI, stroke, invasive cardiovascular procedures, and deaths from other cardiovascular causes increased with longer exposure to HAART, over and above that which could be explained by increasing age alone.[126]

It is also possible that the prevalence of well-known cardiovascular risk factors such as hypertension and smoking varied between the studies published thus far. The HIV Outpatient Study (HOPS), a prospective, observational cohort recruited and followed up since 1992, reported an increased frequency of MI after PI were introduced, although the significance of this association declined when the results were controlled for age and sex, and the presence of hypertension, smoking, and diabetes mellitus.[127] Likewise, a large, open-label, prospective, observational study comparing the incidence of CAD in previously untreated HIV-infected patients who received HAART, with or without protease inhibitors, found a statistically significant 11.5-fold rise in CAD-related events in those patients taking a PI. Twenty-six occurrences of new or unstable angina or fatal and nonfatal MI occurred in 23 patients taking PIs (out of 776 studied) compared with 2 occurrences in the group taking a PI-free regimen (out of 775 studied), for a cumulative annual incidence of CAD-related events of 9.8 per 1,000 patients in the former group and 0.8 per 1,000 patients in the latter ($p < .001$). The risk was particularly high in those individuals who were heavy smokers.[128] Nevertheless, the absolute risk of MI in those taking PIs remains relatively low, and any concerns about precipitating cardiovascular disease should be weighed against the marked benefits obtained with use of PI-containing anti-retroviral therapy.[125]

Why might HIV-infected individuals taking HAART be susceptible to early-onset coronary artery disease? The human immunodeficiency virus itself can precipitate endothelial dysfunction[129] as a result of abnormal expression of cytokines, viral proteins, adhesion molecules, and procoagulant proteins.[45,130] In fact, the first report on myocardial arteriopathy in the absence of classic risk factors for CAD was published in 1987, long before HAART was introduced.[131] A later case report found HIV-1 sequences in the intima and media of the left anterior descending coronary artery of a 32-year-old male with no known cardiovascular risk factors who suffered a fatal myocardial infarction.[130] Grossly, the vessel was eroded and fissured, with dense infiltration by IgA-positive plasma cells and resultant necrosis of the intima visualized microscopically. No thrombi were found.[132] Similarly, Constans and colleagues reported in 1995 that atheromatous plaques of the aorta and cervical and femoral arteries were detected by B-mode ultrasonography more often in HIV-infected patients than in healthy controls matched for cardiovascular risk factors such as sex, age, tobacco consumption, and arterial hypertension.[133] More recent studies have confirmed these findings but reported conflicting results with regard to the importance of PI therapy in the progression of atherosclerotic disease. Maggi and colleagues performed Doppler ultrasonography of the common, internal, and external carotid vessels in 102 patients taking HAART and demonstrated a higher-than-expected prevalence of premature carotid lesion in those taking a PI compared to PI-naïve patients.[134] A year later, Depairon and colleagues visualized the femoral and carotid arteries of 168 HIV-infected individuals but failed to show any association between use of PIs and atherosclerosis, finding instead that the most significant factors in promoting atherosclerosis in these patients were smoking and hyperlipidemia.[135]

Besides the human immunodeficiency virus, infection with cytomegalovirus has been implicated as a possible contributor to coronary vessel atherogenesis and restenosis.[136] As described above, classic risk factors such as hypertension, smoking, dyslipidemia, diabetes mellitus, and family history can contribute to patients' risk of cardiovascular disease as well.[125,137] Finally, a wide range of inflammatory vasculitides such as Behçet's syndrome, Churg-Strauss syndrome, Henoch-Schönlein purpura, Takayasu's arteritis, temporal arteritis, Wegener's granulomatosis, drug-induced hypersensitivity vasculitis, polyarteritis nodosa due to hepatitis B infection, microscopic polyangitis, and Kawasaki-like disease have all been described in HIV-positive individuals.[132,138]

Management of coronary artery disease in patients with HIV infection consists of lifestyle modification (smoking cessation, institution of a vigorous exercise program, and consumption of a healthy diet) and treatment of complicating medical problems (like hypertension, dyslipidemia, glucose intolerance, and hyperhomocysteinemia).[139] Changing the patient's HAART to a regimen that replaces the protease inhibitor ritonavir with nevirapine or efavirenz may be beneficial since these latter drugs are thought to cause an increase in high-density lipoprotein (HDL) cholesterol.[128] Interestingly, Dr. Holmberg's group at the Centers for Disease Control and Prevention recently reexamined data for the HOPS and found that the rate of myocardial infarction declined in 2002 in association with declining use of protease inhibitors and increasing use of statins and other lipid-lowering drugs.[140] In addition, a small randomized trial suggested that antioxidant supplementation with 100 µg of selenium once daily and 30 mg of betacarotene twice daily prevents

increases in the levels of von Willebrand factor and soluble thrombomodulin, both considered markers of endothelial dysfunction.[141] As in non–HIV-infected patients with CAD, coronary angioplasty with or without stent implantation[97,109] and coronary artery bypass grafting[142,143] can be performed safely and alleviate ischemic symptoms in appropriately selected individuals. However, two recent studies imply that persons with HIV infection hospitalized for acute coronary syndrome or MI are more susceptible to restenosis and recurrent infarction following revascularization (utilizing either percutaneous coronary intervention or coronary artery bypass grafting) compared with HIV-negative control patients.[11,144] Although Trachiotis and colleagues raised concern about a possible increase in routine infectious complications following surgery,[145] there is no indication that immunosuppression due to cardiopulmonary bypass accelerates the progression of HIV infection to full-blown AIDS.[145–148] The same group also reported a relatively high rate of needlestick injury, but none of the six medical practitioners so affected developed HIV infection.[145] On a final note, questions have been raised regarding the safety of sildenafil citrate use in patients on PI therapy after a fatal MI was reported in a 47-year-old male taking sildenafil, ritonavir, and saquinavir. The patient described had no cardiac risk factors other than smoking.[149] Because these drugs inhibit the cytochrome P450 isoforms CYP3A4 and CYP2D6 that metabolize sildenafil, it is recommended that patients with erectile dysfunction be started on a lower-than-usual dose of sildenafil (25 mg).[150]

STROKE AND HIV INFECTION

Whereas autopsy studies indicate that cerebral infarction is uncommon in HIV-infected patients in the absence of opportunistic central nervous system infection, lymphoma, or potential sources of emboli,[151–153] retrospective analysis of the Baltimore-Washington Cooperative Young Stroke Study registry found that the adjusted relative risk for either ischemic stroke or intracerebral hemorrhage was 10.4 times higher in individuals with HIV infection than in the general population.[154] As in the situation with coronary artery disease, there is concern that the propensity for stroke may be worsened by protease inhibitor therapy.[155] Other conditions that can predispose to stroke in HIV-infected individuals are listed in Table 21–1.

OTHER THROMBOTIC MANIFESTATIONS OF HIV INFECTION

Unusual thrombotic complications reported in HIV-positive individuals include intracranial venous sinus thrombosis arising in the setting of concurrent CMV infection,[156] primary central nervous system (CNS) B-cell immunoblastic lymphoma,[157] protein S deficiency,[158] and HIV-associated nephropathy

Table 21–1. CAUSES OF STROKE IN HIV-INFECTED INDIVIDUALS[152,208,209]

CNS mass lesions
  Toxoplasmosis
  Lymphoma
Embolic disease
  Infective endocarditis
  Nonbacterial thrombotic endocarditis
  HIV myocarditis with thrombus
Vasculitides
  Viral
    Cytomegalovirus
    Varicella-zoster virus
    Herpes simplex virus
    Human immunodeficiency virus
    Hepatitis B with cryoglobulinemia
  Bacterial
    Mycobacterium tuberculosis
    Syphilis
  Fungal
    Cryptococcosis
    Mucormycosis
    Aspergillosis
    Candida albicans
    Coccidioidomycosis
  Parasitic
    Toxoplasmosis
    Trypanosomiasis
  Other
    Irradiation for CNS lymphoma
    Primary angiitis of the CNS
Coagulation abnormalities
  Protein S deficiency
  Antiphospholipid antibodies
  Disseminated intravascular coagulation
  Thrombotic thrombocytopenic purpura
Injection drug use
  Cocaine
  Heroin
  Hypertension

CNS = central nervous system.

(HIVAN)[49]; central retinal vein occlusion,[159–162] portal vein thrombosis,[25] mesenteric thrombosis,[163] digital ischemia,[3] and limb-threatening arterial thromboses.[11,37,92,98,164] The latter complication has been treated successfully in two reported instances with thrombolysis,[98,164] while insertion of an aorta-bi-iliacal vascular prosthesis was used in one case,[37] and urgent aortofemoral bypass surgery in another.[11]

BLEEDING

Hemorrhage can also be a problem for patients with HIV infection, whether it arises from thrombocytopenia (see below), a congenital disorder such as hemophilia, or gastrointestinal lesions owing to CMV, lymphoma[165] or Kaposi's sarcoma.[166] An increased bleeding tendency was also reported in hemophilia patients soon after the introduction of the first protease inhibitor drugs.[167,168] Although some authors dispute there is an association,[169,170] scattered case reports and occasionally larger series indicate that the most frequent culprit is ritonavir,[171–174] followed by indinavir,[168,175,176] and nelfinavir,[173,176] with amprenavir[177] and lopinavir[174] being implicated most recently. The risk associated with saquinavir seems to be relatively low, perhaps owing to its poor absorption from the gastrointestinal tract.[178] Noted complications due to PI therapy include an increase in joint bleeds, soft tissue bleeding, mucosal bleeding, hemoptysis, hematuria,[175,168] development of a perinephric pseudotumor,[173] and even intracranial bleeding,[177] which was sometimes fatal.[173,174] This higher bleeding propensity is not confined solely to hemophiliacs, however. Nielsen and colleagues reported hypermenorrhea with resultant iron deficiency anemia in four HIV-positive women with previously normal menses following the institution of ritonavir.[179]

The pathophysiology underlying this increased bleeding tendency remains uncertain,[168,175] but platelet dysfunction was seen in three of the six patients in which this was investigated.[171,175,180] It is possible that protease inhibitor–induced inhibition of cytochrome P450 hinders arachidonic acid metabolism, with resultant impairment of platelet function.[177] Whereas bleeding episodes tend to decrease over time and some patients have been successfully rechallenged with either the same or another PI,[168,175,177,178] clinicians caring for patients with hemophilia and other inherited bleeding disorders are urged to caution their patients to monitor themself closely for any untoward bleeding episodes, to consider use of alternative anti-retroviral drugs should bleeding develop, and to consider stopping the PI prior to any planned surgical procedure.[168,175]

THROMBOCYTOPENIA

An association between HIV and low platelet counts was first noted in 1982.[181] The most common cause of HIV-associated thrombocytopenia is now known to be immune thrombocytopenic purpura (ITP), a complication that occurs in 30% or more of patients with AIDS.[182] Although slightly more common in those with advanced HIV infection, ITP most typically arises early in the course of the disease and is seen more frequently in men than women.[1] Unlike the usual form of ITP seen in immunocompetent individuals, patients with HIV-associated ITP commonly have markedly elevated levels of platelet-bound immunoglobulin G (IgG), immunoglobulin M (IgM), and C3C4, as well as circulating polyethylene glycol (PEG)-precipitable serum immune complexes that contain high-affinity IgG directed against an 18–amino acid peptide sequence in platelet glycoprotein IIIa known as GPIIIa-(49-66).[183] This anti–GPIIIa-(49-66) antibody may be induced by HIV glycoprotein 120 but then cross-reacts with platelet GPIIIa,[184] and can be found even in HIV-infected patients who are not thrombocytopenic.[182] Such patients also have relatively increased numbers of CD5+ B cells, which produce IgM rheumatoid factor directed against the Fc portion of IgG,[185] as well as IgM against the F(ab′)$_2$ fragments of anti–GPIIIa-(49-66) antibodies. Individuals with ITP who harbor this latter anti-idiotypic antibody tend to have higher platelet counts, suggesting that symptomatic ITP arises only in those whose dysfunctional immune systems can no longer generate sufficient anti-idiotype antibody to neutralize the circulating anti–GPIIIa-(49-66).[186]

A study of platelet kinetics in 41 HIV-infected thrombocytopenic patients demonstrated that platelet survival is inversely associated with CD4 count, being lower in those with CD4 counts above 200 cells/μL and higher in those with counts below this level.[187] This implies that platelet destruction is more important in patients with higher CD4 counts, whereas decreased platelet production is more important in those with lower CD4 counts. A similar study found that HIV-infected patients have ineffective delivery of viable platelets to the peripheral circulation, despite a sixfold elevation in thrombopoietin levels and a threefold expansion of megakaryocyte mass compared to normal controls.[188] suggesting that HIV-induced apoptosis of megakaryocytes is also an important cause of thrombocytopenia.[189] That direct megakaryocyte infection by HIV occurs is supported by the following: denuded nuclei and ballooning of the peripheral zone of megakaryocyte cytoplasm have been observed by electron microscopy; internalization of HIV particles has been seen in co-culture studies; the presence of the HIV p24 antigen has been shown by immunohistochemical techniques; and expression of HIV RNA has been found using in situ hybridization.[1] Marrow infiltration by infectious organisms or neoplasms, as well as adverse drug effects, can also cause impaired platelet production and thrombocytopenia (Table 21–2).

Although up to 8% of individuals with HIV-associated thrombocytopenia will eventually develop clinically significant bleeding,[190] therapy is not necessary for the majority of patients until the platelet count falls below 30,000/μL.[191] Patients with hemophilia or other coagulopathies should probably receive therapy as soon as their platelet counts fall below 50,000/μL because they have a higher risk of bleeding at baseline.[192,193] Historically, the treatment of choice has been institution of AZT[1]; however, recent studies have shown that HAART is equally effective.[194,195]

HIV-associated ITP can also be treated with glucocorticoids, intravenous IgG (IVIG), intravenous anti-D therapy, splenectomy, danazol, interferon, and vincristine. Glucocorticoids are useful for many patients in the short-term; however, long-term use can cause Cushing's syndrome, an increased risk of fungal infection, and worsening of Kaposi's sarcoma.[1] IVIG induces rapid but unsustained remissions in 71 to 100% of patients[196] but is expensive and difficult to administer on an outpatient basis. Intravenous anti-D therapy is less costly but raises

Table 21–2. THROMBOCYTOPENIA

Decreased Production
  Drugs
    Antiretroviral agents
    Didanosine
    Indinavir
    Ritonavir
    Delavirdine
    Nelfinavir
  Anti-*Pneumocystis carinii* agents
    Trimethoprim-sulfamethoxazole
    Pentamidine
    Pyrimethamine
  Antifungal agents
    Fluconazole
    Amphotericin B
  Antiviral agents
    Ganciclovir
  Antimycobacterial agents
    Rifabutin
    Clarithromycin
  Other
    Alpha-interferon
Deficiencies
  Folate
  Vitamin B$_{12}$
Infection
  HIV
  Parvovirus B19
  Mycobacterium avium complex (MAC)
  Mycobacterium tuberculosis
  Histoplasma capsulatum
  Bartonella henselae (bacillary angiomatosis)
Neoplasia
  Non-Hodgkin's lymphoma
Miscellaneous
  Pre-existing condition

Increased Loss
  Immune thrombocytopenic purpura
  Thrombotic thrombocytopenic purpura
  Hypersplenism
    Infection
    Hemophagocytosis
    Cirrhosis
  Drugs
    Saquinavir
    Interferon

porary reduction in plasma viremia and an increase in absolute CD4 and CD8 counts once these cells are no longer sequestered by the spleen.[199] Splenic irradiation is of negligible benefit, resulting only in partial remissions of brief duration.[200]

Thrombotic microangiopathy (TMA) is also a well-recognized complication of HIV infection, with both hemolytic uremic syndrome (HUS) and thrombotic thrombocytopenic purpura (TTP) being described at various stages of disease. When compared to the latter, HUS is more likely to present at a later stage of HIV infection, to resist treatment, and ultimately to be fatal.[201] It is unclear if HIV-associated TMA is precipitated by endothelial cell damage, as can be seen following exposure to inflammatory cytokines, toxins produced by *Shigella dysenteriae* and *Escherichia coli* O157:H7, CMV infection,[202] or HIV itself.[203] In the two cases of HIV-associated TTP studied thus far,[204,205] persistence of high–molecular-weight von Willebrand factor (VWF) multimers and complete deficiency of VWF-cleaving metalloprotease (ADAMTS-13) were found, but in only 1 case[204] was this due to a demonstrable IgG$_1$ inhibitor of ADAMTS-13. As with patients with idiopathic TTP, plasma exchange is the standard therapy for HIV-associated TMA, but, interestingly, the response may be better in those individuals who have previously undergone splenectomy.[203] While TMA was seen in 1.4% of HIV-infected individuals during the 1980s and early 1990s,[206] recent observational studies suggest that the incidence has declined significantly with the introduction of HAART, such that only 0 to 0.3% of patients are so affected now and usually only with advanced HIV disease.[206,207]

the platelet count above 50,000/μL in only 34% of patients treated and can result in unexpectedly severe hemolysis. However, the duration of response is frequently longer than that seen with IVIG.[197] Splenectomy is also useful and, despite early concerns, does not seem to increase the risk of progression to symptomatic AIDS. A long-term cohort study demonstrated that splenectomized patients were significantly less likely to develop full-blown AIDS and may be less likely to die than those patients who didn't undergo surgery,[198] due in part perhaps to a tem-

REFERENCES

1. Coyle TE. Management of the HIV-infected patient, Part II. Med Clin North Am 1997;81:449–70.
2. Cohen H, Mackie IJ, Anagnostopoulous N, et al. Lupus anticoagulant, anticardiolipin antibodies, and human immunodeficiency virus in haemophilia. J Clin Pathol 1989;42: 629–33.
3. Lafeuillade A, Alessi M-C, Poizot-Martin I, et al. Protein S deficiency and HIV infection [letter]. N Engl J Med 1991; 324:1220.
4. Carson PJ, Goldsmith JC. Atypical pulmonary diseases associated with AIDS. Chest 1991;100:675–7.
5. Becker DM, Saunders TJ, Wispelwey B, Schain DC. Case

report: Venous thromboembolism in AIDS. Am J Med Sci 1992;303:395–7.

6. Maliakkal R, Friedman SA, Sridhar S. Progressive pulmonary thromboembolism in association with HIV disease. NY State J Med 1992;92:403–4.

7. Tanimowo M. Deep vein thrombosis as a manifestation of the acquired immunodeficiency syndrome? A case report. Cent Afr J Med 1996;42:327–8.

8. Howling SJ, Shaw PJ, Miller RF. Acute pulmonary embolism in patients with HIV disease. Sex Transm Infect 1999;75:25–9.

9. Force L, Barrufet P, Herreras Z, Bolibar I. Deep venous thrombosis and megestrol in patients with HIV infection. AIDS. 1999;13(11):1425–6.

10. Winston A, Baker RW, Nelson M, Gazzard B. The use of D-dimers in the diagnosis of occult pulmonary embolism in HIV pulmonary disease—two case reports. Int J STD AIDS 2000;11:675–6.

11. Matetzky S, Domingo M, Kar S, et al. Acute myocardial infarction in human immunodeficiency virus-infected patients. Arch Intern Med 2003;163:457–60.

12. Majluf-Cruz A, Silva-Estrada M, Sanchez-Barboza R, et al. Venous thrombosis among patients with AIDS. Clin Appl Thromb Hemost 2004;10:19–25.

13. Saber AA, Aboolian A, LaRaja RD, et al. HIV/AIDS and the risk of deep vein thrombosis: a study of 45 patients with lower extremity involvement. Am Surg 2001;67:645–7.

14. Fultz SL, McGinnis KA, Skanderson M, et al. Association of venous thromboembolism with human immunodeficiency virus and mortality in veterans. Am J Med 2004;116:420–3.

15. Copur AS, Smith PR, Gomez V, et al. HIV infection is a risk factor for venous thromboembolism. AIDS Patient Care STDS 2002;16:205–9.

16. Sullivan PS, Dworkin MS, Jones JL, et al. Epidemiology of thrombosis in HIV-infected individuals. AIDS 2000;14: 321–4.

17. Wilkes MS, Fortin AH, Felix JC, et al. Value of necropsy in acquired immunodeficiency syndrome. Lancet 1988; 8602:85–8.

18. Afessa B, Green W, Chiao J, Frederick W. Pulmonary complications of HIV infection: autopsy findings. Chest 1990;113:1225–9.

19. Bilgrami S, Cable R, Pisciotto P, et al. Fatal disseminated intravascular coagulation and pulmonary thrombosis following blood transfusion in a patient with severe autoimmune haemolytic anemia and human immunodeficiency virus infection. Transfusion 1994;34:248–52.

20. Lipski DA, Bergamini TM. Upper extremity arterial thrombosis associated with immunohemolytic anemia. Surgery 1996;119:354–5.

21. Saif MW, Bona R, Greenberg B. AIDS and thrombosis: retrospective study of 131 HIV-infected patients. AIDS Patient Care STDS 2001;15:311–20.

22. Saif MW, Morse EE, Greenberg BR. HIV-associated autoimmune haemolytic anemia complicated by pulmonary embolism following a red blood cell transfusion. Conn Med 1998;62:67–70.

23. Shahmanesh M, Brooks J, Shaw PJ, Miller RF. Inferior vena cava filters for HIV-infected patients with pulmonary

embolism and contraindications to anticoagulation. Sex Transm Infect 2000;76:395–7.

24. Jenkins RE, Peters BS, Pinching AJ. Thromboembolic disease in AIDS is associated with cytomegalovirus disease. AIDS 1991;5:1540–2.

25. Carr A, Brown D, Cooper DA. Portal vein thrombosis in patients receiving indinavir, an HIV protease inhibitor [letter]. AIDS 1997;11:1657–8.

26. Koller E, Gibert C, Green L, et al. Thrombotic events associated with megestrol acetate in patients with AIDS cachexia. Nutrition 1999;15:294–8.

27. Vercellotti GM. Effects of viral activation of the vessel wall on inflammation and thrombosis. Blood Coagul Fibrinolysis 1998;9(Suppl 2):S3–6.

28. Uthman I, Tabbarah Z, Gharavi AE. Hughes syndrome associated with cytomegalovirus infection. Lupus 1999;8:775–7.

29. Nieto FJ, Sorlie P, Comstock GW, et al. Cytomegalovirus infection, lipoprotein (a), and hypercoagulability: An atherogenic link? Arterioscler Thromb Vasc Biol 1997;17:1780–5.

30. Schambeck CM, Hinney K, Gleixner J, Keller F. Venous thromboembolism and associated high plasma factor VIII levels: linked to cytomegalovirus infection? [letter]. Thromb Haemost 2000;83:511.

31. Jacobson MC, Dezube BJ, Aboulafia DM. Thrombotic complications in patients infected with HIV in the era of highly active antiretroviral therapy: a case series. Clin Infect Dis 2004;39:1214–22.

32. Sugarman RW, Church JA, Goldsmith JC, Ens GE. Acquired protein S deficiency in children infected with human immunodeficiency virus. Pediatr Infect Dis J 1996;15: 106–11.

33. Erbe M, Rickers V, Bauersachs RM, Lindhoff-Last E. Acquired protein C and protein S deficiency in HIV-infected patients. Clin Appl Thromb Hemost 2003;9: 325–31.

34. Toulon P, Lamine M, Ledjev I, et al. Heparin cofactor II deficiency in patients infected with the human immunodeficiency virus. Thromb Haemost 1993;70:730–5.

35. Lafeuillade A, Alessi MC, Poizot-Martin I, et al. Endothelial cell dysfunction in HIV infection. J Acquir Immune Defic Syndr 1992;5:127–31.

36. Vilaseca MA, Sierra C, Colomé C, et al. Hyperhomocysteinaemia and folate deficiency in human immunodeficiency virus-infected children. Eur J Clin Invest 2001;31: 992–8.

37. Callens S, Florence E, Philippe M, et al. Mixed arterial and venous thromboembolism in a person with HIV infection. Scand J Infect Dis 2003;35:907–8.

38. Laing RB, Brettle RP, Leen CL. Venous thrombosis in HIV infection. Int J STD AIDS 1996;7:82–5.

39. Duerksen DR, Ahmad A, Doweiko J, et al. Risk of symptomatic central venous thrombotic complications in AIDS patients receiving home parenteral nutrition. J Parenter Enteral Nutr 1996;20:302–5.

40. Mathur M, Desai N, Sharma J, et al. Management of a large organized intraatrial catheter-tip thrombus in a child with acquired immunodeficiency syndrome using escalating tissue plasminogen activator infusions. Pediatr Crit Care Med 2006;6:79–82.

41. Smith KJ, Skelton HG, Yeager J, Wagner KF. Cutaneous

thrombosis in human immunodeficiency virus type 1 positive patients and cytomegalovirus viremia [letter]. Arch Dermatol. 1995;131:357–8.

42. Vielhauer V, Schewe CK, Schlöndorff D. Bilateral thrombosis of the internal jugular veins with spasmodic torticollis in a patient with acquired immunodeficiency syndrome and disseminated cytomegalovirus infection [letter]. J Infect 1998;37:90–1.

43. Janier M, Flageul B, Drouet L, et al. Cutaneous and plasma values of von Willebrand factor in AIDS: a marker of endothelial stimulation? J Invest Dermatol 1988;90:703–7.

44. Feffer SE, Fox RL, Orsen MM, et al. Thrombotic tendencies and correlation with clinical status in patients infected with HIV. South Med J 1995;88:1125–30.

45. Seigneur M, Constans J, Blann A, et al. Soluble adhesion molecules and endothelial cell damage in HIV infected patients. Thromb Haemost 1997;77:646–9.

46. Aukrust P, Bjørnsen S, Lunden B, et al. Persistently elevated levels of von Willebrand factor antigen in HIV infection. Downregulation during highly active antiretroviral therapy. Thromb Haemost 2000;84:183–7.

47. Wolf K, Tsakiris, Weber R, et al. Antiretroviral therapy reduces markers of endothelial and coagulation activation in patients infected with human immunodeficiency virus type 1. J Infect Dis 2002;185:456–62.

48. Holme PA, Müller F, Solum NO, et al. Enhanced activation of platelets with abnormal release of RANTES in human immunodeficiency virus type 1 infection. FASEB J 1998;12:79–89.

49. Afsari K, Frank J, Vaksman Y, Nguyen TV. Intracranial venous sinus thrombosis complicating AIDS-associated nephropathy. AIDS Reader 2003;13:143–48.

50. Bissuel F, Berruyer M, Causse X, et al. Acquired protein S deficiency: correlation with advanced disease in HIV-1–infected patients. J Acquir Immune Defic Syndr 1992;5:484–9.

51. Kemkes-Matthes B. Acquired protein S deficiency. Clin Investig 1992;70:529–34.

52. Stahl CP, Wideman CS, Spira TJ, et al. Protein S deficiency in men with long-term human immunodeficiency virus infection. Blood 1993;7:1801–7.

53. Hassell KL, Kressin DC, Neumann A, et al. Correlation of antiphospholipid antibodies and protein S deficiency with thrombosis in HIV-infected men. Blood Coagul Fibrinolysis 1994;5:455–62.

54. Gris J-C, Toulon P, Brun S, et al. The relationship between plasma microparticles, protein S and anticardiolipin antibodies in patients with human immunodeficiency virus infection. Thromb Haemost 1996;76:38–45.

55. Brew BJ, Miller J. Human immunodeficiency virus type 1-related transient neurological deficits. Am J Med 1996;101:257–61.

56. De Larrañga G, Perés S, Puga L, et al. Association between the acquired free protein S deficiency in HIV-infected patients with the lipid profile levels. J Thromb Haemost 2004;2:1195–7.

57. Sorice M, Griggi T, Arcieri P, et al. Protein S and HIV infection. The role of anticardiolipin and anti-protein S antibodies. Thromb Res 1994;73:165–75.

58. Lafeuillade A, Sorice M, Griggi T, et al. Role of autoimmunity in protein S deficiency during HIV-1 infection. Infection 1994;22:201–3.

59. Malia RG, Kitchen S, Greaves M, Preston FE. Inhibition of activate protein C and its cofactor protein S by antiphospholipid antibodies. Br J Haematol 1990;76:101–7.

60. Schved JF, Gris JC, Michard A, et al. Study of the protein S system in HIV-infected patients: acquired protein S deficiency of unsuitable assays. Blood Coagul Fibrinolysis 1992;3:295–301.

61. Culpepper RM, Carr ME. Case report: A novel form of free protein S deficiency in an HIV-positive patient on hemodialysis. Am J Med Sci 1992;303:402–4.

62. Bloom EJ, Abrams DI, Rodger G. Lupus anticoagulant in the acquired immunodeficiency syndrome. JAMA 1986;256:491–3.

63. Kaye BR. Rheumatologic manifestations of infection with human immunodeficiency virus (HIV). Ann Intern Med 1989;111:158–67.

64. Stimmler MM, Quismorio FP Jr, McGehee WG, et al. Anticardiolipin antibodies in acquired immunodeficiency syndrome. Arch Intern Med 1989;149:1833–5.

65. Palomo I, Alarcón M, Sepulveda C, et al. Prevalence of antiphospholipid and antiplatelet antibodies in human immunodeficiency virus (HIV)-infected Chilean patients. J Clin Lab Anal 2003;17:209–15.

66. Canoso RT, Zon LI, Groopman JE. Anticardiolipin antibodies associated with HTLV-III infection. Br J Haematol 1987;65:495–8.

67. Bernard C, Exquis B, Reber G, de Moerloose P. Determination of anticardiolipin and other antibodies in HIV-1–infected patients. J Acquir Immune Defic Syndr 1990;3:536–9.

68. Coll Daroca J, Gutierrez-Cebollada J, Yazbeck H, et al. Anticardiolipin antibodies and acquired immunodeficiency syndrome: prognostic marker or association with HIV infection? Infection 1992;20:140–2.

69. Medina-Rodriguez F, Guzman C, Jara LJ, et al. Rheumatic manifestations in human immunodeficiency virus positive and negative individuals: a study of 2 populations with similar risk factors. J Rheumatol 1993;20:1880–4.

70. Abuaf N, Laperche S, Rajoely B, et al. Autoantibodies to phospholipids and to the coagulation proteins in AIDS. Thromb Haemost 1997;77:856–61.

71. Grünewald T, Burmester G-R, Schüler-Maué E. et al. Antiphospholipid antibodies and CD5+ B cells in HIV infection. Clin Exp Immunol 1999;115:464–71.

72. Ankri A, Bonmarchand M, Coutellier A, et al. Antiphospholipid antibodies are an epiphenomenon in HIV-infected patients. AIDS 1999;13:1282–3.

73. Sedláček D, Ulčová-Gallová Z, Milichovská L, et al. Seven antiphospholipid antibodies in HIV-positive patients: Correlation with clinical course and laboratory findings. Am J Reprod Immunol 2003;50:439–43.

74. Falco M, Sorrenti A, Priori R, et al. Anti-cardiolipin antibodies in HIV infection are true antiphospholipids not associated with antiphospholipid syndrome. Ann Ital Med Int 1993;8:171–4.

75. Panzer S, Stain C, Hartl H, et al. Anticardiolipin antibodies are elevated in HIV-1 infected haemophiliacs but do not

predict for disease progression. Thromb Haemost 1989;61:81–5.

76. Carreno L, Monteagudo I, Lopez-Longo FJ, et al. Anticardiolipin antibodies in pediatric patients with human immunodeficiency virus. J Rheumatol 1994;21:1344–6.

77. Gharavi AE, Sammaritano LR, Wen J, et al. Characteristics of human immuodeficiency virus and chlorpromazine induced antiphospholipid antibodies: effect of beta 2 glycoprotein 1 binding to phospholipid. J Rheumatol 1994; 21:94–9.

78. Weiss L, You JF, Giral P, et al. Anti-cardiolipin antibodies are associated with anti-endothelial cell antibodies but not with anti-beta 2 glycoprotein 1 antibodies in HIV infection. Clin Immunol Immunopathol 1995;77:69–74.

79. González C, Lestón A, Garcia-Berrocal B, et al. Antiphosphatidylserine antibodies in patients with autoimmune diseases and HIV-infected patients: Effects of Tween 20 and relationship with antibodies to β^2-glycoprotein I. J Clin Lab Anal 1999;13:59–64.

80. Petrovas C, Vlachoyiannopoulos PG, Kordossis T, Moutsopoulos HM. Anti-phospholipid antibodies in HIV infection and SLE with or without anti-phospholipid syndrome: Comparisons of phospholipid specificity, avidity and reactivity with β^2-GPI. J Autoimmun 1999;13:347–55.

81. Constans J, Guérin V, Couchouron A, et al. Autoantibodies directed against phospholipids or human β-glycoprotein I in HIV-seropositive patients: relationship with endothelial activation and antimalonic dialdehyde antibodies. Eur J Clin Invest 1998;28:115–22.

82. Silvestris F, Frassanito MA, Cafforio P, et al. Antiphosphatidylserine antibodies in human immunodeficiency virus-1 patients with evidence of T-cell apoptosis and mediated antibody dependent cellular cytotoxicity. Blood 1996;87:5185–95.

83. Shahnaz S, Parikh G, Opran A. Antiphospholipid antibody syndrome manifesting as a deep venous thrombosis and pulmonary embolism in a patients with HIV. Am J Med Sci 2004;327:231–2.

84. Rinaldi R, Manfredi R, Azzimondi G, et al. Recurrent "migraine-like" episodes in patients with HIV disease. Headache 1997;37:443–8.

85. Keeling DM, Birley H, Machin SJ. Multiple transient ischaemic attacks and a mild thrombotic stroke in a HIV-positive patient with anticardiolipin antibodies. Blood Coagul Fibrinolysis 1990;1:333–5.

86. Belmonte MA, Garcia-Portales R, Domenech I, et al. Avascular necrosis of bone in human immunodeficiency virus infection and antiphospholipid antibodies. J Rheumatol 1993;20:1425–8.

87. Ramos-Casals M, Cervera R, Lagrutta M, et al. Clinical features related to antiphospholipid syndrome in patients with chronic viral infections (hepatitis C virus/HIV infection): Description of 82 cases. Clin Infect Dis 2004;38:1009–16.

88. Soweid A, Hajjar R, Hewan-Lowe KO, Gonzalez EB. Skin necrosis indicating antiphospholipid syndrome in patient with AIDS. South Med J 1995;88:786–8.

90. Hassoun A, Al-Kadhimi Z, Cervia J. HIV infection and antiphospholipid antibody: Literature review and link to the antiphospholipid syndrome. AIDS Patient Care STDS 2004;18:333–40.

91. Cappell MS, Simon T, Tiku M. Splenic infarction associated with anticardiolipin antibodies in a patient with acquired immunodeficiency syndrome. Dig Dis Sci 1993;38:1152–5.

92. Witz M, Lehmann J, Korzets. Acute brachial artery thrombosis as the initial manifestation of human immunodeficiency virus infection. Am J Hematol 2000;64:137 9.

93. Tabib A, Greenland T, Mercier I, et al. Coronary lesions in young HIV-positive subjects at necropsy. Lancet 1992; 340:730.

94. Capron L, Kim YU, Laurin C, et al. Atheroembolism in HIV-positive individuals. Lancet 1992;340:1039–40.

95. Paton P, Tabib A, Loire R, Tete R. Coronary artery lesions and human immunodeficiency virus infection. Res Virol 1993;144:225–31.

96. Henry K, Melroe H, Huebsch J, et al. Severe premature coronary artery disease with protease inhibitors [letter]. Lancet 1998;351:1328.

97. Eriksson U, Opravil M, Amann FW, Schaffner A. Is treatment with ritonavir a risk factor for myocardial infarction in HIV-infected patients? [letter]. AIDS 1998;12:2079–80.

98. Behrens G, Schmidt H, Meyer D, et al. Vascular complications associated with the use of HIV protease inhibitors [letter]. Lancet 1998;351:1958.

99. Gallet B, Pulik M, Genet P, et al. Vascular complications associated with the use of HIV protease inhibitors [letter]. Lancet 1998;351:1958–9.

100. Vittecoq D, Escaut L, Monsuez JJ. Vascular complications associated with the use of HIV protease inhibitors [letter]. Lancet 1998;351:1959.

101. Sullivan AK, Nelson MR, Moyle GJ, et al. Coronary artery disease occurring with protease inhibitor therapy. Int J STD AIDS 1998;9:711–2.

102. Karmochkine M, Raguin G. Severe coronary artery disease in a young HIV-infected man with no cardiovascular risk factor who was treated with indinavir [letter]. AIDS 1998;12:2499.

103. Koppel K, Bratt G, Rajs J. Sudden cardiac death in a patient on 2 years of highly active antiretroviral treatment: a case report. AIDS 1999;13:1993–4.

104. Flynn TE, Bricker LE. Myocardial infarction in HIV-infected men receiving protease inhibitors. Ann Intern Med 1999;131:548.

105. Varriale P, Mirzai-tehrane M, Sedighi A. Acute myocardial infarction associated with anabolic steroids in a young HIV-infected patient. Pharmacotherapy 1999;19:881–4.

106. Hayes P, Muller D, Kuchar D. Left main coronary artery disease in a 40-year-old man receiving HIV protease inhibitors. Aust NZ J Med 2000;30:92–3.

107. Friedl AC, Attenhofer J, Schalcher CH, et al. Acceleration of confirmed coronary artery disease among HIV-infected patients on potent antiretroviral therapy [letter]. AIDS 2000;14:2790–2.

108. Muise A, Arbess G. The risk of myocardial infarction in HIV-infected patients receiving HAART: a case report. Int J STD AIDS 2001;12:612–3.

109. Boccara F, Teiger E, Cohen A. Stent implantation for acute left main coronary artery occlusion in an HIV-infected patient on protease inhibitors. J Invasive Cardiol 2002;14:343–6.

110. Escaut L, Monsuez JJ, Chironi G, et al. Coronary artery disease in HIV infected patients. Intensive Care Med

2003;29:969–73.

111. Vittecoq D, Escaut L, Chironi G, et al. Coronary heart disease in HIV-infected patients in the highly active antiretroviral treatment era. AIDS 2003;17 Suppl 1:S70–6.

112. Periard D, Telenti A, Sudre P, et al. Atherogenic dyslipidemias in HIV-infected individuals treated with protease inhibitors. Swiss HIV Cohort Study. Circulation 1999;100:700–5.

113. Tsiodras S, Mantzoros C, Hammer S, et al. Effects of protease inhibitors on hyperglycemia, hyperlipidemia, and lipodystrophy: A 5-year cohort study. Arch Intern Med 2000;160:2050–6.

114. Stein JH, Klein MA, Bellenumeru JL, et al. Use of human immunodeficiency virus-1 protease inhibitors is associated with atherogenic lipoprotein changes and endothelial dysfunction. Circulation 2001;104:257–62.

115. Zhong D, Lu X, Conklin BS, et al. HIV protease inhibitor ritonavir induces cytotoxicity of human endothilial cells. Arterioscler Thromb Vasc Biol 2002;22:1560–6.

116. Laurence J. Vascular complications associated with the use of HIV protease inhibitors [letter]. Lancet 1998;351:1960.

117. Quiros-Roldan E, Torti C, Tinelli C, et al. Risk factors for myocardial infarction in HIV-positive patients. Int J STD AIDS 2005;16:14–8.

118. David MH, Hornung R, Fichtenbaum CJ. Ischemic cardiovascular disease in persons with human immunodeficiency virus infection. Clin Infect Dis 2002;34:98–102.

119. Klein D, Hurley LB, Quesenberry CP Jr, Sidney S. Do protease inhibitors increase the risk for coronary heart disease in patients with HIV-1 infection? J Acquir Immune Defic Syndr 2002;30:471–7.

120. Bozzette SA, Ake CF, Tam HK, et al. Cardiovascular and cerebrovascular events in patients treated for human immunodeficiency virus infection. N Engl J Med 2003;348:702–10.

121. Coplan PM, Nikas A, Japour A, et al. Incidence of myocardial infarction in randomized clinical trials of protease inhibitor-based antiretroviral therapy: An analysis of four different protease inhibitors. AIDS Res Hum Retroviruses 2003;19:449–55.

122. Jütte A, Schwenk A, Franzen C, et al. Increasing morbidity from myocardial infarction during HIV protease inhibitor treatment? [letter]. AIDS 1999;13:1796.

123. Rickerts V, Brodt H, Staszewski S, Stille W. Incidence of myocardial infarctions in HIV-infected patients between 1983 and 1998: the Frankfurt HIV-cohort study. Eur J Med Res 2000;5:329–33.

124. Mary-Krause M, Cotte L, Simon A, et al. Increased risk of myocardial infarction with duration with protease inhibitor therapy in HIV-infected men. AIDS 2003;17:2479–86.

125. Friis-Møller N, Sabin CA, Weber R, et al. Combination antiretroviral therapy and the risk of myocardial infarction. N Engl J Med 2003;349:1993–2003.

126. D'Arminio A, Sabin CA, Phillips AN, et al. Cardio- and cerebrovascular events in HIV-infected persons. AIDS 2004; 18:1811–7.

127. Holmberg SD, Moorman AC, Williamson JM, et al. Protease inhibitors and cardiovascular outcomes in patients with HIV-1. Lancet 2002;360:1747–8.

128. Barbaro G, Di Lorenzo G, Cirelli A, et al. An open-label, prospective, observational study of the incidence of coronary artery disease in patients with HIV infection receiving highly active antiretroviral therapy. Clin Ther 2003;25:2405–18.

129. Chi D, Henry J, Kelley J, et al. The effects of HIV infection on endothelial function. Endothelium 2000;7:223–42.

130. Barbaro G, Barbarini G, Pellicelli A. HIV-associated coronary arteritis in a patient with fatal myocardial infarction [letter]. N Engl J Med 2001;344:1799–1800.

131. Joshi VV, Pawel B, Connor E, et al. Arteriopathy in children with acquired immune deficiency syndrome. Pediatr Pathol 1987;7:261–75.

132. Johnson RM, Barbarini G, Barbaro G. Kawasaki-like syndromes and other vasculitic syndromes in HIV-infected patients. AIDS 2003;17 (Suppl 1):S77–82.

133. Constans J, Marchand JM, Conri C, et al. Asymptomatic atherosclerosis in HIV-positive patients: A case-control ultrasound study. Ann Med 1995;27:683–5.

134. Maggi P, Serio G, Epifani G, et al. Premature lesions of the carotid vessels in HIV-1–infected patients treated with protease inhibitors. AIDS 2000;14:F123–8.

135. Depairon M, Chessex S, Sudre P, et al. Premature atherosclerosis in HIV-infected individuals—focus on protease inhibitor therapy. AIDS 2001;15:329–44.

136. Epstein SE, Speir E, Zhou YF, et al. The role of infection in restenosis and atherosclerosis: focus on cytomegalovirus. Lancet 1996;348(Suppl 1):S13–7.

137. Ball SC. Cardiovascular disease in a patient with AIDS. AIDS Read 2003;13:571–3.

138. Barbaro G. Cardiovascular manifestations of HIV infection. Circulation 2002;106:1420–5.

139. Volberding PA, Murphy RL, Barbaro G, et al. The Pavia consensus statement. AIDS 2003;17(Suppl 1):S170–9.

140. Holmberg SD, Moorman AC, Greenberg AE. Trends in rates of myocardial infarction among patients with HIV [letter]. N Engl J Med 2004;350:730–2.

141. Constans J, Seigneur M, Blann AD, et al. Effect of the antioxidants selenium and beta-carotene on HIV-related endothelium dysfunction. Thrombo Haemost 1998;80: 1015–7.

142. Bittner HB, Fogelson BG. Off-pump coronary artery bypass grafting in a patient with AIDS, acute myocardial infarction, and severe left main coronary artery disease. J Cardiovasc Surg 2003;44:55–7.

143. Varriale P, Saravi G, Hernandez E, Carbon F. Acute myocardial infarction in patients infected with human immunodeficiency virus. Am Heart J 2004;147:55–9.

144. Hsue PY, Giri K, Erickson S, et al. Clinical features of acute coronary syndromes in patients with human immunodeficiency virus infection. Circulation 2004;109:316–9.

145. Trachiotis GD, Alexander EP, Benator D, Gharagozloo F. Cardiac surgery in patients infected with the human immunodeficiency virus. Ann Thorac Surg 2003;76:1114–8.

146. Flum DR, Tyras DH, Wallack MK. Coronary artery bypass grafting in patients with human immunodeficiency virus. J Card Surg 1997;12:98–101.

147. Imanaka K, Takamoto S, Kimura S, et al. Coronary artery bypass grafting in a patient with human immunodeficiency virus. Role of perioperative active anti-retroviral therapy. Jpn Circ J 1999;63:423–4.

148. Frater RW. Cardiac surgery and the human immunodeficiency virus. Semin Thorac Cardiovasc Surg 2000;12:145–7.

149. Hall MCS, Ahmad S. Interaction between sildenafil and HIV-1 combination therapy [letter]. Lancet 1999;353:2071–2.

150. Nandwani R, Gourlay Y. Possible interaction between sildenafil and HIV combination therapy. Lancet 1999;353:840.

151. Berger JR, Harris JO, Gregorios J, Norenberg M. Cerebrovascular disease in AIDS: a case-control study. AIDS 1990;4:239–44.

152. Connor MD, Lammie GA, Bell JE, et al. Cerebral infarction in adult AIDS patients: Observations from the Edinburgh HIV Autopsy Cohort. Stroke 2000;31:2117–26.

153. Evers S, Nabavi D, Rahmann A, et al. Ischemic cerebrovascular events in HIV infection. Cerebrovasc Dis 2003;15:199–205.

154. Cole JW, Pinto AN, Hebel R, et al. Acquired immunodeficiency syndrome and the risk of stroke. Stroke 2004;35:51–6.

155. Menge T, Neumann-Haefelin T, von Giesen H-J, et al. Progressive stroke in an HIV-1–positive patient under protease inhibitors. Eur Neurol 2000;44:252–4.

156. Meyohas MC, Roullet E, Rouzioux C, et al. Cerebral venous thrombosis and dual primary infection with human immunodeficiency virus and cytomegalovirus. J Neurol Neurosurg Psychiatry 1989;52:1010–1.

157. Doberson MJ, Kleinschmidt-DeMasters BK. Superior sagittal sinus thrombosis in a patient with acquired immunodeficiency syndrome. Arch Pathol Lab Med 1994;118:844–6.

158. Iranzo A, Domingo P, Cadafalch J, Sambeat MA. Intracranial venous and dural sinus thrombosis due to protein S deficiency in a patient with AIDS [letter]. J Neurol Neurosurg Psychiatry 1998;64:688.

159. Roberts SP, Haefs TMP. Central retinal vein occlusion in a middle-aged adult with HIV infection. Optom Vis Sci 1992;69:567–9.

160. Friedman SM, Margo CE. Bilateral central retinal vein occlusions in a patient with acquired immunodeficiency syndrome: Clinicopathologic correlation. Arch Ophthalmol 1995;113:1184–8.

161. Mansour AM, Li H, Segal EI. Picture resembling hemicentral retinal vein occlusion in acquired immunodeficiency syndrome: is it related to cytomegalovirus? Ophthalmologica 1996;210:108–11.

162. Park KL, Marx JL, Lopez PF, Rao NA. Noninfectious branch retinal vein occlusion in HIV-positive patients. Retina 1997;17:162–4.

163. Narayanan TS, Narawane NM, Phadke AY, Abraham P. Multiple abdominal venous thrombosis in HIV-seropositive patient. Indian J Gastroenterol 1998;17:105–6.

164. Bush RL, Bianco CC, Bixler T, et al. Spontaneous arterial thrombosis in a patient with human immunodeficiency virus infection: Successful treatment with pharmacomechanical thrombectomy. J Vasc Surg 2003;38:392–5.

165. Bini EJ, Weinshel EH, Falkenstein DB. Risk factors for recurrent bleeding and mortality in human immunodeficiency virus infected patients with acute lower GI hemorrhage. Gastrointest Endosc 1999;49:748–53.

166. Chalasani N, Wilcox CM. Etiology and outcome of lower gastrointestinal bleeding in patients with AIDS. Am J Gastroenterol 1998;93:175–8.

167. Helal A. HIV protease inhibitors and increased bleeding in hemophilia? [letter]. Can Med Assoc J 1997;156:90.

168. Wilde JT, Lee CA, Collins P, et al. Increased bleeding associated with protease inhibitor therapy in HIV-positive patients with bleeding disorders. Br J Haematol 1999;107:556–9.

169. Mandalaki T, Katsarou O, Panagiotopoulou C, Karafoulidou A. Does protease inhibitor treatment induce increased bleeding tendency in haemophilia? Haemophilia 1998;4:766–7.

170. Merry C, McMahon C, Ryan M, et al. Successful use of protease inhibitors in HIV-infected haemophilia patients. Br J Haematol 1998;101:475–9.

171. Ginsburg C, Salmon-Ceron D, Vassilief D, et al. Unusual occurrence of spontaneous haematomas in three asymptomatic HIV-infected haemophilia patients in a few days after the onset of ritonavir treatment. AIDS 1997;11:388–9.

172. Hagerty SL, Ascher DP. Spontaneous bleeding associated with the use of the protease inhibitor ritonavir in a hemophilic patient with human immunodeficiency virus infection. Pediatr Infect Dis J 1998;17:929–30.

173. Hollmig KA, Beck SB, Doll DC. Severe bleeding complications in HIV-positive haemophilic patients. Eur J Med Res 2001;6:112–4.

174. Yazdanpanah Y, Viget N, Cheret A, et al. Increased bleeding in HIV-positive haemophiliac patients treated with lopinavir-ritonavir [letter]. AIDS 2003;17:2397–9.

175. Stanworth SJ, Bolton MJ, Hay CR, Shiach CR. Increased bleeding in HIV-positive haemophiliacs treated with antiretroviral protease inhibitors. Haemophilia 1998;4:109–14.

176. Racoosin JA, Kessler CM. Bleeding episodes in HIV-positive patients taking HIV protease inhibitors: a case series. Haemophilia 1999;5:266–9.

177. Kodoth S, Bakshi S, Seimeca P, et al. Possible linkage of amprenavir with intracranial bleeding in an HIV-infected hemophiliac. AIDS Patient Care STDS 2001;15:347–52.

178. Wilde JT. Protease inhibitor therapy and bleeding. Haemophilia 2000;6:487–90.

179. Nielsen H. Hypermenorrhoea associated with ritonavir. Lancet 1999;353:811–2.

180. Pollmann H, Richter H, Jurgens H. Platelet dysfunction as the cause of spontaneous bleeding in two haemophiliac patients taking HIV protease inhibitors. Thromb Haemost 1998;79:1213–4.

181. Morris L, Distenfeld A, Amorosi E, Karpatkin S. Autoimmune thrombocytopenic purpura in homosexual men. Ann Intern Med 1982;96:714–7.

182. Nardi M, Karpatkin S. Antiidiotype antibody against platelet anti-GPIIIa contributes to the regulation of thrombocytopenia in HIV-1-ITP patients. J Exp Med 2000;191:2093–100.

183. Nardi MA, Liu L-X, Karpatkin S. GPIIIa-(49-66) is a major pathophysiologically relevant antigenic determinant for anti-platelet GPIIIa of HIV-1-related immunologic thrombocytopenia. Proc Natl Acad Sci U S A 1997;94:7589–94.

184. Bettaib A, Fromont P, Louache F, et al. Presence of cross-reactive antibody between human immunodeficiency virus (HIV) and platelet glycoproteins in HIV-related immune thrombocytopenia. Blood 1992;80:162–9.

185. Karpatkin S, Nardi MA, Hymes KB. Sequestration of antiplatelet GpIIIa antibody in rheumatoid factor immune complexes of human immunodeficiency virus 1 thrombo-

cytopenic patients. Proc Natl Acad Sci U S A 1995;92: 2263–7.

186. Karpatkin S, Nardi M, Green D. Platelet and coagulation defects associated with HIV-1 infection. Thromb Haemost 2002;88:389–401.

187. Dominguez A, Gamallo G, Garcia R, et al. Pathophysiology of HIV related thrombocytopenia: an analysis of 41 patients. J Clin Pathol 1994;47:999–1003.

188. Cole JL, Marzec UM, Gunthel CJ, et al. Ineffective platelet production in thrombocytopenic human immunodeficiency virus-infected patients. Blood 1998;91:3239–46.

189. Zauli G, Catani L, Gibellini D, et al. Impaired survival of bone marrow GPIIb/IIIa+ megakaryocytic cells as an additional pathogenetic mechanism of HIV-1-related thrombocytopenia. Br J Haematol 1996;92:711–7.

190. Finazzi G, Mannucci PM, Lazzarin A, et al. Low incidence of bleeding from HIV-related thrombocytopenia in drug addicts and hemophiliacs: implications for therapeutic strategies. Eur J Haematol 1990;45:82–5.

191. Rossi E, Damasio E, Terragna A, et al. HIV-related thrombocytopenia: a therapeutical update. Haematologica 1991; 76:141–9.

192. Ragni MV, Bontempo FA, Myers DJ, et al. Hemorrhagic sequelae of immune thrombocytopenic purpura in human immunodeficiency virus-infected hemophiliacs. Blood 1990;75:1267–72.

193. Fabris F, Mares M, Sartori MT, et al. Long-term treatment of refractory HIV-related immune thrombocytopenia in a patient with haemophilia A. Haematologica 1992;77:79–81.

194. Caso JAA, Mingo CS, Tena JG. Effects of highly active anti-retroviral therapy on thrombocytopenia in patients with HIV infection [letter]. N Engl J Med 1999;341:1239–40.

195. Aboulafia DM, Bundow D, Waide S, et al. Initial observations on the efficacy of highly active antiretroviral therapy in the treatment of HIV-associated autoimmune thrombocytopenia. Am J Med Sci 2000;320:117–23.

196. Majluf-Cruz A, Luna-Castaños G, Huitrón S, Nieto-Cisneros L. Usefulness of a low-dose intravenous immunoglobulin regimen for the treatment of thrombocytopenia associated with AIDS. Am J Hematol 1998;59:127–32.

197. Scaradavou A. HIV-related thrombocytopenia. Blood Rev 2002;16:73–6.

198. Tsoukas CM, Bernard NR, Abrahamowicz M, et al. Effect of splenectomy on slowing human immunodeficiency virus disease progression. Arch Surg 1998;133:25–31.

199. Bernard NF, Chernoff DN, Tsoukas CM. Effect of splenectomy on T-cell subsets and plasma HIV viral titers in HIV-infected patients. J Hum Virol 1998;1:338–45.

200. Blauth J, Fisher S, Henry D, Nichini F. The role of splenic irradiation in treating HIV-associated immune thrombocytopenia. Int J Radiat Oncol Biol Phys 1999;45:457–60.

201. Sutor GC, Schmidt RE, Albrecht H. Thrombotic microangiopathies and HIV infection: Report of two typical cases, features of HUS and TTP, and review of the literature. Infection 1999;27:12–5.

202. Maslo C, Peraldi MN, Desenclos JC, et al. Thrombotic microangiopathy and cytomegalovirus disease in patients infected with human immunodeficiency virus. Clin Infect Dis 1997;24:350–5.

203. Hymes KB, Karpatkin S. Human immunodeficiency virus infection and thrombotic microangiopathy. Semin Hematol 1997;34:117–25.

204. Sahud MA, Claster S, Liu L, et al. Von Willebrand factor-cleaving protease inhibitor in an patient with human immunodeficiency syndrome-associated thrombotic thrombocytopenic purpura. Br J Haematol 2002;116:909–11.

205. Gruszecki AC, Wehrli G, Ragland BD, et al. Management of a patient with HIV infection-induced anemia and thrombocytopenia who presented with thrombotic thrombocytopenic purpura. Am J Hematol 2002;69:228–31.

206. Gervasoni C, Ridolfo AL, Vaccarezza M, et al. Thrombotic microangiopathy in patients with acquired immunodeficiency syndrome before and during the era of introduction of highly active antiretroviral therapy. Clin Infect Dis 2002;35:1534–40.

207. Becker S, Fusco G, Fusco J, et al. HIV-associated thrombotic microangiopathy in the era of highly active antiretroviral therapy: An observational study. Clin Infect Dis 2004;39(Suppl 5):S267–75.

208. Gillams AR, Allen E, Hrieb K, et al. Cerebral infarction in patients with AIDS. Am J Neuroradiol 1997;18:1581–5.

209. Gondim FA, Thomas FP. The relationship between intracranial venous sinus thrombosis and HIV-associated nephropathy [editorial]. AIDS Read 2003;13:146–7.

Index

Page numbers followed by f indicate figure. Page numbers followed by t indicate table.